Visit our website

to find out about other books from W. B. Saunders
and our sister companies in Harcourt Health Sciences

Register free at
www.harcourt-international.com

and you will get

- the latest information on new books, journals and electronic products in your chosen subject areas

- the choice of e-mail or post alerts or both, when there are any new books in your chosen areas

- news of special offers and promotions

- information about products from all Harcourt Health Sciences companies including Baillière Tindall, Churchill Livingstone, Mosby and W. B. Saunders

You will also find an easily searchable catalogue, online ordering, information on our extensive list of journals...and much more!

Visit the Harcourt Health Sciences website today!

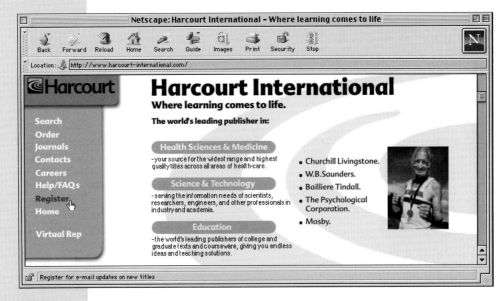

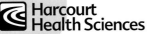

Commissioning Editor/Project Development Manager:
Deborah Russell/Serena Bureau
Project Manager: Hilary Hewitt
Production Manager: Helen Sofio
Design: Barrie Carrr

Veterinary Anaesthesia

TENTH EDITION

L.W. Hall MA, BSc, PhD, Dr (Hons Causa) Utrecht, DVA, DEVC, Hon DACVA, FRCVS

School of Veterinary Medicine,
Cambridge, UK

K.W. Clarke MA, VetMB, DVA, DVetMed, MRCVS

Department of Large Animal Medicine and Surgery
Royal Veterinary College
Hawkshead Lane, North Mimms, Hatfield, Hertfordshire, UK

C.M. Trim BVSc, MRCVS, DVA, DACVA, DECVA

Department of Large Animal Medicine
College of Veterinary Medicine
University of Georgia, Athens, Georgia, USA

 W.B. SAUNDERS

LONDON • EDINBURGH • NEW YORK • PHILADELPHIA • ST LOUIS • SYDNEY • TORONTO • 2001

W. B. Saunders

An imprint of Harcourt Publishers Limited

© Harcourt Publishers Limited 2001

First edition published in 1941 by J.G. Wright
Second edition 1947 (J.G. Wright)
Third edition 1948 (J.G. Wright)
Fourth edition 1957 (J.G. Wright)
Fifth edition 1961 (J.G. Wright and L.W. Hall)
Sixth edition 1966 (L.W. Hall)
Seventh edition 1971 (L.W. Hall), reprinted 1974 and 1976
Eighth edition 1983 (L.W. Hall and K.W. Clarke), reprinted 1985 and 1989
Ninth edition 1991 (L.W. Hall and K.W. Clarke)

ISBN 0 7020 2035 4

Cataloguing in Publication Data:
Catalogue records for this book are available from the British Library and the US Library of Congress.

Note:
Medical knowledge is constantly changing. As new information becomes available, changes in treatment,
procedures, equipment and the use of drugs become necessary. The authors and the publishers have
taken care to ensure that the information given in this text is accurate and up to date. However,
readers are strongly advised to confirm that the information, especially with regard to drug usage,
complies with the latest legislation and standards of practice.

The
publisher's
policy is to use
**paper manufactured
from sustainable forests**

Printed in England

Contents

Preface

This, the 10th edition of *Veterinary Anaesthesia,* is a direct descendant of *Anaesthesia & Narcosis of Animals & Birds* by Sir Frederick Hobday published in 1915 by Baillière, Tindall and Cox. The 1st edition of *Veterinary Anaesthesia,* which had marked similarities to Hobday's book, was written by Professor J.G. Wright and published in 1942. Wright's intention was to 'incorporate in a small volume the present status of knowledge on anaesthesia in the domestic animals'. This he accomplished in 198 small pages with fewer than 100 references to publications – including many to his own work. Since then tremendous advances have been made and now almost every week that passes sees new publications relating to veterinary anaesthesia and its related subjects.Thus, we have had to acknowledge the impossibility of including a comprehensive bibliography in this edition, but we have selected references which should provide a useful introduction to the literature. In addition, we have indicated where attention should be given to material published before computerized databases became available because, despite the increasing complexity of anaesthesia, simple methods also work.

Although extensively revised, the general concepts remain as in previous editions. The aim is still to provide a text for undergraduate veterinary students, a reference work for veterinarians in general practice and laboratory scientists, and a stimulating introduction to the subject for those wishing to specialize in veterinary anaesthesia through the examinations of the Royal College of Veterinary Surgeons, the American College of Veterinary Anesthesiologists and the European College of Veterinary Anaesthesia. Because we believe that clinical anaesthesia encompasses much more than an exercise in applied pharmacology, emphasis is still on the effects of clinically useful doses of drugs and of practical techniques in animal patients, rather than on pharmacological effects demonstrated in healthy experimental animals in laboratories.

We wish to express our appreciation of the invaluable help given by Mrs Lorraine Leonard, librarian of the University of Cambridge Veterinary School, and the librarians at the Royal College of Veterinary Surgeons in tracing older references. Mr Stephen Freane of the Royal Veterinary College gave much assistance with computer-generated figures. Finally, our warmest thanks are due to the publishers for their patience, and especially to Deborah Russell whose encouragement ensured completion of the manuscript.

L.W. Hall
K.W. Clarke
C.M. Trim
2000

Principles and Procedures

General considerations

INTRODUCTION

The clinical discipline concerned with the reversible production of insensibility to pain is known as 'anaesthesia', a term coined by Oliver Wendell Holmes in 1846 to describe a new phenomenon in a single word. It is essentially a practical subject and although becoming increasingly based on science it still retains some of the attributes of an art. In veterinary practice anaesthesia has to satisfy two requirements: (i) the humane handling of animals and (ii) technical efficiency. Humanitarian considerations dictate that gentle handling and restraint should always be employed; these minimize apprehension and protect the struggling animal from possible injury. Technical efficiency is not restricted to facilitation of the procedure to be carried out on the animal, it must also take into account the protection of personnel from bites, scratches or kicks as well as the risks of accidental or deliberate self-injection with dangerous or addictive drugs. Moreover, today it is considered that personnel need protection from the possible harmful effects of breathing low concentrations of inhalation anaesthetic agents.

While anaesthesia has precisely the same meaning as when it was first coined, i.e. the state in which an animal is insensible to pain resulting from the trauma of surgery, it is now used much more widely and can be compared to terms such as 'illness' and 'shock' which are too non-specific to be of real value. Starting with the premise that 'pain is the conscious perception of a noxious stimulus' two conditions may be envisaged: *general anaesthesia* where the animal is unconscious and apparently unaware of its surroundings, and *analgesia* or *local anaesthesia* where the animal, although seemingly aware of its surroundings, shows diminished or no perception of pain.

General anaesthesia is a reversible, controlled drug-induced intoxication of the central nervous system in which the patient neither perceives nor recalls noxious or painful stimuli. Analgesia may be produced by centrally acting drugs such as morphine given in doses insufficient to produce unconsciousness or by substances having a local, transient, selective paralytic action on sensory nerves and nerve endings (local anaesthetics). The analgesia produced by these latter substances may be classified as local or regional, applied as they are by topical application, subdermal or submucous infiltration and by peripheral, paravertebral or spinal perineural injection.

The anaesthetist aims to prevent awareness of pain, provide immobility and, whenever this is needed, relaxation of the skeletal muscles. These objectives must be achieved in such a way that the safety of the patient is not jeopardized during the perianaesthetic period. Many animals fear and resist the restraint necessary for the administration of anaesthetics thereby increasing not only the technical difficulties of administration but also the dangers inseparable from their use. A fully conscious animal forced to breathe a strange and possibly pungent vapour struggles to escape and sympatho-adrenal stimulation greatly increases the risks associated with the induction of anaesthesia. For this reason, veterinary anaesthetists often employ sedative drugs to facilitate the completion of general anaesthesia as well as to overcome the natural fear of restraint inherent in animals and to control any tendency to move suddenly during operations under local analgesia.

In addition, the veterinary anaesthetist must recognize that not only does the response of each species of animal to the various anaesthetics differ due to anatomical and physiological differences, but that there is often a marked variation in response between breeds within each particular species. Another factor which must be considered is that in many parts of the world veterinarians must perform tasks without highly skilled assistance and when employing general anaesthesia, after inducing it themselves, have to depute its maintenance to a nurse or even to a lay assistant. (It must be pointed out that in many countries, including the UK, the delegation of tasks related to anaesthesia to an *untrained* person may in law be considered negligent if a mishap occurs). Thus, the continued development in recent years of safe, simple, easily applied techniques of general anaesthesia and regional analgesia, together with the institution of nurse and anaesthetic technician training programmes, are particularly welcome.

PAIN

CLASSIC TEACHING RELATING TO PAIN

As anaesthesia is invoked to prevent appreciation of pain, any study of the discipline of anaesthesia must be related to an understanding of what constitutes pain. The old classic teaching on pain involved a hard-wired, modality specific, line specific, single pathway which coupled stimulus with pain sensation. Anatomists labelled the axons and nerve cells according to this single relay transmission system. It commenced in the periphery with fine myelinated (Aδ) and unmyelinated (C-fibre) afferents which possessed such high thresholds for stimulation that they only responded to noxious stimuli. Sherrington (1900) termed these structures

'nociceptors' but he realized that impulses in them would not necessarily lead to pain sensation unless the central nervous system accepted them and conveyed them to a pain-perceiving region of the brain. The nociceptor fibres were found to end preferentially on cells in laminae 1, 2 and 5 of the dorsal horn and from there impulses were believed to reach the thalamus by way of spinothalamic fibres which ran in the ventrolateral white matter of the spinal cord. From the thalamus impulses were said to reach a site of pure pain sensation (pain centre) in the association areas of the cerebral cortex.

Afferent mechanisms

In recent years pain studies have resulted in an almost explosive expansion of knowledge relating to pain mechanisms in the body and have shown that these earlier ideas must be abandoned in favour of an interlocking, dynamic series of biological processes which need still further investigation. It is apparent that in the periphery the old picture of fixed property nociceptor cells in damaged tissue passively detecting the products of cell breakdown does not accurately represent what is actually happening. The tissue breakdown products have been shown to have both direct and indirect effects on sensory afferent nerves. The role of unmyelinated sensory fibres themselves in inflammation as proposed by Lewis (1942) is, however, now well established. Leucocytes attracted into damaged tissues secrete cytokines which have both powerful systemic and local effects. Substances such as nerve growth factor synthetized locally in damaged tissue are also involved in pain production (McMahon *et al.*, 1995). The sympathetic nerves play a role in the inflammatory process, new α adrenergic, bradykinin and opiate receptors appear and there are a group of C-fibres which seem to be completely silent in normal tissue but which are activated by ongoing inflammation.

It is now also clear that certain types of pain are produced by afferents with large diameters outside the range of nociceptors. There is evidence that secondary mechanical hyperalgesia, which develops in healthy tissue surrounding injury or in distant tissue to which pain is referred, can be mediated by the thick tactile sensory fibres. These pains are probably provoked by impulses in normal low-threshold afferents entering the central nervous system, where they encounter highly abnormal central nervous circuits that amplify or reroute the signals of normally innocuous events.

The afferent fibres convey information to the central nervous system in two quite different ways. Sensory fibres which have been changed by their contact with damaged or inflamed tissue discharge impulses in a characteristic spatial and temporal pattern. The second way is by transport of chemicals from the tissues along axons towards the dorsal root ganglion. In response to changes in these relatively slowly transported chemicals the chemistry and metabolism of the cytoplasm and cell membrane, including its central terminal arborizations, is altered. This consequently affects the post-synaptic cells of the central nervous system.

Pain and the central nervous system

The first cells of the central nervous system on which the afferents terminate are not exclusively simply relay cells. They form integrated groups with both summation and differentiation functions as well as inhibitory and facilitatory mechanisms. The facilitatory functions appear to become active following noxious inputs and this results in the development of a hyperalgesic state (Treede *et al.*, 1992; Woolf & Doubell, 1994). In addition, there are also powerful inhibitory systems in this region and their failure may contribute to hyperalgesia.

The modulator role of the spinal cord in transmission of nociceptive signals from the periphery to the brain has been known for many years, and new evidence as to the complexity of the system and both the excitatory and inhibitory influence of many different neurotransmitter substances emerges continually (Dickenson, 1995, Marsh *et al.*, 1997). Knowledge of these pathways forms the basis for the provision of pain relief by the epidural or intrathecal administration of analgesic drugs. To date the opioid pathways remain the most important system involved in the production of analgesia at the spinal level, although noradrenaline, the natural ligand acting at α_2 adrenocep-

tors, also has a major role in the spinal modulation of nociception. Opioid receptors and α_2 adrenoceptors are present in laminae 1 and 2 of the dorsal horn, the area involved in the reception and modulation of incoming nociceptive signals, and their density and, in the case of opioid, the proportion of each type of receptor differ at different levels of the spinal cord (Bouchenafa & Livingston, 1987, 1989; Khan *et al.*, 1999). The density of opioid receptors is labile, increasing in response to chronic pain (Brandt & Livingston, 1990; Dickenson, 1995), and changing with age (Marsh *et al.*, 1997).

In both brain and spinal cord, a new receptor has been identified which although sharing a high degree of sequence similarity with opioid receptors is not activated by opioids. This receptor was named the ORL-1 (opioid receptor-like) receptor. Subsequently the endogenous peptide ligand for ORL-1 was identified and named orphanin FQ or nociceptin. This peptide has a widespread distribution throughout the nervous system. Despite its structural similarity to opioid peptides, nociceptin (which has now been synthesized) appears to work through entirely different neurological pathways, and it is thought that these pathways might be involved in the modulation of a broad range of physiological and behavioural functions (Meunier, 1997; Darland & Grandy, 1998). In the midbrain the ORL-1 receptor type has a dense to moderate level of expression in the periaqueductal gray matter, an area known to be involved with nociceptive processing, and where electrical stimulation or opioid agonist agents will produce intense analgesia (Meunier, 1997; Darland & Grandy, 1998). In the spinal cord of the rat, ORL-1 receptors are found in the superficial layers (laminae 1 and 2) of the dorsal horn, in areas similar to those where opioid receptors are located. The density of neurones expressing the ORL-1 receptor varies in different areas of the spinal cord. The most recent work (unpublished results quoted by Darland & Grandy, 1998) suggests that these neurones are internuncial neurones, and do not themselves project forward to the thalamus.

The position of nociceptin in relation to analgesia is still unclear. From the anatomical locations of the ORL-1 receptors it was anticipated that nociceptin would cause analgesia by both spinal and supraspinal mechanisms. In the whole animal, nociceptin does provide analgesia through spinal mechanisms, as intrathecal injection in rats produced a dose-dependent reduction of a spinal nociceptive flexor reflex, and produced behavioural antinocioception in the tail flick test. These effects were not accompanied by sedation or motor impairment, and could not be reversed by antagonists of the opioid, α_2 adrenoceptor agonist or GABA-A receptors, thus suggesting that they acted through a mechanism as yet unknown (Xu *et al.*, 1996). However in rats and mice nociceptin given by intracerebroventricular injection unexpectedly antagonized the analgesic effects of stress, opioids and electroacupuncture, thus suggesting that the supraspinal actions of the peptide were ant-analgesic. The apparent allodynia and hyperalgesia induced by the supraspinal effects of nociceptin can be blocked by another naturally occurring peptide, which has been termed nocistatin (Okuda-Ashitaka *et al.*, 1998; Darland & Grandy, 1998). Despite the complexity of the pathways involving the modulation of pain by nociceptin, interest continues in this field. Recent work has concentrated on the production of antagonists to nociceptin, as theoretically these may provide analgesia by supraspinal mechanisms, and therefore be more suitable as analgesic drugs in the practical situation (Meunier, 1997). When compared with opioid analgesics, a major potential advantage of nociceptin-based compounds is that, to date, they have not been seen to cause behaviour suggestive of euphoria or dysphoria, and therefore have the potential to become analgesics with limited tendency for abuse.

Increased understanding of the activities of the peripheral and first central cells has not been accompanied by similar advances in knowledge of the functioning of the deeper parts of the nervous system. There is considerable new knowledge of the way in which the brainstem exerts a descending control of the receptivity of the dorsal horn cells (Stamford, 1995), but so far there is no understanding of the circumstances in which these controls come into operation. The old idea of a dedicated, localized pain centre is quite untenable because apart from massive excision of the input structures, no discrete lesion in the brain has ever been shown to produce long-lasting analgesia. Thus it is necessary to analyse a distributed system

and until very recently methods to analyse brain systems in a relatively non-invasive manner did not exist.

Investigation of brain systems involved in pain

Even the techniques now available to study activity in the brain have severe limitations. Single photon emission computed tomography (SPECT), positron emission tomography (PET) and functional magnetic resonance imaging (fMRI) provide indirect measures of local brain activity. Direct measures of neural activity can be obtained from magnetoencephalography (MEG) and electroencephalography (EEG). A critical review of all these techniques as applied to human subjects is that of Berman (1995).

SPECT, PET and fMRI measure changes in regional cerebral blood flow (rCBF) and the evidence that links rCBF to increased neural activity as originally proposed by Roy and Sherrington (1890) is now well established. However, as pointed out by Berman (1995) there are important limitations to the usefulness of these techniques. Temporal and spacial resolution are poor, being measured in tens of seconds and several millimetres, while the final images are produced after multiple processing steps on large data sets sometimes obtained by pooling data from several subjects. MEG is limited to the cortical grey matter, the technique is very costly and requires a specially shielded environment because the magnetic fields produced by the brain are of the order of 10^{-13} Tesla, compared with 5×10^{-5} Tesla for the earth's magnetic field. The EEG has well known limitations of complexity due to the difficulties inherent in accurately knowing the shape and conductivity of the different tissues.

It must be said that the application of functional neuroimaging to pain is still of little value to the anaesthetist. There is much disagreement between investigators and the only reliable conclusions seem to be that changes in activity in regions of the di- and telencephalon are associated with pain perception. These facts have been known from other research methods for many years, some of them for more than a century, so that to date imaging methods have done little more than reproduce older findings. However, as these new, relatively or completely non-invasive methods become established they promise to increase our knowledge of cerebral pain mechanisms.

CONTROL OF PAIN

In experimental studies, acute pain behaviour or hyperexcitability of dorsal horn neurones may be eliminated or reduced if the afferent input is prevented from reaching the central nervous system by *pre-injury* local anaesthetic block of afferent fibres or by dampening of the excitability of the central nervous system with opioids *before* it receives an input from nociceptors (Woolf & Wall, 1986; Dickenson & Sullivan, 1987). Similar antinociceptive procedures are less effective when applied *post-injury* (Woolf & Wall, 1986a; Coderre *et al.*, 1990). As a result, the importance of 'timing' of the application of analgesic methods has been suggested as a potential major factor in the treatment of postoperative pain and the experimental studies would indicate a valuable role for pre-emptive analgesia in the prevention of postoperative pain.

In contrast to the experimental findings, several clinical studies in man (the only species where the duration and severity of pain can be relatively easily established) have so far failed to demonstrate any marked superiority of pre-emptive analgesia. Only three studies have been somewhat positive in finding either a delay in request from the patient for additional analgesics or a reduction in the need for postoperative analgesics (Katz *et al.*, 1992; Ejlersen *et al.*, 1992; Richmond *et al.*, 1993). Although it must be recognized that many of the clinical studies have been non-randomized and otherwise poorly designed, there are likely to be good reasons for failure to achieve similar results to those obtained in experimental animals. Although central sensitization may contribute to postoperative pain in humans, surgical trauma differs from the type of stimulus used in most experimental animals. Contrary to a well localized thermal or chemical injury, or brief C-afferent fibre stimulation, the afferent input to the central nervous system during and after surgery is prolonged and extensive with mixed cutaneous, muscular and visceral components. Central stimulation may persist in the postoperative period because of continuing inflammation and hyperalgesia at the site of the wound; the analgesic methods have not been continued into this period. Moreover, conventional postoperative analgesia with local anaesthetics or opioids may not provide total C-afferent block during surgery.

In human subjects it is useful to define pain as that state that disappears when treated for pain. It would, therefore, seem useful to call a drug an analgesic for an animal if it appears to ameliorate the reaction of an animal to what in man would be perceived as pain. However, it is most important to be certain that the treatment has not merely prevented the animal from displaying the sign used by the observer to connote pain in that animal. An extreme example would be to paralyse the animal with a neuromuscular blocking drug. Abolition of a clinical sign may be even more subtle. For example, neurectomy is commonly used to prevent a horse from limping. In man this technique is known to lead to Charcot joints and a deafferentation syndrome, two signs that the unfortunate horse may not be able to exhibit. Even in man, therapy is not a guaranteed test because there are intractable pains that fail to respond to any known therapy. There is no obvious reason to suppose that similar conditions do not exist in animals. Furthermore, because of the differing neurotransmitters and structures and behavioural repertoires it could be that effective analgesics for human subjects are not necessarily effective in all animals (Wall, 1992).

It must be concluded that before clinical recommendations of pre-emptive analgesia can be suggested, well controlled investigations in both animals and man are imperative. In the future, effective pre-emptive analgesia may well be achieved by a multimodal technique, such as a combination of opioids and neural block, or with specific drugs acting at the spinal cord, such as NMDA antagonists, etc. rather than a single modality 'pre-emptive' treatment. There is a need to establish the exact role of post-injury neuroplasticity relative to the magnitude and duration of postoperative pain and to develop simple and reliable methods for clinical measurement of neuroplasticity. It is naive to believe that one analgesic or one single technique will solve the complex problem of postoperative pain. However, research and development of new analgesics acting at the peripheral site of injury, such as the NSAIDs, may lead to a reduction of side effects currently associated with postoperative pain relief. It is now well established that prostaglandins contribute not only to peripheral but also to central sensitization, and that NSAIDs act at peripheral and central sites. Intrathecal administration of NSAIDs results in antinociception in experimental models of central sensitization (Malmberg & Yaksh, 1992; 1992a) and their central action is equally effective whether given before or after the application of the noxious stimulus. This is because they act on intracellular messengers responsible for the maintenance of the persistent nociceptive state in the spinal cord (Coderre & Yashpal, 1994). If the concentration of NSAID in the brain continues to increase for some hours after its administration this could provide analgesia covering much of the immediate postoperative period (Hudspith & Munglani, 1996).

MECHANISMS OF ANAESTHESIA

In 1906 Sherrington stressed the importance of the synapse in central nervous system (CNS) processing. Since then details of synaptic transmission within the CNS have received much attention. Studies have shown that a nerve cell receives information by way of synaptic contacts all over the dendrites and cell body (Fig. 1.1). Impulses travelling in presynaptic fibres progress to the terminal branches to depolarize the nerve endings. This depolarization opens voltage-gated calcium (Ca^{2+}) channels and the influx of calcium into the terminal. The resulting increase in intracellular calcium triggers the exocytotic secretion of transmitter substance from the nerve terminal. The released transmitter diffuses across the synaptic cleft and binds to specific receptor sites on the postsynaptic membrane. Receptor activation results in a change in permeability of the cell membrane to particular ions, which in turn leads to changes in membrane potential and to excitation or inhibition of the postsynaptic neurone depending on the nature of the synapse, i.e. excitatory or inhibitory. This voltage gated activity is generally accepted but it is now known that there is no clear distinc-

tion between voltage modulated channels and ligand gated channels. The demonstration of intermediate forms of ion channels suggests that overall cellular effects are far more complicated than was thought to be the case as little as 25 years ago.

FAST AND SLOW SIGNALLING

The receptors linked directly to ion channels are for fast signalling but synaptic stimulation may result in a more subtle long term modulation of excitability via second messengers. For example, noradrenaline interacts with two different classes of receptors (Pfaffinger & Siegelbaum, 1990). One class activates adenylate cyclase (β adrenoceptors) and the other inhibits adenylate cyclase (α adrenoceptors). Similarly, the response of muscarinic acetylcholine receptors depends on the receptor subtype. M1, M3 and M5 receptors activate phospholipase C and generate diacylglycerol and inositol triphosphate (IP3), while M2 and M4 receptors are associated with inhibition of adenylate cyclase (Fukuda et al., 1989). Many other neurotransmitters, such as dopamine and 5-hydroxytryptamine, are now thought to activate second messenger systems inside the cell.

Both fast and slow synaptic events eventually modulate specific ion channels and alter the level of excitability of postsynaptic neurones. Nerve terminals themselves are subject to modulation by presynaptic axonal contacts by way of presynaptic inhibition (Schmidt, 1971). Also, axons branch and changes in threshold at each branch point may result in different patterns of impulse activity in different nerve branches. Thus, there are both temporal and spatial patterns of neuronal activity in the CNS.

ACTION OF GENERAL ANAESTHETIC AGENTS

At concentrations likely to be found in the brain during surgical anaesthesia general anaesthetics depress excitatory synaptic transmission. The effects of anaesthetics on inhibitory synaptic transmission are more varied and both depression and enhancement of inhibition have been reported. From the above brief account of synaptic processing, it is clear that anaesthetics may act at a number of different sites either enhancing inhibition or depressing excitation at them. Depression of excitation or enhancement of inhibition will reduce transmission through a synaptic relay.

Excitation may be depressed by:

1. Slowing of action potential propagation
2. Enhancement of presynaptic inhibition
3. Depression of release of transmitter substances
4. Depression of the response of postsynaptic receptors
5. Enhancement of postsynaptic inhibition by increased release of inhibitory neurotransmitters
6. Augmentation of the response of postsynaptic receptors to inhibitory neurotransmitters
7. Direct action on postsynaptic neurones to modulate excitability
8. Modulation of the resting cell membrane potential.

It is clear that the action of general anaesthetics is likely to be complex. Moreover, the usual chemical structure/activity relationship seen with most

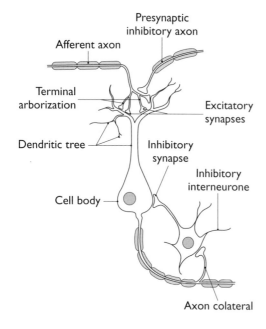

FIG. 1.1 Schematic diagram of the organization of a synaptic relay within the CNS.

bioactive chemicals is conspicuously absent in anaesthetics. There is a very wide range in molecular structure ranging from relatively simple chemicals (e.g. cyclopropane) to complex steroids (e.g. alphaxalone) which may, if conditions are appropriate, lead to a state of anaesthesia. Although convulsants may antagonize some anaesthetics the only effective antagonist for all is very great ambient pressure. Pressure provides a physicochemical barrier to an anaesthetic by action at a putative hydrophobic receptor site: it seems that pressure prevents the normal increase in volume caused by an anaesthetic at the receptor site.

There is still argument over whether anaesthetics have a common mode of action or whether each agent has a unique action, the end result of which is to produce a state of anaesthesia. The simplicity of the idea of a common mode of action is more appealing but is yet to be established. One of the more attractive unifying hypotheses is that voltage sensitive Ca^{2+} channels are the targets for all anaesthetic agents since this cation contributes to the regulation of neuronal excitability and neurotransmitter release through at least three different types of voltage sensitive Ca^{2+} channel (Hirota & Lambert, 1996). However, general anaesthetics differ in their effects on distinct neuronal processes and even their isomers do so, thus a nonspecific unitary mechanism is unlikely.

Natural sleep and general anaesthesia

It is interesting to compare general anaesthesia with natural sleep. Some 40 years have passed since the first recognition of rapid eye movement (REM) sleep (Aserensky & Kleitman, 1953) and the linking of this to Moruzzi and Magoun's earlier finding in 1949 of the arousal-promoting brain stem network – the ascending reticular activating system. Later, in 1962 Jouvet discovered that the pontine reticular formation played a key role in REM sleep generation. It has since been shown that REM sleep is regulated, at least in part, by muscarinic cholinergic receptors of the non-M1 variety localized within the medial pontine reticular formation (Steriade & McCarley, 1990). Animal studies have shown that the injection of minute doses of morphine into the medial pontine reticular formation known to be involved significantly inhibited REM sleep and increased the occurrence of apnoea (Keifer *et al.*, 1992). Even more recently *in vivo* microdialysis studies have shown that systemically administered morphine significantly decreases release of acetylcholine in the medial pontine reticular formation (Lydic *et al.*, 1993). Similar results have been reported for anaesthetic concentrations of the inhalation anaesthetic, halothane (Keifer *et al.*, 1994). Thus, cholinergic neurotransmission in the pontine reticular formation is altered by morphine, halothane and REM sleep. This gives rise to the view that cholinergic transmission in pontine reticular formation may generate some of the phenomena associated with morphine effects and halothane anaesthesia.

Although there are serious reservations about the use of the EEG as an index of anaesthesia (Prys-Roberts, 1987; Hug, 1990; Kulli & Koch, 1991; Kissin, 1993) both halothane and natural sleep produce similar spindles in the cortical EEG suggesting that halothane spindles and natural sleep spindles may be generated by the same thalamocortical mechanisms (Keifer *et al.*, 1994).

Further reseach in this area may prove productive but to date the fact remains that anaesthetics are one of the few groups of drugs which are used clinically without any real understanding of their underlying activity and the reason for their amazing efficacy remains a mystery.

DEPTH OF ANAESTHESIA

Only two years after the first demonstration of general anaesthesia John Snow (1847) stated, quite emphatically, that the point requiring most skill in the administration of anaesthetics is to determine when it has been carried far enough. Snow described five stages of anaesthesia produced by diethyl ether, the last stage in his experiments with animals being characterized by feeble and irregular respiratory movements heralding death – clearly a stage too far. A major problem faced by all anaesthetists since that time is to avoid both 'too light' anaesthesia with the risk of sudden violent movement, and the dangerous 'too deep' stage. Snow suggested guidelines whereby anaesthetists could reduce the risk of either too light or too deep ether anaesthesia. In the First World War the US Army in France was seriously deficient in medical

officers with any experience of anaesthesia and to help the inexperienced doctors avoid some of the dangers Guedel in 1918 devised a scheme involving observation of changes in respiratory rate, limb movement and eye signs which formed the basis of his celebrated 'Signs and Stages of Ether Anaesthesia' which has been included until very recently in all text books of anaesthesia.

The introduction of neuromuscular blocking drugs after World War II completely changed the picture and the emphasis swung from the danger of too deep anaesthesia to that of too light anaesthesia with the risk of conscious awareness and perception of pain. Cullen *et al.* (1972), in an attempt to produce new guidelines indicating depth of anaesthesia, were forced to conclude that it was difficult to categorize the clinical signs of anaesthesia for any one inhalation anaesthetic let alone for inhalation agents in general. Today a very much broader range of different drugs are employed during anaesthesia than were used in the 1970s. These drugs produce a very wide spectrum of quite separate pharmacological actions which include analgesia, amnesia, unconsciousness and relaxation of skeletal muscles as well as suppression of somatic, cardiovascular, respiratory and hormonal responses to surgical stimulation. It is believed from observations in man that loss of conscious awareness is achieved at lighter depths of anaesthesia than are needed to prevent movement.

Electroencephalography (EEG)

The majority of comprehensive studies attempting to monitor the depth of anaesthesia have focussed on the use of the EEG. However, the raw EEG is of very limited value to the clinical anaesthetist because of wide differences in response with different anaesthetics, the long paper runs utilized for recording generating unmanageable amounts of paper, and subjective interpretation of the traces obtained. The fast-moving EEG signals cannot be effectively monitored on visual display unit (VDU) as can the electrocardiogram and in order to simplify the extraction of useful information from complex waveforms a number of methods of compressing, processing and displaying EEG signals have been developed, some of which have been compared by Levy *et al.* (1980) and Stoeckel *et al.* (1981). In attempts to simplify the procedure these techniques have, in many cases, been applied to single channels of EEG rather than the 16 channels normally studied.

It is only possible to describe the EEG changes related to anaesthesia in the most general terms. The earliest changes seen with the induction of anaesthesia are that a previously responsive α rhythm becomes unresponsive and then desynchronized and flattened, becoming replaced with high frequency activity of low or high voltage depending on the agent. Further deepening of anaesthesia is associated with replacement of these waves with slow waves and the slower the frequency the deeper the level of anaesthesia (Mori *et al.*, 1985). Further deepening of anaesthesia produces periods of electrical silence interrupted by bursts of activity. The bursts may be of a few slow waves or with other agents repetitive high voltage spikes or even the 'spike and dome' complexes that characterize epileptic fits. This 'epileptoid' activity has commonly been associated with enflurane but it is charcteristic of ethers (Joas *et al.*, 1971).

Power spectrum analysis

In this technique the EEG signal, after being digitized, is subjected to fast Fourier analysis in which it is separated into a series of sine waves,

the sum of which represents the original signal. Breaking up the original waveform in this way makes it possible to compare one non-standard wave form with another and, in particular, to extract the distribution of components of different frequency within the EEG signal. The power in each frequency band is then derived by squaring the amplitude of each sine wave into which the Fourier Transform has separated the original signal. Power spectrum analysis as a means of monitoring depth of halothane anaesthesia in horses has been reported by Otto and Short (1991).

Considerable ingenuity has been devoted to displaying the three variable data derived from the EEG by power spectrum analysis (Figs 1.2 & 1.3). Methods such as power spectrum analysis demonstrate the relative partitioning of changes associated with depth of anaesthesia as shown in the unprocessed EEG in the general shift to lower frequency but even so they are cumbersome and of limited clinical application. The averaging over time needed for all the various methods is relatively long with a great loss of resolution. Important changes of a transient nature in the EEG such as those associated with arousal and burst suppression may be completely obscured (Bimar & Bellville, 1977). Thus it seems that in the typical clinical environment, in which multiple drugs are administered and clinical end-points are not defined clearly, the success achieved in

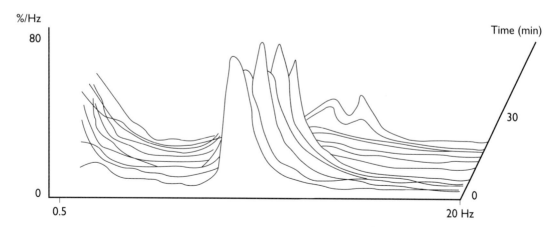

FIG. 1.2 Plot of compressed spectral array of EEG power spectrum. (After Stoeckel & Schwilden, 1987). In this plot it is necessary to suppress the lines behind the hillocks (high power bands) of the plot so that information hidden behind the hillocks is lost. To avoid loss the time axis is at an angle to the other two axes but this only slightly improves the visibility of this lost information.

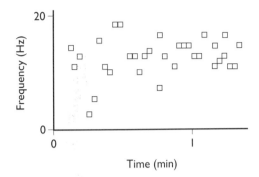

FIG. 1.3 Spectral edge frequency plot. This plot demonstrates the frequency below which lies 95% of the power in the EEG signal. (After Rampil et al., 1980.)

determining the depth of anaesthesia and predicting intraoperative arousal with movement, by study of EEG variables, is limited.

Cerebral function monitoring

A number of methods of analysing the EEG signal have been used in attempts to extract from it a single number which might be related to the depth of anaesthesia. The median frequency and the number of times the signal crosses the isoelectric line in a fixed time have been suggested but have not proved to be useful. The cerebral function analysing monitor (CFAM) of Maynard and Jenkinson (1984) is a development of the cerebral function monitor (CFM) described by Maynard in 1969. The CFM filtered the EEG signal and displayed the average peak voltage on a slowly moving chart to facilitate trend analysis. and was of particular value as a monitor of cerebral perfusion. In the CFAM similar signal processing is employed; after filtering to increase amplitude with frequency and logarithmetic amplitude compression, the frequency distribution is displayed divided into the four conventional EEG frequency bands. This instrument may be used to display transient EEG events and to study evoked potentials. References to the the use of the CFAM are given by Frank and Prior (1987).

Evoked responses

Evoked responses are changes in the EEG produced in the EEG by external stimuli, surgical or otherwise. Anaesthetic depth is a balance between cerebral depression and surgical (or other) stimulation. Thus, cerebral function during anaesthesia is most easily assessed by putting in a stimulus – auditory or somatic or visual – and observing the EEG response. That response can then be compared for amplitude and latency with the response to the same stimulus in the presence of differing brain concentrations of any anaesthetic. Changes in the EEG produced by external stimuli (evoked responses) are not easy to detect because they may be as much as 100 times below normal EEG noise and the technique of signal averaging must be employed. A repetitive stimulus such as clicks in the external ear canal is applied to the subject and an epoch of EEG signal is summated in such a way that the normal EEG signal is cancelled out (because it is random). The evoked response is time-locked to the stimulus and reinforces itself by repetition. The auditory evoked response (AER) is usually summated over 2000 or more epochs, taking 5 to 7 minutes, and this is a limitation of the technique since transient changes may not be detected. The AER can be tracked from its entry into the brain stem via the auditory nerve to the auditory cortex and cortical association areas and the pathway continues to function during quite deep surgical anaesthesia.

There are two ways of producing the AER: the transient method and the steady state method. The middle latency part of the transient response refers to a series of one to three bipolar waves occurring in the first 100 ms after an abrupt auditory event. This middle latency response (MLR) or 'early cortical response' represents processing at the primary auditory cortex and is elicited using clicks at rates near to 10/s. Although rates of as few as 1/s produce larger MLR responses, they take a very long period of signal averaging in order to produce a satisfactory waveform. The transient MLR is promising but the time to produce the response (about 5 min) and difficulties in interpreting the waveforms mean that it is very limited as a clinical tool. In contrast, the steady state method refers to activity in the EEG driven by a train of stimuli delivered at a sufficiently fast rate to cause responses provoked by successive stimuli to overlap. At rates of stimulation near to 40 Hz the amplitude reaches a maximum and with all gen-

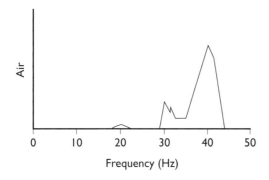

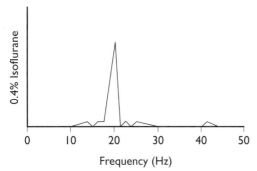

FIG. 1.4 Coherent frequency of the auditory evoked potential. (After Mungliani *et al.*, 1993.) The coherent frequency is derived by a mathematical process which demonstrates the power of the fundamental (which is large compared with the power in the harmonics).

eral anaesthetics the 40 Hz value of the dominant frequency decreases with anaesthetic depth (Mungliani *et al.*, 1993), as illustrated in Fig. 1.4.

Somatosensory evoked potentials (SER or SEP) are usually produced by percutaneous stimulation of a peripheral nerve and the waveform of the evoked potential depends on the site of stimulation and the positions of the cranial electrodes. Again the technique suffers from the time required to obtain a signal; averaging over 4 to 8 minutes may be necessary and this obscures transient EEG changes which may be produced by surgical stimulation.

The effect of surgical stimulation in horses under isoflurane anaesthesia has been examined by Otto & Short (1991). These workers looked at the power spectrum between 1 and 30 Hz and calculated the 80% spectral edge frequency (80% quantile; SEF 80), median power frequency (50% quantile; MED), relative fractional power located in the delta (1 to 4 Hz), theta (4 to 8 Hz), alpha (8 to 13 Hz), beta (13 to 30 Hz) frequency band and the

beta/delta ratio (BD), the theta/delta (T/D) and alpha/delta (A/D) ratio. They concluded that the measured EEG variables A/D ratio, median power frequency and the 80% spectral edge frequency recorded in horses with an end-tidal concentration of 1.7% isoflurane were significantly increased by surgical stimulation, suggesting EEG arousal by this stimulation.

New techniques are now being developed using bandpass digital filtering and automatic peak detection to decrease greatly the time needed for the averaging process (Bertrand *et al.*, 1987). The Bispectral Index (BIS) has been developed by Aspect Medical Systems as a monitor of the state of cortical arousal and gives a number of 0 to 100 depending on the degree of wakefulness of the subject. A low BIS may occur with sleep, anaesthesia and head injury (Driver *et al.*, 1996). The BIS uses both the EEG frequency and phase in its computation but the exact process remains, at the moment, a jealously guarded commercial secret.

More technologies for study of depth of anaesthesia are currently available than at any time in the past but whether any of them will become clinically useful may well be governed by the degree of commercial investment they obtain. To be of use in clinical practice the technology must be presented in monitors that are easy to apply and simple to operate. Many potentially useful technologies will disappear without the balance of academic study and commercial interest being available to assess them (Pomfrett, 1999).

THE 'CLASSIC' SIGNS OF ANAESTHESIA

The so-called 'classic signs' of anaesthesia, such as tabulated in Chapter 2 for convenience of newcomers to the subject and in older textbooks of anaesthesia, were provided by the presence or absence of response of the anaesthetized subject to stimuli provided by the anaesthetist or surgeon. Particular signs of anaesthesia were, therefore, equated with particular anatomical levels or 'planes' of depression of the central nervous system. These signs were often likened to a series of landmarks used to assess the progess made on a journey. Such empirical, traditional methods of assessing the progress of anaesthesia and the anatomical implications that went with these methods incorporated a fallacy, because they took no account of the fact that the changing function of any biological system can only be made in terms of magnitude and time. A depth of unconsciousness is really a particular moment in a continuous temporal stream of biological or neurological phenomena to be interpreted by the magnitude and quality of these phenomena obtaining to that moment.

Use of the term 'depth of anaesthesia' is now so ingrained in common usage that it must be accepted since it probably cannot be eradicated. It is important, however, to realize that it commonly refers to depression of brain function beyond that necessary for the production of 'anaesthesia', i.e. unawareness of surroundings and absence of recall of events.

In general, the volatile anaesthetic agents halothane, enflurane, isoflurane, sevoflurane and desflurane produce a dose-dependent decrease in arterial blood pressure and many veterinary anaesthetists use this depression to assess the depth of anaesthesia. The effect is not so marked during anaesthetic techniques involving the administration of opioid analgesics and nitrous oxide. If the depth of unconsciousness is adequate, surgical stimulation does not cause any change in arterial blood pressure. There are, however, many other factors which influence the arterial blood pressure during surgery such as the circulating blood volume, cardiac output and the influence of drug therapy given before anaesthesia. If ketamine or high doses of opioids are given arterial blood pressure may change very little if the depth of unconsciousness is increased by the administration of higher concentrations of inhalation anaesthetics.

Changes in heart rate alone are a poor guide to changes in the depth of unconsciousness. The heart rate may increase under isoflurane and enflurane anaesthesia due to their direct effect on the myocardium. Arrhythmias are common during light levels of unconsciousness induced by halothane, when they are usually due to increased sympathetic activity. In general, however, tachycardia in the absence of any other cause may be taken to represent inadequate anaesthesia for the procedure being undertaken.

Anaesthetic agents affect respiration in a dose-dependent manner and this was responsible for the original classification of the 'depth of anaesthesia'. In deeply anaesthetized animals tidal and minute volumes are decreased but, depending on the species of animal and on the anaesthetic agents used, respiratory rate may increase before breathing eventually ceases once the animal is close to death. As inadequate anaesthesia also is often indicated by an increase in the rate and/or depth of breathing the unwary may be tempted to administer more anaesthetic agent to the deeply anaesthetized animal in the mistaken impression that awareness is imminent. Laryngospasm, coughing or breath-holding can indicate excessive airway stimulation or inadequate depth of unconsciousness.

All anaesthetic agents, other than the dissociative drugs such as ketamine, cause a dose-related reduction in muscle tone and overdosage produces complete respiratory muscle paralysis. In the absence of complete neuromuscular block produced by neuromuscular blocking drugs the degree of muscle relaxation may, therefore, usually be used as a measure of the depth of anaesthetic-induced unconsciousness. However, even in the presence of muscular paralysis due to clinically effective doses of neuromuscular blockers it is not uncommon to observe movements of facial muscles, swallowing or chewing movements in response to surgical stimulation if the depth of unconsciousness becomes inadequate.

When animals are breathing spontaneously there are several signs which are generally recognized as indicating that the depth of unconsciousness is adequate for the performance of painful procedures, i.e. the animal is unaware of the environment and of the infliction of pain – it is anaesthetized. Sweating (in those animals which do) and lacrimation may both occur if surgical stimulation is intense while the depth of unconsciousness is too light. However, drugs that modify autonomic effects, such as the phenothiazine derivatives (e.g. chlorpromazine or acepromazine) may also modify sweating responses.

Unfortunately, there are many differences between the various species of animal in the signs which are usually used to estimate the depth of unconsciousness. One fairly reliable sign is that of eyeball movement, especially in horses and cattle, although even this may be modified in the presence of certain other drugs, such as the α_2 adrenoceptor agents (see ch. 11 on equine anaesthesia). Fortunately for the animal this test involves inspection only and no touching of the delicate cornea and conjunctiva although it may be necessary to separate the eyelids because these are usually closed. Unless neuromuscular blocking drugs are in use very slow nystagmus in both horses and cattle and downward inclination of the eyeballs in pigs and dogs usually indicates a satisfactory level of unconsciousness and, at this level, breathing should be smooth although its rate and depth may alter depending on the prevailing severity of the surgical stimulation. Nystagmus is also seen in horses just before death from hypoxaemia. Absence of the lash or palpebral reflex (closure of the eyelids in response to light stroking of the eyelashes) is another reasonably reliable guide to satisfactory anaesthesia. In dogs and cats it is safe to assume that if the mouth can be opened without provoking yawning or curling of the tongue, central depression is adequate. In all animals salivation and excessive lacrimation usually indicate a returning awareness.

Disappearance of head shaking or whisker twitching in response to gentle scratching of the inside of the ear pinna is a good sign of unawareness in pigs, cats, rabbits and guinea pigs. Pupil size is a most unreliable guide to unawareness because a dose of an opiate tends to cause constriction of the pupils while atropine causes dilation. The pupils do, however, dilate when an overdose of an anaesthetic has been given or when awareness is imminent.

The experienced anaesthetist relies most of the time on an animal's response to stimuli produced by the surgeon or procedure to indicate adequate depth of unconsciousness. The most effective depth is taken to be that which obliterates the animal's response to pain and/or discomfort without depressing respiratory and circulatory function.

Computer controlled anaesthesia

In general, anaesthetists use 'rules of thumb' when managing the course of anaesthesia. As the anaesthetic administration proceeds, changes in the an-

imal's physiological state are monitored by the anaesthetist who adjusts the rate of administration of intravenous drugs, or the concentration of the administered inhalation anaesthetic, or the lung ventilation, as appropriate for the perceived state of anaesthesia. The extent and direction of the adjustment is determined by this 'rule of thumb' but this does not preclude the provision of safe and effective anaesthesia. Every anaesthetist probably uses some type of rules, but sometimes simple rules are hidden by an aura of profundity designed to enhance the mystique of anaesthesia. A computer may assist in dispelling this mystique.

Given the availability of the necessary hardware and computer software a computer can be used to control the administration of an anaesthetic. It may be programed to respond to a set deviation from some predetermined value measured by a sensor, which is considered by the anaesthetist to be 'normal', by inducing a change in the delivery of an agent. For example, the instructions may be 'If the arterial blood pressure decreases by 10 mmHg then decrease the rate of administration of halothane by 10%'. It is relatively easy to program the computer to do this but a human anaesthetist controlling an anaesthetic administration will not respond in such a precise way. More likely a rule of thumb such as 'If the arterial blood pressure decreases slowly, then the rate of administration of the anaesthetic needs to be decreased a little' will be applied by the anaesthetist. This is because humans have no difficulty in responding to such imprecise information as 'decreases slowly' or 'a little' but there is currently no freely available computer language to describe such imprecise data in such a way that a computer is capable of acting on it.

Accurate control of arterial pressure (or indeed any variable) in any anaesthetized animal imposes the task of frequent monitoring of arterial pressure and adjustments of the rate of anaesthetic administration. Manual methods can lead to poor control with see-sawing values. Automatic closed-loop control of anaesthetic delivery systems, developed to improve the quality of control using standard engineering systems of self-tuning algorithms relying on mathematical models of the cardiovascular system, are not much better because the cardiovascular system is complex. Much of the

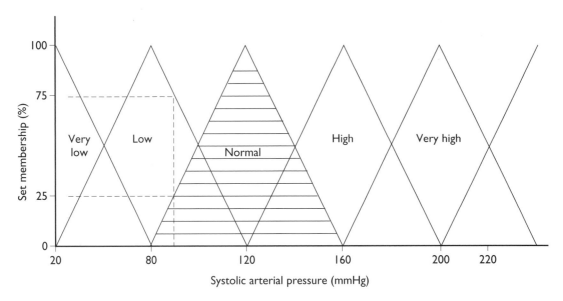

FIG. 1.5 Subdivision of systolic arterial blood pressure into sets using fuzzy logic. The boundaries of each set form a triangle and overlap the boundaries of neighbouring sets. The shaded area shows the extent of the 'normal' set. (After Asbury & Tzabar, 1995.)

complexity arises from the fact that the response is non-linear and involves a time delay before it occurs, while the degree of responsiveness may change with time.

A key to solve this problem was provided by Lofti Zadeh (1965) who coined the term 'fuzzy sets'. This concept says that an item (e.g. a measurement of blood pressure or a blood gas value) can belong simultaneously to several sets to different degrees, from not belonging (or 0% membership) through to totally belonging (or 100% membership) to a set. This principle has been well explained in relation to anaesthesia by Asbury & Tzabar (1995). They point out that a set of mean arterial blood pressure measurements from 20 to 220 mmHg can be assigned into sets such as 'normal', 'very low', 'high', etc. Using classic logic each value then takes on 100% membership of one and only one set. This logic becomes less reasonable when 99 mmHg is interpreted as 'low' but 100 mmHg as 'normal'. When the values are divided into fuzzy sets where the ordinate indicates the extent of membership, each value can belong to one or more sets (but usually two sets). Thus a value of 85 mmHg can be seen as belonging 75% to a set termed 'low' and at the same time 25% to a set termed 'normal' (Fig. 1.5). This gives a way of expressing imprecise information in a form which can be incorporated into a computer program.

Using fuzzy logic control (Ying *et al.*, 1992) which employs a series of rules described in imprecise terms (e.g. 'If the arterial pressure is slightly above the desired range, increase the administration rate of the anaesthetic a little' or 'If the arterial pressure falls catastrophically stop the administration temporarily') leads to much smoother control. These rules would be formulated by questioning an expert anaesthetist so that an engineer can convert the rules and imprecise data into a computer program which fuzzifies the incoming blood pressure data from the measuring device, applies the rules and then calculates a definitive administration rate (defuzzification) and automatically sets it on the anaesthetic delivery system.

The difficulty with fuzzy logic is that its rules have to be extracted from experts who, though perhaps highly efficient in clinical work, do not realize the extent of their own knowledge and particularly how their knowledge is structured. An engineer then needs to optimize the rules and boundaries of fuzzy sets for best performance. In theory, application of fuzzy logic should always result in much smoother and better controlled anaesthesia. The use of fuzzy logic control is likely to grow but its development is both time-consuming and costly.

MINIMAL ALVEOLAR CONCENTRATION (MAC) AND MINIMUM INFUSION RATE (MIR)

Recognition of the problems in establishing that the patient is unconscious at any given moment, coupled with the difficulty of reproducing the same degree of central nervous depression on another occasion, forces the anaesthetist to rely on the concept of minimal alveolar concentration (MAC), sometimes also known as minimal anaesthetic concentration, as proposed by Merkel and Eger (1963). MAC is defined as the alveolar concentration of an anaesthetic that prevents muscular movement in response to a painful stimulus in 50% of the test subjects. If adequate time is allowed for the anaesthetic in the brain to equilibrate with the anaesthetic agent in the blood, the alveolar partial pressure of the anaesthetic (which can be measured) is a reasonably accurate expression of the anaesthetic state. The stimulus, standardized as far as possible, usually consists of tail clamping or an electrical stimulus in animals or surgical incision or an electrical stimulus in man.

The measurement of MAC enables the relative potencies of anaesthetics to be compared, and with the MAC defined as 1.0, the level of central nervous depression can be stated as the ratio of alveolar concentration to the MAC. This reproducible method may be contrasted with the difficulty in using physiological parameters as an indication, or the EEG, which varies according to the agent used.

Although the MAC value represents the anaesthetizing dose for only 50% of subjects the anaesthetist can be reasonably certain that increasing the alveolar concentration to between 1.1 or 1.2 times MAC will ensure satisfactory anaesthesia in the vast majority of individuals because the dose–response curve is relatively steep. In veterinary practice it is also important to note that according to Eger, the variability of MAC is remarkably low between species and is quite constant in any one animal. Finally, it is important to remember that MAC is determined in healthy animals under laboratory conditions in the absence of other drugs and circumstances encountered during clinical anaesthesia which may alter the requirement for anaesthesia. MAC is not affected by the duration of anaesthesia, hyperkalaemia, hypokalaemia, hypercarbia or metabolic acid–base changes. However, MAC is reduced by 8% for every °C reduction in body temperature, by hyponatraemia and with increasing age. In dogs a progressive reduction of halothane MAC has been shown to occur as mean partial pressure is reduced to 50 mmHg. Young animals have high MAC values, and hyperthermia also increases MAC. MAC is measured as vol%, and so is dependent on atmospheric pressure, thus explaining the increased doses of volatile agents required to maintain anaesthesia at high altitudes (Eger, 1974; Quasha et al., 1980).

The accurate control of depth of unconsciousness is more difficult to achieve with intravenous anaesthetic agents. To obtain unconsciousness they must be administered at a rate which produces a concentration of drug in the bloodstream sufficient to result in the required depth of depression of the central nervous system. The concept of minimum infusion rate (MIR) was introduced by Sear and Prys-Roberts in 1970 to define the median effective dose (ED_{50}) of an intravenous anaesthetic agent which would prevent movement in response to surgical incision. Unlike MAC, however, MIR does not necessarily equate with the concentration of the anaesthetic in the blood (Spelina et al., 1986). In veterinary anaesthesia there is a paucity of information relating to the MIR and since there is no way of estimating the concentration of the agent in the blood sufficiently rapidly to enable the anaesthetist to adjust the rate of administration during any operation in the light of the analytical result, its usefulness is questionable. It may be of value in setting infusion rates in computer controlled intravenous anaesthesia but such techniques currently appear to be used infrequently in veterinary practice although it is possible that their use in experimental laboratories is more widespread.

ANAESTHETIC RISK

General anaesthesia and local analgesia do not occur naturally and their induction with drugs

TABLE 1.1 American Society of Anesthesiologists' categories of anaesthetic risk

Category	
Category 1	Normal healthy patient with no detectable disease
Category 2	Slight or moderate systemic disease causing no obvious incapacity
Category 3	Mild to moderate systemic disease causing mild symptoms (e.g. moderate pyrexia, anaemia or hypovolaemia)
Category 4	Extreme systemic disease constituting a threat to life (e.g. toxaemia, uraemia, severe hypovolaemia, cardiac failure)
Category 5	Moribund or dying patients

that even today are never completely devoid of toxicity must constitute a threat to the life of the patient. This can be a major or trivial threat depending on the circumstances, but no owner must ever be assured that anaesthesia does not constitute a risk. When an animal owner raises the question of risk involved in any anaesthetic procedure the veterinarian needs, before replying, to consider:

1. The state of health of the animal. Animals presented for anaesthesia may be fit and healthy or suffering from disease; they may be presented for elective ('cold') surgery or as emergency cases needing immediate attention for obstetrical crises, intractable haemorrhage or thoracic injuries. In the USA the American Society of Anesthesiologists (ASA) has adopted a classification of physical status into categories, an 'E' being added after the number when the case is presented as an emergency (Table 1.1).

This is a useful classification but most importantly it refers only to the physical status of the patient and is not necessarily a classification of risk because additional factors such as its species, breed and temperament contribute to the risk involved for any particular animal. Moreover, the assessment of a patient's 'correct' ASA classification varies between different anaesthetists (Haynes & Lawler, 1995; Wolters et al., 1996).

2. The influence of the surgeon. Inexperienced surgeons may take much longer to perform an operation and by rough technique produce intense and extensive trauma to tissues, thereby causing a greater metabolic disturbance (and increased postoperative pain). Increased danger can also arise when the surgeon is working in the mouth or pharynx in such a way as to make the maintenance of a clear airway difficult, or is working on structures such as the eye or larynx and provoking autonomic reflexes.

3. The influence of available facilities. Crises arising during anaesthesia are usually more easily overcome in a well equipped veterinary hospital than under the primitive conditions which may be encountered on farms.

4. The influence of the anaesthetist. The competence, experience and judgement of the anaesthetist have a profound bearing on the degree of risk to which the patient is exposed. Familarity with anaesthetic techniques leads to greater efficiency and the art of anaesthetic administration is only developed by experience.

GENERAL CONSIDERATIONS IN THE SELECTION OF THE ANAESTHETIC METHOD

The first consideration will be the nature of the operation to be performed, its magnitude, site and duration. In general, the use of local infiltration analgesia may suffice for simple operations such as the incision of superficial abscesses, the excision of small neoplasms, biopsies and the castration of immature animals. Nevertheless, what seems to be a simple interference may have special anaesthetic requirements. Subdermal fibrosis may make local infiltration impossible to effect. Again, the site of the operation in relation to the complexity of the structures in its vicinity may render operation under local analgesia dangerous because of possible movement by the conscious animal, e.g. operations in the vicinity of the eyes.

When adopting general anaesthesia the likely duration of the procedure to be performed will influence the selection of the anaesthetic. Minor, short operations may be performed quite satisfactorily after the intravenous injection of a small dose of an agent such as propofol or thiopental sodium. For longer operations anaesthesia may be induced with an ultra-short acting agent and maintained with an inhalation agent with or without endotracheal intubation. For most major operations under general anaesthesia, preanaesthetic medication ('premedication') will need to be considered, particularly when they are of long duration and the animal must remain quiet and pain-free for several hours after the operation. Undesirable effects of certain agents (e.g. ketamine) may need to be countered by the administration of 'correcting' agents (e.g. α_2 adrenoceptor agonists, atropine). Although sedative premedication may significantly reduce the amount of general anaesthetic which has to be given it may also increase the duration of recovery from anaesthesia. Premedication may be omitted for day-case patients when a rapid return to full awareness is desirable.

The species of animal involved is a pre-eminent consideration in the selection of the anaesthetic method (see later chapters). The anaesthetist will be influenced not only by size and temperament but also by any anatomical or physiological features peculiar to a particular species or breed. Experience indicates that the larger the animal, the greater are the difficulties and dangers associated with the induction and maintenance of general anaesthesia. Methods which are safe and satisfactory for the dog and cat may be quite unsuitable for horses and cattle. In vigorous and heavy creatures the mere upset of locomotor coordination may entail risks, as also may prolonged recumbency.

Individual animals

The variable reaction of the different species of animals, and of individuals, to the various agents administered by anaesthetists will also influence the choice of anaesthetic technique. In addition, factors causing increased susceptibility to the toxic actions of anaesthetic agents must be borne in mind. These include:

1. Prolonged fasting. This, by depleting the glycogen reserves of the liver, greatly reduces its detoxicating power and when using parenterally administered agents in computed doses, allowance must be made for increased susceptibility to them.

2. Diseased conditions. Toxaemia causes degenerative changes in parenchymatous organs, particularly the liver and the heart, and great care

must be taken in giving computed doses of agents to toxaemic subjects. Quite often it is found that a toxaemic animal requires very much less than the 'normal' dose. Toxaemia may also be associated with a slowing of the circulation and unless this is recognized it may lead to gross overdosing of intravenous anaesthetics. In those diseases associated with wasting there is often tachycardia and a soft, friable myocardium; animals suffering from such diseases are, in consequence, liable to develop cardiac failure when subjected to the stress of anaesthesia. It is most important that the presence of a diseased condition is detected before anaesthesia is induced.

EVALUATION OF THE PATIENT BEFORE ANAESTHESIA

It is probable that most veterinary operations are performed on normal, healthy animals. The subjects are generally young and represent good 'anaesthetic risks'. Nevertheless, enquiry should be made to ensure that they are normal and healthy – bright, vigorous and of hearty appetite. Should there be any doubt, operations are best delayed until there is assurance on this point. Many a reputation has been damaged by performing simple operations on young animals which are in the early stages of some acute infectious disease or which possess some congenital abnormality.

When an operation is to be performed for the relief of disease, considerable care must be exercised in assessing the factors which may influence the choice or course of the anaesthetic. Once these are recognized the appropriate type of anaesthesia can be chosen and preoperative measures adopted to diminish or, where possible, prevent complications. The commonest conditions affecting the course of anaesthesia are those involving the cardiovascular and respiratory systems, but the state of the liver and kidneys cannot be ignored.

The owner or attendant should always be asked whether the animal has a cough. A soft, moist cough is associated with airway secretions that may give rise to respiratory obstruction and lung collapse when the cough reflex is suppressed by general anaesthesia. Severe cardiovascular disease may be almost unoticed by the owner and enquiry should be made to determine whether the animal appears to suffer from respiratory distress after exertion, or indeed appears unwilling to take exercise, since these signs may precede other signs of cardiac and respiratory failure by many months or even years. Dyspnoea is generally the first sign of left ventricular failure and a history of excessive thirst may indicate the existence of advanced renal disease, diabetes mellitus or diabetes insipidus.

The actual examination may be restricted to one which is informative yet will not consume too much time nor unduly disturb the animal. While a more complete examination may sometimes be necessary, attention should always be paid to the pulse, the position of the apex beat of the heart, the presence of cardiac thrills, the heart sounds and the jugular venous pressure. Examination of the urine for the presence of albumin and reducing substances may also be useful.

Tachycardia is to be expected in all febrile and in many wasting diseases and under these circumstances is indicative of some myocardial weakness. It can, however, also be due to nervousness and where this is so it is often associaed with rather cold ears and/or feet. Bradycardia may be physiological or it may indicate complete atrioventricular block. In horses atrioventricular block that disappears with exercise is probably of no clinical significance. In all animals the electrocardiogram may be the only way of determining whether bradycardia is physiological or is due to conduction block in the heart.

The jugular venous pressure is also important. When the animal is standing and the head is held so that the neck is at an angle of about 45° to the horizontal, distension of the jugular veins should, in normal animals, be just visible at the base of the neck. When the distension rises above this level, even in the absence of other signs, it indicates an obstruction to the cranial vena cava or a rise in right atrial or ventricular pressures. The commonest cause of a rise in pressure in these chambers is probably right ventricular hypertrophy associated with chronic lung disease although congenital conditions such as atrial septal defects may also be indicated by this sign and it should be remembered that cattle suffering from constrictive pericarditis, or bacterial endocarditis, may have a marked increase in venous pressure.

The presence of a thrill over the heart is always a sign of cardiovascular disease and suggests an increased risk of complications arising during anaesthesia. More detailed cardiological examination is warranted when a cardiac thrill is detected during the preoperative examination.

Auscultation of the heart should never be omitted, particularly when the animal's owner is present because owners expect this to be carried out, but the findings are perhaps only of limited interest to the anaesthetist. The timing of any murmurs should be ascertained by simultaneous palpation of the arterial pulse. Diastolic murmurs are always indicative of heart disease and, while they may be of little importance in relation to cardiac function during anaesthesia, it is unwise to come to this conclusion unless other signs, such as displacement of the apex beat, are absent. Systolic murmurs may or may not indicate the presence of heart disease, but if other signs are absent they are most probably of no significance to the anaesthetist.

Accurate location of the apex beat is possibly the most important single observation in assessing the state of the cardovascular and respiratory systems. It is displaced in most abnormal conditions of the lungs (e.g. pleural effusion, pneumothorax, lung collapse) and in the presence of enlargement of the left ventricle. In the absence of any pulmonary disorder a displaced apex beat indicates cardiac hypertrophy or dilatation.

Oedema in cardiac failure has multiple causes which are not fully understood but include a failing right ventricle and an abnormal renal blood flow that gives rise to secondary aldosteronism and excessive reabsorption of salt and water by the renal tubules. The tissue fluid appears to accumulate in different regions in different species – in horses in the limbs and along the ventral body wall, in cattle it is seen in the brisket region and in dogs and cats the fluid tends to accumulate in the abdominal cavity. The differential diagnosis of peripheral oedema includes renal disease, liver disease and impaired lymphatic drainage.

Pulmonary disorders provide particular hazards for an animal undergoing operation and any examination, no matter how brief, must be designed to disclose their presence or absence. On auscultation attention should be directed towards the length of the expiratory sounds and the discovery of any rhonchi or crepitations. If rhonchi or crepitations are heard excessive sputum is present, and the animal is either suffering from, or has recently suffered, a pulmonary infection. Prolongation of the the expiratory sounds, especially when accompanied by high pitched rhonchi, indicate narrowing of the airways or bronchospasm. Respiratory sounds may be absent in animals with pneumothorax, extensive lung consolidation, or severe emphysema; they are usually faint in moribund animals.

Uneven movements between the two sides of the chest is a reliable sign of pulmonary disease and one which is easily and quickly observed. The animal should be positioned squarely while the examiner stands directly in front of it and then directly behind it. In small animals uneven movement of the two sides of the chest is often better appreciated by palpation rather than by inspection.

The mouth should be examined for the presence of loose teeth which might become dislodged during general anaesthesia and enter the tracheobronchial tree. Other mucous membranes should be inspected for evidence of anaemia, denoted by paleness.

Biochemical tests prior to anaesthesia

The question as to whether preanaesthetic urine and blood analysis should be performed routinely before every elective anaesthetic is controversial. Such tests are essential to confirm or exclude disease conditions suspected as a result of clinical history and examination, but the cost/benefit of their use in animals which appear perfectly healthy can be argued on the basis that the results rarely would alter the anaesthetic protocol to be employed. Urine testing is simple, inexpensive and is particularly important in dogs for in these animals renal disease and previously undiagnosed diabetes mellitus are common. Urine samples may be less readily obtainable from other species of animal. The Association of Veterinary Anaesthetists debated (Spring Meeting, 1998) the question as to the need for routine preanaesthetic checks on haematological and biochemical profiles, and voted that they were unnecessary if the clinical examination was adequate. Although in a very occasional case (e.g. the detection of a partial hepto-portal shunt in a young dog) such tests may detect an unsuspected disease state, in the vast majority of apparently fit healthy animals they constitute an unnecessary expense, and indeed the extra cost involved may prevent an owner from agreeing to continuation of treatment necessary for the wellbeing of the patient.

Provided a brief examination such as that described is carried out thoroughly, and that the examiner has sufficient skill and experience to recognize the significance or lack of significance of the findings, most of the conditions that have a bearing on the wellbeing of an animal in the perioperative period will be brought to light so that appropriate measures can be taken to protect it from harm.

SIGNIFICANCE OF CONDITIONS FOUND BY PREANAESTHETIC EXAMINATION

CARDIOVASCULAR AND RESPIRATORY DISEASE

The cardiovascular and respiratory systems are those which govern the rate at which oxygen can be made available to the tissues of the body. Many years ago Nunn and Freeman drew attention to the crucial fact that this rate is equal to the product of the cardiac output and the oxygen content of the arterial blood. Since the arterial oxygen content approximates to the product of the oxygen saturation and the quantity of oxygen which can be carried by the haemoglobin (about 1.34 ml per g of haemoglobin when fully saturated), the oxygen made available to the body can be expressed by a simple equation:

$$\begin{aligned} \text{Available oxygen} &= \text{cardiac output (ml/min)} \\ \text{(ml/min)} &\quad \times \text{ arterial saturation (\%)} \\ &\quad \times \text{ haemoglobin (g/ml)} \\ &\quad \times 1.34 \end{aligned}$$

This equation, of course, makes no allowance for the small quantity of oxygen which is carried in physical solution in the plasma, but it serves to illustrate the way in which three variables combine to produce an effect which is often greater than is commonly supposed. If any one of the three determining variables on the right-hand side of the equation is changed, the rate at which oxygen is made available to the tissues of the body is altered proportionately. Thus, if the cardiac output is halved, the available oxygen is also halved. If two determinants are lowered simultaneously while the third remains constant, the effect on the available oxygen is the product of the individual changes. For example, if the cardiac output and the haemoglobin concentration are both halved while the arterial oxygen saturation remains at about the normal 95%, only one-quarter of the normal amount of oxygen is made available to the body tissues. If all three variables are reduced the effect is, of course, even more dramatic.

DRUG METABOLISM AND DISEASE STATES

Drugs are usually metabolized through several pathways so that they are changed from fat soluble, active, unexcretable drugs into water soluble, inactive drugs that are able to be excreted by the kidneys and in the bile. Since the mammalian body metabolizes many thousands of compounds every day and has far fewer enzymes, each enzyme metabolizes many substrates. Only very rarely, if ever, will one enzyme metabolize only one substrate. Many things change enzyme function. Mechanisms for enzyme induction are poorly understood, unlike inhibition, which has been much more extensively studied. Enzyme induction is a slow process involving an increased amount of enzyme in the cell over about 24 to 48 hours, whereas inhibition is quick and sometimes occurs after only one dose of an inhibitor. Since enzymes are proteins their concentrations inside cells may be changed by a variety of factors (Fig. 1.6).

There is now an increasing amount of information about how enzymes change in response to one stressful stimulus but it is important to recognize that usually several stimuli exist at the same time in each critically ill animal. Most chemical reactions are sensitive to temperature, speeding up as the temperature increases and slowing with a decrease in temperature, but in spite of this all fevers do not increase the rate of metabolism of drugs: the cause of the fever is important. Infections and pyrogens cause the release of inflammatory mediators which reduce the expres-

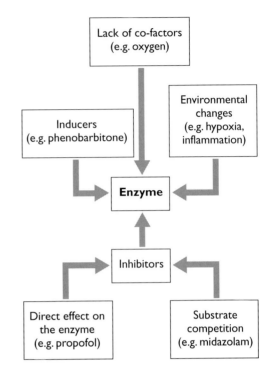

FIG. 1.6 Factors which may change enzyme function.

sion and activity of many enzymes. Non-traumatic stress has been shown to reduce enzyme function, possibly by decreased hepatic blood flow resulting in hypoxaemic induced reduction in metabolizing enzymes. Endogenous corticosteroid secretion as part of the stress response or exogenous steroid given to treat disease will change the expression of drug metabolizing enymes, and metabolic activity also varies with age. The anaesthetist must be aware of these factors so that any increase or decrease in the duration of drug action may be anticipated.

FACTORS AFFECTING TRANSPORT OF DRUGS IN THE BODY

Most drugs are carried in the bloodstream partly bound, usually by electrostatic bonds, to the proteins of the plasma, albumin being far the most important for the majority of agents. Light or moderate protein binding has relatively little effect on drug pharmacokinetics or pharmacodynamics. Heavy protein binding with drugs such as thiopental results in a low free plasma concentration of the drug, which may become progressively augmented as the available binding sites become saturated. The bound drug is, of course, in dynamic equilibrium with free (active) drug in the plasma water. The bonds are generally reversible and conform to the law of mass action:

$$\begin{array}{ccc} [D] & & [P] \\ \text{drug} & + & \text{protein} \end{array} \underset{k_{bf}}{\overset{k_{fb}}{\rightleftharpoons}} \begin{array}{c} [DP] \\ \text{complex} \end{array}$$

The association and dissociation processes take place very quickly, and can generally be taken to be instantaneous. The equilibrium association constant K_A is defined as the ratio of rate constants, and of bound to the product of unbound concentrations:

$$K_A = \frac{k_{fb}}{k_{bf}} = \frac{[DP]}{[D] \times [P]}$$

This simple relationship is often obscured by the fact that one protein molecule may possess several binding sites for any particular drug, which may or may not have the same association constant. It can generally be assumed, however, that so long as the plasma proteins remain unchanged, the ratio of 'free' to 'bound' drug will remain constant. This ratio depends on the nature of the drug molecule. Small, neutral, water soluble drugs will not bind to protein at all but larger lipophilic molecules may exhibit very high binding ratios.

Anaemia is often associated with hypoproteinaemia and this can have marked effects in anaesthesia. In conditions where there is anaemia and hypoalbuminaemia, a greater fraction of a given dose of a drug will be unbound and this will be even greater if other bound drugs have already occupied many of the binding sites. This can result in an increased peak activity of the drug. Liver disease giving rise to hypoalbuminaemia can result in reduced binding of drugs such as morphine so that smaller than normal doses of this analgesic will be effective when pain relief is needed. A rapid intravenous injection of an albumin-bound drug may also lead to increased pharmacological activity because the binding capacity of the albumin in the limited volume of blood with which the drug initially mixes is exceeded and more free (active) drug is presented to the receptor sites. Plasma protein binding enhances alimentary absorption of drugs by lowering the free plasma concentration, thereby increasing the concentration gradient for diffusion from the gut lumen. An apparent exception to the increased activity of drugs in hypoproteinaemic animals is the resistance to tubocurarine seen in cases of liver disease. This is explained by the fact that tubocurarine binds to γ globulin rather than albumin and reversed albumin/globulin ratios are common in hepatic diseases.

Not surprisingly, for a protein with a molecular weight of about 65 000, there are several genetically acquired variants of albumin. Furthermore, the configuration of the albumin molecule also changes during illness and, for example, in renal failure. These changes can be demonstrated by electrophoresis but their significance for the binding of drugs *in vivo* is not known.

RENAL DISEASE

Chronic renal disease is common in dogs, and affected animals cannot produce concentrated urine. Dehydration from any cause deprives the kidneys of sufficient water for excretory purposes (Fig. 1.7). To ensure that these animals receive an adequate fluid intake over the anaesthetic period it is usually necessary to administer fluid by intravenous infusion. A uraemic circle can also be set up in animals suffering from chronic renal disease if the arterial blood pressure is allowed to decrease because of anaesthetic overdose or haemorrhage and renal ischaemia ensues (Fig. 1.8). The maintenance of the circulating fluid volume is most important in all animals with chronic renal disease and it is important that adequate venous access is assured before anaesthesia and operation.

Acute renal failure can be defined as an abrupt decline in renal function with a decrease in glomerular filtration rate (GFR) resulting in the retention of nitrogenous waste products. Acute renal failure is classified into:

(i) Prerenal failure, denoting a disorder in the systemic circulation that causes renal hypoperfusion. Implicit here is that correction of the underlying circulatory disturbance (e.g. by improvement in cardiac function or repletion of volume) restores the GFR. However, prerenal failure is often followed by transition to:

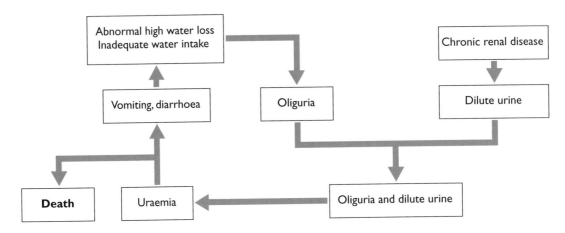

FIG. 1.7 Effect of water deprivation in dogs suffering from chronic renal disease.

(ii) Intrinsic renal failure, where correction of the underlying circulatory impairment does not restore the GFR to normal levels. Intrinsic renal failure generally includes tubular necrosis or the blocking of tubules by cell debris or precipitated proteins and there is no question of unaffected nephrons compensating for failing nephrons as there is in chronic renal failure. Instead all are involved in a massive disturbance of renal function with diversion of blood flow away from the renal cortex towards the medulla and an overall reduction in renal perfusion. There is, however, a potential for complete recovery, whereas chronic renal failure invariably progresses over a variable period of time with no hope of recovery of renal function.

(iii) Postrenal failure (obstructive) is a third possibility.

Excessive reliance on blood pressure maintenance to between the 'autoregulatory range' by infusion or the use of vasoactive drugs overlooks the fact that renal blood flow is labile since the kidneys contribute to the regulation of blood pressure. The incidence of acute renal failure is high after the use of intravenous contrast radiological media, nephrotoxic drugs (e.g. non-steroidal anti-inflammatory drugs, gentamycin, amphotericin). The use of dopamine as a renoprotective agent is controversial; it is said to act as a renal vasodilator but it is probable that the increased renal blood flow when it is given in doses of 2–5 µg/kg/min is due to inotropic effects because other non-dopaminergic inotropic agents have similar effects on renal blood flow.

PREPARATION OF THE PATIENT

Certain operations are performed as emergencies when it is imperative that there shall be no delay and but little preparation of the patient is possible. Amongst these operations are repair of thoracic injuries, the control of severe, persistent haemorrhage, and certain obstetrical interferences where the delivery of a live, healthy neonate is of paramount importance. For all other operations, time and care spent in preoperative preparation are well worthwhile since proper preparation not only improves the patient's chances of survival, but also prevents the complications which might otherwise occur during and after operation. When operations are to be performed on normal, healthy animals, only the minimum of preparation is required before the administration of a general anaesthetic, but operations on dehydrated, anaemic, hypovolaemic or toxic patients should only be undertaken after careful preoperative assessment and preparation.

FOOD AND WATER

Food should be withheld from the animal on the day it is to undergo an elective operation under general anaesthesia. A distended stomach may

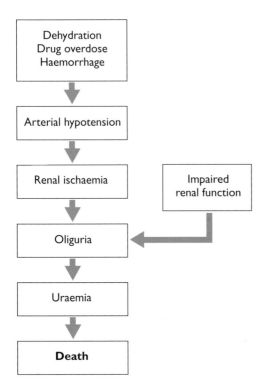

FIG. 1.8 Effect of drug overdose or haemorrhage on arterial blood pressure leading to renal failure and death in the presence of chronic renal disease.

interfere with the free movement of the diaphragm and hinder breathing. In dogs, cats and pigs, a full stomach predisposes to vomiting under anaesthesia. In horses a full stomach may rupture when the horse falls to the ground as unconsciousness is induced. In ruminants, a few hours of starvation will not result in an appreciable reduction in the volume of the fluid content of the rumen but it seems to reduce the rate of fermentation within this organ, thus delaying the development of tympany when eructation is supressed by general anaesthesia.

Excessive fasting exposes the patient to risks almost as great as those associated with lack of preparation and should not be adopted. Any fasting of birds and small mammals is actually life-threatening. Many clinicians are of the opinion that prolonged fasting in horses predisposes to postanaesthetic colic by encouraging gut stasis. In non-ruminants, free access to water should be allowed right up to the time premedication is given, but in ruminants there is some advantage in withholding water for about six hours before abdominal operations because this appears to result in slowing of fermentation in the rumen.

FLUID AND ELECTROLYTES

The water and electrolyte balance of an animal is a most important factor in determining uncomplicated recovery or otherwise after operation. The repair of existing deficits of body fluid, or of one of its components, is complex because of the interrelations between the different electrolytes and the difficulties imposed by the effects of severe sodium depletion on the circulation and renal function.

Fortunately, the majority of animal patients suffer only minor and recent upsets of fluid balance so that infusion with isotonic saline, Hartmann's solution or 5% dextrose, depending on whether sodium depletion or water depletion is the more predominant, is all that is required. An anaesthetic should not be administered to an animal which has a depleted circulating blood volume for the vasodilatation caused by anaesthetic agents may lead to acute circulatory failure, and every effort should be made to repair this deficit by the infusion of blood, plasma or plasma substitute before anaesthesia is induced. In many instances, anaesthesia and operation may be safely postponed until the total fluid deficit is made good and an adequate renal output is achieved, but in cases of intestinal obstruction operation should be carried out as soon as the blood volume has been restored. Attempts to restore the complete extracellular deficit before the intestinal obstruction is relieved result in further loss of fluid into the lumen of the obstructed bowel and, especially in horses, make subsequent operation more difficult. When in doubt about the nature and volume of fluid to be administered, it is as well to remember that, with the exception of toxic conditions and where severe hypotension due to hypovolaemia is present, an animal's condition should not deteriorate further if sufficient fluid is given to cover current losses. These current losses include the inevitable loss of water through the skin and respiratory tract (approximately 20–60 ml/kg/day depending on the age and species of the animal), the urinary and faecal loss, and any abnormal loss such as vomit.

HAEMOGLOBIN LEVEL

As already mentioned on page 21 anaemia may be treated to raise the haemoglobin concentration to more reasonable value before any major premeditated surgery is performed. When operation can be delayed for two or more weeks, the oral or parenteral administration of iron may increase the haemoglobin to an acceptable value, (eg. 10 to 12 g/100 ml blood depending on the species of animal) but when such a delay is inadvisable either the transfusion of red blood cells is indicated or low levels of haemoglobin must be tolerated for their effect of decreasing blood viscosity.

DIABETES MELLITUS

It is sometimes necessary to anaesthetize a dog or cat suffering from diabetes mellitus and if the condition is already under control no serious problems are likely to be encountered. However, if the normal dose of insulin is given, starvation before operation and inappetance afterwards may give rise to hypolgycaemia. There are over 30 commercially available preparations of insulin and they have different durations of action. Short acting insulins (e.g. soluble insulin) have a peak effect at 2 to 4 hours and their effects last for 8 to 12 hours. Medium acting insulins (e.g. semilente) have a peak effect at 6 to 10 hours and activity for up to 24 hours. Long acting insulins have a peak effect at 12 to 15 hours and one dose lasts for at least 36 hours. For this reason it is advisable to switch to purely short acting insulin a few days prior to elective surgery. By doing this, there is effectively no active long acting insulin preparation left on the day of operation and it becomes much easier to control the blood sugar around the perioperative period.

If an emergency operation has to be performed on an uncontrolled diabetic then the condition of the animal requires careful assessment and treatment. Ketonuria is an indication for treatment with gluose and soluble insulin, whilst overbreathing is a sign of severe metabolic acidosis. This must be treated with the infusion of sodium bicarbonate solution but the amount of bicarbonate needed in any particular case can only be calculated with any degree of certainty when the acid–base status is known from laboratory examination of an anaerobically drawn arterial blood sample. In the absence of this data the animal may be treated by infusing 2.5% sodium bicarbonate solution until the overbreathing ceases. Because of the presence of an osmotic diuresis, many uncontrolled diabetics also require treatment for dehydration. The object of management is not to try to correct all disturbances as quickly as possible, so as achieving in an hour or two what normally should take 2 to 3 days. Doing this may produce swings in plasma osmolarity that can be responsible for the development of cerebral oedema. All that is necessary prior to emergency surgery is to correct any hypovolaemia and ensure that the blood glucose level is declining.

INFLUENCE OF PRE-EXISTING DRUG THERAPY

Modern therapeutic agents are often of considerable pharmacological potency and animals presented for anaesthesia may have been exposed to one or more of these. Some may have been given as part of the preoperative management of the animal but whatever the reason for their administration they may modify the animal's response to anaesthetic agents, to surgery and to drugs given before, during and after operation. In some cases drug interactions are predictable and these may form the basis of many of the combinations used in modern anaesthesia, but effects which are unexpected may be dangerous.

In an ideal situation a drug action would occur only at a desired site to produce the sought-after effect. In practice, drugs are much less selective and are prone to produce 'side effects' which have to be anticipated and taken into account whenever the drug is administered. (A 'side effect' may be defined as a response not required clinically, but which occurs when when a drug is used within its therapeutic range.) Apart from these unavoidable side effects which are inherent, adverse reactions to drugs may occur in many different ways which are of importance to the anaesthetist. These include:

1. Overdosage. For some drugs exact dosing may be difficult. Overdosage may be absolute as when an amount greater than the intended dose is given in error, or a drug is given by an inappropriate route, e.g. a normal intramuscular dose may constitute a serious overdose if given intravenously. Relative overdose may be due to an abnormality of the animal; an abnormal sensitivity to digitalis is found in hypokalaemic animals and newborn animals are sensitive to non-depolarizing neuromuscular blocking drugs. The use in dogs and cats of flea collars containing organophosphorus compounds may reduce the plasma cholinesterase and prolong the action of a normal dose of suxamethonium. Overdose manifestations vary from acute to chronic and may produce toxicity by a quantitatively enhanced action which can be an extension of the therapeutic action, e.g. neostigmine in excess for the antagonism of non-depolarizing neuromuscular block. They may also be due to side effects (e.g. morphine producing respiratory depression).

2. Idiosyncrasy. Some animals may have a genetically determined response to a drug which is qualitatively different to that of normal individuals, as in the porcine hyperpyrexia syndrome (porcine malignant hyperthermia).

3. Intolerance. This is exhibiting a qualitatively normal response but to an abnormally low or high dose. It is usually simply explained by the Gaussian distribution of variation in the animal population.

4. Allergy. Allergic responses are, in general, not dose related and the allergy may be due to the drug itself or to the vehicle in which it is presented.The reaction may take a number of forms: shock, asthma or bronchospasm, hepatic congestion from hepatic vein constriction, blood disorders, rashes or pyrexia. Terms such as 'allergic', 'anaphylactic', 'anaphylactoid' or 'hypersensitive' have specific meanings to immunologists but, unfortunately, they are often used interchangeably. Strictly speaking it is inaccurate to use any of these terms until evidence of the immunological basis of a reaction has been established. Many of these reactions are histamine-related but other mediators such as prostaglandins, leucotrienes or kinins may be involved. Some immunologists consider that where either the mediator or the mechanism involved is uncertain, reactions are best described as 'histaminoid' or 'anaphylactoid'.

5. Drug interactions. Despite the importance of drug interactions there is little information in the veterinary literature on this subject. Drug interaction can occur outside the body, as when two drugs are mixed in a a syringe before they are administered, or inside the body after administration by the same or different routes. It is generally unwise to mix products or vehicles in the same syringe or to administer a drug into an intravenous infusion of another drug for this may result in precipitation of one or both drugs or even the formation of new potentially toxic or inactive compounds. The result of the interaction between two drugs inside the body may be an increased or decreased action of one or both or even an effect completely different from the normal action of either drug. The result of interaction may be simply the the sum of the actions of the two drugs $(1 + 1 = 2)$, or greater $(1 + 1 > 2)$, when it is known as synergism. When one agent has no appreciable effect but enhances the response to the other $(0 + 1 > 1)$ the term 'potentiation' is used to describe the effect of the first on the action of the second. An agent may also antagonize the effects of another and the antagonism may be 'chemical' if they form an inactive complex, 'physiological' if they have directly opposing actions although at different sites, or 'competitive' if they compete for the same receptors. Non-competitive antgonism may result from modification by one drug of the transport, biotransformation or excretion of the other. In the liver the non-specific metabolic degradation of many drugs occurs and many different agents have the ability to cause an 'enzyme induction' whilst a few decrease the activity – 'enzyme inhibition'. Analgesics such as phenylbutazone cause enzyme induction and can produce a great increase in the rate of metabolism of substrates. Barbiturate treatment of epilepsy may almost halve the half-life of dexamethasone with a conseqent marked deterioration in the therapeutic effect of this steroidal substance. Competition for binding sites and the displacement of one drug from the bound (inactive) form may lead to increased toxicity. For example, warfarin (which is sometimes used in the management of navicular disease in horses) is displaced by several agents, including the analgesic phenylbutazone, with a resulting risk of haemorrhage.

REFERENCES

Asbury, A.J. and Tzabar, Y. (1995) Fuzzy logic: new ways of thinking for anaesthesia. *British Journal of Anaesthesia* **75**: 1–2.

Aserensky, E. and Kleitman, N. (1953) Regularly occurring periods of eye motility and concomitant phenomena during sleep. *Science* **118**: 273–274.

Berman, J. (1995) Imaging pain in humans. *British Journal of Anaesthesia* **75**: 209–216.

Bertrand, O., Garcia-Larrea, L., Artru, F., Maguire, F. and Pernier, J. (1987) Brain stem monitoring. I. A system for high-rate sequential BAEP recording and feature extraction. *Electroencephalography and Clinical Neurophysiology* **68**: 433–445.

Bimar, J. and Bellville, J.W. (1977) Arousal reactions during anesthesia in man. *Anesthesiology*, **47**: 449–454.

Bouchenafa, O. and Livingston, A. (1987) Autoradiographic localisation of alpha 2 adrenoceptor binding sites in the spinal cord of sheep. *Research in Veterinary Science*, **42**: 382–386.

Bouchenafa, O. and Livingston, A. (1989) Distribution of immunoreactive Met-enkephalin and autoradiographic [3H] DAGO and [3H] DPDPE in the spinal cord of sheep. *Advances in Biological Science* **75**: 289–292.

Brandt, S.A. and Livingston, A. (1990) Receptor changes in the spinal cord of sheep associated with exposure to chronic pain. *Pain* **42**: 323–329.

Coderre, T.J., Vaccarino, A.L. and Melzak, R. (1990) Central nervous system plasticity in the tonic pain response to subcutaneous formalin injection. *Brain Research* **535**: 155–158.

Coderre, T.J. and Yashpal, K. (1994) Intracellular messengers contributing to persistent nociception and hyperalgesia induce by L-glutamate and substance P in the rat formal pain model. *European Journal of Neuroscience*, **6**: 1328–1334.

Cullen, D.J., Egger, E.I.II, Stevens, W. C. et al. (1972) Clinical signs of anesthesia. *Anesthesiology* **36**: 21–36.

Darland, T. and Grandy, D.K. (1998) The orphanin FQ system: an emerging target for the management of pain? *British Journal of Anaesthesia* **81**: 29–38.

Dickenson, A.H. (1995) Spinal cord pharmacology of pain. *British Journal of Anaesthesia* **75**: 193–200.

Dickenson, A.H. and Sullivan, A.F. (1987) Subcutaneous formalin-induced activity of dorsal horn neurones in the rat: differential response to an intrathecal opiate administered pre or post formalin. *Pain* **30**: 349–360.

Driver, I.K., Watson, B.J., Menon, D.K., Aggarwal, S.K. and Jones, J.G. (1996) Bispectral index is a state specific measure of arousal. *British Journal of Anaesthesia*, **77**, 694.

Eger, E.I. (1974) *Anaesthetic Uptake and Action.* Baltimore: Williams and Wilkins,

Ejlersen, E., Andersen, H.B., Eliasen, K. and Mogensen, T.A. (1992) A comparison between pre- and postincisional lidocaine infiltration on postoperative pain. *Anesthesia and Analgesia* **74**: 495–498.

Frank, M. and Prior, P.F. (1987) The cerebral function analysing monitor: principle and potential use. In: Rosen, M. & Lunn, J.N.(eds) *Consciousness, Awareness and Pain in General Anaesthesia.* London: Butterworths, pp 61–71.

Fukuda, K., Kubo, T., Maeda, A., Akiba, I., Bujo, H. *et al.* (1989) Selective effector coupling of muscarinic acetylcholine receptor subtypes. *Trends in Pharmacological Sciences* **10S**: 4–10.

Haynes, S.R. and Lawler, P.G.P. (1995) An assessment of the consistency of ASA physical status classification allocation. *Anaesthesia* **50**: 195–199.

Hirota, K. and Lambert, D.G. (1996) Voltage sensitive Ca^+ channels and anaesthesia. *British Journal of Anaesthesia* **76**: 344–346.

Hug, C.G. (1990) Does opioid 'anaesthesia' exist? *Anesthesia and Analgesia* **73**: 1–4.

Joas, T.A., Stevens, W.C. and Egger E.I. II (1971) Electroencephalographic seizure activity in dogs during anaesthesia. *British Journal of Anaesthesia* **43**: 739–745.

Katz, J., Kavanagh, H., Sandler, A.N., Nierenberg, H., Boylan, J.F., Friedlander, M. and Shaw, B.F. (1992) Preemptive analgesia. Clinical evidence of neuroplasticity contributing to postoperative pain. *Anesthesiology* **77**: 739–746.

Keifer, J.C., Baghdoyan, H.A. and Lydic, R. (1992) Sleep disruption and increased apneas after pontine microinjection of morphine. *Anesthesiology* **77**: 973–983.

Keifer, J.C., Baghdoyan, H.A., Becker, L. and Lydic, R. (1994) Halothane anaesthesia causes decreased acetylcholine release in the pontine reticular formation and increased EEG spindles. *NeuroReport* **5**: 577–580.

Khan, Z.P., Ferguson, C.N. and Jones, R.M. (1999) Alpha 2 adrenoceptor and imidazole agonists – their pharmacology and therapeutic role. *Anaesthesia* **54**: 146–165.

Kissin, I. (1993) General anaesthetic action: An obsolete notion? *Anesthesia and Analgesia* **76**: 215–218.

Kulli, J. and Koch, C. (1991) Does anaesthesia cause loss of consciousness? *Trends in Neuroscience* **14**: 6–10.

Levy,W.J., Shapiro, H.M., Maruchak, G. and Meathe, E. (1980) Automated EEG processing for intraoperative monitoring. *Anesthesiology* **53**: 223–236.

Lewis, T. (1942) *Pain.* New York: Macmillan, ch 1, pp 1–200.

Lydic, R., Keifer, J.C., Baghdoyan, H.A. and Becker, L. (1993) Microdialysis of the pontine reticular formation reveals inhibition of acetylcholine release by morphine. *Anesthesiology* **79**: 1003–1012.

Malmeberg, A.B. and Yaksh, T.L. (1992) Isobolographic and dose-response analyses of the interaction between intrathecal mu and delta agonists: effects of naltrindole and its benzofuran analog (NTB). *Journal of Pharmacology and Experimental Therapeutics.* **263**: 264–275.

Malmbeg, A.B. and Yaksh, T.L. (1992a) Antinoceptive actions of spinal nonsteriodal anti-infalmmatory agents on the formal in test in the rat. *Journal of Pharcacology and Experimental Therapeutics.* **263**: 136–146.

Marsh, D.F., Hatch, D.J. and Fitzgerald, M. (1997) Opioid systems and the newborn. *British Journal of Anaesthesia* **79**: 787–795.

Maynard, D.E. and Jenkinson, J.L. (1984) The cerebral function analysing monitor. *Anaesthesia* **39**: 678–690.

McMahon, S.B., Dmitrieva, N. and Koltzenburg, M. (1995) Visceral pain. *British Journal of Anaesthesia* **75**: 132–144.

Merkel, G. and Eger, E.I. (1963) A comparative study of halothane and halopropane anesthesia. *Anesthesiology* **24**: 346–357.

Meunier, J.C. (1997) Nociceptin, orphanin FQ and the opioid receptor-like ORL1 receptor. *European Journal of Pharmacology* **340**: 1–15.

Mori, K., Shingu, K.,Moti, H. *et al.* (1985) Factors modifying anaesthetic induced EEG activities. In: Stoeckel, H. (ed) *Quantitation, Modelling.*

Moruzzi, G. and Magoun, H.W. (1949) Brainstem reticular formation and activation of the EEG. *Electroencephalography and Neurophysiology* **1**: 455–473.

Mungliani, R., Andrade, J., Sapsford, D.J. , Baddeley, A. and Jones, J.G. (1993) A measure of consciousness and memory during isoflurane administration; the coherent frequency. *British Journal of Anaesthesia* **71**: 633–641.

Okuda-Ashitaka, E., Minami, T., Tachibana, S., Yoshihara, Y., Nischiuchi, Y., Kimura, T. and Ito, S. (1998) Nocistatin, a peptide that blocks nociceptin action on pain transmission. *Nature* **392**: 286–289.

Otto, K. and Short, C.E. (1991) Electroencephalographic power spectrum analysis as a monitor of anesthetic depth in horses. *Veterinary Surgery* **20**, 362–371.

Pfaffinger, P.J. and Siegelbaum, S.A. (1990) K$^+$ channel modulation by G proteins and second messengers. In: Cook, N.S. (ed). see *British Journal of Anaesthesia* (1993) **71**. p 146(**1**): 1–100.

Pomfrett, C.J.D. (1999) Heart rate variability, BIS and 'depth of anaesthesia'. *British Journal of Anaesthesia* **82**: 659–662.

Prys-Roberts, C. (1987) Anaesthesia : A practical or impractical construct? *British Journal of Anaesthesia* **59**: 1341–1345.

Quasha, A.L., Eger, E.I. and Tinker, J.H. (1980) Determination and application of MAC. *Anesthesiology* **53**: 315–334.

Rampil, I.J., Susse, F.J., Smith, N.T., Hoff, R.H. and Flemming, D.C. (1980) Spectral edge frequency – a new correlate of anesthetic depth. *Anesthesiology* , **53**: S12.

Richmond, C.E., Bromley, L.M. and Woolf, C.Ô. (1993) Preoperative morphine pre-empts post operative pain. *Lancet* **342**: 73–76.

Roy, C.S. and Sherrington, C.S. (1890) On the regulation of the blood supply of the brain. *Journal of Physiology* **11**: 85–108.

Schmidt, R.F. (1971) Presynaptic inhibition in the vertebrate central nervous system. *Ergebnisse der Physiologie* **63**: 21–108.

Sear, J.W. and Prys-Roberts, C. (1970) Plasma concentrations of alphaxalone during continuous infusions of althesin. *British Journal of Anaesthesia* **51**: 861–867.

Sherrington, C.S. (1900) Cutaneous sensation. In: *Textbook of Physiology.* Schafer, ch 1, pp 920–1001.

Sherrington, C.S. (1906) *The Integrative Action of the Nervous System.* Hew Haven: Yale University Press, ch 1, pp. 1–200.

Snow J. (1847) On the inhalation of the vapour of ether in surgical operations. London: John Churchill.

Spelina, K.R., Coates, D.P., Monk, C.R., Prys-Roberts, C., Norley, I. and Turtle, M.J. (1986) Dose requirements of propofol by infusion during nitrous oxide anaesthesia in man. *British Journal of Anaesthesia* **58**: 1080.

Stamford, J.A. (1995) Descending control of pain. *British Journal of Anaesthesia* **75**: 217–227.

Steriade, M. and McCarley, R.W. (1990) *Brainstem Control of Wakefulness and Sleep.* London: Plenum Press, ch 1, pp 1–100.

Stoeckel, H., Schwilden, H., Lauren, P. and Schuttler, J. (1981) EEG parameters for evaluation of depth of anaesthesia. *Proceedings of the European Academy of Anaesthesiology* **1**: 73–84.

Stoeckel, H. and Schwilden, H. (1987) Median EEG frequency. In: Rosen, N. and Lunn J.N. (eds) *Consciousness, Awareness and Pain in General Anaesthesia.* London: Butterworths, pp 53–60.

Treede, R.-D., Meyer, R.A., Raja, S.N. and Campbell, J.N. (1992) Peripheral and central mechanisms of cutaneous hyperalgesia. *Progress in Neurobiology* **38**: 397–421.

Wall, P.D. (1992) In: Short, C.E. and Poznak, A. van (eds) *Pain in Animals.* New York: Churchill Livingstone, pp 63–79.

Wolters, U., Wolf, T., Stützer, H. and Schröder, T. (1996) ASA classification and perioperative variables as predictors of postoperative out-come. *British Journal of Anaesthesia* **77**: 217–222.

Woolf, C.J. and Doubell, T.P. (1994) The pathophysiology of chronic pain – increased sensitivity to low threshold Ab-fibre input. *Current Opinion in Neurobiology* **4**: 525–534.

Woolf, C.J. and Wall, P.D. (1986) Morphine-sensitive and morphine-insensitive actions of C-fibre input on the rat spinal cord. *Neuroscience Letters*, **64**: 221–225.

Woolf, C.J. and Wall, P.D. (1986a) Relative effectiveness of C primary afferent fibres of different origins in evoking a prolonged facilitation of the flexor reflex in the rat. *Journal of Neuroscience* **6**: 1433–1442.

Xu, X.J., Hao, J.X. and Weisenfeld-Hallin, Z. (1996) Nociceptin or antinociceptin: potent spinal antinociceptive effect or orphanin FQ/nociceptin in the rat. *NeuroReport* **7**: 2092–2094.

Ying, H., McEarchern, E.D.W., Eddleman, D.W. and Sheppard, L.C. (1992) Fuzzy control of mean aterial pressure in postsurgical patients with sodium nitroprusside infusion. *IEEE Transactions of Biomedical Engineering* **39**, 1060–1070.

Zadeh, L.H. (1965) Fuzzy sets. *Information and Control* **8**: 338–353.

Patient monitoring and clinical measurement

2

INTRODUCTION

From the earliest days of anaesthesia the anaesthetist has monitored the patient's pulse rate, pattern of breathing and general condition. Advances in electronic technology have made reasonably reliable, easily attached, non-invasive monitoring devices available for clinical practice. Observations and measurements of certain parameters before, during, and after anaesthesia provide important data to support the clinical assessment of the animal's condition and improve the chances of survival of the very ill by indicating what treatment is needed, as well as the response to treatment already given.

It is necessary to know what to measure as well as how to measure it and not all anaesthetists may agree on the priority ranking of the monitoring devices available. There can be little doubt that to introduce the full panoply of monitoring equipment for short bloodless procedures on healthy animals may turn a simple anaesthetic administration into a complex one with unnecessary distractions. However, for major surgery, for anaesthesia and surgery of poor-risk patients, and for equine anaesthesia, it would be difficult to defend the failure to use monitoring equipment, especially if it were available.

GENERAL CONSIDERATIONS RELATING TO MONITORING

Anaesthetic mishaps may be caused by mechanical malfunction, disconnection of equipment, or human error. Judgmental error frequently occurs when the anaesthetist is in a hurry and circumvents basic practices and procedures, or when a decision must be made in an emergency. The prevalence of complications may also be associated with inadequate training or experience of the anaesthetist. Knowledge and experience are a function of the nature of the training received and the years of practice, but proper vigilance at all times can only be generated by self-motivation.

Routines should be developed to ensure that each aspect of apparatus function is checked before use. Failure to follow a simple check list in every case features high on the list of causes of anaesthetic disasters. All anaesthetic equipment, including monitoring devices, should be maintained in good functioning order. It should be a matter of course to maintain monitors with a battery back-up fully charged in case of need in an area without a convenient electricity outlet nearby, failure of electricity supply, or the need to disconnect from the main supply to minimize electrical interference with other monitoring equipment.

Proficiency with methods of electronic surveillance must be acquired during minor procedures so that they can be applied properly in circumstances where their use is mandatory (e.g. during major surgery or a cardiovascular crisis). Routine use ensures that probes, sensors, electrodes, etc. can be applied quickly to the animal and increases the likelihood that the information obtained is reliable.

Although current practice is to establish monitoring only after the animal has been anaesthetized, it must be recognised that many complications occur during induction of anaesthesia. Ideally, especially for poor-risk patients, monitoring should begin when the drugs for premedication are administered. Dogs and cats may vomit after administration of an opioid and the quantity and content of the vomit may warn that the animal was fed recently and so may be at risk for regurgitation and pulmonary aspiration of gastric material. Brachycephalic breeds and animals with respiratory problems should always be observed after administration of preanaesthetic drugs because sedation may cause partial or complete airway obstruction or serious respiratory depression. In

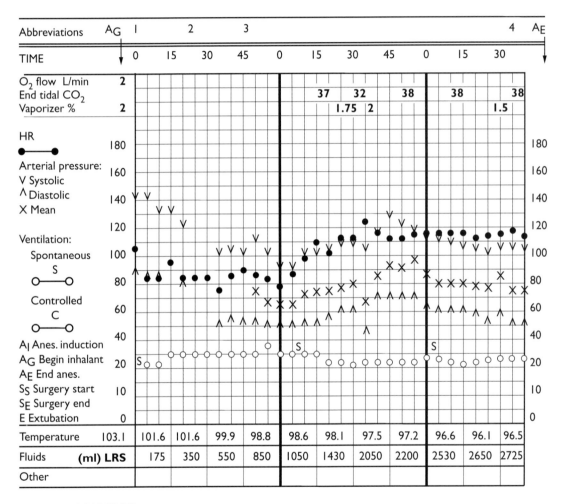

DETAILED COMMENTS:

1. Oxymorphone 1.5mg IV
2. Move to O.R. 1200mg Cefotetan IV
3. Change from indirect to direct arterial BP monitoring
4. Morphine 30mg IM

Fig. 2.1 Anaesthetic record of a 61 kg, 6-year-old female Great Dane anaesthetized for exploratory laparotomy because of torsion of the spleen. Anaesthesia was induced by intravenous administration of ketamine, 200 mg, and diazepam, 10 mg, and maintained with isoflurane. Heart rate, blood pressure and respiratory rate were recorded at regular intervals to facilitate early recognition of adverse trends.

any animal, evaluation of the degree of sedation produced by premedicant drugs may indicate that the anaesthetic plan should be reassessed and either drug doses reduced or additional agents included.

Careful observation of the patient during induction of anaesthesia may allow precise titration of drugs to achieve the desired depth of anaesthesia and ensure early recognition of a complication that requires immediate specific treatment, such as cyanosis, anaphylaxis, or cardiac arrest. Where possible, patients at risk for complications may be attached to specific monitoring equipment before induction of anaesthesia. Appropriate equipment for this would be the electrocardiograph (ECG) and a device for measurement of blood pressure.

Recording drugs, dosages and responses for each patient is essential and provides valuable information for any subsequent time that anaesthesia may be needed. Noting all measurements on an anaesthetic record provides a pictorial description of changes that can be used to predict complications and plan treatment (Fig. 2.1). Retrospective evaluation of difficult cases and of series of records, perhaps of patients with similar surgical procedures, or to compare different anaesthetic protocols, can be used to monitor the anaesthetist's performance and identify difficult situations that require further thought and improved management. For research purposes, data can be acquired into a computer for accurate data summaries.

Monitoring animals during anaesthesia must include observation of behaviour and reflexes and measurement of various physiological parameters at regular intervals to accomplish two objectives. The first objective is to ensure that the animal survives anaesthesia and surgery. The second objective is to obtain information that can be used to adjust anaesthetic administration and management to minimize physiological abnormalities, which is especially important for animals that have already compromized organ systems. The goal is to prevent development of preventable adverse consequences 1 hour, 12 hours, or even 3 days after anaesthesia.

Monitoring should continue into the recovery period to determine the need for additional analgesic drugs and to record serious deviations in body temperature. Mucous membrane colour

should be checked for at least 20 minutes after the animal has been disconnected from oxygen as it may take that long for hypoxaemia to develop in animals that are moderately hypoventilating and breathing air.

A variety of methods using inexpensive or expensive equipment can be used to monitor parameters determined by the species of animal to be anaesthetized and by the abnormalities already present in the patient. Not all monitoring techniques need to be applied to every patient. A recommendation for three levels of monitoring is presented in Table 2.1; level 1 monitoring information should be obtained from all anaesthetized animals, level 2 monitors are affordable and recommended for routine use in some groups of patients, and level 3 monitors individually offer improved monitoring for patients with specific problems.

This chapter will describe the techniques of monitoring using a systems approach, and offer guidelines for interpretation of the information obtained. Further recommendations are given in the chapters devoted to species anaesthesia and the chapter on management of complications.

CLINICAL ASSESSMENT OF THE PATIENT

MONITORING THE CENTRAL NERVOUS SYSTEM

An early attempt at defining depth of anaesthesia through observation of changes in reflexes, muscle tone, and respiration with administration of increased concentration of ether resulted in classification of anaesthesia into four stages (Fig. 2.2). The animal was said to make the transition from consciousness to deep anaesthesia by passing sequentially through Stage I (in which voluntary excitement might be observed), Stage II (when the animal appeared to be unconscious but exhibited involuntary muscle movement, such as limb paddling, and vocalization), Stage III (surgical anaesthesia), and Stage IV (anaesthetic overdose immediately prior to death). Stage III was further divided into Plane 1 (light anaesthesia sufficient only for non-painful procedures), Plane 2 (medium depth anaesthesia employed for most

TABLE 2.1 Prioritization of monitoring

Monitor	Information obtained	Specific use
Level 1 (Basic monitoring)		
• Palpebral and pedal reflexes, eye position	Depth of anaesthesia	All anaesthetized animals
• Respiratory rate and depth of chest or bag excursion	Adequacy of ventilation	All anaesthetized animals
• Oral mucous membrane colour	Oxygenation	All anaesthetized animals
• Heart rate, pulse strength, capillary refill time	Assessment of circulation	All anaesthetized animals
• Temperature	Temperature	Dogs and cats anaesthesia greater than 30 min; all inhalation anaesthesia
Level 2 (Routine use recommended for some patients)		
• Arterial blood pressure measurement (indirect or direct methods)	Blood pressure	All inhalation anaesthesia; cardiovascular disease or depression
• Blood glucose	Blood glucose	Paediatric patients; diabetics; septicaemia; insulinoma
• Electrocardiography	Cardiac rate and rhythm; diagnosis of arrhythmia or cardiac arrest	All inhalation anaesthesia; thoracic trauma or cardiac disease
• Pulse oximetry	Haemoglobin oxygen saturation; pulse rate	Small animals breathing air during anaesthesia; thoracic trauma or pulmonary disease; septicaemia/endotoxaemia
• Urine output, either by expression of urinary bladder or by urethral catheterization	Urine volume produced during anaesthesia; indirect assessment of adequacy of tissue perfusion	Renal disease; some urinary tract surgery; multiorgan failure
Level 3 (Use for specific patients or problems)		
• Anaesthetic gas analyser	Inspired and end-tidal anaesthetic agent concentration; evaluation of depth of inhalation anaesthesia	Any patient on inhalation anaesthetic agent
• Blood gases and pH	$PaCO_2, PaO_2, pH, HCO_3$; base excess/deficit	Suspected hypoventilation or hypoxaemia; measurement of metabolic status
• Capnography	End-tidal carbon dioxide concentration; estimate of adequacy of ventilation; warning of circuit disconnect or cardiac arrest	Suspected hypoventilation during inhalation anaesthesia; patients at risk for complications
• Cardiac output measurement	Cardiac output	Multiorgan failure; research investigations
• Central venous pressure	Adequacy of blood volume	Dehydrated small animal patients; portosystemic shunt
• Electrophysiological diagnostics (electroencephalogram, cortical evoked responses, spectral edge frequency)	Cerebral ischaemia; assessment of depth of anaesthesia	Reliability is being investigated
• Packed cell volume and total protein	Haemodilution and protein concentration	Haemorrhage; large volume infusion of crystalloid solution
• Peripheral nerve stimulator	Neuromuscular transmission	Use of neuromuscular blocking agents

surgical procedures), Plane 3 (deep anaesthesia), and Plane 4 (excessively deep anaesthesia). Although the progression of changes described in Fig. 2.2 are generally accurate representations of the transition from light to deep ether anaesthesia, the rate of changes vary for the newer inhalation agents and are altered by concurrent administration of injectable drugs.

Eye position and reflexes

Eye movements are similar with thiopental, propofol, halothane, and isoflurane in that the eyeball rotates rostroventrally during light and moderate depths of surgical anaesthesia, returning to a central position during deep anaesthesia (Fig. 2.3). Muscle tone is retained during ketamine anaesthesia and the eye remains centrally placed in the orbit in dogs and cats (Fig. 2.4), and only slightly rotated in horses and ruminants. Fine

nystagmus may be present in horses anaesthetised with ketamine (See Chapter 11). The palpebral reflex, which is partial or complete closure of the eyelids (a blink) elicited by a gentle tap at the lateral canthus of the eye or gentle stroking of the eyelashes, is frequently a useful guide to depth of anaesthesia. At a plane of anaesthesia satisfactory for surgery, the palpebral reflex is weak and nystagmus is absent. A brisk palpebral reflex develops when anaesthesia lightens. Ketamine anaesthesia is associated with a brisk palpebral reflex.

A corneal reflex is a similar lid response elicited by gentle pressure on the cornea. The presence of a corneal reflex is no indicator of depth of anaesthesia and may still be present for a short time after cardiac arrest has occurred.

The pedal reflex is frequently tested in dogs, cats and small laboratory animals to determine if depth of anaesthesia is adequate for the start of

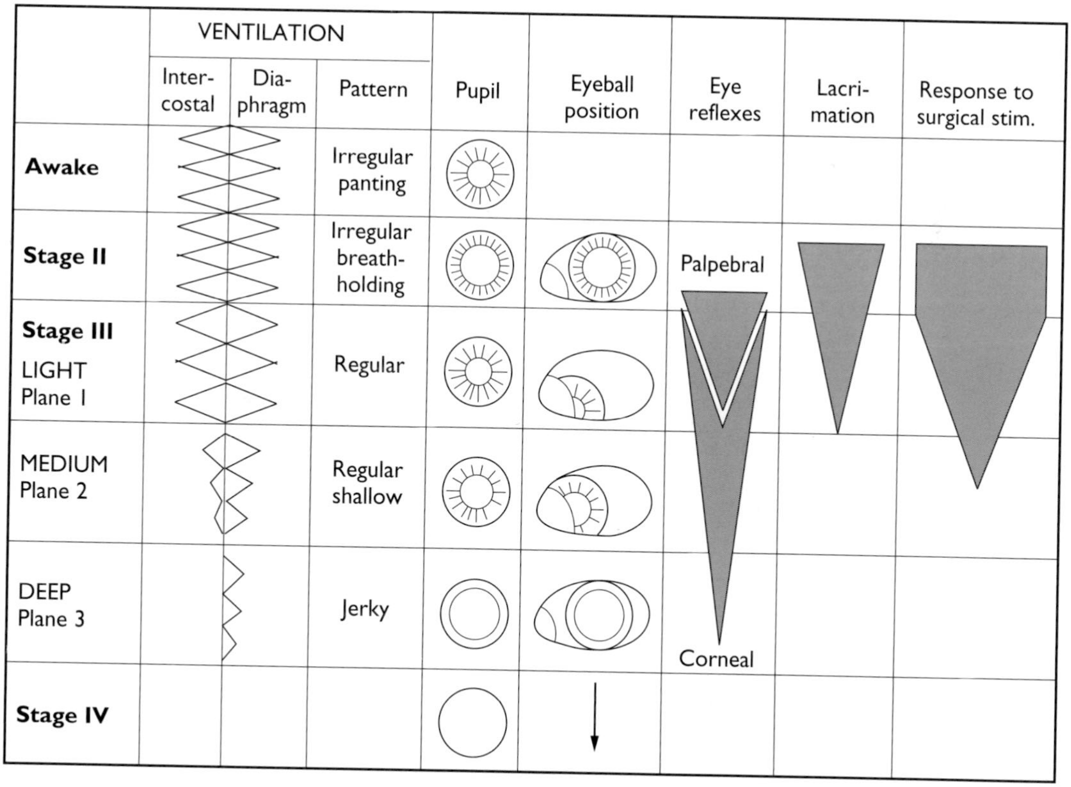

FIG. 2.2 Changes in ventilation and eye signs follow recognized patterns with different stages of inhalation anaesthesia. The progression of these changes will be influenced by inclusion of injectable anaesthetic agents (adapted from Soma, 1971).

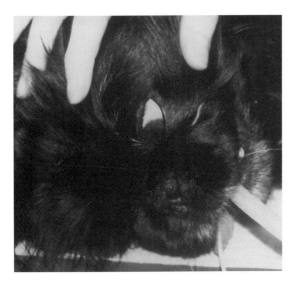

FIG. 2.3 The rostroventral rotation of the eye in this dog is consistent with light and medium planes of halothane or isoflurane anaesthesia.

surgery. Pinching the web between the toes or firm pressure applied to a nail bed will be followed by withdrawal of the limb if anaesthesia is inadequate.

The whisker reflex in cats, where pinching of the pinna elicits a twitch of the whiskers, has been used to assist in titration of pentobarbital to an adequate depth of anaesthesia. After administration of one-third to one-half of the calculated dose

of pentobarbital to facilitate rapid transition through any excitement stage, small increments are administered over several minutes just until the whisker reflex is abolished.

MONITORING OF RESPIRATORY RATE AND CARDIOVASCULAR FUNCTION

Measurements of respiratory rates, heart rates, and blood pressure are not reliable guides to depth of anaesthesia, although increasing the depth of anaesthesia by increasing administration of an anaesthetic agent produces increased respiratory and cardiovascular depression. It is not uncommon for an unstimulated dog anaesthetised with an inhalation agent to have a low arterial blood pressure and yet in the next minute start moving its legs and chewing on the endotracheal tube in response to a skin incision, all accompanied by a dramatic increase in blood pressure. Inhalation agents may elicit different responses, for example, increasing depth of isoflurane anaesthesia may decrease respiratory rates whereas increasing depth of halothane anaesthesia may result in increased respiratory rates. Furthermore, today in a clinical patient, more than one anaesthetic or preanaesthetic agent is generally used and the cardiopulmonary effects are determined by the combination of agents used and the dose rates.

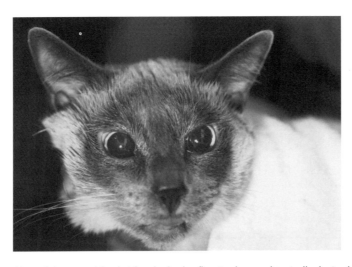

FIG. 2.4 The central position of the eye, with a brisk palpebral reflex, is observed typically during ketamine anaesthesia in cats.

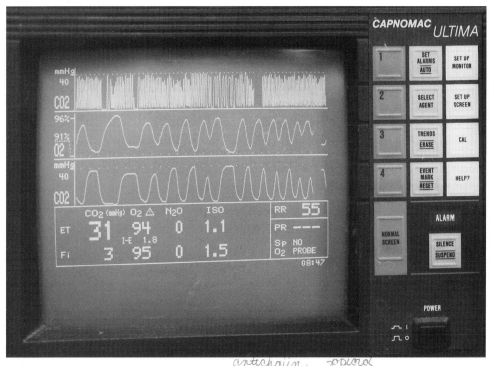

FIG. 2.5 This gas analyser (Capnomac Ultima™, Datex-Engstrom Inc., Tewksbury, Maryland, USA) is monitoring a 27 kg female English Bulldog that was premedicated with glycopyrrolate and butorphanol and anaesthesia induced with propofol. She has been breathing oxygen and isoflurane at a vaporizer setting of 2.5% for 5 minutes. The monitor indicates that the inspired (Fi) isoflurane concentration is less than the vaporizer setting and that the end-tidal (ET) isoflurane concentration is less than MAC value.

Anaesthetic gas analysers

The anaesthetic gas analyser measures the concentration of inhalation anaesthetic agent in inspired and expired gases (Fig. 2.5). The gases are sampled at the junction of the endotracheal tube and breathing circuit either directly in-line or by continuous aspiration of gases at a rate of 150 ml/min to a monitor placed at some distance from the patient. To assess the depth of anaesthesia, the end-tidal concentration of inhalation agent is measured (alveolar concentration is measured at the end of exhalation) and compared with the MAC value for that inhalant anaesthetic and species (Table 2.2). Higher than MAC values will be required to prevent movement in response to surgery, usually 1.2 to 1.5 times MAC, when anaesthesia is maintained almost entirely by inhalation agent. Less than MAC value may be sufficient when analgesia is provided by neuroleptanalgesia, by continuous or intermittent administration of an opioid, or by medetomidine or detomidine. For these animals, the anaesthetic administration must be adjusted according to observation of reflexes and cardiovascular response to surgical stimulus.

It should be noted that the gas analyser also accurately measures inspired anaesthetic concentration, which may be substantially lower than the

TABLE 2.2 **MAC* values for halothane, isoflurane and sevoflurane in several species**			
Anaesthetic agent	**Dogs**	**Cats**	**Horses**
Halothane	0.9	1.1	0.9
Isoflurane	1.4	1.6	1.3
Sevoflurane	2.8	2.6	2.3

* MAC = minimum alveolar concentration of anaesthetic agent required to prevent purposeful movement in 50% of animals in response to a standard painful stimulus.

vaporizer setting in rebreathing systems during anaesthesia in large dogs, horses and ruminants. In the absence of an accurate measure of anaesthetic concentration delivered, administration of an anaesthetic agent may be inadequate despite an apparently adequate vaporizer setting. In a retrospective study of equine anaesthesia, it was found that horses were four times more likely to move during anaesthesia when an anaesthetic agent analyser was not used (C. M. Trim, unpublished observations).

Some monitors using the principles of infrared absorption spectrometry cannot be used for horses or ruminants as they will measure exhaled methane and record the concentration as halothane, for example the Datex Capnomac/Normac (Taylor 1990). Analysers that use higher wavelengths of infrared light should be unaffected by methane (Moens *et al.*, 1991).

Computerized anaesthetic administration

The subject of computerized control of anaesthetic administration has already been discussed in Chapter 1. This control is usually exerted by reference to the changes in the electroencephalogram (EEG) with changes in depth of anaesthesia as determined by clinical signs or end-tidal concentrations of halothane (Otto & Short, 1991; Ekstrom *et al.*, 1993; Johnson *et al.*, 1994). The EEG may be influenced by a variety of factors occurring during anaesthesia, including cerebrocortical depression, hypotension, hypoxaemia, and hypercapnia. Computerized EEG techniques, such as power spectrum analysis (described by 80% or 95% spectral edge frequency), have potential application for monitoring depth of anaesthesia (Otto & Short 1991; Johnson *et al.*, 1994; Otto *et al.*, 1996), but it is most important to recognize the limitations of the raw EEG and its derivatives as discussed in Chapter 1.

MONITORING THE CIRCULATION

The heart rate, tissue perfusion, and blood pressure of all anaesthetized animals should be assessed at frequent regular intervals (Table 2.3).

> **TABLE 2.3 Methods of assessing cardiovascular function in anaesthetized clinical patients**
>
> **Heart rate**
> - Palpation of arterial pulse
> - Oesophageal stethoscope
> - Electrocardiogram
> - Blood pressure monitor
> - Pulse oximeter
>
> **Tissue perfusion**
> - Mucous membrane colour
> - Capillary refill time
> - Blood pressure
> - Bleeding at operative site
> - Observation of intestine colour
> - Urine output
>
> **Arterial blood pressure**
> - Palpation of peripheral pulse
> - Doppler ultrasound method
> - Oscillometric method
> - Arterial catheterization

Heart rate monitors

Heart rates measured before anaesthesia are greatly influenced by the environment. Means (standard deviations, range) of heart rates obtained by palpation from healthy cats at home were 118

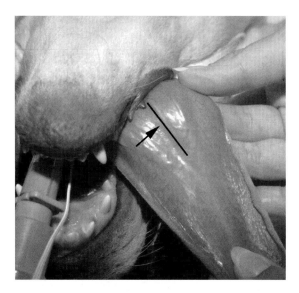

FIG. 2.6 The lingual artery is easily palpated in dogs midline on the ventral surface of the tongue, adjacent to the nerve and between the lingual veins. The arrow in the photograph points to a line drawn adjacent to the lingual artery.

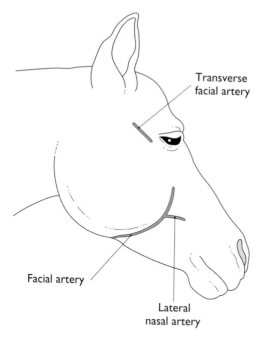

Transverse
facial artery

Facial artery

Lateral
nasal artery

FIG. 2.7 Sites for palpation of arterial pulse or catheter placement for blood pressure measurement in horses.

mean (SD 11, range 80 to 160) beats per minute compared with mean 182 (SD 20, range 142 to 222) when obtained by electrocardiography in the veterinary hospital (Sawyer *et al.*, 1991).

The lowest acceptable heart rates during anaesthesia are controversial, but reasonable guidelines are 55 beats/min for large dogs, 65 beats/min for adult cats, 26 beats/min for horses, and 50 beats/min for cattle. Heart rates should be higher in small breed dogs and much higher in immature animals. It should be remembered that heart rate is a major determinant of cardiac output, consequently, bradycardia should be treated if blood pressure and peripheral perfusion are also decreased.

Heart rate may be counted by palpation of a peripheral arterial pulse, such as the femoral artery in dogs and cats, lingual artery in dogs (Fig. 2.6), facial, median or metatarsal arteries in horses (Fig. 2.7), and femoral, median, or auricular arteries in ruminants and pigs.

Oesophageal stethoscope

The oesophageal stethoscope (Fig. 2.8) is a simple method of monitoring heart rate in dogs and cats. This monitor consists of a tube with a balloon on the end which is passed dorsal to the endotracheal tube and into the oesophagus until the tip is level with the heart. The open end of the tube is connected to an ordinary stethoscope headpiece, to a

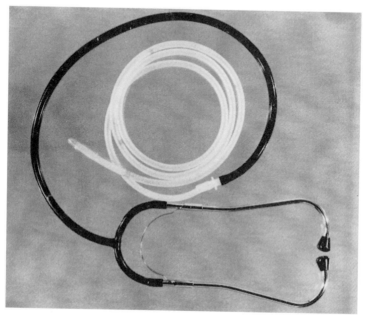

FIG. 2.8 The oesophageal stethoscope. It may be used with a single earpiece or with a conventional stethoscope headpiece. This is a simple and inexpensive monitoring device for heart beat and respiratory activity.

single earpiece that can be worn by the anaesthetist or surgeon, or connected to an amplifier that makes the heart sounds audible throughout the room. This monitor provides only information about heart rate and rhythm; the intensity of sound is not reliably associated with changes in blood pressure or cardiac output. Other electronic oesophageal probes are available to provide heart rate, and some also may produce an ECG and oesophageal temperature.

Electrocardiography

Heart rate and rhythm can be obtained from an electrocardiograph using standard limb leads in small animals, clip electrodes and ECG paste , and selecting ECG Lead II on the oscilloscope (Fig. 2.9A). Poor contact of the electrodes to the skin from hair bunched in the clips, or close proximity to another electrical apparatus, such as the hot water circulating pad, can result in electrical interference that obscures the ECG. The leads should not be placed over the thorax as breathing will move the electrodes and result in a wandering ECG baseline (Fig. 2.9B).

Sinus arrhythmia is abolished when atropine has been administered. Other arrhythmias, for example second degree atrioventricular heart block and premature ventricular contractions, may or may not require specific treatment (see

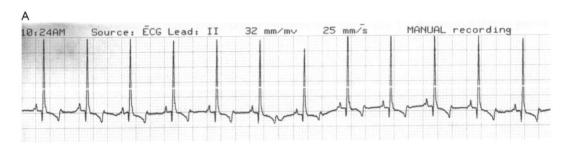

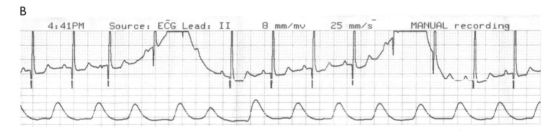

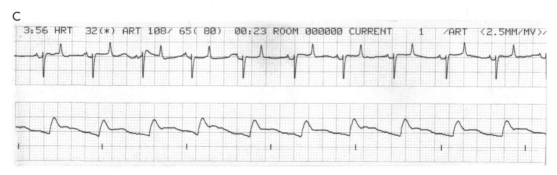

FIG. 2.9 A Normal Lead II ECG from a Labrador anaesthetised with halothane. **B** ECG with a wandering baseline induced by movement of leads as the dog breathes. This dog has a heart rate of 114 beats per minute, systolic arterial pressure of 96 mmHg, diastolic pressure of 46 mmHg, and mean pressure of 61 mmHg. **C** Normal base apex ECG and blood pressure recorded from a horse anaesthetised with isoflurane.

Chapter 20). Dogs with premature ventricular contractions (PVCs) from myocardial ischaemia as a result of a road accident or gastric dilatation and volvulus may be treated with antiarrhythmic drugs before anaesthesia. Rather than completely abolish all arrhythmias, the aim is to monitor blood pressure and tissue perfusion and adjust anaesthetic management to ensure that myocardial and respiratory depression are minimal.

A frequently used monitor lead in equine anaesthesia is the 'base-apex' lead. The right arm electrode is clipped on the neck in the right jugular furrow and the left arm electrode is passed between the forelimbs and clipped at the apex of the heart over the left 5th intercostal space several inches from the midline. The left leg electrode is clipped on the neck or on the shoulder. Good electrical contact is achieved with alcohol or electrode paste. Lead I is selected on the electrocardiograph and the normal configuration includes a negative R wave (Fig. 2.9C). A bifid P wave is frequently observed in the normal equine ECG.

There is a high incidence of sinus arrhythmia and first and second degree atrioventricular (AV) heart block in conscious unsedated horses (Robertson, 1990). In contrast, AV block during anaesthesia is uncommon except when the horse has been premedicated with detomidine, or supplemental intravenous injections of xylazine are given during anaesthesia. The appearance of this arrhythmia during anaesthesia on any other occasion is cause for concern as this rhythm may progress within a few minutes to advanced heart block (P waves only, no ventricular complexes) and cardiac arrest. Atrial fibrillation and VPCs occur rarely but may require specific treatment if associated with hypotension.

Tissue perfusion

Evaluation of tissue perfusion can be done by considering gum or lip mucous membrane colour, the capillary refill time, and the blood pressure. High mean arterial pressure does not guarantee adequate tissue perfusion. For example, when blood pressure increases during anaesthesia in response to a surgical stimulus, cardiac output may be decreased due to increased afterload from peripheral vasoconstriction.

Tissue perfusion is usually decreased when the gums are pale, rather than pink, and the capillary refill time (CRT) exceeds 1.5 seconds, or the mean arterial pressure (MAP) is less than 60 mmHg. When MAP is above 60 mmHg, palpation of the strength of the peripheral pulse and observation of oral membrane colour and CRT should be used to assess adequacy of peripheral perfusion and cardiac output.

Arterial blood pressure

Systolic (SAP), mean (MAP), and diastolic (DAP) arterial pressures in awake healthy animals are approximately 140–160 mmHg, 100–110 mHg, and 85–95 mmHg, respectively. Excepting when premedication has included detomidine or medetomidine or when anaesthesia was induced with ketamine or tiletamine, arterial blood pressure is decreased from the awake value during anaesthesia. Arterial blood pressure is lower in paediatric patients than in mature animals. For example, healthy 5 or 6-day-old foals anaesthetized with isoflurane had an average MAP of 58 mmHg. When the same foals were reanaesthetized 4–5 weeks later, the average MAP had increased to 80 mmHg, with a corresponding decrease in cardiac index (Hodgson et al., 1990).

Hypotension may be defined as a mean arterial pressure of less than 65 mmHg in mature animals. An MAP as low as 60 mmHg may be allowed in dogs and cats provided that the mucous membrane colour is pink and CRT is 1 sec. This combination of values may occur during inhalation anaesthesia at the time of minimal stimulation during preparation of the operative site and before the onset of surgery. MAP is not usually allowed to fall below 65–70 mmHg for any length of time in anaesthetized horses because of the increased risk for postanaesthetic myopathy. When hypotension is documented, appropriate treatment can be instituted, such as decreasing anaesthetic depth or commencing or increasing the intravenous administration of fluids or administration of a vasoactive drug such as dopamine, dobutamine, or ephedrine. The outcome of untreated severe or prolonged hypotension may be unexpected cardiac arrest during anaesthesia or blindness or renal failure after recovery from anaesthesia. In equine practice, consequences also include the potentially fatal syndrome of postanaesthetic myopathy.

An approximate estimate of blood pressure can be made from palpation of a peripheral artery. However, in states associated with vasodilatation, a peripheral pulse can be palpated at pressures as low as 50 mmHg and, in some cases, palpation alone does not suggest the urgency for treatment that is frequently warranted. Furthermore, it is not uncommon for heart rates to be within an accepted normal range while blood pressure is low or decreasing.

Measurement of blood pressure can be made easily; equipment cost varies. The investment in time and money is worthwhile in animals at risk for hypotension, such as small animals and horses anaesthetised with inhalation agents, and in animals with abnormalities likely to give rise to complications during anaesthesia. The least expensive techniques are the Doppler ultrasound technique in dogs and cats, and direct blood pressure measurement using an anaeroid manometer in horses.

Doppler ultrasound for indirect measurement of blood pressure

Hair is first clipped from the skin on the palmar surface of the paw of dogs and cats (Fig. 2.10). A probe covered with contact gel is placed over the artery and taped in place (Fig. 2.11). Ultrasound waves emitted from one of the two piezo-electric crystals embedded in the probe passes through the skin and deeper tissues. A structure which is stationary will reflect sound back to the second crystal without any frequency change (Stegall *et al.*, 1968). Moving objects, such as erythrocytes and the artery wall, will reflect some of the sound at a different frequency (Doppler-shift). The change in frequency can be heard through a loudspeaker as an audible swooshing sound with each pulse.

A cuff is wrapped snugly around an extremity proximal to the probe, in dogs and cats with the centre of the inflatable part of the cuff on the medial aspect of the limb. The cuff is connected to an anaeroid manometer and a bulb for manual inflation of the cuff with air (Fig. 2.12). In horses, the cuff is wrapped around the base of the tail with the

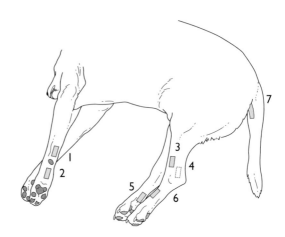

FIG. 2.10 Sites for application of the Doppler probe for indirect measurement of arterial blood pressure in dogs. **1 & 2:** Ulnar artery on the caudal surface of the forelimb, above and below the carpal pad; **3:** cranial tibial artery on the craniolateral surface of the hindlimb; **4 & 5:** saphenous artery on the medial surface of the flexor tendons and on the plantar surface of the paw proximal to the foot pad; **6:** dorsal pedal artery; **7:** coccygeal artery on the ventral surface of the tail.

cuff air bladder centred over the ventral surface of the tail. The probe is taped distal to the cuff over the coccygeal artery in the ventral midline groove. The coccygeal artery can be used for this technique in adult cattle but the results are not reliable. In foals and small ruminants, the probe can be taped over the metatarsal artery on the lateral surface of the hind limb or the common digital artery on the medial side of the forelimb distal to the carpus. The cuff is secured around the limb above the hock or carpus. In pigs, the probe is most reliable when taped over the common digital artery on the caudomedial aspect of the forelimb. The cuff should be placed between the carpus and the elbow but, because of the triangular shape of the forearm, it may be unable to occlude blood flow when inflation of the cuff causes it to slip down over the carpus. The width of the air bladder within the cuff is important for accuracy; a bladder that is too narrow will overestimate blood pressure and one which is too wide will underestimate it. A cuff that is attached too loosely or slips down the extremity and becomes loose, will result in an erroneously high value.

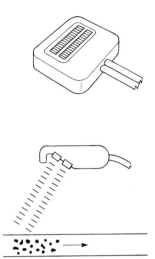

FIG. 2.11 Doppler-shift pulse detector. One piezoelectric crystal emits incident ultrasound signal while the other receives the reflected signal from cells in flowing blood. The frequency shift between the incident and reflected sound is converted to audible sound.

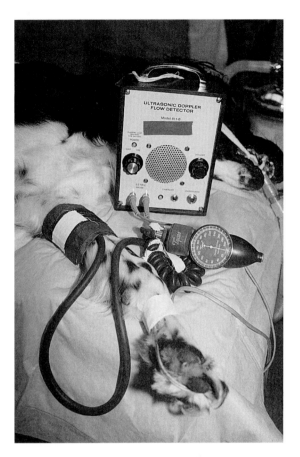

FIG. 2.12 Measurement of arterial pressure in a dog by taping a Doppler probe over an artery distal to the carpal pad so that audible sounds of arterial pulses are emitted from the box. A blood pressure cuff is applied higher up the limb and the anaeroid manometer attached to the cuff is used to identify systolic and diastolic pressures.

To measure blood pressure, the cuff is inflated to above systolic pressure to occlude the artery and no sound is heard. The pressure in the cuff is gradually released until the first sounds of blood flow are detected at systolic pressure. As additional pressure is released from the cuff, diastolic pressure is heard as a change in character of sound from a one or two beat sound to a multiple beat sound, to a muffling of sound, or to a growl. This will occur 15 to 40 mmHg below systolic pressure. The sounds associated with diastolic pressure are well defined in some animals but not at all clear in others. In some animals a first muffling of beat signals may occur 10 to 15 mmHg above the true diastolic pressure. In this event, the second change in beat signal will be more abrupt or distinct. Mean pressure can be calculated as one third of the pulse pressure (systolic–diastolic) plus diastolic pressure.

A decrease in intensity of the pulsing sound, when the attachment and setting have been unchanged, is a reliable indication of decreased blood flow. Furthermore, changes in cardiac rhythm are easily detected by listening to this monitor.

An investigation in cats comparing the Doppler ultrasonic method, using a cuff placed halfway between the carpus and the elbow, with measurements obtained from a femoral artery catheter revealed that the indirect method consistently underestimated the pressure by an average of 14 mmHg (Grandy et al., 1992). Using this technique of measuring blood pressure in mature horses using a cuff width 48% of the circumference of the tail (bladder width 10.4 cm) systolic pressure was underestimated and diastolic pressure overestimated by approximately 9% (Parry et al., 1982). In another investigation, measurements of systolic arterial pressure in horses anaesthetized in dorsal recumbency with halothane using a cuff 41% of the tail circumference was reasonably accurate but in 5% of the horses this technique had an error range of ± 20 mmHg (Bailey et al., 1994).

Oscillometry for indirect measurement of blood pressure

Devices that non-invasively measure peripheral blood pressures using the oscillometric method generally operate by automatically inflating a cuff placed around an extremity (Fig. 2.13). As pressure is released from the cuff, pressure changes occurring within the cuff as a result of adjacent arterial pulsations are detected by a transducer within the monitor. Values for systolic, diastolic, and mean arterial pressures, and heart rate are digitally displayed and the monitor can be programmed to automatically measure at a specific time interval. Artefactual pressure changes induced in the cuff by movement of the extremity, for example, during preparation of the surgical site, will either induce abnormal readings or prevent the monitor from obtaining a measurement.

Published results of comparisons between measurements of blood pressure obtained by indirect and direct methods have identified variability according to the monitor used, cuff size, and site of application of the cuff. The closest correlations between direct and indirect measurements have occurred in anaesthetized dogs, using cuff widths between 40 and 60% of the circumference of the extremity, at systolic pressures greater than 80 mmHg.

An evaluation of the DINAMAP model 1846SX comparing direct measurement of blood pressure from the dorsal pedal artery with measurements obtained from a cuff applied at various sites on the forelimb, hindlimb, and tail determined that the closest correlations were from a cuff on the tail or at a proximal site on the hindlimb (Bodey *et al.*, 1994). The tail cuff delivered the best reproducibility in conscious dogs and although the systolic pressure obtained from the tail cuff was substantially higher than direct values, the tail systolic pressure correlated best with changes in direct blood pressure. In anaesthetized dogs, mean pressures obtained from a cuff applied to a proximal site on the hindlimb were significantly correlated to mean direct pressures, whereas systolic and diastolic pressures were on average 8 and 5 mmHg, respectively, higher than directly measured pressures (Bodey *et al.*, 1994).

Measurements obtained from a DINAMAP model 8100 using a cuff around the metacarpus or metatarsus and cuff width 40–60% of limb circumference were compared with direct measurement of blood pressure from a catheter in the abdominal aorta of medium to large-sized anaesthetized dogs (Sawyer *et al.*, 1991). No differences were found in

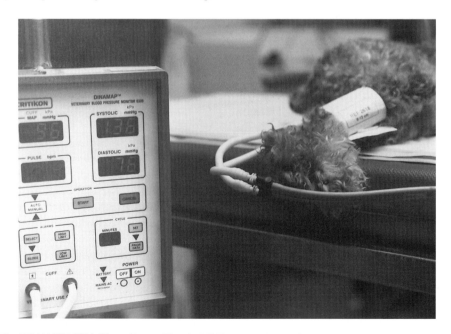

FIG. 2.13 The DINAMAP 8300 (Sharn, Tampa, Florida, USA) utilizes the oscillometric method of measuring arterial blood pressure non-invasively.

measurements recorded from cuffs applied to either forelimb or hindlimb. Differences between indirect and direct measurements were statistically significant but not considered to be clinically significant. In general, indirect pressure measurements were lower than direct measurements and indirect systolic pressure was found to have the most accurate correlation. At systolic pressures of lower than 80 mmHg, indirect pressure measurements were 6 to 15% higher than direct measurements.

In a clinical study of dogs anaesthetized for a variety of soft tissue surgical procedures, indirect measurements of blood pressure using the DINAMAP model 8300 and a cuff around the metatarsus with the arrow directly over the pedal artery were compared with pressures recorded from the dorsal pedal artery in the opposite limb (Meurs *et al.*, 1996). It was concluded that measurements taken at a single point in time varied widely between indirect and direct methods, and that single values do not provide reliable information about changing blood pressure. When five sequential readings over 30 minutes were averaged, this model had a sensitivity of 100% (i.e. the method correctly identified a direct MAP of less than 60 mmHg 100% of the time) in this population of animals, of which 73% were normovolaemic (Meurs *et al.*, 1996). A positive predictive value of 80% was calculated, which indicates that the ability of this method to detect correctly a true MAP of less than 60 mmHg was 80% and that the method incorrectly predicted hypotension 20% of the time.

Six sites for placement of the cuff have been evaluated in anaesthetized cats using the DINAMAP model 8300 (Sawyer, 1992). The greatest accuracy was obtained with the cuff placed between the elbow and carpus with the cuff arrow on the medial side of the limb. An evaluation of the Datascope Passport revealed that this model did not accurately estimate direct blood pressure in cats (Branson *et al.*, 1997).

In horses, the DINAMAP is a commonly used monitor utilizing the oscillometric method of blood pressure measurement. The cuff is wrapped around the tail of mature horses or around the hind limb near the metatarsal artery in foals. The cuff should not be wrapped tightly. Some investigators have recommended that the tail cuff be

placed close to the base of the tail, but in this author's opinion more accurate readings are obtained with the cuff applied approximately 10 cm from the base of the tail, where the tail diameter is constant for the length of the cuff. Early investigations of the DINAMAP confirmed accurate and clinically useful values for arterial pressure using a cuff width 24% of the tail circumference in ponies (Geddes *et al.*, 1977) and 25–35% in horses (Latshaw *et al.*, 1979; Muir *et al.*, 1983). However, measurements were inaccurate at heart rates of less than 25 beats/minute. Our experience using a Model 8300 DINAMAP and a cuff width 35–40% of the tail circumference ratio (child or small adult cuff for a mature horse depending on tail thickness and the amount of hair) has been that the mean arterial blood pressure value obtained from this monitor is usually the same as that obtained by direct blood pressure measurement. Occasionally, the DINAMAP recorded pressures 10 to 20 mmHg higher than the true mean arterial pressure.

In summary, indirect method of measurement of blood pressure provides useful information in most horses, but may produce erroneous values in a small number. Consequently, blood pressure should be measured by direct means whenever

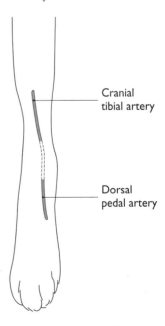

Cranial
tibial artery

Dorsal
pedal artery

FIG. 2.14 Sites for insertion of arterial catheters on the cranial aspect of the right hindlimb of a dog.

possible in horses at risk of developing low blood pressure, for example, during inhalation anaesthesia.

Direct measurement of blood pressure

Measurement of arterial blood pressure directly is accomplished by insertion of a 20 gauge, 22 gauge or, in cats and small dogs, a 24 gauge catheter aseptically into a peripheral artery, usually the dorsal pedal artery, anterior tibial or femoral artery in dogs and cats (Fig. 2.14), the lateral nasal, facial, transverse facial, or metatarsal artery in horses (Fig. 2.7), or an auricular artery in ruminants and pigs (Fig. 2.15). The catheter is connected by saline-filled tubing to either an anaeroid manometer (Fig. 2.16) or an electrical pressure transducer (Fig. 2.17) for measurement of arterial pressure. Either an air gap or a commercially available latex diaphragm (Fig. 2.18) should be maintained next to the anaeroid manometer to prevent saline entering the manometer and to maintain sterility. An optional addition is a continuous flushing device (Fig. 2.19) that can be inserted between the manometer or transducer and the artery. This device is connected to a bag of saline that has been pressurized to 200 mmHg and will deliver 2–4 ml saline/hour to help prevent clotting of blood in the catheter.

The needle of the anaeroid manometer deflects slightly with each beat and the value at the upper

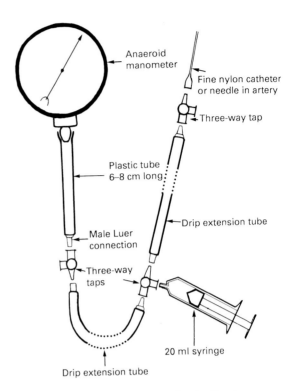

FIG. 2.16 Inexpensive apparatus for the direct measurement of mean arterial blood pressure.

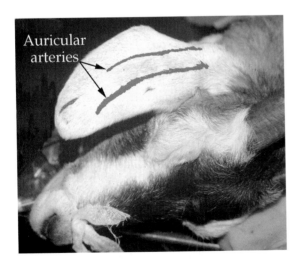

FIG. 2.15 Ink lines have been drawn over the auricular arteries in this goat.

deflection of the needle is slightly less than the values obtained by direct measurement (Riebold & Evans 1985). For accurate measurement, the air–saline junction in the tubing connected to the manometer, or the electrical transducer, are zero reference points and should be placed level with the right atrium or the point of the shoulder when the horse is in dorsal recumbency or level with the sternal manubrium when in lateral recumbency.

The anaeroid manometer costs very little but provides only MAP. The initial cost of an electrocardiograph and blood pressure monitor can be high, however, the electrical transducer does provide much more information, such as digital values for SAP, MAP and DAP, heart rate, and a waveform that can be observed on the oscilloscope or paper printout (Fig. 2.20).

Important advantages of direct measurement of blood pressure are the reliability of measurement and the ability continuously to observe the pressure and immediately detect an abnormality (Fig. 2.21).

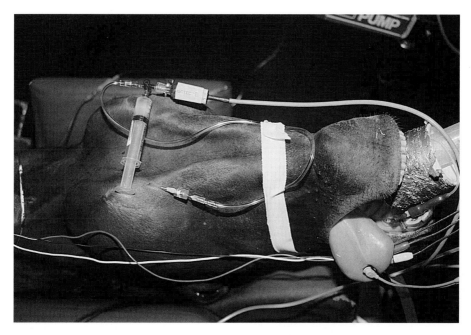

FIG. 2.17 Direct measurement of blood pressure in a horse using a catheter in the facial artery connected by saline-filled tubing to an electrical transducer.

Central venous pressure

The apparatus for measurement of central venous pressure (CVP) can include a commercially-available plastic venous manometer set or be constructed from venous extension tubes and a centimetre ruler (Fig. 2.22). A catheter of sufficient length is introduced into the jugular vein and advanced until its tip lies in the cranial vena cava. The distance the catheter tip has to be introduced is, initially, estimated by measurement of length, but once the catheter is connected to the manometer its position may be adjusted until the level of fluid in the manometer tube moves in time with the animal's respiratory movements. In dogs and cats the introduction of a catheter into the jugular vein is often greatly facilitated by laying the animal on its side and extending its head and neck over a pillow or sandbag. If the catheter is to be left in position for a long time it is kept patent with a drip infusion or the catheter is kept filled with heparin-saline solution (10 units/ml) between measurements. Readings may be taken at any time. If an intravenous drip is used it is turned full on and the stopcock manipulated first to fill the manometer tube from the bag or bottle and then to connect the manometer tube to the catheter. The fall of fluid in the manometer is observed and should be 'step-like' in response to respiratory pressure changes. The central venous pressure is read off when fluid fall ceases.

Venous pressures being low, the margin of error introduced by inaccuracies in obtaining a suitable reference point to represent zero pressure may be clinically significant. Whatever apparatus is used, the zero of the scale should be carefully located, either by placing the patient and manometer in close proximity or by using a spirit level to ensure accuracy. The ideal reference point is the mean pressure in the right atrium but for practical purposes the most appropriate is the sternal manubrium which is easily located and is related to the position of the right atrium in all animals, irrespective of body position. Measurements of CVP are not significantly affected by positioning the animal in right or left recumbency or by catheter size, although oscillations are more easily observed with a 16 gauge catheter (Oakley *et al.*, 1997).

CVP is used in the evaluation of adequacy of blood volume, with the normal range being 0 to 5 cm H_2O in small animals. Hypovolaemia is

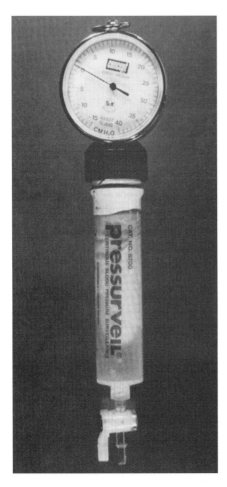

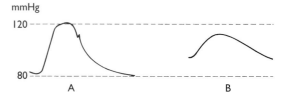

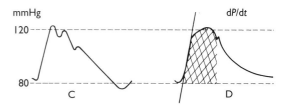

FIG. 2.20 Waveforms from direct measurement of the arterial pressure. **A** Good trace. **B** Recording of the same pressure but with excessive damping, systolic pressure low, diastolic pressure high, mean arterial pressure unchanged. **C** Recording of same pressures but with resonance, systolic pressure apparently increased while diastolic pressure reduced, mean pressure unchanged. **D** Illustration of how left ventricular contractility may be estimated from the rate of rise of pressure during early systole (dP/dt) while the shaded area gives an index of stroke volume.

indicated when the CVP is less than $0\,cmH_2O$. An increase in pressure above $12\,cmH_2O$ may be caused by fluid overload or cardiac failure.

Left atrial pressure (pulmonary artery wedge pressure)

Left heart failure may precede that of the right side and precipitate pulmonary oedema without a rise in central venous pressure. The pulmonary artery

FIG. 2.18 Pressure transfer unit in which a latex diaphragm isolates the anaeroid manometer from the fluid-filled catheter line. These units are presterilized and disposable.

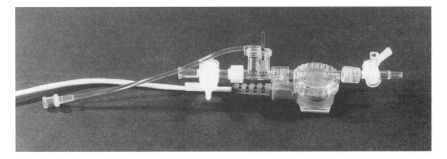

FIG. 2.19 Continuous infusion valve for attachment to a pressure transducer. A pressurized bag of intravenous fluid is connected to the plastic tube to give a continuous infusion of 3 ml per hour. With this particular version, rapid flushing of the manometer line is achieved by pulling the rubber tag on top of the valve.

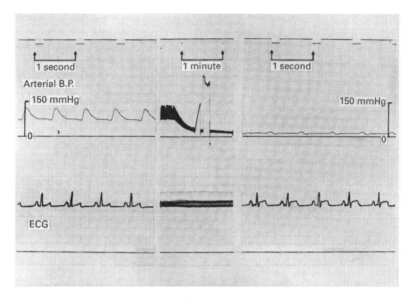

FIG. 2.21 Top: pressure trace from a dog's femoral artery. Bottom: Lead II electrocardiogram. Circulatory failure from an overdose of pentobarbital. Note that while the pressure trace shows the circulation to be ineffective, the ECG trace is little different from normal – heart rate monitors relying on the QRS complex for detection of the heart beat would, under these circumstances, show an unchanged heart rate and in the absence of a blood pressure record encourage the erroneous belief that all was well with the circulatory system.

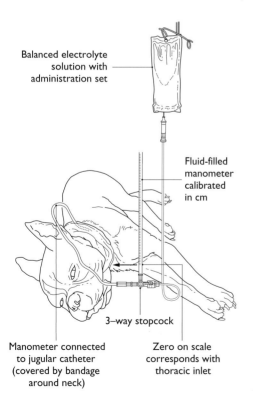

FIG. 2.22 Schematic diagram of the apparatus for measurement of central venous pressure.

wedge pressure (PAWP) is used as a measure of the left atrial filling pressure. A balloon-tip catheter is introduced into the jugular vein and its tip advanced into the heart. Inflation of the balloon with 0.5 ml air facilitates floating the catheter in the bloodstream into the pulmonary artery and then the catheter can be advanced until the tip is wedged in a small pulmonary vessel. The measurement is made using the same apparatus as is used for the measurement of central venous pressure or using an electrical pressure transducer. Care must be taken to ensure that vessel occlusion is not maintained between measurements or pulmonary infarction may occur. If a balloon catheter is used the balloon should only be inflated while measurements are made and if a simple catheter is used it should be slightly withdrawn from the wedged position between measurements.

Cardiac output

The measurement of cardiac output is not one which is routinely carried out in clinical anaesthesia. For research purposes it may be determined by invasive methods such as the direct or indirect

Fick estimations, dye (indocyanine green) or thermal dilution. Modern non-invasive methods include Doppler shift measurements, including colour Doppler displays, but the cost of the necessary apparatus renders them impracticable for most veterinary purposes.

Blood loss

Monitoring blood loss should include measuring the volume of blood aspirated from a body cavity, estimating free blood on drapes around the surgical site, and counting blood-soaked gauze swabs. The volume of blood lost on the swabs may be estimated or the swabs weighed and, after the weight of the same number of dry gauze swabs has been subtracted, applying the formula that 1 g weight equals 1 ml blood. Measurement of packed cell volume is not useful in acute blood loss as this value will not change initially. Once large volumes of balanced electrolyte solution have been infused the packed cell volume and total protein concentrations will decrease. When evaluating packed cell volume changes it is important to consider that anaesthesia *per se* will result in sequestration of red blood cells in the spleen and decrease the packed cell volume by up to 20%.

In the conscious animal, loss of blood volume is initially compensated for by increased heart rate and cardiac contractility, together with peripheral vasoconstriction. These physiological responses are blunted or abolished during anaesthesia. Consequently, the significance of the blood loss may not be appreciated owing to maintenance of a normal heart rate. Furthermore, it should be remembered that when mean arterial pressure is decreasing in response to haemorrhage, cardiac output decreases to a greater extent (Fig. 2.23) (Weiskopf *et al.*, 1981).

Measurement of arterial pressure is an important step in the management of blood loss as oxygen delivery to tissues is impaired when mean arterial pressure decreases below 60 mmHg. The potential impact of blood loss on the patient may be evaluated better by assessing the volume of blood loss against the total blood volume. The blood volume varies between species and is usually assessed in mature animals as 86 ml/kg body weight in dogs, 56 ml/kg in cats, 72 ml/kg in

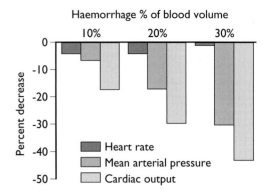

FIG. 2.23 Cardiovascular responses to graded hemorrhage in five isoflurane-anaesthetized dogs. Results are presented as percent change from values measured before blood loss (adapted from Weiskopf *et al.*, 1981).

draught horses and ponies, 100 ml/kg in Thoroughbreds and Arabians, 60 ml/kg in sheep.

Blood volume of paediatric patients may be 50% greater than the blood volume of the mature animal. The percentage of this volume that the animal can lose before circulatory shock ensues depends to a large extent on the physical status of the patient, the depth of anaesthesia, and the support treatment provided. The maximum blood loss allowed before giving a blood transfusion is usually 20% of the estimated blood volume, however, in some animals up to 40% of the total blood volume may be lost without onset of hypotension or hypoxia if the patient has no major preanaesthetic illness, is ventilated with oxygen, the depth of anaesthesia is lightened, balanced electrolyte solution is infused intravenously, and vasoactive drugs are administered as needed.

MONITORING THE RESPIRATORY SYSTEM

Visual observation of respiratory rate and depth of breathing is a basic estimate of adequacy of breathing. The respiratory rate may be counted by observation of chest movement or movement of the reservoir bag on the anaesthesia machine. The excursion of the chest, abdomen, or bag should be observed to gain an impression of the depth of breathing. In general, except possibly in horses, a spontaneous rate of 6 breaths/min or less constitutes respiratory depression. Respiratory rates of 10 breaths/min or greater may provide adequate ventilation but the breaths may be shallow and result in hypoventilation. Chest wall movement with no corresponding movement of the bag is common with complete respiratory obstruction.

Rate monitors and apnoea alarms

Rate monitors and apnoea alarms may use a thermistor either connected to the endotracheal tube or placed in front of a dog's nose. The thermistor detects temperature differences between inspired and exhaled gases to produce a signal that drives a digital rate meter to make a noise which varies in intensity or pitch in time with the animal's breathing. An alarm sounds if a constant gas temperature is detected. Like the oesophageal stethoscope that counts only heart rate, the respiratory rate monitor registers rate only and not adequacy of ventilation.

Tidal and minute volume monitors

The volume of each breath (tidal volume) and the volume of gas inhaled or exhaled per minute (minute volume) can be measured in small animals by attaching a gas meter such as a Wright's respirometer within the circle circuit or to the endotracheal tube. The respirometer has a low resistance to breathing and is reasonably accurate over volumes ranging from 4 l/min to 15 l/min but under-reads below 4 l/min. Gas meters sufficiently large for adult horses are not routinely utilised but domestic dry-gasmeters can be incorporated in large animal breathing systems.

Measurement of arterial pH and blood gas tensions

Measurement of the partial pressure of carbon dioxide ($PaCO_2$) in a sample of arterial blood by blood gas analysis is the best monitor of ventilation. Arterial blood may be collected from any peripheral artery used for blood pressure measurement. A small amount of 1:1000 heparin should be drawn into a 3 ml syringe using a 25 gauge needle and the plunger withdrawn to wash the inside of the syringe with heparin. Excess heparin is then squirted from the syringe leaving only syringe dead space filled with heparin and no bubbles. A 1–2 ml sample of blood is collected from most

animals. A micro technique using 0.2 ml blood drawn into a 1 ml syringe can be used for very small animals.

The blood sample should be collected anaerobically slowly over several respiratory cycles and without aspirating any air bubbles. After expressing a drop of blood and any bubbles from the needle, the syringe should be sealed either with a special cap or by inserting the tip of the needle into a rubber stopper. The syringe should be inverted several times to mix the blood with the heparin. If the sample is not analysed immediately, the syringe should be immersed in a container containing ice and water. The temperature of the animal should be measured at the time of sampling.

The blood sample is then introduced into equipment incorporating electrodes measuring pH, PCO_2 and PO_2. The machine may use the measured values to compute bicarbonate (HCO_3), total CO_2 (TCO_2), base excess (BE) and oxygen saturation (SaO_2). The patient's temperature is entered into the blood gas analyser for appropriate adjustment of pH and PO_2. The patient's haemoglobin concentration must be known for an accurate measure of base excess. Fully automated pH and blood gas analysers are highly accurate but expensive. Portable and less expensive equipment is available, for example, StatPal® (PPG

TABLE 2.4 Normal values for pH, $PaCO_2$, and PaO_2 in mature conscious unsedated animals. Values for $PaCO_2$, and PaO_2 given as pKa (mmHg)

Species	pHa	$PaCO_2$	PaO_2	References
Dogs	7.40	4.67 (35)	13.6 (102)	Horwitz et al., 1969
Cats	7.34	4.5 (34)	13.7 (100)	Middleton et al., 1981
Horses	7.38	5.0–6.1 (38–46)	13.5 (100)	Steffey et al., 1987; Clarke et al., 1991; Wagner et al., 1991; Wan et al., 1992
Cattle	7.40	5.28 (39)	12.0 (89)	Gallivan et al., 1989
Sheep	7.48	4.4 (33)	12.3 (92)	Wanner & Reinhart, 1978
Goats	7.45	5.48 (41)	12.6 (95)	Foster et al., 1981

Industries, Inc., La Jolla, California, USA) and i-STAT (Sensor Devices, Inc., Waukesha, Wisconsin, USA), although the cost of individual analyses is higher.

Normal values for $PaCO_2$ in conscious unsedated animals are given in Table 2.4. Increased $PaCO_2$ (hypercapnia) is a direct consequence of hypoventilation and commonly occurs during anaesthesia. $PaCO_2$ values exceeding 8 kPa (60 mmHg) are indicative of significant respiratory depression. A decrease in $PaCO_2$ (hypocapnia) is due to increased ventilation. A PaO_2 less than 2.6 kPa (20 mmHg) causes cerebral vasoconstriction and cerebral hypoxia.

Hypercapnia in dogs and cats, particularly during halothane anaesthesia, may be associated with arrhythmias such as premature ventricular depolarizations. In these animals intermittent positive pressure ventilation (IPPV) will result in normal cardiac rhythm within a few minutes. Hypercapnia in horses during anaesthesia may cause stimulation of the sympathetic nervous system, increased blood pressure and cardiac output (Wagner et al., 1990; Khanna et al., 1995). Adverse effects of hypercapnia are observed in some horses as tachycardia of 60–70 beats/min, or hypotension caused by decreased myocardial contractility. These abnormalities are corrected within 5–10 minutes by initiating controlled ventilation. More frequently, the effects of hypoventilation during inhalation anaesthesia are manifested as an inadequate depth of anaesthesia despite a vaporiser setting that should provide a sufficient depth of anaesthesia. In these animals, controlled ventilation expands the lungs, thereby improving uptake of anaesthetic agent and resulting in increased depth of anaesthesia.

Arterial oxygenation can be monitored by direct measurement of the partial pressure of oxygen in a sample of arterial blood (PaO_2) or indirectly by attaching a sensor to the tongue, for example, and measuring oxygen saturation of arterial blood (pulse oximetry). PaO_2 values are influenced by the inspired oxygen tension (P_IO_2), adequacy of ventilation, cardiac output, and blood pressure. A PaO_2 of 12–14.6 kPa (90–110 mmHg) is normal in unsedated animals at sea level and PaO_2 values less than 8 kPa (60 mmHg) constitute hypoxaemia.

The maximum possible PaO_2 is governed by the PiO_2 and animals breathing oxygen may have PaO_2 values up to five times greater than when breathing air. The partial pressure of oxygen at the alveolar level (PAO_2) can be calculated from the following formula:

$$PAO_2 = [(\text{barometric pressure} - P_{\text{water vapour}}) \times \text{FIO}_2] - PaCO_2,$$

where the value for water vapour is 6.25 kPa (47 mmHg) and FIO_2 is the fractional concentration of oxygen in inspired gas. Values for PAO_2 greater than 53.2 kPa (400 mmHg) are expected in healthy dogs breathing oxygen. Horses and ruminants are subject to lung collapse during recumbency and anaesthesia and, consequently, ventilation and perfusion are mismatched within the lung, resulting in a lower PaO_2.

Hypoxaemia may develop in dogs and cats during anaesthesia or recovery as a result of hypoventilation when breathing air. This situation is most likely to occur in old animals, animals with hypotension, pneumothorax, pulmonary disease, CNS depression from metabolic disease, or after administration of opioids. Hypoxaemia may also develop during general anaesthesia as a result of severe lung collapse. Patients at greatest risk are small animals during thoracotomy or repair of a ruptured diaphragm, foals with pneumonia and horses with abdominal distension from pregnancy or colic. Cyanosis may be suspected but is not always obvious, especially in horses. Monitoring by blood gas analysis or pulse oximetry will confirm low PaO_2 or SaO_2.

Pulse oximetry

Pulse oximetry is a non-invasive method of continuously measuring haemoglobin oxygen - saturation (SpO_2). The sensor consists of light-emitting diodes (LEDs) that emit light in the red (660 nm) and infrared (940 nm) wavelengths and a photodetector that measures the amount of light that has been transmitted through tissues (Tremper & Barker, 1990). The principles of measurement are based on the different light absorption spectra of oxyhaemoglobin and reduced haemoglobin, and the detection of a pulsatile signal.

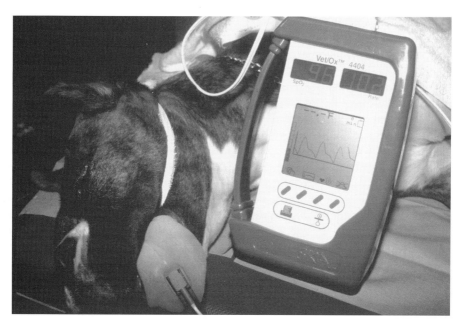

FIG. 2.24 Pulse oximeter (Heska Corporation, Fort Collins, Colorado, USA) showing the dog's heart rate and haemoglobin oxygen saturation in waveform and as a digital number.

Pulse oximeters display a digital record of pulse rate, with an audible beep, and some monitors display the oxygen saturation waveform (Fig. 2.24). A limit for acceptable saturation can be entered into the monitor, allowing an alarm to sound when lower values are sensed. The pulse rate displayed on the oximeter must correspond to the rate obtained by palpation or ECG, and the sensor be in position for at least 30 seconds, before the measurement can be assumed to be accurate. The shape of the sensor, thickness of tissue placed within the sensor, the presence of pigment and hair, and movement of the patient, can be responsible for the oximeter failing to measure oxygen saturation. It may be impossible to obtain a reading from a pulse oximeter when peripheral vasoconstriction is severe, for example, after administration of medetomidine in dogs or patients in circulatory shock.

Arterial oxygen saturation (SaO_2) is the percent of haemoglobin saturated with oxygen. The relationship between PaO_2 and SaO_2 is not linear because haemoglobin changes its affinity for oxygen at increasing levels of saturation, and the association is further altered by pH and temperature of the blood (Fig. 2.25). Oxygen delivery to tissues is defined by the oxygen content (oxygen combined with haemoglobin and dissolved in plasma) and the cardiac output, although oxygen delivery to an individual organ is influenced by the blood flow to that specific organ. Hypoxia is inadequate tissue oxygenation caused by low arterial oxygen content or inadequate blood flow. An animal with a low haemoglobin will have low blood oxygen content despite PaO_2 and SaO_2 being within

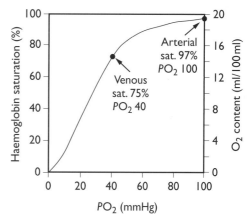

FIG. 2.25 Graph depicting the relationship between PaO_2, haemoglobin oxygen saturation SaO_2, and oxygen content.

their normal ranges. Anaesthetic management of anaemic patients should, therefore, include administration of 100% inspired oxygen and cardiovascular support.

A pulse oximeter detects inadequate blood oxygenation, which should be taken as an indication to supplement the animal's inspired oxygen concentration and to search for the cause. A pulse oximeter is a valuable monitor for animals anaesthetized with injectable anaesthetic agents and breathing air, or during inhalation anaesthesia in patients with pulmonary disease or traumatic pulmonary contusions or pneumothorax, and during thoracotomy or major surgery in the cranial abdomen. It is also important to keep track of oxygenation in animals during recovery from anaesthesia, in patients with partial airway obstruction, or when ventilation is depressed or impaired by systemic opioid administration or residual pneumothorax after thoracotomy or ruptured diaphragm repair.

The pulse oximeter is particularly valuable because it provides an immediate monitor of decreased oxygen saturation, so that corrective treatment can be initiated before respiratory or cardiovascular failure develops. Evaluation of the patient should take into account the fact that the pulse oximeter does not measure carbon dioxide concentration or blood pressure and may continue to read satisfactorily in the presence of hypotension. However, it can provide a warning of a severe decrease in tissue blood flow caused by hypotension or decreased cardiac output by abruptly failing to obtain a signal. Loss of signal may also occur spontaneously with no change in the patient's condition and measurement is restored by changing the position of the probe. Compression of the base of the tongue between the endotracheal tube and the jaw may decrease blood flow and signal acquisition from a probe clipped to the tongue.

Different body sites in dogs have been evaluated for accuracy of measurement of SaO_2. In one investigation, a multisite clip probe placed on the lip, tongue, toe web, and the tip of the tail gave accurate and reliable estimations of SaO_2 values during conditions of full haemoglobin saturation and moderate haemoglobin desaturation (92%) (Huss et al., 1995). In this study, the human finger probe

was accurate only when placed on the dog's lip and when haemoglobin saturation was complete. The lip was found to be the best site in conscious animals. Another study of conscious dogs in an intensive care unit found that a circumferential pulse oximeter probe around a digit or the metatarsus produced excellent correlations between pulse oximeter and SaO_2 values (Fairman, 1993). An evaluation of the Ohmeda Biox 3700 with a human ear probe applied to the tongue provided an accurate evaluation of SaO_2 (Jacobson et al., 1992). The pulse oximeter underestimated SaO_2 at higher saturations and overestimated SaO_2 at saturations < 70%. However, as the authors pointed out, detection of hypoxaemia is more important than measurement of the exact degree of hypoxaemia. In our experience, a rectal sensor is useful for monitoring oxygenation in dogs and cats recovering from anaesthesia.

Different monitors, types of sensors, and alternatives sites for measurement have been evaluated in horses (Whitehair et al., 1990; Chaffin et al., 1996). The Ohmeda Biox 3700 pulse oximeter and the Physio-Control Lifestat 1600 pulse oximeter were evaluated in mature horses using the human ear lobe probe (Whitehair et al., 1990). Measurements were obtained from the tongue and the ear, with the most accurate measurements obtained from the tongue; the oximeters failed to detect a pulse at the nostril, lip, or vulva. The results revealed that both oximeters tended to underestimate saturation by 3.7%, with 95% of the oxygen saturation values within 1 percent above or 8 percent below SaO_2 (Whitehair et al, 1990). The Nellcor N-200 pulse oximeter was evaluated in anaesthetized foals using a fingertip probe (Durasensor DS-100A) (Chaffin et al., 1996). Attachment of the probe to the tongue or ear of the foals slightly underestimated SaO_2 within the range of 80–100% saturation. In our experience, a sensor applied to the Schneiderian membrane in the nostrils yields the most accurate results in horses.

Reflectance pulse oximeters detect changes in absorption of light reflected from tissues, rather than transmitted through tissues as just described (Watney et al., 1993; Chaffin et al., 1996). Attachment of a reflectance probe designed for the human forehead to the ventral surface of the base

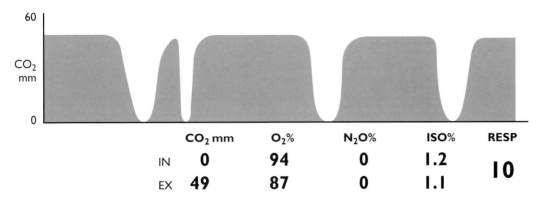

	CO₂ mm	O₂%	N₂O%	ISO%	RESP
IN	0	94	0	1.2	10
EX	49	87	0	1.1	

FIG. 2.26 Capnograph (redrawn) from a foal anaesthetized with isoflurane and an end-tidal concentration of 1.1%. The foal is breathing spontaneously at 10 breaths per minute and the end-tidal concentration of carbon dioxide is 6.5 kPa (49 mmHg), confirming a degree of hypoventilation.

of the tail in foals had 100% sensitivity for detecting $SaO_2 < 90\%$ but consistently underestimated the actual value (Chaffin *et al.*, 1996). Therefore, this probesite combination will incorrectly identify some foals as being hypoxaemic.

Capnography

Capnography indirectly estimates $PaCO_2$ by measuring the concentration of CO_2 in expired gas. Capnography is also useful for diagnosis of mechanical problems in anaesthetic circuits, airway obstruction, and cardiogenic shock. Gas is aspirated from the endotracheal tube or Y-piece (Matthews *et al.*, 1990) and the capnometer measures CO_2 concentration by infrared absorption (Fig. 2.5). Gases leaving the analyser should be directed back into the anaesthetic circuit or into the scavenging system. The capnometer provides breath-by-breath numerical values for carbon dioxide concentration and some monitors display the CO_2 waveform (capnograph). The upward slope of the waveform represents expiration and the highest value is the end-tidal CO_2 (E_TCO_2). The downward slope occurs during inspiration and the inspiratory baseline should be zero (Fig. 2.26).

Falsely low measurements of E_TCO_2 may occur with the use of non-rebreathing circuits, because the high gas flow results in dilution of expired gases, and in animals with very small tidal volumes or that are panting. Bumps and dips in the expiratory plateau may be caused by spontaneous respiratory efforts, heart beats, and movements of

the animal by the surgeon. Changes in E_TCO_2 or waveform are useful indicators of significant alteration in physiological status or equipment malfunction (Table 2.5). A sudden decrease in E_TCO_2 is cause for concern and the patient and equipment should be checked for hypotension, cardiac arrest, or equipment leaks and disconnection. Exhaled water vapour condenses in the sampling tubing and water trap but when water enters the monitor unpredictable and bizarre values are obtained.

Significant correlation between E_TCO_2 and $PaCO_2$ has been recorded in dogs and horses, with the $PaCO_2$ exceeding the E_TCO_2 by 1.00–4.65 kPa

TABLE 2.5 **Troubleshooting the capnogram**
Unexpectedly low E_TCO₂
Cardiac arrest
Sampling line disconnected or broken
Endotracheal tube cuff deflated
Tidal volume too small
Failure to read zero on inspiration (rebreathing)
Large apparatus deadspace
Exhausted soda lime
Expiratory valve on circle stuck in open position
Breathing rapid and shallow
Prolonged inspiratory or expiratory slope
Slow inspiratory time
Obstruction or crack in the sampling line
Gas sampling rate too slow
Leak around connection to circle or tracheal tube
Lung disease

(1–35 mmHg) depending on the degree of pulmonary shunting and lung collapse. $E_T CO_2$ values exceeding 6.7 kPa (50 mmHg) represent increased $PaCO_2$ and significant hypoventilation. However, when $E_T CO_2$ is normal, $PaCO_2$ may be normal or increased and when $E_T CO_2$ is low, $PaCO_2$ may be low, normal or increased. Therefore, if blood gas analysis is available one direct measurement of $PaCO_2$ is advisable when the $E_T CO_2$ value is normal or low, particularly in dogs with pulmonary disease or during thoracotomy, and anaesthetized horses at risk for severe lung collapse, such as colic patients or foals.

The difference between $PaCO_2$ and $E_T CO_2$ is usually less in dogs than in horses. In a group of mechanically ventilated dogs in intensive care, the $E_T CO_2$ was on average 0.67 kPa (5 mmHg) less than $PaCO_2$ (Hendricks & King, 1994). Nonetheless, there was sufficient variation to conclude that although high $E_T CO_2$ confirms the presence of hypoventilation, some patients may be erroneously identified as having adequate ventilation. In anaesthetized healthy mature horses an average difference of 1.6 kPa (12 mmHg), range 0–4.3 kPa (0–32 mmHg) was recorded during halothane (Cribb, 1988; Moens, 1989) and 1.9 kPa (14 mmHg) during isoflurane anaesthesia (Cribb, 1988). A stronger correlation between $E_T CO_2$ and $PaCO_2$ was identified during halothane compared with isoflurane anaesthesia (Meyer & Short, 1985; Cribb, 1988). No significant increase in $PaCO_2$ – $E_T CO_2$ difference was recorded with increased duration of anaesthesia (Cribb, 1988; Moens,1989). In one study of 110 horses, the $PaCO_2$–$E_T CO_2$ difference was greater in heavier horses and was increased when horses were in dorsal recumbency compared with lateral recumbency (Moens, 1989). A mean $PaCO_2$–$E_T CO_2$ difference of 1.8 ± 0.9 kPa (13.4 ± 6.9 mmHg; range 0–37.5 mmHg) was measured in 125 horses anaesthetized with isoflurane in dorsal recumbency for colic surgery (Trim, 1998). Spontaneously breathing foals anaesthetized with isoflurane had a mean $PaCO_2$–$E_T CO_2$ difference in the first hour of anaesthesia of 0.9 kPa (7 mmHg) which increased over 90 minutes of anaesthesia to 1.7 kPa (13 mmHg), coincident with an increase in $PaCO_2$ (Geiser & Rohrbach, 1992). These authors were unable accurately to predict $PaCO_2$ from $E_T CO_2$ and emphasized the limitations of capnometry in spontaneously breathing anaesthetized foals (Geiser & Rohrbach, 1992).

Monitoring acid–base status

The values for HCO_3 and TCO_2 calculated from the measured values for pH and $PaCO_2$ are influenced by both metabolic and respiratory physiological functions and both values are increased by hypercapnia. The base excess value is obtained by a calculation that defines the metabolic status by eliminating deviations of the respiratory component from normal. Zero base excess is neither acidotic nor alkalotic. Positive base excess describes a metabolic alkalosis and a negative base excess (base deficit) defines a metabolic acidosis. The metabolic status of a healthy animal is influenced by its diet and, in general, carnivores usually have a mild metabolic acidosis and herbivores a metabolic alkalosis. An approximate estimate of severity of acid–base changes can be obtained from the guideline that a 5 mmol/l change from normal is a mild deviation, a 10 mmol/l change is a moderate deviation, and a 15 mmol/l deviation is severe.

Chemical determination of TCO_2 in serum or plasma is often used as an estimate of blood bicarbonate concentration and acid–base status of patients when blood gas analysis is unavailable. However, the values obtained using auto-analysers may be significantly different from that obtained by calculation from pH and PCO_2. Errors arise from differences in handling the samples, such as exposure to air, underfilling of blood collection tubes, delay in analysis, and changing reagents. A combination of these factors may result in lowering the TCO_2 by as much as 5.3 mmol/l in canine blood and 4.6 mmol/l in feline blood. This degree of inaccuracy might result in erroneous assumptions and affect clinical decisions.

Acid–base evaluation has always used the Van Slyke technique as the 'gold standard' measurement but more recently a very similar approach has been available in the form of a simple kit, intended for use with serum (the 'Harleco' system), which, when correctly used, is capable of high precision by clinical standards, allowing TCO_2 status to be determined with reasonable confidence from samples of venous whole blood (Groutides & Michell, 1988).

Monitoring body temperature

In the normal animal, body heat is unevenly distributed with the core temperature being 2–4°C higher than the peripheral. General anaesthesia inhibits vasoconstriction, allowing generalized redistribution of body heat. An additional decrease in body temperature occurs as heat is lost to the environment by exposure to cold operating room conditions, skin preparation with cold solutions, and abdominal surgical exposure. Furthermore, anaesthetics inhibit thermoregulation, vasoconstriction, and shivering, thereby decreasing the thresholds for cold responses. Administration of unwarmed iv. fluid contributes substantially to the decrease in body temperature.

Hypothermia

Hypothermia, (35°C; 96°F), may develop in animals anaesthetized in a cool environment. A decrease in temperature of 1–3°C below normal has been demonstrated to provide substantial protection against cerebral ischaemia and hypoxaemia in anaesthetised dogs (Wass *et al.*, 1995). However, life-threatening cardiovascular depression may develop when the temperature decreases below 32.8°C (91°F). Perioperative hypothermia is associated with several other significant adverse effects (Table 2.6) (Carli *et al.*, 1991; Sheffield *et al.*, 1994; Kurz *et al.*, 1996).

Rectal or oesophageal temperature should be monitored at regular intervals during inhalation anaesthesia, during protracted total intravenous anaesthesia, and during recovery from anaesthe-

---

TABLE 2.6 Adverse effects of perianaesthetic hypothermia

Impaired cardiovascular function
Hypoventilation
Decreased metabolism and detoxification of anaesthetic drugs
Weakness during recovery from anaesthesia
Decreased resistance to infection
Increased incidence of surgical wound infection
Increased postoperative protein catabolism

---

sia. Small animals can be insulated from a cool environment by a variety of methods, including plastic covered foam pads and hot water circulating pads to lie on, and wrapping of extremities with towels or plastic insulation. Heat loss from the respiratory tract may be minimized by ensuring that the inspired air remains warm and humidified. This can be accomplished by employing rebreathing circuits and low flow administration, or by attachment of a humidifier to the endotracheal connexion of the anaesthetic circuit. Heat loss in small cats and dogs is effectively limited by insertion of a low-volume passive humidifier (e.g. Humid-Vent®, Gibeck) between the endotracheal tube and the anaesthetic circuit. The water vapour in exhaled gases condenses on the humidifier so that the inhaled air is moistened and warmed.

Fluids to be administered iv. should be warm, either in the bag or bottle by storage in an incubator or at the time of administration by attaching a warming block to the administration line. Active skin warming of the limbs may be the most effective method of preventing heat loss (Cabell *et al.*, 1997). This can be accomplished by application of hot water or hot air circulating devices, or warmed towels and gel-filled packs.

Special care should be taken to avoid skin sloughing from burns caused by application of devices that are too hot. Electrical heating pads and packs heated in a microwave oven are frequently to blame for tissue damage. It should also be remembered that warming devices placed over the site of an intramuscular injection, or an opioid-filled patch applied to the skin, may alter local blood flow and speed absorption of the drug.

Hyperthermia

Increased body temperature is occasionally measured in anaesthetized animals. Hyperthermia developing in dogs and cats is most often caused by either excessive application of heat in an attempt to prevent hypothermia or by a pyrogenic reaction to a bacterial infection, a contaminant in iv. fluids, or drugs. Other causes of intraoperative hyperthermia are loss of central nervous system temperature regulation, thyrotoxicosis, or phaeochromocytoma. Rarely, hyperthermia is a manifestation of the malignant hyperthermia syndrome (MH) which is a life-threatening hyper-metabolic condition triggered by stress and certain anaesthetic agents.

Hyperthermia (40.5 °C; 105 °F) quite frequently develops in cats during recovery from anaesthesia that included administration of tiletamine-zolaze-pam. In these animals, the increase in temperature is associated with increased muscle activity such as paddling, uncoordinated movements, or pur-poseful movements directed at restraints or band-ages. Treatment that is usually effective includes directing a flow of air over the cat from a fan placed outside the cage and providing sedation, for example, butorphanol, 0.2 mg/kg i.m., with or without acepromazine, 0.05–0.1 mg/kg i.m.

Malignant hyperthermia

Malignant hyperthermia (MH) occurs most fre-quently during anaesthesia of human beings and pigs (McGrath, 1986; Roewer *et al.*, 1995), but has been reported to occur in dogs (O'Brien *et al.*, 1990; Nelson, 1991), cats (Bellah *et al.*, 1989), and horses (Manley *et al.*, 1983; Klein *et al.*, 1989). Clinical signs of MH in pigs (p.366) usually include an increase in temperature, increased respiratory rate and depth, increased $E_T CO_2$ and $PaCO_2$, metabolic acidosis, tachycardia, hypertension, and arrhyth-mias. Purple blotches may be observed in the skin of the abdomen and snout. The soda lime canister on the anaesthesia machine may be-come excessively hot to touch and the absorbent changes colour rapidly, reflecting massive carbon dioxide production. Rigidity of the jaw and limb muscles may be observed as the condition pro-gresses. The animal dies unless the condition is treated early.

The clinical appearance of dogs developing MH during anaesthesia may differ from pigs. Tachy-cardia may not be a feature, skeletal muscle rigidi-ty may not occur, and rectal temperature may not increase until the syndrome is well estab-lished (Nelson, 1991). The earliest signs may be related to increased CO_2 production. These signs include an increased respiratory rate and depth, rapid changing of soda lime colour, a hot soda lime canister, and increased $E_T CO_2$ in the absence of hypoventilation or malfunctioning one-way valves. Increased respiratory rate would be the

only one of these signs present in a dog that was merely overheated.

The clinical picture of MH in horses is not clear cut. Abnormal measurements may not be observed for some time after induction of anaesthesia. Observed signs may be suggestive that the horse is in a light plane of anaesthesia, however, the earliest changes are usually increased $PaCO_2$ and $E_T CO_2$. Heart rates may be mildly elevated and arterial blood pressure is often within the normal range for inhalation anaesthesia (Manley *et al.*, 1983; Klein *et al.*, 1989). Changes in anaesthetic management may permit the horse to survive anaesthesia but severe rhabdomyolysis developing during recovery from anaesthesia may necessitate euthanasia.

Monitoring urine volume

The urinary output depends on the renal blood flow which, in turn, depends on cardiac output and circulating blood volume, and thus it is a relat-ively sensitive indicator of the circulatory state during anaesthesia. Measurement of urine pro-duction is advisable in animals with severe chronic renal disease, renal failure, or circulatory failure from non-renal causes. The urinary bladder may be catheterized using aseptic technique before anaesthesia or after induction of anaesthesia, and the catheter connected to a plastic bag for continu-ous collection of urine.

Urine output of less than 1 ml/kg/hour is inad-equate and an indication for treatment. In event of inadequate urine flow, the anaesthetist should first check that the catheter is not blocked by mucus or a blood clot and that urine is not pooling in the bladder and cannot drain because of the relation-ship between the catheter tip and positioning of the animal.

Monitoring blood glucose

Clinical signs of hypoglycaemia may not be obvi-ous during anaesthesia and the condition may go unrecognized. Consequences of hypoglycaemia are coma, hypotension, or prolonged recovery from anaesthesia with depression, weakness, or even seizures.

Animals at risk for developing hypoglycaemia during anaesthesia include paediatric patients, diabetics, and animals with hepatic disease, portosystemic shunt, insulinoma, and septicaemia or endotoxaemia. Occasionally, healthy adult sheep, goats, and even horses develop hypoglycaemia which manifests as a prolonged or weak recovery from anaesthesia. Routine monitoring of patients at risk for hypoglycaemia should include measurement of blood glucose at the start and the end of anaesthesia. Blood glucose can be determined rapidly using reagent strips and a glucometer. Animals with low blood glucose concentrations initially or those undergoing major or prolonged surgery, should have their blood glucose monitored at approximately 1 hour intervals during anaesthesia.

Patients at risk for hypoglycemia should be given 5% dextrose in water (D5W) as part of the intraoperative i.v. fluid therapy. D5W should be infused at a rate of 2–5 ml/kg/hour to maintain blood glucose between 5.5–11.0 mmol/l (100 and 200 mg/dl). Balanced electrolyte solution should also be infused at the usual rate of 5–10 ml/kg/hour.

Monitoring neuromuscular blockade

The mechanical response to nerve stimulation (i.e. muscular contraction) may be observed following the application of supramaximal single, tetanic or 'train-of-four' electrical stimuli to a suitable peripheral motor nerve, usually a foot twitch in response to stimulation of the peroneal, tibial, or ulnar nerves. During general anaesthesia the response obtained may be influenced by the anaesthetic agents and any neuromuscular blocking drugs which have been used. Details about neuromuscular blocking drugs and the monitoring technique are given in Chapter 7.

MONITORING OF EQUIPMENT

Before any anaesthetic is administered all equipment likely to be used should be carefully checked. It is essential to ensure that the O_2 supply will be adequate, the circuit is free from leaks and that the correct volatile anaesthetic is in the vaporizer. If soda lime is to be used its freshness should be checked by blowing CO_2 through a small portion and testing to see whether this causes it to get hot.

The colour indicator incorporated in many brands of soda lime cannot be relied upon to indicate freshness.

Interruption in the supply of O_2 to the patient is one of the most serious events which can occur during anaesthesia and many anaesthesic machines incorporate warning devices which sound alarms if the O_2 supply fails. However, when a rebreathing circuit is being used, the delivery of O_2 in the fresh gas supply does not always ensure that the inspired gases will contain sufficient O_2 to support life. Dilution of the O_2 in a rebreathing system is particularly likely to occur in the early stages of anaesthesia when denitrogenation of the patient is taking place, or when N_2O is used with low total flow rates of fresh gas. Measurement devices are available which can be used to demonstrate to the anaesthetist that the patient is receiving an adequate concentration of O_2 (Fig. 2.5).

Inspired and end-tidal concentrations of volatile anaesthetics can be measured by sampling gases from the endotracheal tube connector, as described earlier in this chapter. In addition to providing information on the concentration of the volatile anaesthetic agent in the patient, the analyser acts as a monitor of the accuracy of output of the vaporizers.

REFERENCES

Bailey, J.E., Dunlop, C.I., Chapman, P.L., *et al.* (1994) Indirect Doppler ultrasonic measurement of arterial blood pressure results in a large measurement error in dorsally recumbent anaesthetised horses. *Equine Veterinary Journal* **26**(1): 70–73.

Bellah, J.R., Robertson, S.A, Buergelt, C.D. and McGavin A.D. (1989) Suspected malignant hyperthermia after halothane anesthesia in a cat. *Veterinary Surgery* **18**(6): 483–488.

Bodey, A.R., Young, L.E., Bartram, D.H., Diamond, M.J. and Michell, A.R. (1994) A comparison of direct and indirect (oscillometric) measurements of arterial blood pressure in anaesthetised dogs, using tail and limb cuffs. *Research in Veterinary Science* **57**: 265–269.

Branson, K.R., Wagner-Mann, C.C. and Mann, F.A. (1997) Evaluation of an oscillometric blood pressure monitor on anesthetized cats and the effect of cuff placement and fur on accuracy. *Veterinary Surgery* **26**, 347–353.

Cabell, L.W., Perkowski, S.Z., Gregor, T. and Smith, G.K. (1997) The effects of active peripheral skin warming on perioperative hypothermia in dogs. *Veterinary Surgery* **26**: 79–85.

Carli, F., Webster J., Pearson M., *et al.* (1991) Postoperative protein metabolism: effect of nursing elderly patients for 24 h after abdominal surgery in a thermoneutral environment. *British Journal of Anaesthesia* **66**: 292–299.

Chaffin, M.K., Mathews, N.S., Cohen, N.D. and Carter, G.K. (1996) Evaluation of pulse oximetry in anaesthetised foals using multiple combinations of transducer type and transducer attachment site. *Equine Veterinary Journal* **28**(6): 437–445.

Clarke, K.W., England, G.C.W. and Goosens, L. (1991) Sedative and cardiovascular effects of romifidine, alone and in combination with butorphanol, in the horse. *Journal of Veterinary Anaesthesia*, **18**: 25–29.

Cribb, P.H. (1988) Capnographic monitoring during anesthesia with controlled ventilation in the horse. *Veterinary Surgery* **17**(1): 48–52.

Ekstrom, P.M., Short, C.E. and Geimer, T.R. (1993) Electroencephalography of detomidine-ketamine-halothane and detomidine-ketamine-isoflurane anesthetized horses during orthopedic surgery: a comparison. *Veterinary Surgery* **22**(5): 414–418.

Fairman, N. (1993) Evaluation of pulse oximetry as a continuous monitoring technique in critically ill dogs in the small animal intensive care unit. *Veterinary Emergency and Critical Care* **2**(2): 50–56.

Forster, H.V., Bisgard, G.E. and Klein, J.P.(1981) Effect of peripheral chemoreceptor denervation on acclimatization of goats during hypoxia. *Journal of Applied Physiology* **50**(2): 392–398.

Gallivan, J.G., McDonell, W.N. and Forrest, J.B. (1989) Comparative ventilation and gas exchange in the horse and cow. *Research in Veterinary Science* **46**(3): 331–336.

Geddes, L.A., Chaffee, V., Whistler, S.J., Bourland, J.D. and Tacker, W.A. (1977) Indirect mean blood pressure in the anesthetized pony. *American Journal of Veterinary Science* **38**(12): 2055–2057.

Geiser, D.R. and Rohrbach, B.W. (1992) Use of end-tidal CO_2 tension to predict arterial CO_2 values in isoflurane-anesthetized equine neonates. *American Journal of Veterinary Research* **53**(9): 1617–1621.

Grandy, J.L., Dunlop, C.I., Hodgson, D.S., Curtis, C.R. and Chapman, P.L. (1992) Evaluation of the doppler ultrasonic method of measuring systolic arterial blood pressure in cats. *American Journal of Veterinary Research* **53**(7): 1166–1169.

Groutides, C. and Michell, A.R. (1988). A method for assessment of of acid-base disturbances. *Clinical Insight*, **3**: 209–210.

Hendricks, J.C. and King, L.G. (1994) Practicality, usefulness, and limits of end-tidal carbon dioxide monitoring in critical small animal patients. *Journal of Veterinary Emergency and Critical Care* **4**: 29–39.

Hodgson, D.S., Dunlop, C.I., Chapman, P.L. and Steffey, E.P. (1990) Cardiopulmonary effects of isoflurane in foals (abstract). *Veterinary Surgery* **19**: 316.

Horwitz, L.D., Bishop, V.S., Stone, H.L. and Stegall, H.F. (1969) Cardiovascular effects of low-oxygen atmospheres in conscious and anaesthetized dogs. *Journal of Applied Physiology*, **27**(3): 370–373.

Huss, B.T., Anderson, M.A., Branson, K.R., Wagner-Mann, C.C. and Mann, F.A. (1995) Evaluation of pulse oximeter probes and probe placement in healthy dogs. *Journal of the American Animal Hospital Association* **31**(1): 9–14.

Jacobson, J.D., Miller, M.W., Matthews, N.S., Hartsfield, S.M. and Knauer, K.W. (1992) Evaluation of accuracy of pulse oximetry in dogs. *American Journal of Veterinary Research* **53**(4): 537–540.

Johnson, C.B., Young, S.S. and Taylor, P.M. (1994) Analysis of the frequency spectrum of the equine electroencephalogram during halothane anaesthesia. *Research in Veterinary Science* **56**(3): 373–378.

Khanna, A.K., McDonell, W.N., Dyson, D.H. and Taylor, P.M. (1995) Cardiopulmonary effects of hypercapnia during controlled intermittent positive pressure ventilation in the horse. *Canadian Journal of Veterinary Research* **59**: 213–221.

Klein, L., Ailes, N., Fackelman, G., Kellon, E. and Rosenberg, H. (1989) Postanesthetic equine myopathy suggestive of malignant hyperthermia. A case report. *Veterinary Surgery* **18**(6): 479–482.

Kurz, A., Sessler, D.I. and Lenhardt, R. (1996) Perioperative normothermia to reduce the incidence of surgical-wound infection and shorten hospitalization. *New England Journal of Medicine* **334**(19): 1209–1215.

Latshaw, H., Fessler, J.F., Whistler, S.J. and Geddes, L.A. (1979) Indirect measurement of mean blood pressure in the normotensive and hypotensive horse. *Equine Veterinary Journal* **11**: 191–194.

Manley, S.V., Kelly, A.B. and Hodgson, D. (1983) Malignant hyperthermia-like reactions in three anesthetized horses. *Journal of the American Veterinary Medical Association* **183**: 85–89.

Matthews, N.S., Hartsfield, S.M., Cornick, J.L. and Jacobson, J.D. (1990) A comparison of end-tidal halothane concentration measurement at different locations in the horse. *Veterinary Surgery* **19**: 317 (Abstract).

McGrath, C. (1986) Malignant hyperthermia. *Seminars in Veterinary Medicine and Surgery (Small animal)* **1**: 238–244.

Meurs, K.M., Miller, M.W. and Slater, M.R. (1996) Comparison of the indirect oscillometric and direct arterial methods for blood pressure measurements in anesthetized dogs. *Journal of the American Animal Hospital Asociation* **32**: 471–475.

Meyer, R.E. and Short, C.E. (1985) Arterial to end-tidal CO_2 tension and alveolar dead space in halothane- or isoflurane-anesthetized ponies. *American Journal of Veterinary Research* **46**: 597–599.

Middleton, D.J., Ilkiw, J.E. and Watson, A.D.J. (1981) Arterial and venous blood gas tensions in clinically healthy cats. *American Journal of Veterinary Research* **42**(9): 1609–1611.

Moens, Y. (1989) Arterial-alveolar carbon dioxide tension difference and aveolar dead space in halothane anaesthetised horses. *Equine Veterinary Journal* **21**(4): 282–284.

Moens, Y., Gootjes, P. and Lagerweij, E. (1991) The influence of methane on the infrared measurement of halothane in the horse. *Journal of Veterinary Anaesthesia* **18**: 4–7.

Muir, W.W., Wade, A. and Grospitch, B. (1983) Automatic noninvasive sphygmomanometry in horses. *Journal of the American Veterinary Medical Association* **182**(11): 1230–1233.

Nelson, T.E. (1991) Malignant hyperthermia in dogs. *Journal of the American Veterinary Medical Association* **198**(6): 989–994.

O'Brien, P.J., Pook, H.A., Klip, A. *et al.* (1990) Canine stress syndrome/malignant hyperthermia susceptibility: calcium-hemostasis defect in muscle and lymphocytes. *Research in Veterinary Science* **48**: 124–128.

Oakley, R.E., Olivier, B., Eyster, G.E. and Hauptman, J.G. (1997) Experimental evaluation of central venous pressure monitoring in the dog. *Journal of the American Animal Hospital Asociation* **33**: 77–82.

Otto, K.A. and Short, C.E. (1991) Electroencephalographic power spectrum analysis as a monitor of anesthetic depth in horses. *Veterinary Surgery* **20**(5): 362–371.

Otto, K.A., Voigt, S., Piepenbrock, S., Deegan, E. and Short, C.E. (1996) Differences in quantitated electroencephalographic variables during surgical stimulation of horses anesthetized with isoflurane. *Veterinary Surgery* **25**: 249–255.

Parry, B.W., McCarthy, M.A., Anderson, G.A. and Gay, C.C. (1982) Correct occlusive bladder width for indirect blood pressure measurement in horses. *American Journal of Veterinary Research* **43**: 50–54.

Riebold, T.W. and Evans, A.T. (1985) Blood pressure measurements in the anesthetized horse: comparison of four methods. *Veterinary Surgery* **14**(4): 332–337.

Robertson, S.A. (1990) Practical use of ECG in the horse. *In Practice* **12**(2): 59–67.

Roewer, N., Dziadzka, A., Greim, C.A., Kraas, E. and Schulteamesch, J. (1995) Cardiovascular and metabolic responses to anesthetic-induced malignant hyperthermia in swine. *Anesthesiology* **83**: 141–159.

Sawyer, D.C. (1992) Indirect blood pressure measurements in dogs, cats and horses: correlation with direct arterial pressures and site of measurement. In: *Proceedings of the XXVII World Small Animal Veterinary Association Congress*. Rome, Italy, 1992, pp 93–98.

Sawyer, D.C, Brown M., Striler E.L., Durham, R.A., Langham, M.A. and Rech, R. H. (1991) Comparison of direct and indirect blood pressure measurement in anesthetized dogs. *Laboratory Animal Science* **41**(2): 134–138.

Sheffield, C.W., Sessler D.I. and Hunt, T.K. (1994) Mild hypothermia during isoflurane anesthesia decreases resistance to E. coli dermal infection in guinea pigs. *Acta Anaesthesiologica Scandinavica* **38**(3): 201–205.

Soma, L.R. (1971) Depth of General Anaesthesia. In: Soma, L.R. (ed.) *Textbook of Veterinary Anaesthesia*. Baltimore: Williams & Wilkins Company, pp 178–187.

Steffey, E.P., Dunlop, C.I., Farver, T.B., Woliner, M.J. and Schultz, L.J. (1987) Cardiovascular and respiratory measurements in awake and isoflurane-anesthetized horses. *American Journal of Veterinary Rearch* **48**(1): 7–12.

Stegall, H.E., Kardon, M.B. and Kemmerer, W.T. (1968) Indirect measurement of arterial blood pressure by Doppler ultrasonic sphygmomanometry. *Journal of Applied Physiology* **25**(1): 793–798.

Taylor, P.M. (1990) Interference with the Datex Normac anaesthetic agent monitor for halothane in horses and sheep. *Journal of the Association of Veterinary Anaesthetists* **17**: 32–34.

Tremper, K.K. and Barker, S.J. (1990) Monitoring of oxygen. In: Lake, C.L. (ed) *Clinical Monitoring*. Philadelphia: W. B. Saunders Company, pp 283–313.

Trim, C.M. (1998) Monitoring during anaesthesia: techniques and interpretation. *Equine Veterinary Education* (4): 207–218.

Wagner, A.E., Bednarski, R.M. and Muir, W.W. (1990) Hemodynamic effects of carbon dioxide during intermittent positive-pressure ventilation in horses. *American Journal of Veterinary Research* **51**(12): 1922–1929.

Wagner, A.E., Muir, W.W. and Hinchcliff K.W. (1991) Cardiovascular effects of xylazine and detomidine in horses. *American Journal of Veterinary Research* **52**(5): 651–657.

Wan, P.Y., Trim, C.M. and Mueller, P.O.E. (1992) Xylazine-ketamine and detomidine-tiletamine-zolazepam anesthesia in horses. *Veterinary Surgery* **21**(4): 312–318.

Wanner A. and Reinhart, M.E. (1978) Respiratory mechanics in conscious sheep: response to methacholine. *Journal of Applied Physiology* **44**(3): 479–482.

Wass, C.T., Lanier, W.L., Hofer, R.E., Scheithauer, B.W. and Andrews, A.G. (1995) Temperature changes of > 1 or =1 °C alter functional neurologic outcome and histopathology in a canine model of complete cerebral ischemia. *Anesthesiology* **83**(2): 325–335.

Watney, G.C.G., Norman, W.M., Schumacher, J.P. and Beck, E. (1993) Accuracy of a reflectance pulse oximeter in anesthetized horses. *American Journal of Veterinary Research* **54**(4): 497–501.

Weiskopf, R.B., Townsley, M.I., Riordan, K.K., Chadwick, K., Baysinger, M. and Mahoney, E. (1981) Comparison of cardiopulmonary responses to graded hemorrhage during enflurane, halothane, isoflurane, and ketamine anesthesia. *Anesthesia and Analgesia* **60**: 481–491.

Whitehair, K.J., Watney, G.C.G., Leith, D.E. and DeBowes, R.M. (1990) Pulse oximetry in horses. *Veterinary Surgery* **19**(3): 243–248.

Introduction to general anaesthesia: pharmacodynamics and pharmacokinetics

3

INTRODUCTION

The term *pharmacodynamics* refers to the relationship between drug concentration and its clinical or pharmacological effect, while *pharmacokinetics* refers to the mathematical description of the various processes relating to drug movement from the site of its administration, followed by distribution to the tissues and, finally, elimination from the body. To paraphrase, pharmacokinetics is 'what the body does to the drug' whereas pharmacodynamics is 'what the drug does to the body'. They cannot be regarded as separate processes for drugs produce effects *in vivo* which alter their own kinetic and dynamic profiles, for example by means of acute haemodynamic effects and increased or decreased end-organ sensitivity by 'up' or 'down' receptor regulation (Fig. 3.1).

In the account of the pharmacokinetics of inhaled drugs which follows frequent reference is made to tensions, solubilities and concentrations of gases in solution. These terms may perhaps be best explained by considering specific examples.

THE TENSIONS OF AGENT DISSOLVED IN A LIQUID

This is the pressure of the agent in the gas with which the liquid should be in equilibrium. A liquid and a gas, or two liquids, are in equilibrium if, when separated by a permeable membrane, there is no exchange between them. The statement that 'the tension of nitrous oxide in the blood is 50.5 kPa (380 mmHg)' means that if a sample of blood were placed in an ambient atmosphere containing nitrous oxide at a concentration of 50% v/v (and, therefore according to Dalton's law, exerting a partial pressure of 50.5 kPa (380 mmHg) there would be no movement of nitrous oxide into or out of the blood. 'Tension' is a term used by physiologists and anaesthetists, while physicists speak of 'partial pressure'.

SOLUBILITY COEFFICIENTS OF GASES

At any given temperature the mass of a gas dissolved in a solution, i.e. its concentration in the solution, varies directly with its tension (Henry's law) and is governed by the solubility of the gas in the particular solvent. The solubility of anaesthetics varies widely and, therefore, at any one tension, the quantities of the different anaesthetics in the solvent are not equal. The solubility of anaesthetics in the blood and tissues are best expressed in terms of their partition, or distribution, coefficients. For example, the blood–gas partition coefficient of nitrous oxide is 0.47. This means that when blood and alveolar air containing nitrous oxide at a given tension are in equilibrium, there will be 47 parts of nitrous oxide per unit volume (say per litre) of blood for every 100 parts of nitrous oxide per unit volume (litre) of alveolar air. In general, the partition coefficient of a gas at a stated temperature is

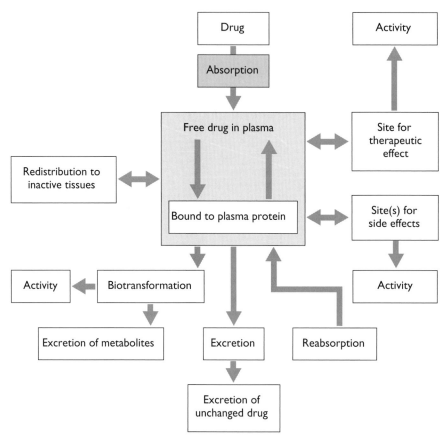

FIG. 3.1 Pathways for the uptake, distribution and elimination from the body of an active drug.

the ratio, at equilibrium, of the gas's concentration on the two sides of a diffusing membrane or interface.

Tissue solubility does not necessarily correlate with blood–gas solubility. The newer volatile agents (e.g. isoflurane, desflurane, sevoflurane) may have a low blood–gas partition coefficient but their brain–blood partition coefficient is not necesssarily lowered to the same extent. The brain–blood partition coefficient can be estimated by dividing the brain–gas with the blood–gas partition coefficient. The brain–blood partition co-efficients for halothane, enflurane, isoflurane and desflurane calculate to be 1.86, 1.73, 1.67 and 1.27, respectively. Hence desflurane has a more rapid uptake in the brain tissue. For simplicity, in many theoretical calculations it is often assumed that in the brain and all other tissues (except fat) gases have very nearly the same solubility as they have in blood because their tissue–blood partition co-efficients are sufficiently close in unity.

CONCENTRATION OF A GAS IN SOLUTION

The concentration of a gas in solution may be expressed in a variety of ways including :

1. The volume of gas which can be extracted from a unit of volume of solution under standard conditions (v/v)
2. The weight of dissolved gas per unit volume of solvent (w/v)
3. The molar concentration, i.e. the number of gram–molecules of gas per litre of solvent. The molar concentration is the most useful – equimolar solutions of gases of different molecular weights contain equal concentrations of molecules. This would not be so if their concentrations in terms of w/v were equal.

PHARMACOKINETICS OF INHALED ANAESTHETICS

Inhaled anaesthetics have a pharmacokinetic profile which results in ease in controlling the depth of anaesthesia as a result of rapid uptake and elimination: a knowledge of this profile can facilitate their use in clinical practice. They cannot be introduced into the brain without at the same time being distributed through the entire body, and this distribution exerts a controlling influence over the rate of the uptake or elimination of the anaesthetic by brain tissue. Although with some agents there may be some metabolism, all the gaseous and volatile substances used as anaesthetics may be regarded as essentially inert gases as far as uptake and elimination are concerned.

UPTAKE OF INHALED ANAESTHETICS

If some factors are reduced to their simplest possible terms, and certain assumptions are made, it is possible to give approximate predictions relating to inert gas exchange in the body (Bourne, 1964). These predictions are sufficiently realistic for practical purposes and serve to illustrate the main principles involved. Once these are understood more elaborate expositions found elsewhere (Eger, 1974, 1990; Mapleson, 1989) should become reasonably easy to follow.

For simplicity, the physiological variables such as cardiac output and tidal volume must be assumed to be unaffected by the presence of the gas, and to remain uniform throughout the administration. Allowance cannot be made for alterations in the tidal volume as administration proceeds. The blood supply to the grey matter of the brain must be assumed to be uniform and the gas to be evenly distributed throughout the grey matter. Finally, although in practice anaesthetics are seldom administered in this way, the anaesthetic must be assumed to be given at a fixed inspired concentration, and, what is more, it must be assumed that no rebreathing of gases occurs.

The tensions of the gas in the alveolar blood and tissues all tend to move towards inspired tension (Kety, 1951) but a number of processes, each of which proceeds at its own rate, intervene to delay

the eventual saturation of the tissues. The tension of the gas in the brain follows, with a slight delay, its tension in the alveolar air. Since both the rate of induction and recovery from inhalation anaesthesia are governed by the rate of change of the tension of the anaesthetic in the brain, and this in turn is governed by the rate of change of tension in the alveoli, the factors which determine the anaesthetic tension in the alveoli are obviously of very great importance.

The rate at which the tension of an anaesthetic in the alveolar air approaches its tension in the inspired air depends on the pulmonary ventilation, the uptake of the anaesthetic by the blood and tissues and the inspired concentration. First, by means of pulmonary ventilation the gas is inhaled, diluted with functional residual air, and enters the alveoli. This is where diffusion occurs and normally the alveolar gas equilibrates almost immediately with the pulmonary blood which is then distributed throughout the body. A second diffusion process occurs across the capillary membranes of the tissues into the interstitial fluid and from there through the cell membranes into the cells themselves. Venous blood leaving the tissues is in equilibrium with the tissue tension. The blood from the tissues returns to the lungs, still carrying some of its original content of anaesthetic, and is again equilibrated with alveolar gas which now

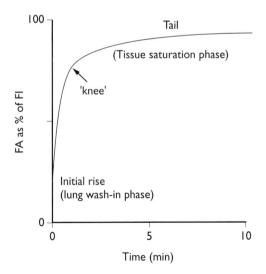

FIG. 3.2 Typical alveolar tension curve for an inert gas inhaled at a fixed concentration from a non-rebreathing system.

contains a slightly higher tension of the anaesthetic. It is in this manner that the alveolar (or arterial) and venous (or tissue) tensions of the anaesthetic in question gradually, and in that order, rise towards eventual equilibrium with the inspired tension.

As this complex process proceeds, the tension of the anaesthetic in the alveolar air increases continuously, but not at a uniform rate. Plotted against time, alveolar tension rises in a curve that is, in general, the same for every inert gas (Fig. 3.2). This curve tails off and slopes gradually upwards until, after several hours or even days, depending on the anaesthetic in question, complete equilibrium is reached. The steep initial rise represents movement of anaesthetic into the lungs, i.e. the pulmonary *wash-in* phase. The slowly rising tail represents more gradual tissue saturation. The change from steep part of the curve to the tail marks the point at which lung wash-in gives place to tissue saturation as the most important influence. The tail can be very long if the anaesthetic in question has a very high fat/blood partition coefficient.

BLOOD SOLUBILITY AND ALVEOLAR TENSION

The shape of curve obtained with any given anaesthetic depends on a number of factors. These include such things as minute volume of respiration; the functional residual capacity of the lungs; the cardiac output and the blood flow to the main anaesthetic absorbing bulk of the body – muscles and fat. However, one physical property of the anaesthetic itself is considerably more important than all of these factors – the solubility of the anaesthetic in the blood. This is the factor which determines the height of the 'knee' in the alveolar uptake curve. With anaesthetics of low blood solubility the knee is high; with high solubility the knee is low. This may be illustrated by consideration of the hypothetical extremes of solubility.

A totally insoluble gas would not diffuse into the pulmonary blood and would not be carried in it away from the lungs. If such a gas were inhaled at a constant inspired tension in a non-rebreathing system, its alveolar tension would increase exponentially as lung washout proceeded until, after a

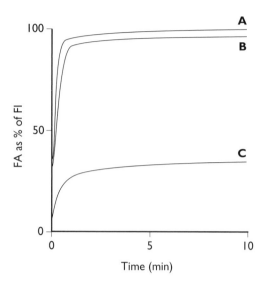

FIG. 3.3 Alveolar tension curves for a totally insoluble gas, **A** of low solubility, **B** (nitrous oxide) and a gas of extremely high solubility, **C** all breathed at a constant inspired concentration from a non-rebreathing system.

very short time, alveolar tension equalled inspired tension (Fig. 3.3). The curve obtained would be all initial rise and there would be no tail. Such a gas could not ever be an anaesthetic, since none would ever reach the brain.

A gas of extremely low blood solubility (Fig. 3.3, curve B) would give an almost identical curve. The loss into the pulmonary blood stream of only a minute amount of the gas contained in the lungs at any moment would bring the tension of the gas in the blood into equilibrium with that in the alveolar air. The capacity of the blood for such a gas would be extremely small. Likewise, the capacity of the entire body tissue (with the possible exception of fat) would be small, since as already pointed out, the tissue–blood partition coefficients of most anaesthetics are close to unity. If such an agent, even when given at the highest permissible concentration of 80% with 20% of oxygen only produced a faint depression of the central nervous system, it could nevertheless be looked upon as a very active agent because it would be deriving its effect through the presence in the brain of only a minute trace.

At the other hypothetical extreme would be a gas of very nearly infinite solubility in blood. All but a very small fraction of the gas in the lungs at

TABLE 3.1 Partition coefficients of some inhalation anaesthesics at 37 °C					
Partition coefficient	**Desflurane**	**Isoflurane**	**Sevoflurane**	**Enflurane**	**Halothane**
Blood–gas	0.42	1.40	0.60	2.00	1.94
Tissue–blood:					
Brain	1.29	1.57	1.70	2.70	1.94
Heart	1.29	1.61	1.78	1.15	1.84
Liver	1.31	1.75	1.85	3.70	2.07
Muscle	1.02	1.92	3.13	2.20	3.38
Fat	27.20	44.90	47.59	83.00	51.10

any one moment would dissolve in the pulmonary blood as soon as the blood arrived at the alveoli. The capacity of the blood and body tissues for such a gas would be vast. The alveoli tension curve (Fig. 3.3, C) would be very flat, with virtually no rapid initial rise and a very slowly rising tail. Given enough time for full equilibrium, it might be possible to achieve very deep anaesthesia by using a minute inspired tension but of course, in one sense the gas would be a very weak anaesthetic, since its concentration in the brain would be enormous.

Ranging between these hypothetical extremes of solubility are the gaseous and volatile anaesthetics. Their solubilities in blood and tissues for man and some animals (figures taken from various sources but mainly from data sheets) are shown in Table 3.1. The effect of the different solubilities on the alveolar tension when the agents are administered at a constant inspired tension are shown in Fig. 3.4.

THE TENSION OF ANAESTHETIC AGENTS IN BRAIN TISSUE

In addition to the alveolar tensions, the anaesthetist is also concerned with the tension of anaesthetic agents in the grey matter of the brain. In the lungs (unless pathological changes are present) diffusion from the alveolar air to the blood is almost instantaneous, so that for theoretical purposes the tension in the arterial blood leaving the lungs can be regarded as equal to the tension in the alveolar air. Only when the body has become absolutely saturated does the arterial tension equal the tissue tension. During the saturation process, and after the administration is stopped, the tissue tension is accurately represented by the tension of the agent in the venous blood leaving that tissue. This lags behind the arterial tension by an amount which depends mainly upon the blood supply to the tissue. Fatty tissues are exceptions to this rule, for in them the relative solubilities play an important part. In organs with a rich blood supply such as the brain and heart, the venous tension rises quite quickly to the arterial tension. After about 20 minutes (in man) with anaesthetics whose solubility in grey matter is about equal to that in blood, or perhaps 40 minutes in the case of agents like halothane which are a little more soluble in grey matter, arterial and grey matter tensions, during uptake and during elimination, are almost equal (Fig. 3.3).

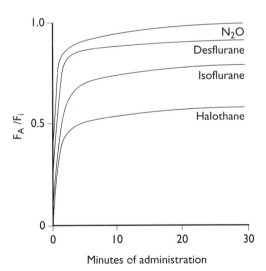

FIG.3.4 Increase in alveolar tension (FA) towards inspired tension (FI) during administration at a fixed concentration in a non-rebreathing system. Effect of blood solubility. The curves are not drawn accurately and only represent approximate, relative curves.

It follows from these considerations that if a gas has a low blood solubility, any change in its tension in the alveolar air is quickly reflected in the grey matter in the brain, whereas if the blood solubility is high there will be a considerable delay because the whole body will act as a very large buffer. Thus, with an inhalation anaesthetic, the speed with which induction of anaesthesia can be carried out (when the inspired tension is kept constant) is governed by the solubility of the anaesthetic in the blood. Low solubility (e.g. desflurane) favours rapid induction, whereas high blood solubility (methoxyflurane) leads to slow induction. The important point to note here is, of course, that so far all arguments have been based on the assumption that the inspired concentration is maintained constant. In fact, alteration of the inspired tension can do much to overcome the slow induction with agents of high blood solubility. For example, if in animals methoxyflurane were given at concentrations which would give satisfactory anaesthesia afer full equilibration, induction might take many hours. It would be a very long time before the animal even lost consciousness. The difficulty is, of course in practice, overcome by starting the administration not with this concentration, but with one which is much higher and which would, if administered indefinitely, kill the animal. As the desired level of anaesthesia is reached the inspired concentration is gradually reduced. Even so, induction with a very soluble agent such as methoxyflurane is slow.

It is in fact standard practice to hasten induction of anaesthesia in this way. However, the maximum concentration which can be administered is limited by the volatility of the anaesthetic, and its pungency. Many anaesthetics are so pungent or irritant that they cannot be inhaled in high concentrations.

RECOVERY FROM ANAESTHESIA

When the administration of the anaesthetic is terminated, its concentration in the inspired air cannot be reduced (*wash-out* phase) to below zero. Although the full buffering effect of the body tissues will not be seen after accelerated inductions and brief administration (those tissues with a poor blood supply or high tissue–blood partition coefficient will then be only very incompletely saturated), elimination of the more soluble anaesthetics will take time and recovery will be slow. Low blood solubility leads to rapid elimination of anaesthetics like desflurane and rapid recovery from anaesthesia.

At the end of anaesthesia the volume of nitrous oxide eliminated causes the minute volume of expiration to exceed the inspired volume and this outpouring of nitrous oxide dilutes the alveolar content of oxygen. If the animal is breathing room air, the alveolar oxygen tension can fall to low levels, resulting in a severe reduction in PaO_2. This phenomenon, called '*diffusion hypoxia*' can also happen if nitrous oxide is cut off during anaesthesia. Theoretically, it can happen with any agent, but it is unlikely to have any ill effects with very soluble agents such as methoxyflurane, because of the small volumes involved and the slow excretion of the agent. The danger is greatest if two insoluble agents (e.g. nitrous oxide and desflurane) are administered together.

SPEED OF UPTAKE AND ELIMINATION RELATED TO SAFETY OF INHALATION AGENTS

Blood solubility is not only important as a factor influencing the speed of induction and recovery. It has wider implications; it determines (in an inverse manner) the extent to which tissue tensions keep pace with alterations in inspired tension and thus it controls the rate at which anaesthesia can be deepened or lightened. With a very soluble agent such as diethyl ether or methoxyflurane no sudden change in tissue tension is possible; if gross overdosage is given the anaesthetist has plenty of time in which to observe the signs of deepening unconsciousness and to reduce the strength of the inhaled mixture. With an anaesthetic of low blood solubility such as desflurane, however, increase in tissue tension follows very quickly after an increase in the inspired tension; anaesthesia may deepen rapidly and a gross overdose may result. It is, therefore, very important with the less soluble anaesthetics to consider carefully the factors that favour the giving of an overdose, the chief of which must be volatility and potency.

Volatility

Volatility governs the potential strength of the inspired mixture for obviously the more volatile the anaesthetic the greater the risk of its being administered at a high concentration. Gaseous anaesthetics and liquid anaesthetics which have low boiling points are, therefore, potentially dangerous. Because gases are passed through flowmeters the danger is, in their case, rather less, since the anaesthetist has an accuracy of control only possible with volatile liquids by the use of special, often expensive vaporizers.

Potency

Potency determines the magnitude of a possible overdose. With a weak anaesthetic such as nitrous oxide overdose is imposssible; if it were not for lack of oxygen, nitrous oxide could be given at 100% concentration without danger. However, a concentration of 80% of an agent which was fully effective when given at a concentration of say 5% would constitute gross overdosage. This is, of course, self-evident, but as has been pointed out by Bourne (1964), anaesthetists have in the past paid insufficient attention to the precise meaning and measurement of potency, so that there is much confusion. An acceptable definition of potency would do much to clarify thought relating to safety of inhalation anaesthetics.

UPTAKE AND ELIMINATION OF INHALATION ANAESTHETICS IN CLINICAL PRACTICE

The various assumptions made for the purpose of theoretical or mathematical predictions of inhalational anaesthetic uptake and elimination cannot be made in everyday practice. Many of the factors which have to be regarded as constant if any mathematical prediction is to be made, do, in fact, vary considerably during the course of anaesthesia. These factors include the tidal volume; the physiological dead-space; the functional residual capacity (FRC – that volume of gas in the lungs which dilutes each single breath of anaesthetic); the thickness and permeability of the alveolar–capillary membrane; the cardiac output and pulmonary blood flow (which may be different, especially in pathological conditions of the lungs); regional variations in ventilation/perfusion relationships in the lungs; the blood flow through the tissues of the body; the partition coefficients of the anaesthetic between the gaseous or vapour state and lung tissue or blood, and between blood and the body tissues; and the blood flow diffusion coefficient and diffusion distance for each of the tissues of the body.

In addition the anaesthetics themselves may modify many of the variables as administration proceeds. For example, most anaesthetics depress breathing and reduce the cardiac output. Considerations such as these indicate only too clearly why it is not yet possible to give a complete account of the uptake and elimination of inhalation anaesthetics as encountered in clinical practice.

OTHER FACTORS AFFECTING INHALATION ANAESTHETIC ADMINISTRATION

(1)   The vaporizer

The output or concentration delivered from a vaporizer can be calculated but they are usually calibrated manually by the manufacturer. Modern vaporizers are capable of delivering very accurate concentrations but there are several factors that can influence the concentration of a volatile agent in the gas mixture leaving the vaporizer (Fig. 3.5). Older vaporizers were inaccurate at low gas flow rates but most are, today, stable for flows of 100 ml to 5000 ml/min. The vapour pressure of the volatile anaesthetic in the vaporizing chamber is temperature dependent and most modern vaporizers have temperature compensating mechanisms to correct for this so that output is constant for a wide temperature range.

Vaporizers are usually calibrated for a specific carrier gas (mostly air or oxygen). When switching from pure oxygen as the carrier gas to a mixture of nitrous oxide and oxygen, some nitrous oxide dissolves in the volatile liquid anaesthetic in the vaporizing chamber and thus the total amount of gas leaving the chamber decreases, causing an overall decrease in the concentration of the volatile agent. When nitrous oxide is switched off, the dissolved nitrous oxide evaporates from the liquid

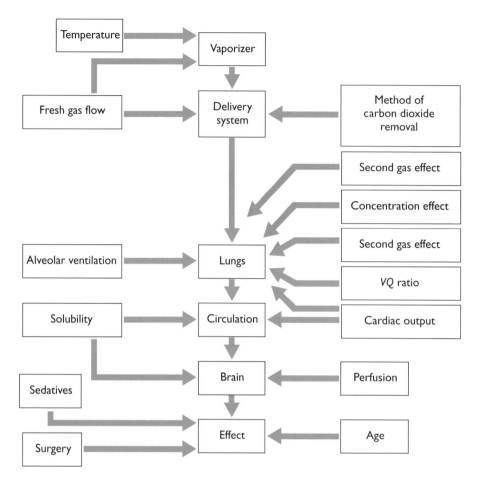

FIG. 3.5 The concentration cascade between the vaporizer and the brain tissue and some factors which influence it.

volatile anaesthetic agent, resulting in an increased flow through the vaporizing chamber and, therefore, an increase in the delivered concentration. This effect can lead to an error of 20–30% depending on the fresh gas flow (Lin, 1980).

(2) The breathing system

The fresh gas that flows into the breathing system (circuit) is diluted by the expired alveolar gas, causing a difference between the concentration of the inflowing gas and the concentration which is actually inspired. The lower the fresh gas flow rates the greater this difference becomes. Absorption by tubing and any absorbent used to remove carbon dioxide, as well as high anaesthetic uptake by the animal, may also increase this difference. At the beginning of anaesthesia soda lime behaves like a 'molecular sieve' with saturable characteristics. Later a quasi-steady state occurs and anaesthetic agents dissove in accordance with their partial pressure. Wet soda lime absorbs much less of volatile anaesthetics than when it is dry because the 'molecular sieve' is occupied by water. A variable amount of the anaesthetic may be absorbed in the tubing of the breathing system. There is a large difference between materials and polycarbon is more inert in this respect than teflon.

In a circle system the fresh gas utilization will vary widely depending on the arrangement of the system components. An arrangement with the spill-off valve between the fresh gas inlet and the lungs will result in a lower fresh gas utilization. Better characteristics with greater utilization are found where the spill-off valve closes during inspiration and is as close to the lungs as possible.

(3)   The lungs

Depending on how much fresh gas reaches the lungs and how much anaesthetic is carried away in the arterialized blood there will be a variable concentration difference between the inspired and arterial concentrations of the anaesthetic. The inspired concentration of the agent is the easiest parameter to be changed by the anaesthetist in order to influence the uptake and elimination of the anaesthetic.

With higher alveolar ventilation there is a more rapid increase in the alveolar uptake curve. During spontaneous ventilation, the animal is to some extent protected against overdosage because volatile anaesthetics depress ventilation and consequently, due to negative feed back, the speed of uptake is reduced. The relative ventilatory depressant effects of some inhaled agents are: nitrous oxide < halothane (Bahlman *et al.*, 1972) < isoflurane (Fourcade *et al.*, 1971) < enflurane (Calverley *et al.*, 1978).

During spontaneous ventilation the alveolar tension of halothane or isoflurane cannot increase to more than 23 mmHg regardless of the inspired concentration because of the resultant ventilatory depression (Munson *et al.*, 1973).

Nitrous oxide, because it can be given in high concentration, increases alveolar ventilation and thus its own uptake via the *concentration effect*, in particular when the animal is hypoventilated and highly soluble agents are used (Eger, 1963). For example, if halothane is used in low concentrations, its uptake is increased as well (*second gas effect*) due to the additional inspiratory inflow by the concentration effect of the nitrous oxide (Epstein *et al.*, 1964).

(4)   Cardiac output

Cardiac output is another major determinant of inhaled anaesthetic uptake. The higher the cardiac output the more anaesthetic agent is removed from the alveolar gas and the slower is the rise in alveolar concentration. The volatile anaesthetic agents all depress cardiac output and while with spontaneous ventilation a protective negative feed back exists with respect to high concentrations, the reverse is true for the circulation because due to

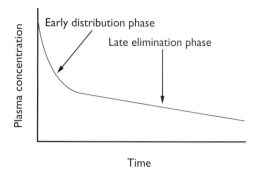

FIG. 3.6 Plasma concentration versus time relationship following rapid intravenous administration of a drug such as propofol, illustrating the rapid decline in plasma drug concentration during the early distributional (α) phase and the much slower decline in the terminal (β) elimination phase.

the depressed circulation less of the agent is removed from the alveoli so that alveolar concentration rises more rapidly.

PHARMACOKINETICS OF INTRAVENOUS ANAESTHETICS

The pharmacokinetics of the intravenous agents, i.e. the processes by which drug concentrations at effector sites are achieved, maintained and diminished after intravenous injection, is of increasing importance today because of the use of computer models to study drug uptake and elimination, and the use of microprocessors to control anaesthetic administration. For a more detailed account of their pharmacokinetics than follows here reference should be made to standard textbooks of pharmacology (e.g. Dean, 1987; Pratt & Taylor, 1990).

Pharmacokinetic variables commonly reported for intravenous or otherwise parenterally administered drugs are total apparent volume of distribution, total elimination clearance, and elimination half-life.

TOTAL APPARENT VOLUME OF DISTRIBUTION

The total apparent volume of distribution (V_d) relates the amount of drug in the body to the plasma or blood concentration:

$$V_d = \text{amount of drug/drug concentration.}$$

A frequently reported total volume of distribution is the volume of distribution at steady state, V_{dss}, the total apparent volume a drug would have if it were in equilibrium with all body tissues. Another commonly reported, and usually larger, total volume of distribution is $V_{d\beta}$ which, together with elimination clearance (Cl_E), determines the elimination half-life.

In theory, a volume of distribution is measured by injecting a known quantity of the drug and, after allowing an adequate period of time for it to distribute, determining its concentration (both free and combined) in the plasma . In practice the equilibrium necessary is seldom attained because before it is complete the opposing processes of metabolism or excretion come into operation.

A knowledge of the apparent volume of distribution makes it possible to calculate the doses to be administered initially and subsequently to achieve desired concentrations in the blood and tissues.

TOTAL ELIMINATION CLEARANCE (Cl_E) AND ELIMINATION HALF-LIFE ($t_{1/2\beta}$)

Cl_E is an independent variable relating the rate of irreversible drug removal from the body to the plasma or blood concentration:

$$Cl_E = \text{rate of elimination} / \text{drug concentration}$$

Thus, Cl_E is the sum of the elimination clearances of all the organs and tissues of the body, principally the liver and the kidneys. The elimination half-life, $t_{1/2\beta}$, is a dependent variable and is the time required for the amount of drug in the body to decrease by one-half:

$$t_{1/2\beta} = \ln 2 \times V_{d\beta} / Cl_E$$
$$\text{or, } t_{1/2\beta} = 0.693 \times V_{d\beta} / Cl_E.$$

These pharmacokinetic variables can be useful for drugs with a rapid onset of action, such as intravenously administered propofol, but they do not provide a complete description of their pharmacokinetics. The total volume of distribution is not realized until after extensive drug distribution and redistribution has occurred. Thus, predicted early drug concentrations based on the dose and V_{dss} will be very low. Although elimination clearance begins from the time the drug arrives at the clearing organs, the relatively slow decline in drug concentrations due to elimination clearance becomes a significant factor in the relationship of plasma (or blood) concentration with time only after the inital rapid decline due to the distribution and redistribution phase is over (Fig. 3.6).

It is now appreciated that the offset of clinical effect is not simply a function of half-life. It may be affected by the rate of equilibration between plasma and effector site and duration of infusion. Hughes *et al.* (1992) proposed the use of context-sensitive half-time ($t_{1/2 \text{ context}}$) and defined this as the time for the plasma conentration to decrease by 50% after termination of an i.v. infusion designed to maintain a constant plasma concentration. Context refers to the duration of infusion. They demonstrated that context-sensitive half-lines of commonly used i.v. anaesthetic agents and opioids could differ markedly from elimination half-lives and were dependent on duration of infusion.

COMPARTMENTAL MODELS

Drugs injected into a vein are distributed directly in the blood stream to the brain and the other tissues of the body. Those given by the alimentary route (by mouth or high into the rectum) must first be absorbed into the blood and they then pass through the liver before reaching the central nervous system. Passage through the liver (the *'first pass'*) is avoided if the drugs are given via the mucous membranes of the nose, the terminal rectum, or sublingually, so that administration of suitable drugs by these routes renders the effective dose similar to that needed by the intravenous route. Elimination of these drugs from the body is not a reversal of the process of absorption; they are broken down, mostly in the liver, and are then excreted mainly by the kidneys.

When a drug is administered by intravenous injection the onset and duration of its effect depend on the distribution to the tissues, tissue binding and access to those tissues where the pharmacological effect takes place, interaction with receptor sites, and elimination by various routes (Fig. 3.1). Since the body is composed of innumerable tissue zones, each with a unique blend of perfusion, binding affinity, etc. for the drug, quantification of the whole process is nearly impossible unless some gross simplifications can be made. For any particular drug the body can be thought of as comprising one or more *compartments*, each of which can be considered as a space throughout which the substance is uniformly distributed and has uniform kinetics of distribution or transport (Sheppard, 1948).

Secondary dispersion of highly lipid-soluble drugs such as the intravenous anasthetic agents occurs as they cross cell membranes and the limiting factor to this process is the rate at which they are delivered to the cells – the blood flow to the tissues. Thus, organs with a rapid blood flow (e.g. brain, heart, liver, kidney) initially receive a high concentration of the drug but, with time, this is depleted as the agent redistributes into moderately and slowly perfused tissues (the muscles and fat, respectively). The greater the lipid solubility of the drug the more rapid its redistribution but even charged drugs can be redistributed. Redistribution also means that repeated doses of the drug can exert prolonged effects due to the gradual passage over an extended period from saturated sites where it is inactive, back into the plasma. Plasma and the organs where blood flow is rapid can be taken to represent one 'compartment', while moderately and poorly perfused tissues represent second and third compartments.

The one compartment model

When drugs behave as if they were distributed into a single uniform compartment excretion takes place according to *'first order'* kinetics, i.e. in any time period a constant proportion of the remaining drug will be eliminated; the elimination rate is proportional to the concentration. When a drug concentration decreases in this constant proportion manner, the concentration curve can be defined by a simple exponential equation:

$$C/C^0 = e^{-kt}$$

where C = drug concentration at time t; C^0 = drug concentration at time 0 (i.e. immediately after i.v. administration); k = a constant; t = time elapsed; and e = the base of the natural logarithm (2.718).

Taking the natural logarithm of both sides of the equation, a linear equation results :

$$\ln (C/C^0) = -kt \text{ or } \ln (C/C^0)/t = -k.$$

Thus, the natural logarithm of the proportion by which C has decreased to time is a constant (k)

which has the dimension of rate and will be stated in reciprocal units (t^{-1}). From this it follows that a graph of $\ln(C/C^0)$ against time will yield a straight line, of gradient –k. In practice, very few drugs behave according to one compartment kinetics, since some initial redistribution from the circulation to other tissues is almost inevitable. The majority of drugs can be regarded as obeying what are known as *zero order* or *first order kinetics*.

A *zero order process* is one which occurs at a constant rate and is, therefore, independent of the quantity of drug present at the particular sites of absorption or removal. A zero order process requires a large excess of drug available on the entry side (e.g. intravenous infusion) or, on the removal side, a system of limited capacity.

A *first order process* is considered to be the most common for both drug absorption and elimination. In a first order process the rate of the reaction is exponentially related to the amount of drug available. In other words, a constant *fraction* of the drug is absorbed or eliminated in constant time. The rate constants (k_{ab} and k_{el}) are measurements of these fractions since they represent the fraction of the drug present which is absorbed or eliminated in unit time (usually in 1 minute or 1 hour).

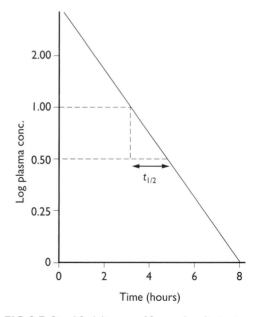

FIG. 3.7 Simplified diagram of first order elimination from the plasma of an intravenous drug. The plot of log plasma concentration versus time is linear.

A very simplified example of a first order elimination is shown in Fig. 3.7 where the natural logarithm (ln) of the plasma concentration of a drug given by a single intravenous injection is plotted against time. Under these conditions a plot of ln plasma concentration versus time is linear. The time taken for the plasma concentration to halve ($t_{1/2}$) is known as the plasma half-life. V_d can be calculated for the initial concentration (i.e. that at zero time) and from this, by assuming V_d to be constant over the whole time period (which, in practice, it seldom is), the clearance from the plasma can be calculated. A more accurate method assumes (usually incorrectly) that the clearance from the plasma is a constant fraction of the instantaneous level, thus:

$$\text{Plasma clearance } (C_1) = \frac{\text{Original dose}}{\text{Area under curve to complete elimination.}}$$

The area under the curve (AUC) is obtained from a graph of the actual (not log concentration) against time. A drug with a high C_1 will have a lower AUC than one with a lower C_1 given at the same dose. A drug given to an animal with a reduced C_1 resulting from disease will have a higher AUC than the same drug administered to an animal with a normal C_1. It follows from this that the diseased animal will be exposed to a higher drug concentration for a longer period of time and greater and more persistent drug effects can be produced unless the dose of the drug is reduced.

What is known as 'the plateau principle' applies when a drug undergoes zero order absorption and first order elimination. Under these conditions it can be shown that when the concentration of the drug being administered is changed, the time taken to reach a steady state (plateau) level is determined solely by the reciprocal of k_{el}. The height of the plateau reached depends on the concentration of the drug administered and when this height is attained the amount of drug given is reduced to maintain it. Similar principles apply when a loading dose is followed by subsequent doses to maintain this level (Fig. 3.8). About 97% of a drug will be eliminated from the plasma in about $5 \times t_{1/2}$ (i.e. 50% + 25% + 12.5% + 6.25% + 3.125%).

The two compartment model

Frequently, the serial plasma concentrations after the intravenous administration of a drug show an initial rapid decay (the α phase), followed by a linear decline (the β phase) when plotted on the same semi-logarithmic axes. The curve of best fit is a biexponential decay, which is characteristic of drug concentration in the central compartment (V_1) of a two compartment system where the drug is assumed to enter V_1, from which it is also elim-

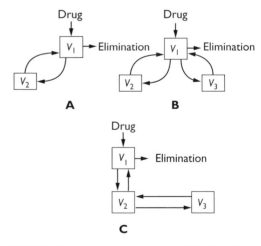

FIG. 3.9 **A** Two compartment model. **B** Mamillary three compartment model. **C** Catenary three compartment model. In the mamillary three compartment model both V_2 and V_3 exchange with V_1, whereas in the catenary model V_3 is 'deep' to V_2 and is not connected in any way to V_1. This catenary model has been proposed for some drug metabolites and has characteristics of its own.

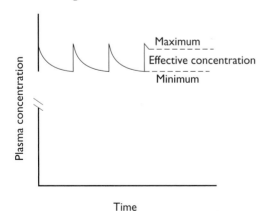

FIG. 3.8 Intermittent intravenous dosage to maintain an effective anaesthetic concentration. Single compartment model.

inated. A second peripheral compartment (V_2) receives drug by redistribution from V_1 but elimination of the drug does *not* take place except by transfer back to V_1 (Fig. 3.9).

In the two compartment model the half-life is expressed as $t_{1/2\beta}$ which makes it clear that it is limited to the β (elimination) phase of the decay, but it depends on both elimination and distribution rates so that it cannot be regarded as a direct indicator of elimination rate.

The multi-compartment model

A three compartment model has been used to explain a curve of declining drug concentration which does not fit in a conveniently bi-exponential fashion and better fits a three-exponential equation. However, great care must be exercised when expanding the number of terms, since the 'degrees of freedom' in the regression equations are progressively reduced, thus widening the confidence interval for the line. In other words, although a more complex curve may fit measured concentration points better, the *probability* of it being correct diminishes. There are two types of three compartment models. In one, the 'mamillary' model, both peripheral compartments (V_2 and V_3) connect to the central compartment (V_1). For some drug metabolites a different, 'catenary', model has been proposed where V_3 is 'deep' to V_2, but is not connected to V_1 and has quite different characteristics.

Rarely can a plasma decay curve be defined so precisely as to permit justification of more than three exponential terms. Moreover, the compartments cannot be equated with true anatomical volumes. The use of 'perfusion models' overcomes many difficulties to some extent, but these require much more information. The perfusion model takes a number of anatomically defined compartments and, by consideration of their volumes, blood flow rates through them and tissue/blood partition coefficients computes the movement of drug between them. Although the distribution of cardiac output in the anaesthetized horse (Staddon *et al.*, 1979) and the solubility of halothane in equine tissues have been studied (Webb & Weaver, 1981) there is little other relevant information in the veterinary literature. Moreover, the tissue/blood partition coefficients vary widely

because of the wide range of solubilities in the various tissues. Thus, the perfusion model is limited by the number of identifiable tissues or organs for which reliable data are available.

PRACTICAL METHODS OF DRUG DELIVERY DURING INTRAVENOUS ANAESTHESIA

It is now generally agreed that it is possible to improve the titration of intravenous drugs by administering continuous variable rate infusions rather than by injecting intermittent bolus doses. Continuous infusion is the logical extension of the more traditional incremental bolus dose method which inevitably leads to fluctuations in blood (and hence brain) concentrations that follow each bolus dose (Fig. 3.8). To achieve an effective blood concentration rapidly, it is necessary to administer a 'loading dose', just as with inhalation anaesthesia it is usually necessary to start with a high inspired concentration. Similarly, as with the inhalation anaesthetics, it is necessary to reduce the dose administered to maintain this effective concentration.

In practice, intravenous infusions are generally titrated on an empirical basis depending on the response of the animal to the infusion rate. However, the aim for the future is to predict the dosage requirements from pharmacokinetic data. The smaller the loading dose, the greater the initial maintenance infusion rate needed because the amount of drug infused must be equal to that which is removed from the brain by both distribution and elimination processes. With time, distribution assumes less importance, and the infusion rate required to maintain any given blood concentration becomes solely dependent on the elimination rate. Thus, the infusion rate needed to maintain a given concentration in the body decreases as a function of the infusion period. Considerations of this nature have led to the establishment of two or three stages in computer controlled infusion regimens following a loading dose or inital high infusion rate.

Ideally, the anaesthetist would like to know the concentration of the anaesthetic agent attained and maintained at its site of effect (i.e. the brain) but, as may be guessed from the above considerations, this is rarely possible. All that can be said is that

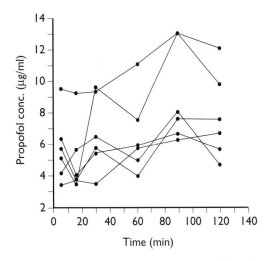

FIG. 3.10 Blood propofol concentrations (μg/ml) in 6 dogs (beagles) after an induction dose of 7 mg/kg followed by an infusion of 0.4 mg/kg/min, illustrating the tendency of blood concentrations to rise when the infusion rate is kept constant throughout 120 minutes of anaesthesia.

the plasma or blood drug concentration is *often* related to, and is a valid measure of, the required quantity so that $t_{1/2}$ is, usually, the paramount determinant of dose frequency when intermittent administration is practised. The main difficulties in devising suitable computer controlled infusion regimens for the induction and maintenance of intravenous anaesthesia arise from the variable response of individual subjects (Fig. 3.10). The future of computer-controlled infusions for administering intravenous anaesthetics will depend on their safety, reliability, cost-effectiveness and 'user friendliness'.

The clinical anaesthetist may be forgiven for feeling that the sources of variation are so legion that in the case of many drugs used in anaesthetic practice it is better to titrate dose against response rather than attempt to predict the correct dose on theoretical grounds. This is a somewhat regressive pharmacologic approach to the administration of intravenous agents but, at the moment, it certainly offers a simpler model for everyday use. Even using this approach, a clear understanding of the ways in which the animal's 'drug model' may be modified by physiological or pathological changes makes it possible to anticipate variations in drug requirements and, therefore, titrate with greater skill and delicacy.

REFERENCES

Bahlman, S.H., Eger, E.I. II, Halsy, M.J., *et al.* (1972) The cardiovascular effects of halothane in man during spontaneous ventilation. *Anesthesiology* **36**(5): 494–502.

Bourne, J.G. (1964) Uptake , elimination and potency of the inhalational anaesthetics. *Anaesthesia* **19**: 12–32.

Calverley, R.K., Smith, N.T., Jones, C.W., Prys-Roberts, C. and Eger, E.I. II (1978) Ventilatory and cardiovascular effects of enflurane anesthesia during spontaneous ventilation in man. *Anesthesia and Analgesia*, **54**(6), 610–618.

Dean, P.M. (1987) *Molecular Foundations of Drug Receptor Interaction.* Cambridge: Cambridge University Press.

Eger, E.I. II (1963) Effect of inspired anesthetic concentration on the rate of rise of alveolar concentration. *Anesthesiology* **24**: 153–157.

Eger, E.I. II (1974) *Anesthetic Uptake and Action.* Baltimore : Williams and Wilkins.

Eger, E.I. II (1990) Uptake and distribution. In: Miller, R.D. (ed) *Anesthesia*, 3rd Ed New York: Churchill Livingstone, pp 85–104.

Epstein, R.M., Rackow, H., Salanitre, E. and Wolf, G.L. (1964) Influence of the concentration effect on the uptake of anesthetic mixtures: the second gas effect. *Anesthesiology* **25**: 364–371.

Fourcade, H.E., Stevens, W.C., Larson, C.P. *et al.* (1971) The ventilatory effects of forane, a new inhaled anesthetic. *Anesthesiology* **35**(1): 26–31.

Hughes, M.A., Glass, P.S.A. and Jacobs, J.R. (1992) Context-sensitive half-time in multicompartment pharmacokinetic models for intravenous anaesthetic drugs. *Anesthesiology* **76**(3): 334–341.

Kety, S.S. (1951) The theory and applications of the exchange of inert gas at the lungs and tissues. *Pharmacological Reviews (Baltimore)* **3**: 1–41.

Lin, C.Y. (1980) Assessment of vaporizer performance in low-flow and closed-circuit anesthesia. *Anesthesia and Analgesia* **59**: 359–366.

Mapleson, W.W. (1989) Pharmacokinetics of inhalational anaesthetics. In: Nunn, Utting and Brown (eds) *General Anaesthesia*, 5th edn. London: Nunn, Utting & Brown, pp. 44–59.

Munson, E.S., Eger, E.I. II and Bowers, D.L. (1973) Effects of anaesthetic-depressed ventilation and cardiac output on anesthetic uptake: a computer nonlinear simulation. *Anesthesiology* **38**(3): 251–259.

Pratt, W.B. and Taylor, P. (1990) *Principles of Drug Action: the Basis of Pharmacology*, 3rd edn. Edinburgh: Churchill-Livingstone.

Sheppard, C.W. (1948) The theory of the study of transfers within a multi-compartment system. *Journal of Applied Physics* **19**: 70–76.

Staddon, G.E., Weaver, B.M.Q. and Webb, A.I. (1979) Distribution of cardiac output in anaesthetized horses. *Research in Veterinary Science* **27**(1): 38–45.

Webb, A.I. and Weaver, B.M.Q. (1981) Solubility of halothane in equine tissues at 37 °C. *British Journal of Anaesthesia* **53**(5): 479–486.

Principles of sedation, analgesia and premedication

4

INTRODUCTION

There is considerable confusion concerning the terminology applied to sedative, tranquillizing and hypnotic drugs, and no single classification is completely satisfactory. However, the following definitions are commonly used and almost universally recognized:

- A *hypnotic* is a depressant of the central nervous system which enables the animal to go to sleep more easily, or a drug used to intensify the depth of sleep. They are rarely used in veterinary medicine because the state of sleep, from which the animal is easily aroused by minor stimulation such as noise, is seldom recognizable.

- A *sedative* is a drug which relieves anxiety and as a result tends to make it easier for the patient to rest or sleep – in fact they are usually associated with drowsiness. Many drugs fall into both the sedative and the hypnotic categories, the differentiation usually being related to dose. They are best considered as one group, exemplified by chloral hydrate or xylazine where low doses cause drowsiness and higher doses cause sleep.

- A *tranquillizer* (or *ataractic*) is a drug with a predominant action in relieving anxiety without producing undue sedation. They affect mood or behaviour but in recent years the terms have become unpopular (Tobin & Ballard, 1979) and indeed the classification of tranquillizers as 'major' and 'minor' suggested by the World Health Organization is now rarely used. Instead,

in pharmacological texts (Booth, 1988), classification is based on medical clinical uses of the drugs. Thus, three categories are recognized: *antianxiety* drugs (or *anxiolytics*), *antipsychotic* drugs and the classic *sedative/hypnotics*. Benzodiazepines are considered to be both anxiolytics and sedative/hypnotics. Drugs now classified as antipsychotic are those previously termed *neuroleptics*. They reduce psychomotor agitation, curiosity and apparent aggressiveness in animals, exerting their effects by blocking dopamine-mediated responses in the central nervous system. Overdose causes marked extrapyramidal symptoms and parkinsonian-type tremor (Lees, 1979, 1979a; Vickers *et al.*, 1984). Drugs of the butyrophenone and phenothiazine groups are now categorized as antipsychotics. The term 'tranquillizer' is still loosely used in clinical anaesthesia to cover both the anxiolytics and antipsychotics (Dundee & Wyant, 1989), and will continue to be used in places in this and later chapters.

The multiplicity of definitions is confusing and understanding of the major actions of the drugs is more important than being able to categorize them, for with this understanding it is possible to appreciate the limitations of the drugs in use. For example, if drugs such as the benzodiazepines are used for premedication they will not quieten the animal, but may make it more difficult to handle by removing its inhibitions, so that vicious animals become more likely to bite or kick, and even friendly animals may become uncontrollable. By reducing nervousness, phenothiazine derivatives may make an animal more liable to sleep, but will not make the vicious animal easier to handle, no matter what dose is given.

Effective sedation depends on the careful selection of the drug appropriate for the procedure, the species of animal, its temperament and condition, and must allow for possible side effects. Where sedation is to control an animal so that it may undergo surgery under local analgesia, comparatively high doses of drugs may be used, but where sedation fails to be adequate, resort may have to be made to drug combinations or to general anaesthesia. Where 'sedative' and 'tranquillizing' drugs are used for premedication, low doses are usually utilized and their effect on the subsequent depth and duration of anaesthesia must be taken into account. In all cases it is important that the animal is left undisturbed for an adequate period of time after administration of the sedative because stimulation during the onset of the drug's action may prevent the full effect from developing. To sedate an animal that is in pain a suitable analgesic must be used, possibly in combination with a sedative drug, because most sedative drugs themselves have little or no analgesic activity and may cause exaggerated reactions to painful stimulation.

During the past two decades major pharmacological advances have been made in the recognition of specific drug receptor sites and of the actions resulting from their stimulation or blockade. These advances have been followed by synthesis of potent drugs which act as agonists or as antagonists at such sites. Where receptors are involved in sedation and anaesthesia, these advances have included a better understanding of the actions of existing drugs, availability of newer and more potent agonist drugs, and of antagonists enabling the reversal of some sedative agent effects.

SEDATION

PHENOTHIAZINE DERIVATIVES

Drugs of this group are classified as antipsychotic drugs (or in older terminology 'neuroleptics'). All have a wide range of central and peripheral effects, but the degree of activity in different pharmacological actions varies from one compound to another. These actions and side effects have been well reviewed (Tobin & Ballard, 1979; Lees, 1979, 1979a).

Being dopamine antagonists, they have calming and mood-altering (antipsychotic?) effects, and also a powerful antiemetic action, particularly against opioid induced vomiting. The degree of sedation produced varies markedly between drugs. For many uses in medical practice sedation is an unwanted side effect, but in veterinary medicine the phenothiazine derivatives are used primarily for this purpose. In general, they do not have analgesic activity, although methotrimeprazine is claimed to be a powerful analgesic in man. Their major cardiovascular side effects are related to their ability to block α_1 adrenoceptors, and thus having an anti-adrenaline effect. This results in marked arterial hypotension primarily due to peripheral vasodilatation, and a decrease in packed cell volume caused by splenic dilatation. They exert an antiarrhythmic effect on the heart (Muir et al., 1975; Muir, 1981) which was originally thought to be due to a quinidine action on the cardiac membrane (Lees, 1979, 1979a), but has more recently been suggested as being caused by a blocking action on the cardiac α-arrhythmic receptors (Maze et al., 1985; Dresel, 1985). They have a spasmolytic action on the gut although, at least in horses, gut motility is not reduced (J. Davis, personal communication 1990). However, as they cause relaxation of the cardiac sphincter, in ruminants they increase the chance of regurgitation should an animal become recumbent. They have varying degrees of antihistamine activity and also produce a partial cholinergic block. All phenothiazine derivatives cause a fall in body temperature partly due to increased heat loss through dilated cutaneous vessels and partly through resetting of thermoregulatory mechanisms. In spite of all their side effects the phenothiazines are well tolerated by the majority of normovolaemic animals.

Although promethazine is used as an antihistamine, the most commonly used phenothiazine today in the UK, North America and Australasia is acepromazine, but other derivatives such as chlorpromazine, promazine and propiopromazine are used in some European and other countries.

Acepromazine

Acepromazine is the 2-acetyl derivative of promazine and has the chemical name 2–acetyl-10-(3-dimethylaminopropyl) phenothiazine; it is prepared as the maleate, a yellow crystalline solid. The drug has marked sedative properties, which are responsible for its popularity in veterinary medicine. Like all phenothiazine drugs, with low doses there are effects on behaviour, and as the dose is increased sedation occurs but the dose–response curve rapidly reaches a plateau after which higher doses do not increase, but only lengthen sedation, and increase side effects (Tobin & Ballard, 1979). Further increase in doses may cause excitement and extrapyramidal signs. In many animals sedation may be achieved with i.m. doses as low as 0.03 mg/kg although the drug has been used safely at ten times this dose when prolonged effects were required. A calming effect on the behaviour of excitable animals can be seen at doses even below 0.03 mg/kg, making acepromazine, particularly, a drug liable to abuse especially in the equine sporting field. The length of action is prolonged. Clinically obvious sedation lasts 4–6 hours after doses of 0.2 mg/kg, but in horses Parry and coworkers (1982) considered that there were detectable residual effects for 12 hours after doses of 0.1 mg/kg, and for 16–24 hours after 0.15 mg/kg i.m. Owners of giant breeds of dog often complain that their animals are sedated for several days following acepromazine administration, but scientific substantiation of these reports is not available.

In practice, the dose is chosen in relation to the length of sedation required and the purpose for which it is needed. However, the drug cannot be relied upon to give sedation in all animals; some individuals fail to become sedated and, in these, other drugs or drug combinations must be employed. Excitement reactions are rare but have been reported following i.v. (Tobin & Ballard, 1979) or i.m. injection of the drug (MacKenzie & Snow, 1977). Other central effects of acepromazine include hypothermia and a moderate antiemetic effect. Acepromazine is said to reduce the threshold at which epileptiform seizures occur but it is claimed that in man the phenothiazine derivatives have an anticonvulsant effect. It is difficult to reconcile these two statements but in veterinary medicine it seems to be generally agreed that acepromazine should be avoided in animals with a history of fits or which are in danger of convulsions for any reason (e.g. after myelography).

In all species of animal acepromazine causes a dose related fall in arterial blood pressure and this property has been particularly well documented in the horse (Kerr *et al.*, 1972a; Glen, 1973; Muir & Hamlin, 1975; Parry *et al.*, 1982). This property is thought to be mediated through vasodilatation brought about by peripheral α_1 adrenoceptor block. In most fit and healthy animals the lowering of blood pressure is well tolerated but in shocked or hypovolaemic animals a precipitous and even fatal fall in arterial pressure can occur. The effects of clinical dose rates of acepromazine on heart rate are generally minimal, most investigators having found a slight rise (MacKenzie & Snow, 1977; Kerr *et al.*, 1972a; Parry *et al.*, 1982) or no change (Muir *et al.*, 1979). However, Popovic *et al.* (1972) reported that in dogs doses of 0.1 mg/kg i.m. acepromazine caused bradycardia and even sinoatrial arrest, and atrioventricular block has been noted in horses (L.W. Hall, unpublished observations). These differences in reports could be due to the route of administration, dose (0.1 mg/kg is high compared with doses usually used in clinical practice), or individual animal sensitivity. Changes in cardiac output appear to be minimal (Maze *et al.*, 1985). Acepromazine has antiarrhythmic effects and protects against adrenaline induced fibrillation (Muir *et al.*, 1981) and this property must be an advantage when this drug is used for preanaesthetic medication.

Fainting and cardiovascular collapse has been reported to occur occasionally in all species of animal following the use of even low doses of acepromazine. In some cases it may have been due to administration to a hypovolaemic animal but in others it has not been explained. Some strains of Boxer dogs are renowned for collapsing after a very small dose of acepromazine given by any route, and it has been suggested that this may be due to orthostatic hypotension or to vasovagal syncope.

Clinical doses have little effect on respiration and although sedated animals may breathe more slowly the minute volume of respiration is usually unchanged (Muir *et al.*, 1975; Tobin & Ballard, 1979; Parry *et al.*, 1982).

Acepromazine has little antihistamine activity but has a powerful spasmolytic effect on smooth muscle including that of the gut. It is metabolized in the liver and both conjugated and non-conjugated metabolites are excreted in the urine. The drug causes paralysis of the retractor penis muscle and protrusion of the flaccid penis from the prepuce in bulls and stallions; it was often given to facilitate examination of the penis. In horses, however, physical damage to the dangling penis may result in swelling and failure of the organ to return within the prepuce when the drug action ceases. This event, which may eventually necessitate amputation of the penis, has been reported as occurring in horses following the use of several phenothiazine derivatives.

Priapism has been reported in stallions following the use of acepromazine as part of the neuroleptanalgesic mixture 'Large Animal Immobilon' (Pearson & Weaver, 1978). In most reports the stallion was being castrated but priapism has been encountered in other circumstances, for example immediately after induction of anaesthesia with an intravenous barbiturate in acepromazine premedicated horses (Lucke & Sanson, 1972). Current speculation is that priapism and flaccid protrusion of the penis is due to acepromazine blockade of central and peripheral adrenergic and dopaminergic receptors but the therapeutic administration of catecholamines and anticholinergics has found limited success. However, Wilson *et al.* (1991) have reported two cases of priapism in adult horses where detumescence followed the administration of 8 mg of benztropine mesylate (a drug used in the treatment of Parkinson disease) which is believed to be a central anticholinergic. It is of interest that Edwards and Clarke (unpublished observations) have encountered three cases of priapism in horses undergoing surgery for relief of colic which had *not* been given acepromazine.

As both priapism and flaccid paralysis with subsequent physical injury are equally calamitous in valuable breeding stallions the manufacturers specifically contraindicate the drug in these animals. Members attending a meeting of the Association of Veterinary Anaesthetists held in the UK discussed the use of acepromazine in some

detail and their conclusion was that, despite the possible side effects involving the equine penis, the drug remained a useful sedative in male horses. It was, however, recommended that only minimal doses of acepromazine should be administered, preferably by i.m. rather than i.v. injection, and in the event of priapism or prolonged prolapse of the flaccid penis, the condition ought to be treated quickly and efficiently (Jones, 1979). The penis must be supported to prevent or reduce swelling and the application of ice packs together with massage and manual compression may also be of help.

In the UK acepromazine is available as 2% and 10% solutions for injection, and for oral use in dogs and cats as tablets of 5 and 20 mg. The injectable forms are non-irritant and are effective by i.v., i.m. and s.c. routes. Following i.v. injection sedation is usually obvious within 5 minutes but in some cases the full effects may not be apparent for 20 minutes and when the drug is used for premedication by this route at least this period should be allowed to elapse before anaesthetic agents are given. Maximal effects are seen 30–45 minutes after i.m. and s.c. injection. It has been claimed that absorption from s.c. sites is poor and the fact that, at least in small animals, it works very well when given s.c., may indicate that even the minimum recommended doses are larger than necessary. Given by the oral route, absorption, and therefore its effects, are very variable and much higher doses need to be administered (e.g. 1–3 mg/kg in dogs and cats).

Very small doses have been used to treat behavioural problems in dogs and horses but the dose required in any individual case can only be found by trial and error. Its antiemetic properties make it a useful drug for the prevention of motion sickness in dogs and cats and its spasmolytic properties have led to its use in spasmodic colic in horses. It has been very widely used in all species of animal as a sedative and premedicant, as well as in combination with etorphine as 'Large Animal Immobilon'.

Parenteral doses of acepromazine for sedative and premedicant purposes in most domestic animals are in the range of 0.025 to 0.100 mg/kg, the lower doses being used by the i.v. route. Higher doses of up to 0.2 mg/kg may be used safely by i.m. injection. Recommended doses for specific purposes will be discussed in the chapters relating to the individual species of animal.

Propionylpromazine

Propionylpromazine, 10-(3-dimethyl amino-propyl)-2-propionylphenothiazine, has been widely used on the Continent of Europe and in Scandinavia for sedation and premedication of both small and large animal patients. Its actions, the sedation it produces and its side effects are very similar to those of acepromazine. In horses it is used in doses of 0.15–0.25 mg/kg and in dogs the dose ranges from 0.2–0.3 mg/kg. It has also been widely used in combination with methadone.

Chlorpromazine

This compound, 2-chloro-10-(3-dimethylamino-propyl) phenothiazine hydrochloride, was used extensively in veterinary practice but has largely been replaced by acepromazine and propionylpro-mazine. Its actions and side effects are similar to those of acepromazine, but it is less potent (doses of up to 1 mg/kg were used in all species of animal), has a longer duration of action and produces less sedation. It is particularly unreliable in horses, giving rise to what appears to be a state of panic due the muscle weakness it supposedly causes. It is still widely used in human medicine for its antipsychotic actions as in psychotic patients its weak sedative properties constitute a desirable feature.

Promazine

This is 10-(3-dimethylaminopropyl) phenothiazine hydrochloride and has actions similar to those of chlorpromazine but is claimed to give better sedation with fewer side effects. For premedication it was administered at doses of up to 1 mg/kg but it is seldom used today.

Methotrimeprazine

This is a typical phenothiazine but it is also a potent analgesic, having a potency about 0.7 times that of morphine. In veterinary practice in the UK it has been combined with etorphine as the neuroleptanalgesic mixture 'Small Animal Immobilon'.

Promethazine

This drug, 10-(2-dimethylaminopropyl) phenothiazine hydrochloride, was probably the first phenothiazine derivative to be used in veterinary anaesthesia. Solutions of this drug are irritant to the tissues and when used for premedication should be injected deeply in a large muscle mass 40–60 minutes before anaesthesia. In emergencies the drug can be given, after dilution with isotonic saline, by very slow i.v. injection. Rapid i.v. injection causes a profound fall in arterial blood pressure which may be fatal in shocked or hypovolaemic animals.

Promethazine is used in veterinary medicine primarily for its potent antihistamine activity; it is employed for premedication prior to the administration of anaesthetic drugs which cause histamine release.

BUTYROPHENONES

In man the butyrophenone group of compounds were classed as major tranquillizers (neuroleptics) but they can cause very unpleasant side effects, including hallucinations, mental agitation, and even feelings of aggression. These side effects are often not obvious to an observer and only become known when a human patient recovers from the drug and complains, often bitterly, about the experience. The incidence of these side effects is dose related and increases with increase of dose. Overdose results in dystonic reactions. We do not know whether the subjective effects produced in animals are similar to those known to occur in man, but the unpredictable aggressive behaviour shown by some animals when under the influence suggests they may be.

Cardiovascular and respiratory effects of the butyrophenones are minimal, although slight arterial hypotension may result from α adrenergic blockade. They are potent antiemetics, acting on the chemoemetic trigger zone to prevent drug-induced vomiting, such as may be caused by opioid analgesics. It is this latter property which makes the butyrophenones the drug of choice for the neuroleptic component of neuroleptanalgesia.

From experience of their use in man it seems doubtful whether the butyrophenones should ever be used on their own as tranquillizing agents, but in veterinary medicine they have been used in this way as well as in neuroleptanalgesic combinations. It may be that blocking of central dopaminergic and noradrenergic activity is responsible for their ability to suppress evidence of opioid-induced excitement.

Azaperone

Azaperone, 4'-fluoro-4 [4-(2 pyridyl)-1-piperazinyl] butyrophenone, is a drug licenced in the UK for use in pigs where its i.m. administration produces a good, dose-related sedative effect up to the maximum recommended dose for clinical use (4 mg/kg). Pigs may show excitement during the first 20 minutes following injection, particularly if disturbed during this period. Intravenous administration of this drug frequently results in a vigorous excitement phase.

Azaperone in clinical doses has minimal effects on respiration, such effect as there is being that of slight stimulation (Clarke, 1969). Clarke also reported a consistent small fall in arterial blood pressure following the i.m. injection of 0.3–3.5 mg/kg of the drug. The effect is presumably due to the α adrenergic block common to all butyrophenones. Reductions in cardiac output and heart rate in pigs were reported by MacKenzie and Snow (1977) to be clinically insignificant.

Azaperone is widely used both as a sedative and as a premedicant in pigs. In anaesthesia, given prior to the use of metomidate, it is a useful premedicant (p.368). It is also sold directly to farmers to be used to sedate pigs before transportation, and to prevent fighting following the mixing of calves or pigs in one pen. When azaperone is used as a sedative or premedication for vaginal delivery of piglets or for caesarian section, the piglets may appear sleepy for some hours after delivery. However, provided they are kept warm they breathe well and there is usually no problem due to this sleepiness.

In horses i.m. doses of 0.4–0.8 mg/kg can sometimes give good sedation (Aitken & Sanford, 1972) but some horses develop muscle tremors and sweat profusely (Lees & Serrano, 1976) and, in practice, azaperone often proves unsatisfactory. Should an excitement reaction be encountered an extremely dangerous situation arises in which injury to the horse and/or its handlers could occur (Dodman & Waterman, 1979). Although Dodman and Waterman suggest that the cause of excitement may be a reaction to the ataxia produced, the fact that pigs show a similar reaction, coupled with the known central nervous effect in man, suggests that the excitement is due to a direct effect of the drug. Thus, its use in horses cannot be recommended.

Droperidol

Droperidol is a potent neuroleptic agent with an action of 6–8 hours duration. It is an extremely potent antiemetic and is said to antagonize the respiratory depressant effects of morphine-like compounds by increasing the sensitivity of the respiratory centre to carbon dioxide. Although it was claimed that extrapyramidal side effects were rare, they are produced by overdosing – but are sometimes delayed for up to 24 hours after administration of the drug. Doses of 0.1–0.4 mg/kg give useful sedation in pigs for 2–5 hours. However, in pigs droperidol has largely been superseded by the less expensive azaperone. Its main use was in neuroleptanalgesia techniques when combined with fentanyl (p.369), but more recently 0.5 mg/kg has been used with 0.3 mg/kg midazolam, both given i.m., to produce dependable sedation.

Fluanisone

This is 4'-fluoro-4-[4-(o-methoxy)phenyl]-1-piperazinyl) butyrophenone. It was used for neuroleptanalgesic techniques in many laboratory animals.

BENZODIAZEPINES

Chlordiazepoxide was first introduced in 1955 and since this time drugs of the benzodiazepine group have been widely used in human and veterinary medicine, although their veterinary applications appear to have been more limited. In man, drugs of this group are utilized to provide:

1. an anti-anxiety action
2. sedation and hypnosis
3. anticonvulsant effects
4. muscle relaxation
5. retrograde amnesia.

A very wide range of different compounds now exist which are employed for one or more of these effects, these compounds differing primarily in bioavailability, permissible route of administration and length of action.

Benzodiazepine compounds exert their main sedative effects through depression of the limbic system, and their muscle relaxing properties through inhibition of the internuncial neurones at spinal levels. Their action is thought to be through stimulation of specific benzodiazepine (BZ) receptors, and there are as many as six variants of BZ sites (Doble & Martin, 1992). The ligand interactions with BZ sites are unusual in that three categories of action can be identified. Agents which increase γ amino butyric acid (GABA) binding and also GABA-induced chloride currents, are regarded as agonists. Others reduce both GABA binding and GABA- induced chloride flux; they are known as inverse agonists and are believed to be responsible for anxiety and convulsions as well as having analeptic properties. A third group, the genuine antagonists of both agonists and inverse agonists, bind but have no efficacy at the site; flumazanil is the drug of this type.

GABA is now well validated as one of the two major inhibitory amino acid transmitters in the central nervous system, the other being glycine (Bloom, 1996). Glycine performs this inhibitory function in the spinal cord, brain stem and retina, whereas GABA is found in the cerebrum and cerebellum. Two types of GABA receptors are recognized and both these $GABA_A$ and $GABA_B$ receptors are found at pre- and postsynaptic sites. $GABA_A$ receptors have at least eight interacting binding sites (Sieghart, 1992). Benzodiazepines potentiate the actions of GABA at the $GABA_A$ receptor and they do so by increasing the frequency of Cl^- channel opening. Ligand binding studies have shown high affinity binding sites for benzodiazepines associated with GABA and there

is a reciprocal interaction by which GABA and the benzodiazepines each increase the binding of the other agent. There is a very good correlation between the binding affinities of benzodiazepines to this site and their clinical potencies and it is, therefore, assumed that this is the site at which they produce their main effects. *In vitro*, sevoflurane at concentrations found in clinical anaesthesia activates both $GABA_A$ and $GABA_B$ mediated inhibitions in the hippocampus (Hirota & Roth, 1997)

It is very difficult if not impossible to induce anaesthesia with benzodiazepine drugs in fit healthy animals (Lees, 1979, 1979a), although they do combine with almost any other central nervous depressant drug to give anaesthesia. It is in combinations with such drugs as the opioids that they are generally employed. Certainly, when used for premedication at subanaesthetic doses, they do markedly reduce the dose required of subsequent anaesthetic agents, but when they are used in many combinations their advantage of causing minimal cardiovascular and respiratory effects may be lost (Dundee & Wyant, 1989).

Most benzodiazepines have a high oral bioavailability and many can also be given by the i.m. and i.v. routes. Their action when given i.v. is not within one circulation time; there are marked differences between individuals in sensitivity and it may take several minutes for maximal effects to become apparent. Metabolism is in the liver and in many instances metabolites are as active or more active than the parent compound; actions therefore tend to be prolonged. In fit animals they do not, on their own, cause sedation and indeed their anxiolytic properties may result in animals becoming uncontrollable – a phenomenon also noted in people (Dundee & Wyant, 1989).

They are used in combination with other drugs to produce sedation and analgesia for intensive care and to counteract the convulsant and hallucinatory properties of ketamine. In a variety of animals benzodiazepines have the property of stimulating appetite (Van Miet *et al.*, 1989). Diazepam has been particularly widely used for this in cats showing anorexia following illness and doses of up to 1 mg/kg have been claimed to be successful in restoring normal feeding habits. However, in debilitated cats i.v. doses of 0.05–0.1 mg/kg are usually adequate and doses of 0.4 mg/kg should not be exceeded if deep sedation is not to result.

Of the available benzodiazepine drugs, diazepam, midazolam, climazolam and zolazepam have been most utilized in veterinary anaesthesia.

Diazepam

Diazepam is probably the most widely used of the benzodiazepines. It is, like all other compounds of this group, insoluble in water and solutions for injections contain solvents such as propylene glycol, ethanol, and sodium benzoate in benzoic acid. Intravenous injection may give rise to thrombophlebitis and this is thought to be due to the solvents rather than to diazepam itself. An emulsion specially prepared for i.v. injection is claimed to be non-irritant to veins, but the bioavailability of this preparation is reduced compared with that of other formulations. Because of the problems of solubility diazepam should not be diluted with water or mixed with solutions of other drugs.

The effects of diazepam in domestic animals are not well documented. A rise in plasma concentration, coupled with a return of clinical effects, occurs 6–8 hours after administration and is thought to be due to enterohepatic recycling of the drug and/or its metabolites (Dundee & Wyant, 1989). Premedication with diazepam increases the length of action of other anaesthetic agents and the drug is particularly useful prior to ketamine anaesthesia to reduce the hallucinations which seem to be associated with this dissociative anaesthetic agent.

The sedative and hypnotic effects of diazepam appear to be minimal or absent in fit, healthy dogs and attempts to use it for hypnosis or as an i.v. induction agent have been unsuccessful because, used alone in healthy animals, it often induces excitement. At clinical dosage rates diazepam has no significant effect on the circulation or respiratory activity but does produce some muscular relaxation due to its action at internuncial neurones. It has very low toxicity and large doses given to dogs for prolonged periods do not produce any changes in liver or kidney function.

Diazepam has a major role in veterinary practice in the control of convulsions of any origin. Averill (1970) recommends that dogs in status epilepticus should be given 5 mg by slow i.v. injection, followed if necessary by a further 5 mg, and more recently doses of 10–35 mg have been recommended for this purpose. In dogs and cats the drug has been used both for premedication as a preventative measure and postoperatively to control convulsions caused by radiographic techniques involving the introduction of contrast media into the spinal canal. Convulsions of toxic origin in cats have also been treated successfully with the drug.

The use of diazepam as a premedicant, sedative and tranquillizer is less well documented. Oral doses of up to 5 mg per day have been used in dogs to control behavioural problems without producing unwanted sedation. It has been used for premedication prior to the use of ketamine in dogs and horses (Short, 1981, 1981a), and during anaesthesia to abolish ketamine-induced convulsions in cats (Reid & Frank, 1972). In the postoperative period, provided pain has been relieved by the appropriate use of analgesic agents, diazepam may be given i.v. in doses of up to 1 mg/kg/hour to control restlessness and facilitate the carrying out of necessary nursing.

Diazepam alone has not been widely used in large animals and in horses its muscle relaxing properties may be associated with induced panic (Muir et al., 1982; Rehm & Schatzmann, 1984). It may, however, be used as part of a protocol of general anaesthesia.

Midazolam

Midazolam, (8-chloro-6 (2-flurophenol)-1–methyl-4H imidazo (1,5-a) (1,4)) benzodiazepine is a water soluble compound yielding a solution with a pH of 3.5. Above pH values of 4.0 the chemical configuration of the molecule changes so that it becomes lipid soluble. The aqueous solution is not painful on i.v. injection and does not cause thrombophlebitis. It is metabolized in the liver and in man its half-life is considerably shorter than that of diazepam thus it is less cumulative and recovery is more rapid. These properties have led to its being used for i.v. sedation and 'induction of anaesthesia'. Like most benzodiazepines it has minimal respiratory and cardiovascular effects and in combination with opioids has been widely used in man for cardiac surgery (Dundee & Wyant, 1989).

Although literature relating to its use is sparse, midazolam has been used fairly extensively in small animal patients, especially with ketamine in cats (Chambers & Dobson, 1989). The combination of midazolam (0.25 mg/kg) and metaclopramide (3.3 mg/kg) will produce good sedation in pigs even though neither drug on its own will produce sedation in these animals. Again in pigs, midazolam (0.3 mg/kg) has been used by i.m. injection with droperidol (0.5 mg/kg) to produce excellent sedation.

Climazolam

Climazolam is a potent benzodiazepine which, following i.v. administration, has a very rapid onset of effect. It has been used in a wide variety of animals including cattle, sheep, horses and dogs (Rehm & Schatzmann, 1984; Erhardt et al., 1986; Komar & Mouallem, 1988). In cattle, 5 mg/kg orally cause sedation and ataxia but much lower doses by the i.v. or i.m. routes give useful sedation. Horses, however, panic (presumably from the feeling of muscle weakness) and the drug is contraindicated on its own for these animals, although it is useful in anaesthetic combinations, being particularly effective for use with ketamine (Rehm & Schatzmann, 1984). Climazolam (1.0–1.5 mg/kg) has also been used in combination with fentanyl (5–15 µg/kg) for anaesthesia in the dog (Erhardt et al., 1986).

Zolazepam

This drug is claimed to have marked hypnotic effects in man. It is now being used in animals combined, in a fixed ratio, with the dissociative agent, tiletamine (Rehm & Schatzmann, 1984). This combination ('Telazol', Parke Davis), produces respiratory depression and periods of excitement occur during recovery.

Flumazenil (benzodiazepine antagonist)

Originally developed for the treatment of overdose in man, flumazenil is a potent and specific benzodiazepine antagonist and in medical practice is now being widely employed to reverse midazolam sedation in 'day case' patients.

Flumazenil has been reported to reverse diazepam or climazolam sedation in sheep and cattle (Rhem & Schatzmann, 1984) and has also been used in combination with naloxone to reverse climazolam/fentanyl combination anaesthesia (Erhardt et al., 1986). Although to date the veterinary use of flumazenil has been limited (Gross et al., 1992; Tranquilli et al., 1992) there is no reason why it should not be employed in any situation where it may become necessary to reverse the effects of a benzodiazepine drug.

α_2 ADRENOCEPTOR AGONISTS

Xylazine has been used as a sedative in animals since 1968 (Sagner et al., 1968, 1968a) but at that time the mechanisms of its complex actions and side effects were not understood. When it was described as 'both excitatory and inhibitory of adrenergic and cholinergic neurones' (Kronberg et al., 1966) this statement appeared more than a little confusing. A similar drug, clonidine, was originally used in man for its powers of peripheral vasoconstriction but later became (and still is) used as an antihypertensive (Schmidtt, 1977).

These actions and the correctness of the above description only became explicable when Langer (1974) suggested the existence of receptor sites situated presynaptically on the noradrenergic neurones which, when stimulated by noradrenaline, inhibited the further release of this transmitter, thus forming a negative feedback mechanism. Langer suggested further that these presynaptic inhibitory receptors differed from the previously recognized α adrenoceptors and should therefore be termed α_2 adrenoceptors. There is now convincing evidence for the presence of postsynaptic and presynaptic α_2 adrenoceptors in both central and peripheral sites. The distinction between α_1, and α_2 adrenoceptors is made on sensitivity to specific agonist and antagonists. Adrenaline and noradrenaline stimulate both types. For α_1 adrenoceptors, phenylephrine and methoxamine are considered to be fairly specific agonists and prazosin to be a specific antagonist. Classically, for pharmacological tests clonidine is considered a specific α_2 adrenoceptor agonist and yohimbine and idazoxan antagonists. However, very few drugs are absolutely specific in their actions and the vast majority can only be described as showing selectivity, thus at higher doses the alternative α receptors may also be stimulated or blocked, a factor possibly explaining some of the side effects and aberrant reactions occasionally seen with their clinical use.

Characteristic adrenergic responses are predicated by the structure of the α_2 adrenoceptors which is similar to many other neurotransmitter receptors including the other adrenergic (α_1, β), muscarinic, opioid and dopamine receptors. Each of these receptors consists of a single polypeptide chain which meanders back and forth through the cell membrane. The intramembranous portion of each adrenergic receptor is hydrophobic and all are similar in structure; from this it can be inferred that they are the site which recognizes noradrenaline, the common neurotransmitter for each of the adrenergic receptors. By way of contrast, the cytoplasmic adrenergic receptor proteins show much difference in structure and especially in their 'contact regions' for the many guanine nucleotide binding proteins (G proteins). At least four different G proteins couple to the α_2 adrenoceptors. Moreover, biological molecular probes have shown that at least three different α_2 isoreceptors exist (Bylund, 1988). These are defined by the location of the gene for the receptor on the chromosome, being either α_2c_2, α_2c_4, or α_2c_{10}. It is also possible to divide the α_2 adrenoceptors at the level of intracellular second messenger systems. For example, the postsynaptic α_2 adrenoceptors in vascular smooth muscle and the presynaptic α_2 adrenoceptors on peripheral sympathetic nerve endings utilize different transduction mechanisms (Nichols *et al.*, 1988). Finally it is now recognized that there are species differences in the location, distribution and type of α_2 receptors.

As the presynaptic α_2 adrenoceptors inhibit noradrenaline release, it might be expected that the action of agonists would be the opposite of the classic effects of sympathetic stimulation. However, where postsynaptic α_2 adrenoceptors exist they often exert a stimulating action similar to that exerted by α_1 adrenoceptors at the same site. The major central and peripheral actions most relevant to anaesthetic practice of stimulation of

TABLE 4.1 **Results of α_2 adrenoceptor stimulation**	
CNS	Sedation, analgesia, hypotension, bradycardia
CVS	Peripheral vasoconstriction → initial hypertension. Central bradycardia and vasomotor depression → hypotension
Gut	Relaxation, decreased motility
Salivation	Decreased
Gastric secretion	Reduced
Uterus	Stimulation
Hormones	Reduced release of insulin, renin and antidiuretic hormone (ADH)
Eyes	Mydriasis, decreased intraocular pressure
Platelets	Aggregation

After Livingstone, Nolan & Waterman (1986)

the α_2 adrenoceptors are summarized in Table 4.1 and the clinical effects seen with drugs which are agonist at this site are the result of the balance of these actions.

Clinical actions of α_2 adrenoceptor agonist drugs

In recent years many new potent and highly selective α_2 adrenoceptor agonists have been developed for both medical and veterinary use. In veterinary practice the major drugs used are xylazine, detomidine, medetomidine and romifidine; clonidine, although primarily used in medical practice, has also been studied in animals in some detail.

The major actions and side effects of all these drugs are similar, although there may be differences in length of action and in the extent and significance of some of the side effects seen. There are variations between the drugs in their specificity for α_2 and α_1 receptors and this explains some of the differences in observed clinical effects. There is also marked variation in species sensitivity to their actions. For example, cattle are approximately 10 times more sensitive to xylazine than horses or dogs, but are equally sensitive to medetomidine as dogs, and equally or less sensitive to detomidine than horses. Pigs appear very resistant to all the drugs so far tested. Generalized comparisons of their potency are meaningless except in the context of a stated species of animal.

The α_2 adrenoceptor agonist drugs are used primarily for their central effect of profound sedation (even of hypnosis in some species of animal) but they also give analgesia through both spinal and central actions even in subsedative doses (Vainio *et al.*, 1986; Nolan *et al.*, 1986; Scheinin & Macdonald, 1989). This is not surprising because α_2 adrenoceptors and opioid receptors share similar regions of the brain and even some of the same neurones. Binding of either α_2 adrenergic or μ opioid receptor agonists results in activation of the same transduction systems (the membrane associated G proteins).

The major side effects of α_2 adrenoceptor agonists are on the cardiovascular system. Although the majority of investigations have been into the actions of xylazine, the evidence to date with the newer compounds suggests that their actions are, in the main, similar. In all species there is marked bradycardia due to central stimulation and mediated through the vagus nerves. The effects on arterial blood pressure depend on the relative effects of the central and peripheral stimulation. There is often an initial hypertensive phase, the extent and duration of which depend on the particular drug, its dose, route of administration, and the species of animal concerned, followed by a more prolonged period of arterial hypotension, again dependent on the drug and the species of animal. Cardiac output falls (but the drugs seem to have little direct action on the myocardium) and the circulation appears to be slowed. The exact state of the peripheral circulation is more complicated and dose dependent. During the early phase of arterial hypertension with bradycardia, peripheral resistance is increased, presumably through shut down of blood vessels. How long this poor peripheral perfusion lasts is difficult to ascertain and probably depends on the species of animal, the drug and the dose used, because in the hypotensive phase peripheral resistance is said to be reduced.

The bradycardia, which can be severe, has given rise to much discussion. Many authorities have recommended medication with anticholinergics prior to sedation with these drugs to prevent the fall in heart rate but recent evidence has thrown doubt on the soundness of this advice. To be effective the anticholinergic must be given an adequate time prior to the α_2 adrenoceptor agonist; arrhythmias or tachycardia often result and the hypertensive phase of the agonist's action may be enhanced in the absence of bradycardia. In cats it has been shown that anticholinergics further decrease cardiac output, presumably due to the resulting tachycardia preventing adequate filling of the heart during diastole (Dunkle *et al.*, 1986), but this does not necessarily apply in larger animals. Work involving continuous recording of the ECG has shown the pulse rates of normal sleeping dogs (Hall *et al.*, 1991) and horses (Hall, unpublished data) to drop to values similar to those seen in animals sedated by α_2 adrenoceptor agonists. The bradycardia in the sedated animal can be overridden by toxaemia or by the administration of some anaesthetics. Thus, the use of anticholinergics remains controversial and more study of the possible combinations is necessary before an informed judgement of their use can be made.

The question of the possible direct effects of α_2 adrenoceptor agonists on the myocardium is also an open one. There have been reports of animals which were in a very excited state at the time of xylazine administration suffering sudden cardiac arrest and the suggestion has been made that this drug might sensitize the heart to adrenaline induced arrhythmias. Indeed Muir and Piper (1977) showed this to be the case in halothane anaesthetized dogs but failed to show the same effect in horses. It must be noted here that pharmacological studies have failed to demonstrate α_2 adrenoceptors in the heart but their presence in the coronary vessels has been established.

Respiratory effects appear to differ between species of animal. Although with doses which cause deep sedation in dogs, cats and horses, respiratory rates may be reduced, there is no serious fall in PaO_2 (Hsu, 1985; Dunkle *et al.*, 1986). In ruminants tachypnoea may occur, breathing appears to require a considerable effort and the PaO_2 shows desaturation of the haemoglobin (DeMoor & Desmet, 1971; Raptopoulos *et al.*, 1985; Nolan *et al.*, 1986). This hypoxaemia does not seem to be due to changes in blood pressure or in ventilation and, indeed, has been shown to occur following clonidine injection in anaesthetized artificially ventilated sheep (Eisenach, 1988). Thus, intrapulmonary mechanisms have been postulated as the cause, hypoxaemia being accompanied by a marked increase in intrapulmonary shunt. Xylazine causes a marked increase in airway resistance in sheep (Nolan & Waterman, 1985) but not in cattle (Watney, 1986).

All α_2 adrenoceptor agonist drugs cause an increase in urination, thought to be through inhibition of ADH release, but when high doses are used, diuresis is possibly assisted by hyperglycaemia. Gut motility ceases almost completely. These side effects must be taken into account when these drugs are used to facilitate investigations such as barium meals and glucose tolerance tests. Another important side effect of α_2 adrenoceptor agonists is that many (but not all) cause significant uterine stimulation and their administration is, therefore, contraindicated in very early or late pregnancy for they may induce abortion.

In doses which produce clinical sedation most of these drugs cause hypothermia but the mechanism by which this is produced appears to differ between drugs and species of animal. Xylazine induced hypothermia has been shown to be antagonized by idazoxan whilst clonidine induced hypothermia is intensified by this antagonist (Livingstone et al., 1984). In rats, low doses of detomidine cause hypothermia which can be reversed by yohimbine (Virtanen, 1986) but higher doses cause hyperthermia probably due to an α_1 adrenoceptor-stimulating action.

When α_2 adrenoceptor agonists are used for premedication they greatly reduce the dose requirements of inhalation anaesthetics (Virtanen, 1986) or intravenous agents. They also combine with opioids to produce deep sedation or even anaesthesia.

Xylazine

Xylazine, 2-(2,6-dimethylphenylamino)-4H-5,5 dihydro-1,3-thiazine, was enthusiastically received as a sedative and over the past 20 years it has maintained its popularity as a generally reliable sedative and premedicant in a wide range of animal species (Clarke & Hall, 1969). The drug is a typical α_2 adrenoceptor agonist and exerts its effects accordingly. However, there are marked variations in susceptibility to it between the various species of domestic animals. Horses, dogs and cats require 10 times the dose needed in cattle and even then the degree of sedation achieved in horses is considerably less. Pigs are even more resistant than horses (Sagner et al., 1968, 1968a). It is possible that lesser variations in sensitivity may occur in breeds within a single species and that this might contribute to the occasional failure of the drug to produce sedation.

Xylazine can be given by i.v., i.m. or s.c. injection although the s.c. route is not very reliable. Injections are non-irritant although minor temporary swellings have been reported at the site of i.m. injection of concentrated solutions in horses. Although never proved by laboratory testing, most users of the drug are satisfied that the potency of available commercial solutions decreases with age, and that this deterioration is enhanced by increased environmental temperature (Van Dieten, 1988, personal communication).

In horses the drug is usually used in doses that enable the animal to remain standing (although with marked ataxia), but in ruminants and small animals sedation is dose dependent and higher doses are used which may cause recumbency, unconsciousness and a state close to general anaesthesia. After these high doses sedation is very prolonged and is accompanied by marked cardiovascular and respiratory depression, i.e. they constitute overdoses. The sedative effects of xylazine appear to be synergistic with a variety of analgesic, sedative and anaesthetic drugs and such combinations are much preferable to overdoses of xylazine for the production of sedation.

Although the drug can be a potent analgesic, claims as to the degree of analgesia achieved at clinical dose rates are conflicting. Sedative doses appear to produce a short period of intense analgesia in horses – there is considerable experimental and clinical evidence that it produces excellent analgesia in equine colic (Lowe, 1978). However, others (Clarke & Hall, 1969; Tronicke & Vocke, 1970) have found that horses deeply sedated with xylazine may respond violently to manipulations or even attempts to inject local analgesics. It may be that such reactions are a response to touch rather than pain as non-painful procedures such as hair clipping or placing a radiographic plate may cause a horse to respond with a well directed kick.

Cattle and small animals do not show this marked response to touch. Analgesia is not adequate for minor surgery and in cats Arbeiter *et al.* (1972) found that even massive doses of xylazine sufficient to cause prolonged unconsciousness were inadequate to abolish all reaction to painful stimuli in the majority of animals. Thus, despite the undoubted analgesic properties of the drug, in the opinion of the authors where surgery is to be performed local analgesia must be used to supplement its effects.

The cardiovascular effects of xylazine are typical of this group of drugs and appear to be similar in all species of animal (Clarke & Hall, 1969; Garner *et al.*, 1971; Haskins *et al.*, 1986). An initial rise in arterial blood pressure following its i.v. injection as a bolus is short lived and the pressure then falls to 10 to 20% below initial resting levels. The hypertensive phase is not always evident after i.m. injection, possibly because of reduced peak blood concentrations of the drug.

Cardiac output falls due to bradycardia and heart block is usually observed. The advisability of using anticholinergic drugs to counteract bradycardia is disputed (Kerr *et al.*, 1972; Hsu, 1985). Pronounced hypertension associated with the bradycardia can usually be avoided by using minimal doses and i.m. or slow i.v. injection. Xylazine appears to have little direct effect on the myocardium but causes a dose related depression of respiration. Falls in PaO_2 are species specific, being particularly severe in ruminants, while the muscle relaxing properties make the drug contraindicated in animals suffering from upper airway obstruction.

Other side effects of xylazine include: muscle twitching when sedation is deep; sweating in horses at the time sedation is diminishing; vomiting at the onset of sedation in dogs and cats; hypergylcaemia; decreased intraocular pressure and gut motility and increased urine production. Xylazine also causes uterine contractions and should not be used in late pregnancy for it may induce premature labour. Increase in uterine tone may contraindicate it in cattle or horses receiving ovum transplants since this may reduce the chance of implantation.

Xylazine has proved to be a very safe sedative in a wide variety of animals but some serious reactions have been reported. There have been reports of violent excitement or collapse in horses associated with its intravenous injection. Some of these mishaps may have been due to inadvertent intra-arterial injection, but it is probable that a few have been genuine drug reactions. Fainting through extreme bradycardia has been suggested as a possible cause of collapse, but this is unlikely because the greatest bradycardia is coupled with arterial hypertension. Deaths have also been reported in cattle and the problems of recumbency in ruminants must be increased by the hypoxaemia caused by α_2 adrenoceptor agonists. The advent of the opportunity to limit the duration of recumbency by the reversal of sedation with drugs such as atipamezole should increase the safety of xylazine in these animals. In small animals deaths have mainly resulted from the use of xylazine for premedication.

In most species of animal, xylazine is a useful drug for premedication prior to induction of anaesthesia with one of a wide variety of agents. Its use greatly reduces the dose of anaesthetic required, and although the reduction can often be predicted from the degree of sedation achieved it may still be present in animals which have responded poorly to the drug. In heavily sedated animals circulation is slowed, the effects of subsequent anaesthetic agents is delayed and overdose of the anaesthetic may result. Thus, particular care is needed when this sedative is followed by i.v. agents such as the barbiturates, Saffan or propofol. Xylazine is particularly useful in combination with ketamine for its muscle relaxing properties help to reduce the rigidity caused by the dissociative agent and for many years xylazine/ketamine combinations have proved useful in a wide range of animal species (Muir *et al.*, 1977; 1978; Butera *et al.*, 1978; Brouwer *et al.*, 1980; Hall & Taylor, 1981; Waterman, 1981).

Detomidine

Detomidine, 4-(2,3-dimethylphenyl)methyl-1H-imidazole hydrochloride, is an imidazole derivative which has been developed as a sedative/analgesic for animals. It is supplied in multi-dose bottles at a concentration of 10 mg/ml and may be given by the i.v. and i.m. routes. It is not effective if given orally, but is when administered sublingually because it is readily absorbed through mucous membranes. In a variety of laboratory animals its sedative potency has been shown to be of a similar order to that of clonidine and approximately 10 times (Virtanen, 1986) that of xylazine. (These relative potencies are not necessarily the same in domestic animals for in cattle, unlike xylazine, it is no more potent than it is in horses).

The properties of detomidine are well documented in *Acta Veterinaria Scandinavica*, Supplement 82/1986 (20 papers). Its analgesic powers have been shown in a number of pain models and it is particularly effective as an analgesic in equine colic (Virtanen, 1985; Clarke, 1988; Jochle *et al.*, 1989). Cardiovascular changes are typical of an α_2 adrenoceptor agonist in that there is a marked bradycardia and following doses of 20μg/kg arterial blood pressure is elevated for about 15 minutes but falls significantly below control values within 45 minutes of injection of the drug (Clarke & Taylor, 1987; Sarazan *et al.*, 1989). Higher doses of the drug are followed by more prolonged arterial hypertension but as yet there have been no investigations into whether this is followed by prolonged hypotension. Work to date in horses shows that arterial pressure during anaesthesia after detomidine premedication appears to be dependent on the anaesthetic agents used (Clarke, 1988). Like xylazine, detomidine causes a minimal fall in equine PaO_2 (Clarke, 1988), but marked hypoxaemia in sheep (Waterman *et al.*, 1986). In horses, other side effects include muscular twitching, sweating, piloerection, hyperglycaemia, a marked diuresis and reduced gut motility. Side effects increase in frequency and duration with increased dose.

One difference between xylazine and detomidine appears to be in their effects on the uterus. Whereas xylazine appears to have marked ecbolic effects, detomidine, at i.v. doses of 20μg/kg, slows electrical activity in the pregnant bovine uterus, although 40–60μg/kg causes an increase in electrical activity (Jedruch & Gajewski, 1986).

Detomidine is primarily used as a sedative for horses. In early work doses between 10 and 300 μg/kg were employed, horses remaining standing after the highest doses, although sedation and side effects (bradycardia, arterial hypertension, ataxia, sweating, piloerection, muscle tremor and diuresis) were unacceptably prolonged. This early work serves to demonstrate the very high therapeutic index of the drug as subsequent clinical experience has shown that i.v. doses of 10 to 20μg/kg give adequate sedation for about an hour with much more limited side effects (Clarke & Taylor, 1987). Its action is prolonged in the presence of abnormal liver function, even when this is not clinically apparent (Chambers *et al.*, 1996). The drug has also been widely used in horses for premedication prior to induction of anaesthesia with agents such as ketamine, thiopental and propofol (Taylor & Clarke, 1985; Clarke *et al.*, 1986). A more detailed description of the effects and uses of detomidine in horses is given in Chapter 11.

The doses of detomidine required in cattle appear to be similar to those in horses. Again, early experimental work suggested that high doses were needed for adequate sedation but subsequent trials have shown that doses of up to 30μg/kg are satisfactory. In the authors' experience, doses of 10μg/kg i.v. produce sedation in cattle very similar to that seen in horses, i.e. cattle remain standing but show marked ataxia. The relative lack of hypnotic effect with detomidine means that cattle are more likely to remain standing than after xylazine and this probably led to the initial misapprehension that cattle required higher doses. Low doses of detomidine may be used safely in early and late pregnancy in cattle (Chapter 18).

Medetomidine

This compound, 4-(1-(2,3-dimethylphenyl) ethyl)-1H-imadazole, is a very potent, efficacious and selective agonist for α_2 adrenoreceptors in the central and peripheral nervous system (Virtanen *et al.*, 1988). The preparation that has been used in veterinary anaesthesia is a mixture of two sterioisomers and contains 1mg/ml of the racaemic mixture. The dextrorotatory isomer, which is used in man as a premedicant and anxiolytic (Scheinin *et al.*, 1987; MacDonald *et al.*, 1988), is the active component.

Apart from the required actions of sedation, hypnosis and analgesia (Stenberg *et al.*, 1987) medetomidine has the usual marked cardiovascular effects of this group of drugs (bradycardia, arterial hypertension followed by hypotension and reduced cardiac output). Its actions in dogs and cats have been well reviewed by Cullen (1996).

In most animals medetomidine slows respiration (Clarke & England, 1989). Nevertheless, at normal sedative doses in non-ruminant animals the $PaCO_2$ does not rise to an excessive level (Vainio, 1989; Cullen & Reynoldson, 1993) and there is less depression of the ventilatory response to CO_2 than is commonly seen in anaesthetized animals. However, cyanosis has been reported in up to one third of dogs sedated with medetomidine (Clarke & England, 1989; Vaha-Vahe, 1989; Sap & Hellebrekers, 1993). This cyanosis is not associated with a lowered arterial PaO_2 or an oxygen saturation below 95% and has been attributed to a slow tissue blood flow with increased oxygen extraction leading to cyanosis from venous desaturation.

It has not yet been established whether medetomidine is safe for use in pregnant animals but in bitches the electrical activity of the uterine muscle is depressed at doses of 20 μg/kg, while at higher doses (40–60 μg/kg) there is an initial increase in this activity for some 5–7 minutes followed by depression; pregnant bitches do not abort (Jedruch & Gajewski, 1989). Medetomidine markedly reduces the MAC of volatile agents given subsequently for anaesthesia and a similar synergism must be expected with i.v. agents whenever medetomidine premedication is used.

The solution is non-irritant and can be administered by s.c., i.m. or i.v. injection. Intravenous injection gives the fastest and most reliable results and vomiting is less common than with other routes of administration. Vomiting occurs in 10 to 20% of dogs and 50 to 65% of cats given i.m. medetomidine and although some sedation may be evident within 5 minutes maximal sedation is not achieved until 20 minutes have elapsed. Although medetomidine is ineffective when given by mouth, as it is inactivated by passage through the liver, it is readily absorbed through mucous membranes and can be administered effectively sublingually.

Following its administration in the dog, the animal rapidly becomes ataxic then stands quietly with its head down. Vomiting may occur at this time, but tends to be of short-lived duration compared with that induced by xylazine. Next, the dogs becomes recumbent but even if apparently very deeply sedated it can be made to arise and walk around in an ataxic manner before resuming recumbency. Muscle twitching may occur, being most marked in most deeply sedated animals. In the medium sized dog, maximal sedation is achieved with i.m. doses of 40 μg/kg (or half these doses by i.v. injection), higher doses lengthening the duration of sedation but up to 80 μg/kg also contributing to further analgesia. Smaller animals appear more resistant to the effects so that it has been suggested that doses should be calculated on the basis of μg/unit body surface area rather than on body weight. Sedation is less effective in noisy or disturbing surroundings but, once sedated, dogs are not usually responsive to sound. All the other typical side effects such as vomiting, muscular twitching, hypothermia, decreased gut movement and hyperglycaemia, have been noted (Vainio et al., 1986; Clarke & England, 1989).

In cats higher doses (80 to 150 μg/kg i.m.) are needed to produce sedation. Sedation is usually excellent but the animals are capable of being aroused. The i.v. use of medetomidine in cats has apparently not been widely explored.

The drug has been widely used in combination with other drugs to prolong recumbency. In the dog opioids have proved to be successful (Clarke & England, 1988) but the most popular combinations have been with ketamine, even 1 to 2 mg/kg of ketamine being adequate to ensure prolongation of recumbency.

Medetomidine has been used in sheep and cattle; i.v. doses of 10 to 20 μg/kg causing sedation similar to that seen after 0.1 to 0.2 mg/kg of xylazine (Clarke & England, unpublished observations). In wild animals higher doses are required and the drug has usually been used in combination with ketamine when administered by dart gun for immobilization. Indeed, medetomidine/ketamine combinations have been found to provide excellent immobilization and relaxation in a wide range of species of animals, while the ability to reverse the sedation with α_2 adrenoceptor antagonists has proved to be particularly useful (Jalenka, 1989, 1989a).

The drug has also been used in many rodents and other laboratory animals and there is marked variation in susceptibility to its effects, the guinea pig being most resistant. Once again, combinations with ketamine are more effective than the sedative alone.

Romifidine

This drug, developed from clonidine, has typical α_2 adrenoceptor agonist effects. It has undergone clinical trials in Germany, Switzerland and the UK as a sedative (Clarke *et al.*, 1991) and premedicant (Young, 1992) for horses. Maximal sedation is achieved with i.v. doses of 80 μg/kg. When compared in horses given i.v. xylazine (1 mg/kg) or detomidine (20 μg/kg) it produces less ataxia and the head is not lowered to the same extent, but response to imposed stimuli is reduced to the same degree by all three drugs. At these doses, the duration of effect is longest with romifidine, the horses remaining quieter than normal for some considerable time after obvious sedation has waned. Romifidine produces a marked increase in urine production over 90 minutes accompanied by an increase in sodium and glucose excretion while creatinine clearance remains constant (Gasthuys *et al.*, 1996).

In dogs, recovery from romifidine is rapid (Michelsen, 1996) but the liver contributes very little to its overall clearance from the body (Chism & Rickert, 1996).

α_2 ADRENOCEPTOR ANTAGONISTS

The central and peripheral effects of the α_2 adrenoceptor agonists can be reversed by the use of equally specific antagonists. The antagonists used include yohimbine (Hsu *et al.*, 1989), idazoxan (Docherty *et al.*, 1987; Hsu *et al.*, 1989), tolazoline (Hsu *et al.*, 1987) and atipamezole (Clarke & England, 1988; Kock *et al.*, 1989), the most potent and specific being atipamezole.

The ability to awaken xylazine or detomidine-sedated subjects has proved to be particularly useful in wild animals where prolonged sedation may be fatal (Kock *et al.*, 1989), and in domestic ruminants (Thompson *et al.*, 1989) where prolonged recumbency is again unwelcome. Also, in some clinical situations the α_2 adrenoceptor antagonists are useful in small animal practice.

When using antagonists in the clinical situation it is necessary to consider the pharmacokinetics of the drugs involved, because if the antagonist is eliminated faster than the agonist, resedation will occur; this is most serious in wild animals which are not under observation and vulnerable to predators. The dose rates of antagonist drugs for reversing sedation will obviously vary with the dose of sedative used and the elapsed time after its administration. With all antagonists investigated, higher doses are required to reverse cardiopulmonary effects than to reverse sedation (Hsu *et al.*, 1989; Vainio & Vaha-Vahe, 1989). The situation is complicated by the fact that there may be species differences in antagonistic effects and it is, therefore, very difficult to be certain of the exact dose of antagonist necessary in any particular case. For this reason it is important that no side effects occur should the antagonist be overdosed. Convulsions have occasionally been reported after yohimbine, idazoxan and atipamezole but in most reports ketamine, which is not influenced by the α_2 adrenoceptor antagonists, was part of the sedative combination used and may have been the cause of this side effect.

Of the α_2 adrenoceptor antagonists, yohimbine and atipamazole are the most commonly used in veterinary practice. Numerous studies have demonstrated the effectiveness of yohimbine in antagonizing α_2 agonist induced sedation and analgesia in laboratory animals, dogs and cats (Holmberg & Gershon, 1961; Hsu, 1983). Doses of 0.1 mg/kg have generally been employed to reverse xylazine sedation in small animals; high doses have caused excitement in dogs (Paddleford, 1988). Yohimbine has sometimes been used in combination with 4-aminopyridine, a drug which releases acetylcholine and other neurotransmitters from presynaptic nerve endings, but the combination appears to have no advantages over the use of the antagonist alone.

Atipamezole has mainly been used to reverse medetomidine sedation in dogs (Clarke & England, 1988; Vainio & Vaha-Vahe, 1989), cats (Virtanen, 1989) and wild animals. Serious relapse into sedation has not been noted, although following low doses of the drug animals have been described as appearing 'tired' for some hours. Overdose of atipamezole does not appear to cause problems in most species of animal, injection into the unsedated dog (Clarke & England 1988) causing mild muscular tremors but little else and convulsions have never been noted in the absence of ketamine. However, although atipamezole appears to have little effect in unsedated cats, when used to reverse medetomidine sedation a few cats have been described as being 'over-reversed' but overt excitement has not been seen. Atipamezole has also been shown to be effective in reversing detomidine sedation in horses, and xylazine sedation in wild animals, sheep and cattle.

Tolazoline (Tolazine, Lloyd Laboratories, Iowa) is used in doses of 4 mg/kg to antagonize the effects of xylazine in horses. The rate of i.v. administration needs to be controlled to approximately 100 mg/min. It is a mixed α_1 and α_2 adrenergic receptor antagonist and also has a direct peripheral vasodilator action. Temporary side effects, which usually last not more than 1 to 2 hours, include increases in blood pressure, tachycardia, peripheral vasodilatation and sweating.

TAMERIDONE

Tameridone, a purine alkyl piperidine derivative, has undergone extensive clinical and pharmacological investigations in cattle where i.v. doses of 0.05 mg/kg or i.m. doses of 0.1–0.2 mg/kg produce good sedation for 90–120 minutes. Sedation appears to be dose dependent in depth and takes longer to appear than sedation after xylazine administration. The drug appears to be equally effective in all breeds of cattle but cows at full term undergoing caesarian section appear to be unduly sensitive, i.v. doses of 0.03 mg/kg readily causing recumbency. In the USA tameridone has been tried extensively for the capture and transport of wild ruminant animals but the results have been variable – doses and depth of sedation achieved differ between species of animal.

ANALGESIA

Although an animal may be deemed to be unconscious during general anaesthesia and, therefore, incapable of appreciating pain, there is now evidence that the use of analgesic drugs before and during general anaesthesia assists in obtaining a smooth, pain-free recovery. All general anesthetics undoubtedly have an intrinsic analgesic action but further analgesia can be provided by four main methods:

1. Use of local analgesics
2. Use of α_2 adrenoceptor agonists
3. Use of non-steroidal anti-inflammatory drugs (NSAIDs)
4. Use of opioid drugs.

Local analgesics, particularly the long acting group of drugs, e.g. bupivacaine, used during surgery may also provide outstanding postoperative analgesia. These drugs are discussed in more detail in Chapter 10. α_2 Adrenoceptor agonists, discussed above, when used parenterally at analgesic doses will also cause deep sedation (which is not always a disadvantage in the postoperative period) and bradycardia. In man, and increasingly in animals, these α_2 adrenoceptor agonists are now being administered epidurally to limit their side effects.

With all of these drugs, there is now convincing evidence that they are more effective if administered before pain becomes manifest (Mitchell & Smith, 1989).

NON-STEROIDAL ANTI-INFLAMMATORY DRUGS (NSAIDs)

These agents act primarily by inhibiting prostaglandin release at the site of trauma and by reducing inflammation and swelling – themselves a major source of postoperative pain. Details of the very large number of NSAIDs, their uses, limitations and toxicity are beyond the scope of this book but are well reviewed in current standard pharmacological texts. With due care, they can make a most useful contribution to postoperative analgesia.

Salicylate

Acetylsalicylate ('Aspirin') was one of the first NSAIDs used in veterinary medicine and still has a place, particularly for postoperative pain and discomfort in small animals. It acts as an analgesic both centrally and peripherally. It is said to cause gastric irritation due, in part, to ion trapping (ion trapping occurs when an ion passes through a membrane and encounters a different pH from which it has difficulty in escaping). By this mechanism the concentration of aspirin within a cell may contribute to the gastric irritation because aspirin which is absorbed in the stomach at the intracellular pH of approximately 7.4 reverts to the ionized form which can only slowly cross from the cells into the blood plasma (aspirin $pK_a = 3.4$ so that the ionized concentration is 10^4 times that of the unionized amount). The so-called 'soluble' aspirins are certainly solutions at about neutral pH, i.e. when dissolved in water, but precipitate a considerable proportion of the drug in the acid medium of the gastric juice. 'Buffered' aspirin preparations reduce ion trapping by decreasing gastric absorption. In the alkaline medium of the small intestine the aqueous solubility of aspirin increases and although the unionized form of the drug is present in much lower proportion, most of the absorption into the bloodstream occurs due to the larger absorptive surface and the greater time spent in this part of the gastrointestinal tract. Plasma content is chiefly (due to rapid hydrolysis in blood and liver) in the form of sodium salicylate which is heavily protein bound.

There is little evidence of clinical harm caused by aspirin irritation of the canine or feline stomach apart from one isolated report of buffered aspirin causing massive gastric haemorrhage in a Greyhound (Shaw *et al.*, 1997). By diminishing platelet aggregation it has a small, clinically insignificant, effect in prolonging blood coagulation.

Dogs can quite safely be given 10 mg orally per day and cats 5 mg per day by the same route (Davis & Donnelly, 1968). It may be given preoperatively, or after the first 48 to 72 hours postoperatively when the most severe postoperative pain has waned.

Phenylbutazone

Phenylbutazone is a favourite drug of horse owners wishing to alleviate minor degrees of lameness as an alternative to euthanasia. Veterinary anaesthetists may use this drug as an analgesic anti-inflammatory in the treatment of equine postanaesthetic rhabdomyolysis in i.v. doses of 4 mg/kg. In dogs i.v. injections or oral administration of up to 20 mg/kg (100 and 200 mg tablets are available in the UK) are used for the treatment of

pain and may be given daily in divided doses every 8 hours for not more than one week.

The drug is highly protein bound and should not be administered with other highly protein bound drugs for this can lead to toxic effects. It should not be administered to cats (Christianson, 1980) and since in all animals it produces many side effects which are likely to be severe if the usual therapeutic dose is exceeded many authorities consider this drug to be obsolescent.

Flunixin

Flunixin in i.v. doses of 1.1 mg/kg is used in horses suffering from colic for its antiendotoxic and visceral pain relieving properties. Doses should not be repeated more than twice. Consequently, many animals presented for surgical treatment of colic will have received the drug prior to surgery. Its safety in pregnant mares has not been demonstrated. The drug in tablet form is also used in dogs for the control of postoperative pain and inflammation at a dose of 1 mg/kg for up to three days. Side effects in dogs include vomiting and diarrhoea and it should not be administered to pregnant bitches. Its pharmacokinetics and pharmacodynamics in cats have been reported by Lees and Taylor (1991).

Ketoprofen

Ketoprofen is used in horses, dogs and cats. It is said to be approximately 15 times more potent than phenylbutazone and 30 times more potent than aspirin. The i.v. dose for horses is 2.2 mg/kg, once daily, in dogs it is 2 mg/kg by the i.v., i.m. or s.c. routes, and in cats (s.c.) 2 mg/kg is given, in each case for not more than three days.

In common with other NSAIDs it is not permitted by the racing authorities of Great Britain and Ireland to be used at the time of racing and ketoprofen or its conjugates can be detected in urine for up to 10 days after its administration ceases.

Carprofen

Carprofen is the latest NSAID to be introduced into veterinary practice. It does not appear to act by inhibition of cyclo-oxgenase or lipoxygenase (McKellar *et al.*, 1990) as the earlier NSAIDs do. The side effects of these drugs generally result from inhibition of prostaglandin formation by this mechanism, so carprofen promises to have fewer side effects than the other drugs.

In horses carprofen is used as a single i.v. dose of 0.7 mg/kg (1 ml/70 kg) which may be repeated after 24 hours or followed with oral therapy for up to five days. In dogs, the drug is given before or immediately after induction of general anaesthesia in i.v. or s.c. doses of 4 mg/kg for 'pre-emptive analgesia'. Clinical evidence in dogs suggests that only a single dose of carprofen is required in the first 24 hours perioperatively; if analgesia is needed after this, half the initial dose may be given for not more than seven days. Its analgesic activity in cats has been described by Lascelles *et al.*, (1995) who found that i.m. pethidine (meperidine) in doses of 10 mg/kg produced significantly better postoperative analgesia for up to two hours postoperatively but from 2 to 20 hours postoperatively the reverse was true and 4 mg/kg carprofen provided significantly better pain relief.

OPIOID ANALGESICS

Opioids have been used as painkillers in man for at least 2000 years and the refined and processed extracts, morphine and heroin, still have a major role as analgesics. There is now a wide range of both naturally occurring and synthetic opioids, so that the clinician has an enormous range of choice. The principal reason for employing opioids is to provide analgesia but some are used as cough suppressants. Unfortunately, these drugs have a wide range of side effects, the most important of which is probably respiratory depression. Even more unfortunately, in man these drugs cause euphoria and addiction, rendering them liable to abuse and resulting in controls on their use. Abuse is not a feature of their use in veterinary patients but they have other undesirable side effects, including the production of nausea and vomiting (in dogs), constipation, pruritis and in some cases dysphoria. Whilst in dogs they invariably cause sedation, in cats and horses higher doses cause excitement, although clinical doses can be used quite safely in these species of animal, being particularly unlikely to produce excitement when pain is present.

The use of nalorphine as an antidote to morphine poisoning in man was first reported in 1951 and since then other agents which antagonize the effects of morphine have been produced. Many of these have partial agonist activity, sufficient for them to be used as analgesics, and often they are less liable to abuse and, therefore, have fewer controls over their use. Pure antagonists, such as naloxone, will reverse the effects of morphine at doses which have no intrinsic activity when given alone.

In recent years the discovery of specific receptor sites of action for the opioids (first suggested by Martin *et al.*, 1976) and the identification in the central nervous system of endogenous ligands such as encephalins, endorphins and dynorphin which act at these receptors, has led to better understanding of the multiple actions of agonist and partial agonist opioid drugs, as well as providing the possibility of the development of more specific drugs with fewer side effects. On the basis of response to specific drugs Martin *et al.* initially postulated the existence of three opioid receptors receptors, termed μ, κ and σ.

Other multiple receptors have since been postulated and it is now accepted that the one known as the δ receptor is of importance. Table 4.2 shows receptor selectivity of some opioid analgesics. Many authorities now do not consider the σ receptor to be a true opioid receptor. The actions which are suggested to occur on activation of these

TABLE 4.2 Receptor selectivity (agonist and antagonist) of some opioid drugs

Drug	μ receptor	κ receptor	δ receptor
Buprenorphine	+++	?	?
Butorphanol	++	++	−
Diprenorphine	++	++	++
Fentanyl	+++	−	−
Methadone	+++	−	−
Morphine	+++	+/−	−
Naloxone	+++	+	+
Nalbuphine	+++	+	−
Pentazocine	++	+	+
Pethidine	++	−	−
Remifentanil	+++	−	−
Sufentanil	+++	+	+

various receptors have been the subject of very many reviews and Table 4.3 summarizes, in a very simplified form, the suggested actions following stimulation of the receptors as gleaned from these reviews.

The cloning of receptor sites, with the identification of a large number of variations, has led to a re-classification in which the classical receptors are now termed OP_1 (previously the δ receptor), OP_2, (κ) and OP_3. (μ). However, as this classification is as yet unfamiliar in anaesthetic use, the original terminology will continue to be used in this book.

It is thought that analgesia results primarily from stimulation of the μ and κ receptors while stimulation of the δ receptors modulates the effects at the μ receptors.

Drugs classified as pure agonists, e.g. morphine, cause analgesia by stimulation of the μ and κ receptors, although they may have actions elsewhere. Naloxone is antagonistic at all receptors where it is active. The partial agonist/antagonist drugs show a range of activity. Some may act as agonists at one type of receptor whilst antagonizing at another; some have partial agonist actions at a single type of receptor, low doses stimulating the receptor but higher doses antagonizing this effect. Unfortunately, in intact animals, unlike in pharmacological preparations, responses may not be so clear cut. For example, butorphanol is said to have no μ activity but it induces a 'walking' response in horses, which is said to be a μ effect (Tobin *et al.*, 1979). Nevertheless, despite discrepancies, a knowledge of the range of activity at different receptors is helpful in arriving at an understanding of the actions, side effects and reversibility of the wide range of opioids available for clinical use.

Increasing the dose of pure agonist drugs increases analgesia but, unfortunately, also increases respiratory depression. Moreover, all the drugs which have potent μ agonist activity appear to have effects which give rise to abuse by humans. It has been suggested that there are μ_1 and μ_2 receptors, stimulation of μ_1 resulting in analgesia whilst μ_2 stimulation leads to respiratory depression and abuse. Meptazinol was claimed to be a pure μ_1 agonist (Sanford, 1948) but this drug does not appear to have lived up to early expectations and is now thought to act also by other mechanisms.

Partial agonists have a limit to the analgesia they can produce, increasing doses sometimes antagonizing the analgesia of lower doses (i.e. the dose–response curve is bell-shaped). However, the respiratory depression produced by the partial agonists is also limited, maximal depression reaching a plateau at high doses. Unfortunately, the maximal respiratory depression produced may still be of some clinical significance. Partial agonist drugs are less liable to human abuse, primarily because many produce unpleasant dysphoric and hallucinatory effects. Psychomimetic and hallucinatory effects have generally been considered signs of σ receptor stimulation. Recently, pure κ agonists have become available and it was hoped that these drugs would have the analgesic advantages of an opioid agonist without causing respiratory depression or having a major potential for abuse. Regrettably, all the drugs available to date cause unacceptable dysphoria in man and as a result it is now postulated that some of the actions attributed to σ receptor stimulation may in fact be a property of κ receptor stimulation. As animals cannot complain of dysphoric or hallucinatory experiences it behoves veterinarians to exercise care when using drugs likely to cause such effects.

General actions of opioid agonists in animals

At least in man, it seems that the euphoric effects of morphine-like drugs contribute to the analgesia

TABLE 4.3 **Actions suggested to occur on stimulation of opioid receptors**	
Receptor	**Suggested action**
μ	Spinal and supraspinal analgesia
	Respiratory depression
	Euphoria
	Nausea and Vomiting
	Changes in gut motility
	Miosis
	Addiction
	Sedation
κ	Supraspinal analgesia
	Sedation
	Addiction (mild)
	Miosis
	Dysphoria and psychomimetic effects
δ	analgesia
σ	Dysphoria and psychomimetic effects
	Mydriasis

they produce, patients being unconcerned by any residual pain. Whether this is also true in animals can only remain a speculation. The pure agonists produce dose-dependent respiratory depression but it must be emphasized that in chest pain low doses may improve respiratory activity through the analgesic effect. In ambulatory humans, dogs and cats, morphine and some other opioid agonists cause vomiting and as they also produce marked depression of the cough reflex care must be taken to ensure that inhalation of vomit does not occur. Opioid agonists increase the tone of the gut, particularly of the sphincters, and decrease transit time, causing constipation. Their use is generally contraindicated for biliary or ureteric pain as they cause spasm of the bile and ureteric ducts. Cerebrospinal fluid pressure is elevated, so their use is also contraindicated in head injuries. The pure agonist drugs' effects of causing tolerance and addiction in man results in their being subject to tight statutory controls.

In humans, dogs and rabbits, opioid agonists tend to cause central nervous depression whilst in cats and horses excitement may predominate. This species difference reflects in many of the properties of the drugs. High doses of morphine will sedate dogs, but not horses or cats. Opioid agonists generally cause miosis, and do so in the dog, but generalized excitement in horses and cats may sometimes be accompanied by mydriasis. The effects on the cardiovascular system are very variable and depend on the drug, its dose and the species of animal concerned. In general, however, at high doses they cause bradycardia, thought to be mediated via vagal mechanisms, and this is regularly seen in dogs. They have minimal direct effect on the heart and their effects on arterial blood pressure may be very variable. Release of histamine by morphine and pethidine may cause arterial hypotension in dogs. Opioid agonists usually cause arterial hypertension and tachycardia in horses – presumably manifestations of the excitement reaction although under some circumstances bradycardia can occur (Muir *et al.*, 1978; Clarke & Paton, 1988). High doses of opioids produce muscle rigidity in all species of animals, including dogs.

It must be emphasized again that the presence or absence of pain can have a major influence on the response to opioids, and horses and cats in pain when these drugs are given may show no adverse reactions to doses which would cause excitement in normal animals.

Use and choice of opioid analgesics

Opioid drugs may be used to provide analgesia before, during and after surgery as well as in combination with sedative drugs for 'chemical control'. The choice of opioid will depend on the degree of analgesia needed, the speed of onset of the drug's action and the length of action required, as well as on the side effects that can be tolerated in the circumstances. When analgesia is needed during surgery, an opioid with a fairly long action may be used for premedication (e.g. morphine or buprenorphine), or a short acting drug such as fentanyl or alfentanil given during surgery. Where potent agonists such as fentanyl or alfentanil are used to provide a major component of anaesthesia for surgery, respiratory depression may be severe and respiratory support with intermittent positive pressure ventilation of the lungs and oxygen supplementation will be necessary. A similar degree of respiratory depression during the recovery period is unacceptable if less support is available. As all opioids cross the placenta, care must be taken if they are used at parturition, although naloxone may be used to antagonize respiratory depression in the neonate.

Dysphoric or hallucinatory effects will not be a problem during general anaesthesia and are often prevented in conscious animals by the use of sedatives, but may cause distress if drugs causing these effects are given to unsedated, ambulatory animals. Because opioids often have a synergistic depressant action in combination with sedatives or anaesthetics, doses (particularly of the more potent agents) may need to be reduced when combinations of these drugs are used. The use of partial agonist drugs was encouraged by their freedom from statutory controls in many countries, but now in the USA pentazocine, butorphanol and buprenorphine are all FDA controlled and in the UK buprenorphine and pentazocine are controlled drugs while butorphanol is a prescription-only medicine.

Epidural opioids

Opioids, including morphine, oxymorphone, fentanyl, sufentanil and butorphanol have been used by the epidural route in order to try to achieve analgesia without central and respiratory depression during and after surgery. There are differences in receptor pharmacology and extrapolation from human experience may be unwise. In man, respiratory depression may occur and is sometimes seriously delayed, but this does not seem to be a clinical problem in dogs. Another common side effect is pruritis in 67–100% of patients, although only serious in 1–10% (Morgan, 1989). Epidural opioids administered through indwelling catheters may have a role to play in the provision of prolonged analgesia but in veterinary practice maintaining asepsis in the management of indwelling epidural catheters can present problems. When they are used by epidural injection care must be taken to ensure that the solution does not contain a preservative, for this may damage nerves.

OPIOID AGONISTS

Morphine

Morphine, the principal alkaloid found in opium (the partially dried latex from the unripe capsule of *Papaver somniferum*) is still the 'gold standard' against which other analgesics are assessed. As the alkaloid itself is insoluble in water, it is supplied as a water soluble salt, usually the sulphate or hydrochloride. Because of its euphoric properties in man it is strongly addictive and its use is, therefore, subject to controls.

Its major properties are those of producing analgesia, respiratory depression and constipation. Small doses have minimal effects on the cardiovascular system but higher doses may cause bradycardia and hypotension in dogs. In these animals histamine release may contribute to its hypotensive action. In horses, hypertension may occur with minimal changes in heart rate (Muir *et al.*, 1978).

Doses of 0.1 to 0.3 mg/kg by intramuscular injection will usually provide good analgesia in most species of animal if they are in pain when the drug is given, but in cats it may be safer to restrict

the dose to 0.1 mg/kg. Excitement reactions, bradycardia and histamine release are more common when the drug is given by the intravenous route and even after intravenous injection analgesia may not become apparent for some 15 minutes.

Papaveretum

The mixture of drugs now marketed as papaveretum contains morphine, papaverine and codeine and is currently available in two strengths. This combination differs from that sold previous to 1993 under the Trade name, 'Omnopon' which also contained a number of other morphine alkaloids. In veterinary anaesthesia, the advantage of 'Omnopon' over morphine alone was that it caused less vomiting in ambulatory dogs. 'Omnopon' was commonly used with hyoscine in the preparation 'Omnopon-Scopolamine', which contained 20 mg of the alkaloids with 0.4 mg of hyoscine ('Scopolamine') per ml. The combination was a time-honoured premedication in medical anaesthesia, and a 1 ml vial of the 'Omnopon-Scopolamine' mixture with 3 mg of acepromazine was useful to sedate and control vicious dogs. The authors have no experience with the current preparation of papaveretum, but it is probable that it will be equally effective as a canine sedative when combined with hyoscine (still available in the UK as Scopolamine) and acepromazine.

Pethidine

Pethidine ('meperidine' in North America) is only 1/10 th as potent as morphine and although its primary actions are typical of agonist opioids it also appears to have atropine-like properties. Unlike morphine, it appears to relax intestinal spasm and so is particularly useful in equine spasmodic colic. It rarely, if ever, causes vomiting in dogs or cats and has little effect on the cough reflex. Doses given by i.m. injection have little effect on arterial blood pressure but pethidine is a potent histamine liberator and because of this its i.v. injection can result in severe hypotension in dogs.

In large animals doses of 1 mg/kg by i.m. injection and in dogs 1–2 mg/kg produce generally satisfactory analgesia. In cats i.m. doses of 10–20 mg per cat may be given. Pethidine appears to have a short half life in animals (Alexander & Collett, 1974; Kalthum & Waterman, 1988) and these doses only give effective pain relief for 1.5 to 2 hours.

Methadone

Methadone is a synthetic agonist, approximately equipotent to morphine in terms of analgesia, although it produces less sedation in dogs and more ataxia in horses. It is less likely to cause anaphylactoid reactions than is pethidine. It has been widely used in horses at i.v. or i.m. doses of 0.1 mg/kg, higher doses carrying an increased risk of ataxia and excitement. The dose for the dog is generally accepted to be 0.25 mg/kg.

Methadone has frequently been used in dogs and horses as part of sedative/opioid combinations. A preparation used on the Continent of Europe, 'Polamivet', contains 2.5 mg of the laevorotatory isomer together with 0.125 mg of an atropine-like compound, diphenylpiperidonoethylacetamide hydrochloride, per ml of solution and this mixture is widely used in combination with the phenothiazine derivative, propionyl promazine, 'Combelen', for sedation of horses and dogs.

Fentanyl

This drug is about 50 times as potent as morphine. It is a pure agonist capable of producing a high level of analgesia, sufficient to allow surgery (Tobin *et al.*, 1979). Effective following i.v. injection, it is also rapidly absorbed across mucous membranes. Following i.v. injection it is effective in 4–7 minutes and, although claimed to be short acting (15 to 20 minutes) this is largely due to redistribution in the body so that cumulative effects occur with prolonged or high dosages.

The pharmacology of fentanyl in animals has been well described (Tobin *et al.*, 1979; Sanford, 1984). In dogs, rats and primates it produces sedation and myosis, whilst in mice, cats and horses it causes excitement with mydriasis. Horses show a very marked locomotor response, pacing increasing with dosage, yet they show very little ataxia (Tobin *et al.*, 1979). As with all opioid agonists, analgesia is accompanied by respiratory depression and when the drug is used in dogs during

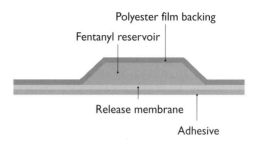

FIG. 4.1 Diagrammatic section through a fentanyl patch (fentanyl transdermal system; Duragesic, Janssen).

general anaesthesia IPPV is usually necessary if the dose used exceeds 0.2 mg/kg. Fentanyl has little effect on the cardiovascular system but usually causes some slowing of the pulse. Occasionally severe bradycardia occurs, necessitating the administration of anticholinergics.

In veterinary practice, fentanyl was initially used as part of neuroleptanalgesic mixtures for dogs (Marsboom & Mortelmans, 1964) but it is now popular in balanced anaesthesia techniques and for postoperative analgesia in intensive care. In man, the use of adequate doses of opioids such as fentanyl has been shown to reduce the stress and catabolic responses to anaesthesia and surgery, and to reduce morbidity. There is some evidence to indicate that a similar reduction in stress response occurs in animal patients given these analgesics during surgery.

A recent development has been the availability of cutaneous patches for the continuous, controlled administration of fentanyl (Fig. 4.1) and although there is still some debate about the best way to employ them they are apparently being used on dogs and cats in the USA. In the UK they are available for use in man (Janssen-Cilag Ltd., Saunderton, High Wycombe, Bucks, HP14 4HJ) and designed to release 25 μg/hour, 50 μg/hour, 75 μg/hour and 100 μg/hour.

They all produce a skin depot of the drug so that fentanyl continues to be absorbed into the circulation for some time after removal of the patch. There was concern that drug abuse might be encouraged by the use of these patches in canine outpatients, however, recommended disposal of the patch after its removal from the skin entails no more than folding it over and discarding into the household trash bin. Their use in animals is not licenced but, in the future, they may make the provision of postoperative analgesia for day case surgery easier to ensure. Egger *et al.*(1998) recommended that because of inter-individual and intra-individual variation in plasma fentanyl concentrations obtained from the use of 50, 75 and 100 µg/hour patches, they should be applied 24 hours before the anticipated time that analgesia will be required.

Alfentanil

This fentanyl derivative is only one-quarter as potent an analgesic as fentanyl itself but has the advantage of being rapidly effective (1 to 2 minutes following i.v. injection). It has been claimed to be shorter acting although studies of its pharmacokinetics in dogs throw some doubt on this since it has been shown to be more cumulative following repeated doses. Alfentanil plasma levels decay triphasically in dogs ($t_{1/2}\beta = 104$ minutes), and less than 1% of the drug is excreted unchanged as alfentanil, metabolism into a large number of inactive metabolites being rapid (Heykants *et al.*, 1982). Analgesia is accompanied by respiratory depression and very severe bradycardia may occur (Arndt *et al.*, 1986).

In dogs alfentanil may be used to reduce the induction dose of an i.v. anaesthetic although this may entail production of several minutes of apnoea. For example, mixing 10 µg/kg of alfentanil with 0.3 or 0.6 mg of atropine and injecting this mixture some 30 seconds before injecting propofol can reduce the dose of propofol needed to induce anaesthesia to less than 2 mg/kg, but apnoea of up to three minutes duration may occur (Chambers, 1989). Similar results follow when alfentanil at this dose is used prior to the injection of thiopental. However, with these i.v. anaesthetics apnoea is not nearly so prolonged when the alfentanil dose is reduced to 5 µg/kg, while there is still a desirable reduction in the dose of anaesthetic needed to allow endotracheal intubation. Alfentanil is now often used in intermittent doses to provide an 'analgesic element' in anaesthetized dogs about to be subjected to intense surgical stimulation but in spontaneously breathing animals the individual doses should not exceed 5 µg/kg if there are no facilities for prolonged IPPV of the lungs.

In Munich, Erhardt has used etomidate/alfentanil (Erhardt, 1984; Erhardt *et al.*; 1985, 1985a) to

produce short periods of anaesthesia followed by a rapid recovery in a wide range of species.

Remifentanil

Remifentanil is a fentanyl derivative with an ester linkage which is rapidly broken down by non-specific tissue and plasma esterases and is responsible for its unique characteristics. It is a pure µ agonist (James *et al.*, 1991) and the EEG effects of remifentanil are similar to those of other opioids in dogs (Hoffman *et al.*, 1993). Clearance is unlikely to be dependent on renal or hepatic function and because *in vitro* it is a poor substrate for butyrylcholinesterases (pseudocholinesterases), its clearance should be unaffected by cholinesterase deficiency induced by anticholinesterase flea collars. Currently, remifentanil is formulated in glycine, an inhibitory neurotransmitter, and consequently it should not be given by spinal or extradural injection.

Rapid biotransformation to minimally active metabolites should be associated with a short, predictable duration of action with no accumulation of effect on repeated dosing or with continuous infusion. Its effects are antagonized by naloxone and its potency is similar to that of fentanyl, and 15 to 30 times that of alfentanil. Bolus i.v. injection is said to cause a reduction of about 20% in mean arterial blood pressure and heart rate, but more detailed haemodynamic investigations are awaited. Recovery from remifentanil anaesthesia is said to be much more rapid than for any other opioid studied to date, especially after continuous infusions maintained for six or more hours (Michelsen *et al.*, 1996).

To date there are no reports of the clinical use of remifentanil in veterinary practice. It may be that it will be used widely (perhaps in place of nitrous oxide during general anaesthesia) because of its predictability, short duration of action and easily reversible effects, but its exact niche in veterinary anaesthesia remains to be seen.

Other fentanyl derivatives

Sufentanil, lofentanil and carfentanil

Sufentanil is approximately 10 times as potent as fentanyl, while lofentanil has a very potent and exceptionally long lasting effect. Neither of these drugs has been used extensively in veterinary medicine. Carfentanil is one of the most potent opioids known. It is said to be 3–8 times as potent as etorphine and has proved to be useful in elephants (Bengis *et al.*, 1985), although at the concentrations used it is a dangerous drug to handle since it is rapidly absorbed across mucous membranes. An antagonist drug suitable for use in humans should be readily available whenever carfentanil is used.

Etorphine

Etorphine is a very potent derivative of morphine which is claimed to be effective in a dose of about 0.5 mg per 500 kg. It appears to have all the properties of morphine but equipotent doses cause more respiratory depression. Its very great potency constitutes its sole advantage in that an effective dose for a very large animal can be dissolved in a small volume of solvent, enabling it to be used in dart gun projectiles for immoblizing wild game animals. In anaesthetic practice this very same potency makes it a difficult drug to handle and constitutes a hazard to the anaesthetist.

Etorphine is an extremely long acting compound and recovery from its effects is also delayed by enterohepatic recycling. Its action is usually terminated by the use of diprenorphine, a specific antagonist, but relapse into deep sedation may occur. The drug has the highly undesirable property of producing stimulation of the central nervous system before depressing it and this results in a period of excitement. In an attempt to overcome this, etorphine is marketed in fixed ratio combinations with phenothizine tranquillizers ('Large Animal Immobilon' with acepromazine and 'Small Animal Immobilon' with methotrimeprazine). Should accidental self-administration occur, death can result if the antidote is not readily available.

Buprenorphine

Buprenorphine is a partial agonist that is popular as a premedicant and postoperative analgesic in cats, dogs and laboratory animal where it is used by the i.v., i.m. and s.c. routes. Although in man it is given in the form of a sublingual tablet, sublingual absorption is difficult to achieve in animals and oral administration is ineffective as the drug is broken down during first pass through the liver.

This drug is unusual in that its association and dissociation with receptors is very slow. Thus, even after i.v. injection it has a prolonged onset of action (30 minutes or longer), a fact often forgotten in its use. Its long duration of action (known to be about eight hours in man) is due to its slow dissociation from receptors and analgesia remains long after it can no longer be detected in the blood by most assay methods. This tight binding to receptors means that its actions are very difficult to reverse with naloxone, although pretreatment with naloxone will prevent its effects. Should respiratory depression result from the use of buprenorphine it should be treated with IPPV of the lungs, or with non-specific respiratory stimulants such as doxapram.

The analgesic dose–response curve is bell-shaped, higher doses antagonizing analgesia already produced by lower doses but higher doses do not antagonize the respiratory depression once this has reached a plateau. In the authors' experience serious respiratory depression is rare with the usual clinical doses but as its onset may be delayed, when it does occur, it is important that any animal given the drug remains under close observation for at least two hours after its administration. On its own, in clinical doses, it does not appear to cause sedation, or to cause excitement in susceptible species of animal, but its use towards the end of surgery slows recovery from anaesthesia. Its effects on the cardiovascular system are minimal.

Doses used in dogs and cats vary from 6 to 10 µg/kg and in horses the authors have found it an effective analgesic at doses of 6 µg/kg for orthopaedic cases. However, the bell-shaped nature of the dose–response curve must be considered and if these doses are inadequate for pain relief, they may be followed by doses of a pure agonist drug. Buprenorphine has also been extensively used with α_2 adrenoceptor agonists in sedative combinations.

The popularity of the drug in the UK has undoubtedly been due to its prolonged length of action, that it provides better analgesia than can be obtained with other partial agonists and, until recently, its freedom from control under the Misuse of Drugs Act 1971.

Butorphanol

In the UK this drug is currently not subject to controls under the Misuse of Drugs Act 1971. It is used in cats, dogs and horses for analgesia and in sedative combinations with α_2 adrenoceptor agonists. Butorphanol is also used in dogs for its antitussive effect. In dogs and horses it is said to have minimal effects on the cardiovascular system (Trim, 1983; Robertson *et al.*, 1981) but caution may be in order here for in man it causes increased pulmonary vascular resistance and, at high doses, hypertension, so it is not recommended for patients with cardiovascular disease.

In experimental horses it has been used in doses of 0.1 to 0.4 mg/kg but the higher doses caused restlessness and apparent dysphoria (Kalpravidh *et al.*, 1984) and the dose currently used clinically is 0.02 to 0.1 mg/kg by i.v. injection, which seems to be particularly effective for the relief of mild colic. However, in the authors' experience even this dose may induce walking behaviour in unrestrained animals.

Doses of 0.1 to 0.5 mg/kg by i.m. or s.c. injection have been found to give effective analgesia for up to four hours in both dogs and cats (Paddleford, 1988). In experimental studies visceral analgesia was found to be superior to somatic analgesia, and lower doses superior to higher doses, possibly indicating that, like buprenorphine, the dose–response curve is bell shaped. Butorphanol may be given orally for analgesia although doses 5–10 times those by injection are required to produce an equivalent effect.

Pentazocine

In man this partial agonist has lost its earlier popularity due to producing a high incidence of dysphoria and hallucinatory responses, coupled with causing a marked increase in pulmonary vascular resistance. Moreover, because of its abuse potential, in the UK it is controlled under the Misuse of Drugs Act 1971. Although it is impossible to assess dysphoria in animals most veterinarians with

extensive experience of pentazocine have seen signs they associate with such an effect, particularly following high doses.

Despite these problems pentazocine has been quite widely used in veterinary practice, doses of 1 to 3 mg/kg being said give to three hours of pain relief (Taylor & Houlton, 1984; Sawyer & Rech, 1987; Paddleford, 1988). Pentazocine can be given orally but first pass liver metabolism means that high doses are necessary. In the experimental horse colic model doses of 0.5 to 4.0 mg/kg have been tested, the higher doses giving rise to ataxia and muscle tremors. The recommended dose for the relief of colic pains in horses is 0.33 mg/kg i.v., followed 15 minutes later by a similar i.m. dose.

Nalbuphine

Although this drug has minimal cardiovascular effects and appears to cause few dysphoric reactions, it has a low ceiling of analgesia and is not recommended for relief of severe pain. In experimental dogs it has been found that doses of 0.75 mg/kg give reasonable visceral analgesia; somatic analgesia is poor and analgesia is always inferior to that provided by butorphanol. As part of a sedative combination for use in horses, in the doses employed for this, nalbuphine alone produces no discernible unwanted effects in pain-free horses.

SEQUENTIAL ANALGESIA

Sequential analgesia is a term introduced to describe the use of partial agonists subsequent to pure agonists (usually fentanyl) in an attempt to reverse residual respiratory depression whilst maintaining analgesia. First attempted with pentazocine, buprenorphine, butorphanol and nalbuphine have also been used for this purpose (Mitchell & Smith, 1989). On theoretical grounds buprenorphine should be the least efficient and nalbuphine the most because of their μ agonist and antagonist properties (Table 4.2), and nalbuphine has been widely recommended for use in man for this purpose. In laboratory practice, buprenorphine has been used to reverse the effects of high dose fentanyl (Flecknell, *et al.*, 1989).

The idea of agonist/antagonist analgesia is not new for many years ago a combination of pethidine together with its antagonist levallorphan was marketed, but was found to produce no less respiratory depression than pethidine alone at equianalgesic doses. It is clear that the final outcome of sequential analgesia must be the result of a delicate balance of activities at the various receptors and the 'reversing' drugs must be given with great care according to the need of the individual patient.

OPIOID ANTAGONISTS

Pure antagonists

Naloxone

Naloxone is a pure antagonist at all opioid receptors and so will reverse the effect of all opioid agonists but it is less effective against partial agonists. In man, reversal of opioid actions with naloxone is sometimes accompanied by tachycardia but there are no reports of this in the veterinary literature. The drug is fairly short acting and its effects may wear off before those of the previously administered agonist so that repeated doses may be needed. This is particularly important in veterinary medicine where large and frequent doses of naloxone are necessary to counter the accidental self-administration of the potent long acting agent, etorphine.

Naloxone given to an animal that has not received an opioid may temporarily alter its behaviour and it has been claimed that it is effective in stopping horses crib-biting (Booth, 1988). Naloxone is thought by some to have a role in the treatment of shock (Booth, 1988).

Naltrexone

Naltrexone is a long acting derivative of naloxone and although not apparently often used in veterinary practice it could prove useful should a long acting pure antagonist be required.

Partial agonists used as antagonists

Some partial agonists, which either give poor analgesia or produce dysphoria sufficient to preclude their use as analgesics, are used *for* their antagonistic properties. Nalorphine was the first to be used as an opioid antagonist but has now been superseded by naloxone. Diprenorphine is marketed as a specific antagonist of etorphine and in animals it appears to be very efficient in this role. However as it causes hallucinations in man it is only licensed for use in animals and in medical practice naloxone remains the drug of choice for countering the effects of etorphine.

SEDATIVE–OPIOID COMBINATIONS

When opioids are combined with sedative drugs, synergism seems to occur, sedation and analgesia being greater than that capable of being achieved by either drug alone. The use of the sedative will often also prevent any excitement effects that might occur with the opioid alone. There is nothing new about the use of such combinations, veterinarians having used them for many years to make animals more manageable (Amadon & Craige, 1936). The range of sedative/opioid mixtures in use for sedation and control of animals is now enormous, α_2 adrenoceptor agonists, neuroleptic agents and benzodiazepines all having been combined with a wide variety of agonist and partial agonist opioids. Depth of sedation achieved depends primarily on the opioid employed, partial agonists or less potent agonist combinations producing sedation whereas large doses of potent opioids such as fentanyl or alfentanil can achieve anaesthesia. Unfortunately, severe respiratory depression may accompany the use of these high dose opioid techniques. Suitable combinations for sedation, control and anaesthesia in each species of animal are given in later chapters of this book.

The term neuroleptanalgesia has been used to describe the combination of opioids with phenothiazines or butyrophenones (neuroleptics). The principles of their use are the same as outlined above for any sedative/opioid combination but the neuroleptic agents have the specific property of reducing opioid-induced vomiting in dogs. Neuroleptic techniques can be used in two ways. At comparatively low opioid dose rates they can be used for control, or as premedication before general anaesthesia; at higher dose rates they can

TABLE 4.4 Composition of some commercially available neuroleptanalgesic mixtures

Commercial name	Analgesic	Neuroleptic
Thalamonal	Fentanyl 0.05 mg/ml	Droperidol 20 mg/ml
Hypnorm	Fentanyl 0.315 mg/kg	Fluanisone 10 mg/ml
Immobilon SA	Etorphine 0.074 mg/ml	Methotrimeprazine 18 mg/ml
Immobilon LA	Etorphine 2.45 mg/ml	Acepromazine 10 mg/ml

be used to produce sufficient depression of the central nervous system to enable surgery to be performed. This latter use is sometimes termed 'neuroleptanaesthesia' and was the way in which the technique was first used in veterinary medicine (Marsboom & Mortelmans, 1964), but it is associated with profound respiratory depression and should not be used unless facilities for respiratory support are available.

To obtain the best results the neuroleptic should be administered first and, when it is fully effective, the analgesic should be given to produce the desired result. In veterinary medicine, however, for convenience it is usual to employ commercially available fixed ratios of the two drugs and it must be accepted that this ratio may not be optimal for any particular animal.

The composition of commercially available mixtures of fentanyl/butyrophenone tranquillizer are given in Table 4.4. All have similar properties and may be considered together. They are used in dogs, primates and rodents, but they are contraindicated in cats because fentanyl may cause violent excitement in these animals. They are usually used to produce deep sedation with profound analgesia sufficient for procedures such as endoscopy, or the lancing of a superficial abscess, but are inadequate for major surgery. The rationale for using the short acting fentanyl with long acting butyrophenones is not obvious, but the combination appears effective.

Fentanyl has been used with fluanisone for neuroleptanalgesia in a 1:50 mixture (Fluanisone Comp.). Given at a dosage level of 0.1 mg/kg of fentanyl with 5 mg/kg of fluanisone by slow i.v. injection it produced a short period of anaesthesia after short and mild excitement. Recovery was slow, the time varying from 2 to 10 hours before recovery to full consciousness. Respiratory effects are variable, with both hyperpnoea and respiratory depression occurring. The advantages of the mixture include ease of administration, wide safety margin, quiet postoperative state, reversibility with narcotic antagonists (such as naloxone), and tolerance by animals in poor physical condition. Disadvantages include variable response in certain breeds, the spontaneous movements which occur, the need to employ nitrous oxide or local analgesia when major surgery is to be performed, and the possibility of respiratory depression.

Fentanyl has also been used in the UK in combination with fluanisone, as the preparation 'Hypnorm'. Diarrhoea has been reported to follow the administration of this mixture in over 24% of canine patients.

The effects of fentanyl with fluanisone and fentanyl with droperidol in pigs have been studied but neither mixture produced better sedation than droperidol alone.

The results obtained by neuroleptanalgesic techniques are more impressive in monkeys. In these animals the technique may offer distinct advantages over the more conventional methods of anaesthesia especially when skilled assistance is not available.

'IMMOBILON'

'Immobilon' is marketed for both small and large animal use, the concentrations of etorphine and the tranquillizer in each preparation being as shown in Table 4.4. At the doses recommended by the manufacturers the preparations cause intense central nervous depression with considerable analgesia, allowing major surgery to be carried out. When surgery is completed it was recommended that the effects of the etorphine (but not of the phenothiazine tranquillizer) be reversed by the use of the specific antagonist ('Revivon'). LA Revivon contains 3.0 mg/ml and SM Revivon 0.272 mg/ml of diprenorphine.

The effects of 'Immobilon' in horses are what might be expected to follow such high doses of an opiate drug in this species of animal. Intramuscular injection regularly leads to excitement during induction; after i.v. injection the horse becomes recumbent within one minute and although excitement may occur it is much less marked. Once recumbent, intense muscular activity makes the animal very stiff and violent continuous tremors occur. The muscles relax somewhat after about 20 minutes. Blood pressure and heart rate increase to very high levels but respiration is severely depressed. Following the i.v. injection of 'Revivon' most horses regain the standing position within a few minutes. Occasionally, horses become excited shortly after standing and a further excitement phase may occur several hours later due to enterohepatic recycling of the etorphine. The disadvantages associated with the use of 'Immobilon' in domestic animals far outweigh the advantages.

'Immobilon' and other etorphine-containing mixtures have been extensively used for the capture of wild game. Although generally used as 'knockdown' doses, as in horses, they are also commonly used at lower dose rates whereby the animals (elephants and giraffes) became sedated but remain standing. 'Immobilon' is not recommended for wild felidae (nor domestic cats!).

In man etorphine is extremely potent and the use of 'Immobilon' constitutes a danger to the anaesthetist and assistants. Should an accident occur, naloxone is recommended as the drug of choice for treatment of human beings, but several doses may be needed to maintain respiration until medical help can be obtained.

ANTICHOLINERGIC AGENTS

Anticholinergic agents are widely used in anaesthesia to antagonize the muscarinic effects of acetylcholine and thus to block transmission at parasympathetic postganglionic nerve endings. The main purposes are:

1. To reduce salivation and bronchial secretions
2. To block the effects of impulses in the vagus nerves
3. To block certain of the effects produced by drugs which stimulate the parasympathetic system.

The reduction of salivation and bronchial secretion is necessary if irritant volatile anaesthetics such as ether are used, but it is not essential with modern halogenated anaesthetics like halothane and isoflurane. However, in small dogs and in cats, even a little secretion may be enough to give rise to significant respiratory obstruction and in such small patients it is arguably advisable to administer anticholinergics before any anaesthetic. Ruminants produce large quantities of saliva but anticholinergic drugs merely make their saliva more viscid and thick and more likely to create respiratory obstruction, so these drugs should not be used.

Some drugs, in particular the α_2 adrenoceptor agonists and, in high doses, the opioids, can cause marked vagus-mediated bradycardia. Also, under light anaesthesia, surgery of the head and neck is prone to trigger vagal reflexes, and the horse, dog and cat seem to be most at risk from these disturbances. In cats the oculocardiac reflex is well known to result in bradycardia and even cardiac arrest; stimulation of the nose or other similarly sensitive structures can have the same effect or cause laryngospasm. In horses, stimulation about the head and neck can produce sudden cardiac arrest without a prior warning of bradycardia.

Anticholinesterase drugs such as neostigmine are used to antagonize the block produced by competitive neuromuscular blocking drugs and their use must be preceded or combined with one of the anticholinergic drugs to block the muscarinic effects of the released acetylcholine. Also, the depolarizing agent suxamethonium has effects similar to those of acetylcholine and, at least in dogs and cats, an anticholinergic 'cover' should be employed when this relaxant is used.

In recent years the advisability of routine premedication with anticholinergic drugs has been questioned. These drugs certainly have side effects and the tachycardia they induce may be undesirable when it reduces stroke volume or cardiac output. Disturbance of vision may cause a cat or horse to panic. Reduced gut motility may cause colic in horses. In man, considerable discomfort results from dry mouth in the postoperative period and, presumably, this may also be the case in animals. These disadvantages must be weighed against the advantages already mentioned.

Current practice, where ether is not to be used, seems to be not to use anticholinergic drugs for routine premedication, but to reserve them for corrective measures should bradycardia occur during the course of the anaesthetic. This, of course, assumes that monitoring is adequate to detect the bradycardia. However, it must be remembered that following i.v. injection atropine may cause further bradycardia through a central effect before blocking at the vagal endings and increasing the heart rate. Thus, it can be argued that in dogs, cats and pigs the i.m. use of atropine before induction of anaesthesia is preferable to waiting for bradycardia and heart block to appear during the course of anaesthesia and correction by i.v. administration. The use of i.v. atropine or glycopyrrolate to correct some drug-induced bradycardias has been shown to be associated with further bradycardia and heart block (Richards *et al.*, 1989). Thus, the decision to include an anticholinergic agent in premedication may be based on the species of animal concerned, its size, the drugs to be used for and during anaesthesia, the likelihood of complications from bradycardia or vagal reflexes, the level of monitoring in use and any specific contraindications. The main contraindications are in conditions associated with tachycardia and in certain forms of glaucoma which are aggravated by dilatation of the pupil.

Atropine

Atropine, the most important of the alkaloids obtained from *Atropa belladonna* (deadly nightshade), is used in anaesthesia as its water-soluble sulphate. Its metabolism is not the same in all species of animal. When administered to dogs, atropine disappears very rapidly from the bloodstream. Part of the dose is excreted unchanged in the urine, part appears in the urine as tropine and the remainder is apparently broken down in the body to as yet unidentified substances. In cats, atropine is hydrolyzed by either of two esterases which are found in large quantities in the liver and kidneys. These esterases are also found in rabbits and rats.

Atropine inhibits transmission of postganglionic cholinergic nerve impulses to effector cells but inhibition is not equally effective all over the body and atropine has less effect upon the urinary bladder and intestines than upon the heart and salivary glands.

The drug has unpredictable effects on the central nervous system. Certain cerebral and medullary functions are initially stimulated then later depressed, so that the final outcome depends on the dose used and the route of administration. Clinical doses may produce an initial slowing of the heart due to stimulation of vagal centres in the brain before its peripheral anticholinergic effects occur. Atropine overdose causes a 'central cholinergic effect' with fluctuations between hyperexcitability and depression. Although atropine is, in general, a very safe drug with a wide therapeutic margin, occasional cases have been reported where an individual person or animal has appeared unduly sensitive to the central effects.

The main action of the drug is on the heart rate, which usually increases due to peripheral inhibition of the cardiac vagus: the initial slowing due to central action is only seen before the onset of peripheral inhibition. Arterial blood pressure is usually unchanged, but if already depressed by vagal activity due to reflex or drug action (e.g. halothane) it will be raised by the administration of atropine. In man, an increase in the incidence of cardiac arrythmias has been observed during anaesthesia following atropine premedication, but K. W. Clarke (unpublished observations) found that atropine reduced the incidence of ventricular extrasystoles in cats anaesthetized with a variety of halogenated volatile anaesthetics. Cardiac arrhythmias (e.g. bigeminy) in dogs previously attributed to atropine were probably due to barbiturates and are often seen in the absence of atropine.

The minute volume of respiration is slightly increased due to central stimulation. Bronchial musculature is relaxed and bronchial secretions are reduced. Both anatomical and physiological dead space are increased by atropine (Nunn & Bergman, 1964). Studies in dogs at the Cambridge Veterinary School and elsewhere have not shown any hypoxaemia attributable to atropine administration.

Atropine has marked ocular effects. Mydriasis results from the local or systemic administration of atropine. Except in dogs, where the parenteral administration of clinical doses of atropine does not alter pupillary size, the mydriasis may interfere with the so-called 'ocular signs' of anaesthesia. The ocular effects also result in visual disturbances and animals so effected must be approached with great caution as they may have problems in judging distances. This is particularly important in horses and cats as both these animals tend to panic in response to sudden movements which they do not see clearly.

Although atropine reduces muscle tone in the gastrointestinal tract, at the doses used for premedication this effect is minimal. The passage of barium meals along the gut of the dog is not appreciably slowed by atropine premedication but it is possible that the incidence of postanaesthetic colic in horses is increased by the use of this drug.

Because of the different ways in which they metabolize the drug, the effectiveness of a given dose varies according to the species of animal but its therapeutic index is such that a wide range of doses can be recommended. In dogs, doses from 0.02 to 0.05 mg/kg are employed, while in cats doses of up to 0.3 mg (approximately 0.1 mg/kg for an adult cat for example) are perfectly safe. Pigs may be given 0.3 to 1.8 mg according to size. The exact dose is largely determined by the fact that, at least in the UK, atropine sulphate for injection is still supplied in a solution of 0.6 mg/ml – a legacy of earlier days when doses were measured in grains. A large animal preparation containing 10 mg/ml is now available, and this enables horses to be given doses between 10 and 60 mg much more conveniently than was previously possible.

To neutralize the muscarinic effects of anticholinesterases such as neostigmine, in cats, dogs and pigs 0.6 to 1.2 mg of atropine are given slowly i.v. 2 to 5 minutes before these agents are injected, or else mixed in the syringe and injected with the anticholinesterase. In horses doses of 10 mg appear to be adequate for this purpose.

Glycopyrrolate

Glycopyrrolate is a quaternary ammonium anticholinergic agent with powerful and prolonged anti-sialagogue activity. As an anti-sialagogue it is about five times as potent as atropine. In man, clinical doses have an almost selective effect on salivary and sweat gland secretion. Cardiovascular stability is excellent, there being little change in heart rate, and there is a reduction in cardiac arrhythmias compared with their incidence after atropine. This cardiovascular stability was thought to make it particularly useful for combination with anticholinesterases for antagonizing the effects of non-depolarizing neuromuscular blocking agents and, indeed, as glycopyrrolate is claimed to have a more rapid onset of action than atropine, a preparation of neostigmine with glycopyrrolate is available for this purpose. However, work on anaesthetized human patients showed no difference in the cardiovascular effects of atropine and glycopyrrolate other than in the time of onset of action – glycopyrrolate taking 2 to 3 minutes to become effective following i.v. injection (Short & Miller, 1978).

Glycopyrrolate has now been used widely in veterinary practice in doses of 0.01 to 0.02 mg/kg (Short et al., 1974). However, although it has been satisfactory in preventing excessive salivation and bradycardia, it has proved disappointingly similar to atropine in its effects on the heart rate (Richards et al., 1989). A comparison of atropine given i.v. at doses of 0.02 to 0.04 mg/kg with i.v. glycopyrrolate (0.02 and 0.01 mg/kg) in dogs with drug-induced bradycardia showed that both agents caused a high incidence of cardiac arrhythmia, including atrioventricular block, during the first three minutes after injection. This is surprising since glycopyrrolate does not readily cross the blood–brain barrier and suggests that arrhythmias may be due to mechanisms other than central stimulation.

The fact that the drug does not readily cross the blood–brain barrier means that it has little central action, producing less effect on vision than other anticholinergic agents and thus it could be the anticholinergic of choice in horses and cats.

Hyoscine

Hyoscine is an alkaloid resembling atropine, found in the same group of plants but usually obtained from the shrub henbane (*Hyoscyamus niger*). The peripheral actions of hyoscine resemble those of atropine. However, its relative potency at different sites differs from atropine. It is a more potent anti-sialagogue but less effective as a vagolytic so that its effect on heart rate is less than that of atropine when they are given in equipotent doses for their drying effects. The central effects of hyoscine are greater than those of atropine and in horses it may produce considerable excitement. In general, although hyoscine is used in man (in spite of its propensity to cause hallucination) as a depressant of nervous activity, it is not suitable for this purpose in animals. It has been used as the hydrobromide for premedication in dogs in doses of 0.2 to 0.4 mg and it is often used with paraveretum.

PREMEDICATION

Preanaesthetic medication or 'premedication' helps both the anaesthetist and the animal, for it makes induction and maintenance of anaesthesia easier for the anaesthetist while at the same time rendering the experience safer and more comfortable for the patient. It implies the administration, usually before, but sometimes at or immediately after, the induction of anaesthesia, of sedatives, anxiolytics and analgesics, with or without anticholinergics.

The classic aims of premedication are :

1. To relieve anxiety thus apprehension, fear and resistance to anaesthesia.
2. To counteract unwanted side effects of agents used in anaesthesia. Effects which may require modification depend on the species of animal and on the drugs used; they include vomiting (mainly in dogs and cats), poor quality of recovery, bradycardia, salivation and excessive muscle tone.
3. To reduce the dose of anaesthetic. In many, but not all cases, drug combinations may have a lower incidence of side effects than a high dose of the anaesthetic would have on its own.
4. To provide extra analgesia.

The use of anticholinergic agents for premedication has been discussed in the previous section. Analgesic agents are essential if the patient is in pain in the preoperative period, but even when pain is absent, analgesics may increase preoperative sedation, reduce the dose of anaesthetic needed, contribute to analgesia during surgery and even, if sufficiently long acting, contribute to analgesia postoperatively. The use of long acting analgesics such as buprenorphine is particularly popular for the contribution they make to all stages of the anaesthetic process. Very potent but short acting opioids such as fentanyl and alfentanil will reduce the dose of anaesthetic required, but their short action means that further analgesia must be provided during recovery.

The sedative and anxiolytic drugs play the major role in premedication, improving the quality of anaesthesia and recovery, contributing to anaesthesia and, in some cases counteracting unwanted side effects such as the muscle rigidity produced by ketamine. By calming the animal in the preoperative period, the necessary clipping and cleaning is made more pleasant for both the animal and nursing staff. Moreover, by controlling emotional disturbance the release of catecholamines is reduced, thus decreasing the chance of adrenaline-induced cardiac arrhythmias, smoothing the course of anaesthesia and (usually) ensuring a quiet recovery.

The degree of activity of the central nervous system at the time when anaesthesia is induced determines the amount of anaesthetic which has to be administered to produce surgical anaesthesia. This activity is lowered by wasting disease, senility and surgical shock and increased by pain, fear, fever and conditions such as thyrotoxicosis. Sedatives and analgesics decrease the irritability of the central nervous system and thereby enhance the effects of the anaesthetic agents. In general, the depressant effects of the drugs used in premedication summate with those of the anaesthetic and unless this is clearly understood overdosage may occur. Most sedative drugs depress respiration, and if given in large doses before anaesthetics which also produce respiratory depression (e.g. thiopental sodium or halothane), respiratory failure may occur before surgical anaesthesia is attained. Premedication must, therefore, be regarded as an integral part of the whole anaesthetic technique and never as an isolated event.

The type of sedative drug chosen for premedication will depend on a variety of factors. Phenothiazine derivatives such as acepromazine are good anxiolytics and reduce the incidence of vomiting. Their use usually results in a calm, but delayed, recovery and delayed recovery is usually to be avoided in horses and ruminants for in these animals prolonged recumbency gives rise to problems. To prevent recovery being unacceptably delayed, doses of the phenothiazine derivatives used for premedication should be below those recommended for simply sedating animals when anaesthesia is not contemplated. Phenothiazine drugs undoubtedly increase the chance of regurgitation at induction of general anaesthesia in ruminants.

The α_2 adrenoceptor agonists have a major effect in reducing the dose of subsequent anaesthetic required; doses at the lower end of the dosage range provide profound sedation and are useful in the animal which is particularly difficult to handle. They also provide some degree of muscle relaxation and are especially effective in counteracting the muscle tension associated with the use of drugs such as ketamine.

Benzodiazepines provide little obvious preoperative sedation but their muscle relaxing properties are useful when drugs such as ketamine are to be used and they reduce the dose of subsequent anaesthetic needed.

Often, more than one sedative drug is used in premedication. For example, α_2 adrenoceptor agonists and benzodiazepines may be combined prior to the use of ketamine. However, such polypharmacy must be used with care, as many such combinations have synergistic activity and it is easy to administer an overdose of anaesthetic agents given subsequently.

For premedication, drugs can be given by any one or more of the usual routes of drug administration. The choice is governed both by the nature of the drug to be used and the time which is available before anaesthesia is to be induced. If there is plenty of time the drugs may be given sublingually, by mouth or into the rectum. The rectal route is not very satisfactory and is only used when for some reason the others are impracticable, but the sublingual route is surprisingly effective for the α_2 adrenoceptor agonists, making it possible to subdue vicious animals by using a syringe to squirt the drug into the animal's open mouth. If only 5 to 10 minutes will elapse before anaesthesia is to be induced, then the i.v. route must be employed. It is always as well to ensure that the preliminary medication exerts its full effects before the administration of a general anaesthetic is begun, otherwise respiratory depression and even respiratory failure may occur even during light anaesthesia.

In the past it was fairly simple to define the limits of premedication and when anaesthesia began. Today, with the wide range of different types of drugs available, such distinctions are no longer clear. Neuroleptanalgesic techniques may enable surgery to be carried out without further resort to general anaesthetic agents. Dissociative agents such as ketamine may be regarded as being drugs for premedication or for the induction of general anaesthesia. Hypnotics (e.g. chloral hydrate or pentobarbital sodium) may be used at low doses for sedation, or at higher doses to produce hypnosis or even anaesthesia. In clinical practice, exact definitions of terminology are unimportant as long as the anaesthetist clearly understands the role played by each drug used, be it 'premedicant', 'dissociative agent' or 'anaesthetic', in the total process in bringing the animal to a state suitable for the performance of surgery, examination, or whatever else is required. Anxiolytics, sedatives, hypnotics and analgesics all have their place in this process. In any particular case, the choice of drugs, their dose and route of administration, gives the anaesthetist the opportunity to demonstrate artistry as well as scientific knowledge.

REFERENCES

Aitken, M.M. and Sanford, J. (1972) Comparative assessment of tranquillizers in the horse. *Proceedings of the Association of Veterinary Anaesthetists of Great Britain and Ireland* 3: 20–28.

Alexander, F. and Collet, R.A. (1974) Pethidine in the horse. *Research in Veterinary Science* 17: 136–137.

Amadon, R.S. and Craige, A.H. (1936) Observations on the use of bulbocapnine as a soporific in horses. *Journal of the American Veterinary Medical Association* 41: 737–754.

Arbieter, K., Szekely, H. and Lorin, D. (1972)*Veterinary. Medical Reviews. (Leverkusen)* 3:248.

Arndt, J.O., Bednarski, B. and Parasher, C. (1986) Alfentanil's analgesic, respiratory and cardiovascular actions in relation to dose and plasma concentration in unanesthetized dogs. *Anesthesiology* 64 (3):345.

Averill, D.R. (1970) Treatment of status epilepticus in dogs with diazepam sodium. *Journal of the American Veterinary Medical Association* 56: 432–434.

Bengis, R.G., de Vos, V. and van Niekerk, J. (1985) Immobilisation of the African Elephant. *Proceedings of the 2nd International Congress of Veterinary Anaesthesia*: 142–143.

Bloom, F.E. (1996) Neurotransmission and the central nervous system. Chapter 12 in the Pharmacological basis of Therapeutics. (Eds) Hardman, J.G. and Limind, L.E. New York, McGraw-Hill.

Booth, N.H. (1988) *Veterinary Pharmacology and Therapeutics*, 6th edn. Ames: Iowa University Press, ch. 15.

Brouwer, G.J., Hall, L.W. and Kutchel, T.R. (1980) Intravenous anaesthesia in horses after xylazine premedication. *Veterinary Record* **107** (11): 241–245.

Butera, T.S., Moore, J.N., Garner, H.E., Amend, J.F., Clarke, L.L. and Hatfield, D.G. (1978) Diazepam/xylazine combination for short-term anesthesia in the horse. *Veterinary Medicine/Small. Animal Clinician* **73** (4):490–499.

Bylund, D.B. (1988) Subtypes of alpha-2 adrenoceptors: pharmacological and molecular biological evidence converge. *Trends in Pharmacological Sciences* **9** (10): 356–361.

Chambers, J.P. (1989) Induction of anaesthesia in dogs with alfentanil and propofol. *Journal of the Association of Veterinary Anaesthetists of Great Britain and & Ireland* **16**: 14.

Chambers, J.P. and Dobson, J.M. (1989) A midazolam and ketamine combination as a sedative in cats. *Journal of the Association of Veterinary Anaesthetists of Great Britain and Ireland* **16**: 53–54.

Chambers, J.P., Waterman, A.E., Livingston, A. and Goodship, A.E. (1996) Prolonged action of detomidine in Thoroughbred horses with abnormal liver function. *Journal of the Association of Veterinary Anaesthetists of Great Britain and Ireland* **23**: 27–28.

Chism, J.P. and Rickert, D.E. (1996) The pharmacokinetics and exra-hepatic clearance of remifentanil, a short acting opioid agonist, in male beagle dogs during constant rate infusions. *Drug Metabolism and Disposition*, **24**(1): 34–40.

Christiansen, G. (1980) The toxicity of selected therapeutic agents used in cats. *Veterinary Medicine and Small Animal Clinician* **75**: 1133–1137.

Clarke, K.W. (1969) Effects of azaperone on the blood pressure and pulmonary ventilation in pigs. *Veterinary Record* **85**: 649–651.

Clarke, K.W. (1988) Clinical pharmacology of detomidine in the horse. Academic dissertation. London: University of London.

Clarke, K.W. and England, G.C.W.(1988) Behavioural effects of medetomidine/opioid combinations in the dog. *Advances in Veterinary Anaesthesia (Brisbane)*: 104–114.

Clarke, K.W. and England, G.C.W. (1989) Medetomidine, a new sedative-analgesic for use in the dog and its reversal with atipamezole. *Journal of Small Animal Practice* **30**: 343–348.

Clarke, K.W., England, G.C.W. and Goosens, L. (1991.) Sedative and cardiovascular effects of romifidine alone and in combination with butorphanol in the horse. *Journal of Veterinary Anaesthesia* **18**: 25–29.

Clarke, K.W. and Hall, L.W. (1969) Xylazine – a new sedative for horses and cattle. *Veterinary Record* **85** (19): 512–517.

Clarke, K.W. and Paton, B.S. (1988) Combined use of detomidine with opiates in the horse. *Equine Veterinary Journal* **20**(5): 331–334.

Clarke, K.W. and Taylor, P.M. (1985) Detomidine as a premedicant in the horse. *Journal of the Association of Veterinary Anaesthetists* **14**: 29–32.

Clarke, K.W. and Taylor, P.M. (1987) Detomidine: a new sedative for horses. *Equine Veterinary Journal* **18**: 366–370.

Clarke, K.W., Taylor, P.M. and Watkins, S.B. (1986) Detomidine/ketamine anaesthesia in the horse. *Acta Veterinaria Scandinavica* **82**: 167–179.

Cullen, L.K. (1996) Medetomidine sedation in dogs and cats: a review of its pharmacology, antagonism and dose. *British Veterinary Journal* **152**: 519–535.

Cullen, L.K., Reynoldson, J.A. (1993) Xylazine or medetomidine premedication before propofol anaesthesia. *Veterinary Record* **132**: 378–383.

Davis, L.E., Donnelly, E.J. (1968) Analgesic drugs in the cat. *Journal of the American Veterinary Medical Association* **153**: 1161–1167.

DeMoor, A. and Desmet, P. (1971) *Veterinary Medicine Reviews (Leverkusen)*: 163.

Doble, A. and Martin, A. (1992) Multiple benzodiazepine receptors – no reason for anxiety. *Trends in Pharmacological Science* **13** (2): 76–81.

Docherty, T.J., Ballinger, J.A., McDonell, W.N., Pascoe, P.J. and Valliant, A.E. (1987) Antagonism of xylazine induced sedation by idazoxan in calves. *Canadian Journal of Veterinary Research* **51**: 244.

Dodman, N.H. and Waterman, A.E. (1979) Paradoxical excitement following the intravenous administration of azaperone in the horse. *Equine Veterinary Journal* **11**: 33–35.

Dresel, P.E. (1985) Cardiac alpha receptors and arrhythmias. *Anesthesiology* **63**: 582–583.

Dundee, J.W. and Wyant, G.M. (1989) *Intravenous Anaesthesia*. Edinburgh: Churchill Livingstone.

Dunkle, N., Moise, N.J., Scarlettg-Kranz, J. and Short, C.E. (1986) Cardiac performance in cats after administration of xylazine or xylazine + glycopyrrolate: echocardiographic evaluations. *American Journal of Veterinary Research*. **47**: 2212–2216.

Egger, C.M., Duke, T, Archer, J. and Cribb, P.H. (1998) Comparison of plasma fentanyl concentrations by using three transdermal fentanyl patch sizes in dogs. *Veterinary Surgery*, **27**(2): 159–166.

Eisenach, J.C. (1988) Intravenous clonidine produces hypoxia by a peripheral alpha-2 adrenergic mechanism. *Journal of Pharmacology and Experimental Therapeutics* **244**: 247–252.

England, G.C.W., Clarke, K.W. and Goossens, L. (1992). A comparison of the sedative effect of three alpha 2 adrenoceptor agonists, romifidine, detomidine and xylazine, in the horse. *Journal of Veterinary Pharmacology and Therapeutics* 15: 194–201.

Erhardt, W. (1984) Anesthesia procedures in the rabbit. *Tierarztl Prax* 12: 391–402.

Erhardt, W. (1984) *Proceedings of the 15th Congress of European Society of Veterinary Surgery.* p. 11.

Erhardt, W., Kostlin, R., Seiler, R., Tonzer, G., Tielebier-Langenscheidt, B., Limmer, R., Pfeiffer, U., Blumel, G. (1985) Respiratory functional hypoxia in ruminants under general anesthesia *Tierarztl Prax* **Suppl 1**: 45–49.

Erhardt, W., Seiler, R., Riedl, V., Aschenbrenner, G., Blumel, G (1985a) Ultrashort hypnoanalgesia with alfentanyl and etomidate in the dog–circulatory and respiratory studies *Berl Munch Tierarztl Wochenschr* **98**: 413–417.

Erhardt, W., Stephen, M., Schatzmann, U. *et al.* (1986) Reversal of anaesthesia by simultaneously administered benzodiazepine and opioid antagonists in the dog. *Journal of the Association of Veterinary Anaesthetists* 14: 90–99.

Flecknell, P.A., Liles, J.H., Wootton, R. (1989) Reversal of fentanyl/fluanisone neuroleptanalgesia in the rabbit using mixed agonist/antagonist opioids. *Laboratory Animal Science* 23: 147–155.

Garner, H.E., Amend, J.F. and Rosborough, J.P. (1971.) Effects of Bay Va 1470 on cardiovascular parameters in ponies. *Veterinary Medicine and Small Animal Clinician* **66**: 1016–1021.

Gasthuys, F., Martens, A., Goosens, L. and De Moor, A. A. (1996) Quantitative and qualitative study of the diuretic effects of romifidine in the horse. *Journal of Veterinary Anaesthesia.* 23(1): 6–10.

Glen, J.B. (1973) Dissociative anaesthesia. *Proceedings of the Association of Veterinary. Anaesthetists* 4: 71–76.

Gross M.E., Tranquilli, W.J., Thurmon, J.C., Benson, G.J. and Olson, W.A. (1992) Yohimbine/flumazenil antagonism of hemodynamic alterations induced by a combination of midazolam, xylazine and butorphanol in dogs. *Journal of the American Veterinary Medical Association,* **201**: 1887–1890.

Hall, L.W., Dunn, J.K., Delaney, M., Shapiro, L.M. (1991) Ambulatory electrocardiography in dogs. *Veterinary Record* **129**: 213–216.

Hall, L.W. and Taylor, P.M. (1981) Clinical trial of xylazine with ketamine in equine anaesthesia. *Veterinary Record* **108**: 489–493.

Haskins, S.C., Patz, J.D. and Farver, T.B. (1986) Xylazine and xylazine-ketamine in dogs. *American Journal of Veterinary Research* 47: 636–641.

Heykants, J., Meuldermans, W. and Michiels, M. (1982) *Proceedings of the VIth European Congress of Anaesthesiology, London.*

Hill, D.R., Bowery, N.G. (1981) 3H-baclofen and 3H-GABA bind to bicuculline-insensitive GABA B sites in rat brain. *Nature* 290 (5802): 149–152.

Hirota, K. and Roth, S.H. (1977) Sevoflurane modulates both GABAa and GABAb receptors in area CA1 of rat hippocampus. *British Journal of Anaesthesia.* **78**: 60–65.

Hoffman, W.E., Cunningham, F., Jameds, M.K., Baughman, V.L. and Albrecht, R.F. (1993) Effects of remifentanil, a new short-acting opioid, on cerebral flow, brain electrical activity and intracranial pressure in dogs anaesthetized with isoflurane and nitrous oxide. *Anesthesiology* **79**: 107–113.

Holmberg, G. and Gershon, J. (1961)Autonomic and psychic effects of yohimbine hydrochloride. *Psychopharmacology* 2: 93–106.

Hsu, W.H. (1983) Antagonism of xylazine-induced CNS depression by yohimbine in cats. *Californian Veterinarian* **37**(7): 19–21.

Hsu, W.H. (1985) Effects of atropine on xylazine-pentobarbital anesthesia in dogs: prelminary study. *American Journal of Veterinary Research* **46**: 856–858.

Hsu, W.H., Schaffer, D.D. and Hanson, C.E. (1987) Effects of tolazoline and yohimbine on xylazine-induced central nervous system depression, bradycardia and tachypnea in sheep. *Journal of the American Veterinary Medical Association* **190**: 423–426.

Hsu, W.H., Hanson, C.E., Hembrough, F.B. and Schaffer, D.D. (1989) Effects of idazoxan, tolazoline and yohimbine on xylazine- induced respiratory changes and central nervous depression in ewes. *American Journal of Veterinary Research* **50** (9): 1570–1573.

Jalenka, H.H. (1989) The use of medetomidine, medetomidine- ketamine combinations and atipamezole at Helsinki Zoo – a review of 240 cases. *Acta Veterinaria Scandinavica* **Suppl 85**: 193–198.

Jalenka, H.H. (1989a) Evaluation and comparison of two ketamine-based immobilization techniques in snow leopards. *Journal of Zoo and Wildlife Medicine* **20**(2): 163–169.

James, M.K., Feldman, P.L. and Schuster, S.V.(1991) Opioid receptor activity of GI87084B, a novel ultra-short acting analgesic, in isolated tissues. *Journal of Pharmacology and Experimental Therapeutics* **259**(2): 712–718.

Jedruch, J. and Gajewski, Z. (1986) The effect of detomidine hydrochloride, Domosedan, on the electrical activity of the uterus in cows. *Acta Veterinaria Scandinavica.* **82** (Suppl.): 189.

Jedruch, J., Gajewski, Z. and Ratajska-Michalzak, K. (1989) Uterine motor responses to an alpha 2 adrenergic agonist, medetomidinehydrochloride in bitches during the end of gestation and the post-partum period. *Acta Veterinaria Scandinavica* **Suppl 85**: 129–134.

Jochle, W., Moore, J.M., Brown, J., Baker, G.J., Lowe, J.E., Fubini, S., Reeves, M.T., Watkins, J.P. and White, N.A. (1989) Comparison of detomidine, butorphanol, flunixin meglumine and xylazine in clinical cases of equine colic. *Equine Veterinary Journal* (Suppl.) **7**: 111–116.

Jones, R.S. (1979) Acepromazine in male horses. *Veterinary Record* **105**: 405.

Kalpravidh, M., Lumb, W.V., Wright, M. and Heath, R.B. (1984) Effects of butorphanol, flunixin, levorphanol, morphine and xylazine in ponies. *American Journal of Veterinary Research* **45**: 217.

Kalthum, W. and Waterman, A.E. (1988) The pharmacokinetics of pethidine in the dog. *Journal of Association of Veterinary Anaesthetists* **15**: 39–41.

Kerr, D.D., Jones, E.W., Holbert, M.S. and Huggins, K. (1972a) Comparison of the effects of xylazine and acetylpromazine maleate in the horse. *American Journal of Veterinary Research* **33**: 777–784.

Kerr, D.D., Jones, E.W., Huggins, K. and Edwards, W.C. (1972) Sedative and other effects of xylazine given intravenously to horses. *American Journal of Veterinary. Research* **33**: 525–532.

Kock, R.A., Jago, M., Gulland, F.M.D. and Lewis, J. (1989) The use of two novel alpha 2 adrenoceptor antagonists idazoxan and its analogue RX821002A in zoo and wildlife animals. *Journal of the Association of Veterinary Anaesthetists* **16**: 4–10.

Komar, E. and Mouallem, H. (1988) Climaxolam as a sedative in sheep. *Journal of the Association of Veterinary Anaesthetists.* **15**: 127–133.

Kronberg, G., Oberdorf, A., Hoffmeister, F. and Wirth, W. (1966) Adrenergich-cholinergische neuronenhemmstoffe. *Naturwissenschaften* **53**: 502.

Langer, S.Z. (1974) Presynaptic regulation of catecholamine release. *Biochemical Pharmacology.* **23**(13): 1793–8000.

Lascelles, B.D.X., Cripps, P., Mirchandani, S. and Waterman, A.E. (1995) Carprofen as an analgesic for postoperative pain in cats: dose titration and assessment of efficacy in comparison to pethidine hydrochloride. *Journal of Small Animal Practice* **36**(12): 535–541.

Lees, P. (1979) Chemical Restraint of Large Animals. Chapter 21 in *Pharmacological Basis of Small Animal Medicine.* Edited Bogan, J.A., Lees, P. and Yoxall, A.T. London. Blackwell Scientific Publications: Oxford, UK.

Lees, P. (1979a) *Pharmacological Basis of Small Animal Medicine.* Oxford: Blackwell Scientific Publications.

Lees, P. and Serrano, L. (1976) Effects of azaperone on cardiovascular and respiratory functions in the horse. *British Journal of Pharmacology.* **56**(3): 263–269.

Lees, P. and Taylor, P.M. (1991) Pharmacodynamics and pharmacokinetics of flunixin in the cat. *British Veterinary Journal* **147**(4): 298–305.

Livingstone, A., Low, J. and Morris, B. (1984) Effects of clonidine and xylazine on body temperature in the rat. *British Journal of Pharmacology* **81**(1): 189–193.

Livingston, A., Nolan, A. and Waterman, A., (1986/87). The pharmacology of the alpha 2 adrenergic agonist drugs. *Journal of the Association of Veterinary Anaesthetists* **14**: 3–10.

Lowe, J.E. (1978) Xylazine, pentazocine, meperidine and dipyrone for the relief of balloon induced equine colic; a double blind comparative evaluation. *Journal of Equine Medicine and Surgery* **2** (6): 286–291.

Lucke, J.N. and Sansom, J. (1979) Penile erection in the horse after acepromazine. *Veterinary Record* **104**: 21–22.

MacDonald, E., Ruskoaho, H. Scheinin, M. and Virtanen, R. (1988) Therapeutic applications of drugs acting on alpha-adrenoceptors. *Annals of Clinical Research* **20**: 298–310.

Marsboom, R. and Mortelmans, J. (1964) *Small Animal Anaesthesia.* Oxford: Pergamon Press.

Martin, W.R., Eades, C.C., Thompson, J.A., Huppler, R.E. and Gilbert, P.E. (1976) The effects of morphine and nalorphine-like drugs in the independent and morphine-dependent chronic spinal dog. *Journal of Pharmacology and Experimental Therapeutics* **197**(3): 517–532.

Maze, M., Hayward, E. and Gaba, D.M. (1985) Alpha 1-adrenergic blockade raises epinephrine-arrhythmia threshold in halothane- anesthetized dogs in a dose-dependent fashion. *Anesthesiology* **63**: 611–615

McKellar, Q.A., Pearson, T., Bogan, J.A., Galbraith, E.A., Lees, P. and Tiberghien, M.P. (1990) Pharmacokinetics, tolerance and serum thromboxane inhibition of carprofen in the dog. *Journal of Small Animal Practice* **31**: 443–448.

Mackenzie, G. and Snow, D.H. (1977) An evaluation of chemical restraining agents. *Veterinary Record* **101**: 30–33.

Michelsen, L.G., Salmenperå, M., Hug, C.C. Szlam and Vandermeer, D. (1996) Anaesthetic potency of remifentanil in dogs. *Anesthesiology* **84**: 865–872.

Mitchell, R.W.D. and Smith, G. (1989) The control of acute postoperative pain. *British Journal of Anaesthesia* **63**: 147–153.

Morgan, M. (1989) The rational use of intrathecal and extradural opioids. *British Journal of Anaesthesia* **63**: 165–188.

Muir, W.W. (1981) Drugs used to produce standing chemical restraint in horses. *Veterinary Clinics of North America* **3**: 17–44.

Muir, W.W. and Hamlin, R.L. (1975) Effects of acetylpromazine on ventilatory variables in the horse. *American Journal of Veterinary Research* **36**: 1439–1442.

Muir, W.W. and Piper, F.S. (1977) Effect of xylazine on indices of myocardial contractility in the dog. *American Journal of Veterinary Research* **38**: 931–934.

Muir, W.W., Sasms, R.A., Hoffman, R.H. and Noonan, J.S.(1982) Pharmacodynamic and pharmacokinetic properties of diazepam in horses. *American Journal of Veterinary Research.* **43**(10): 1756–1762.

Muir, W.W., Skarda, R.T., Milne, D.W. (1977) Evaluation of xylazine and ketamine hydrochloride for anesthesia in horses. *American Journal of Veterinary Research* **38**: 195–201.

Muir, W.W., Skarda, R.T. and Sheehan, W.C. (1978) Evaluation of xylazine, guaifenesin and ketamine hydrochloride for restraint in horses. *American Journal of Veterinary Research.* **39**: 1274–1278.

Muir, W.W., Skarda, R.T. and Sheehan, W.C. (1979) Hemodynamic and respiratory effects of a xylazine-acetylpromazine drug combination in horses. *American Journal of Veterinary Research* **36**: 1299–1303.

Muir, W.W., Werner, L.L. and Hamlin, R.L. (1975) Effects of xylazine and acetylpromazine upon induced ventricular fibrillation in dogs anesthetized with thiamylal and halothane. *American Journal of Veterinary Research* **36**: 1299–1303.

Nichols, A.J., Motley, E.D. and Ruffolo, R.R. (1988) Differential effects of pertussis toxin on the pre- and postjunctional alpha-2-adrenoceptors in the cardiovascular system of the pithed rat. *European Journal of Pharmacology* **145**: 345–349.

Nolan, A.M. and Waterman, A.E. (1985) Preliminary results of a study on the effects of xylazine on airway pressure in the sheep's lung. *Journal of the Association of Veterinary Anaesthetists* **13**: 122–123.

Nolan, A.M., Waterman, A.E. and Livingston, A. (1986) The analgesic activity of alpha-2 adrenoceptor agonists in sheep: A comparison with opioids. *Journal of the Association of Veterinary Anaesthetists* **14**: 14–15.

Nunn, J.F. and Bergman, N.A. (1964) The effect of atropine on pulmonary gas exchange. *British Journal of Anaesthesia.* **36**: 68–73.

Paddleford, R.R. (1988) *Manual of Small Animal Anaesthesia.* Edinburgh: Churchill Livingstone.

Parry, B.W., Anderson, G.A. and Gay, C.C. (1982) Hypotension in the horse induced by acepromazine maleate. *Australian Veterinary Journal* **59**: 148–152.

Pearson, H. and Weaver, B.M.Q. (1978) Priapism after sedation, neuroleptanalgesia and anaesthesia in the horse. *Equine Veterinary Journal* **10**: 85–90.

Popovic, N.A., Mullane, J.E. and Yhap, M.D. (1972) Effects of acetylpromazine maleate on certain cardiorespiratory responses in dogs. *American Journal of Veterinary Research* **33**: 1819–1824.

Raptopoulos, D., Koutinas, A., Moustardis, N. and Papasteriadis, A. (1985) The effect of xylazine or xylazine plus atropine on blood gases in sheep. *Proceedings of the 2nd International Congress of Veterinary Anaesthesia* pp 201–202.

Rehm, W. F. and Schatzmann, U. (1984) Benzodiazepines as sedatives for large animals. *Journal of the Association of Veterinary Anaesthetists* **12**: 93–106.

Reid, J.S. and Frank, R.J. (1972) Prevention of undesirable side reactions of ketamine anesthesia in cats. *Journal of the American Animal Hospitals Association* **8** (2): 115–119.

Richards, D.L.S., Clutton, R.E. and Boyd, C. (1989). Electrocardiographic findings following intravenous glycopyrrolate to sedate dogs: a comparison with atropine. *Journal of the Association of Veterinary Anaesthetists* **16**: 46–50.

Robertson, J.T., Muir, W.W. and Sams, R. (1981) Cardiopulmonary effects of butorphanol tartrate in horses. *American Journal of Veterinary Research.* **42**: 41–44

Sagner, Von G., Hoffmeister, F. and Kronberg, G. (1968) Pharmakologische grundlagen eines neuartigen praparates fur die analgesie *Deutsche Teirarztliche Wochenschrift* **22**: 565–572.

Sagner, Von G., Hoffmeister, F. and Kronberg, G. (1968a) *Deutsche. Teirarztliche Wochenschrift* **22**: 565.

Sanford, J. (1984) Meptazinol – a new analgesic agent. *Journal of the Association of Veterinary Anaesthetists* **12**: 48–60.

Sap, R. and Hellebrekers, L.J. (1993) Medetomidine/propofol anaesthesia for gastroduodenal endoscopy in dogs. *Journal of Veterinary Anaesthesia* **20**: 100–102.

Sarazan, R.D., Starke, W.A., Krause, G.F. and Garner, H.E. (1989) The cardiovascular effects of detomidine, a new alpha2–adrenoceptor agonist, in the conscious pony. *Journal of Veterinary Pharmacology and Therapeutics.* **12**(4): 378–388.

Sawyer, D.C. and Rech, R.H. (1987) Analgesia and behavioral effects of butorphanol, nalbuphine and pentazocine in cats. *Journal of the American Animal Hospitals Association* **23**: 438–446.

Scheinin, N. and Macdonald, E. (1989) An introduction to the pharmacology of alpha-2 adrenoceptors in the central nervous system. *Acta Veterinaria Scandinavica* **85** (Suppl.): 11–19.

Scheinin, M., Kallid, A., Koulu, M., Viikkari, J. and Scheinin, H. (1987) Sedative and cardiovascular effects of medetomidine, a novel selective alpha2 -adrenoceptor agonist in healthy volunteers. *British Journal of Clinical Pharmacology* **24** (4): 443–451.

Schmidtt, H. (1977) The pharmacology of clonidine and related products Chapter 7 in: Antihypertensive agents, Ed Gross, Berlin, Springer-Verlag.

Shaw, N., Burrows, C.F. and King, R.R. (1997) Massive gastric hemorrhage induced by buffered aspirin in a greyhound. *Journal of the American Animal Hospitals Association,* **33**: 215–219.

Short, C.E. (1981) Intravenous anesthesia. *Veterinary Clinics of North America*: In Equine Anaesthesia (ed. E.P. Steffey. Philadelphia J.B. Saunders, pp. 195–208.

Short, C.E. (1981a) In: Steffey, E.P. (ed) *Veterinary Clinics of North America: Equine Anaesthesia* Philadelphia: WB Saunders, p. 205.

Short, C.E., Paddleford, R.R. and Cloy, D. (1974) Glycopyrrolate for prevention of pulmonary complications during anesthesia. *Modern Veterinary Practice* **55**(3): 194–196.

Sieghart, W. (1992) GABA receptors: ligand gated chloride channels modulated by multiple drug binding sites. *Trends in Pharmacological Science* **13**: 446–450.

Stenberg, D., Salven, P. and Mettinen, M.V.J. (1987) Sedative action of the alpha-2 agonist medetomidine in cats. *Journal of Veterinary Pharmacology and Therapeutics* **10**: 319–323.

Taylor, P.M. and Clarke, K.W. (1985) Detomidine as a premedicant in the horse. *Journal of the Association of Veterinary Anaesthetists* **14**: 29–32.

Taylor, P.M. and Houlton, J.E.F. (1984) Post-operative analgesia in the dog: a comparison of morphine, buprenorphine and pentazocine. *Journal of Small Animal Practice* **25**: 437–451.

Thompson, J.R., Hsu, W.H., Kersting, K.W. (1989) Antagonistic effect of idazoxan on xylazine-induced central nervous system depression and bradycardia in calves. *American Journal of Veterinary Research* **50**: 734–736.

Tobin, T. and Ballard, S. (1979) Pharmacological Review – the phenothiazine tranquilizers. *Journal of Equine Medicine and Surgery*. **3**: 460–466.

Tobin, T., Combie, J., Schults, T. and Dougherty, J. (1979) The pharmacology of narcotic analgesics in the horse. III Characteristics of the locomotor effects of fentanyl and apomorphine. *Journal of Equine Medicine and Surgery* **3**: 284–288.

Tranquilli, W.J., Lemke, K.A., Williams, L.L. *et al*. (1992) Flumazenil efficacy in reversing diazepam or midazolam overdose in the dog. *Journal of Veterinary Anaesthesia* **19**: 65–68.

Trim, C.M. (1983) Cardiopulmonary effects of butorphanol tartrate in dogs. *American Journal of Veterinary Research* **44**: 329–331.

Tronicke, R. and Vocke, G. (1970) Contributions to the use of the preparation Rompun as a sedative and for anaesthetic premedication in the horse, *Veterinary Medical Reviews (Leverkusen)*: 247–254.

Vaha-Vahe, T. (1989) The clinical efficacy of medetomidine. *Acta Veterinaria Scandinavica* **Suppl 85**: 151–154.

Vainio, O. (1989) Introduction to the clinical pharmacology of medetomidine. *Acta Veterinaria Scandinavica* **Suppl 85**: 85–88.

Vainio, O. and Vahe-Vahe, T. (1989) Reversal of medetomidine sedation by atipamezole in dogs. *Journal of Veterinary Pharmacology and Therapeutics* **13**: 15–22.

Vainio, O., Palmu, L., Virtanen, R. and Wecksell, J. (1986) Medetomidine: A new sedative and anlagesic drug for dogs and cats. *Journal of the Association of Veterinary Anaesthetists* **14**: 53–55.

Van Miet, A., Koot, M. and Van Duin, C. (1989) Appetite modulating drugs in dwarf goats, with special emphasis on benzodiazapine induced hyperphagia and its antagonism by flumazenil & R15–3505. *Journal of Veterinary Pharmacology andTherapeutics* **12**: 147–156.

Vickers, M.D., Schneider, H. and Wood-Smith, F.G. (1984) *Drugs in Anaesthetic Practice*, 6th edn.

Virtanen, G. (1985) Evaluation of the alpha1 and alpha2 adrenoceptor effects of detomidine. *European Journal of Pharmacology* **108**: 163–169.

Virtanen, R. (1986) Pharmacology of detomidine and other alpha2 adrenoceptor agonists in the brain. *Acta Veterinaria Scandinavica* **82** (Suppl.): 35–46.

Virtanen, R. (1989) Pharmacological profiles of medetomidine and its antagonist atipamezole. *Acta Veterinaria Scandinavica*. **85** (Suppl.): 29–37.

Virtanen, R., Savola, J.M., Saano, V., Nyman, L. (1988) Characterization of the selectivity, specificity and potency of medetomidine as an alpha 2-adrenoceptor agonist. *European Journal of Pharmacology* **150**: 9–14

Waterman, A.E. (1981) Preliminary observations on the use of a combination of xylazine and ketamine hydrochloride in calves. *Veterinary Record* **109**: 464–467.

Waterman, A.E., Nolan, A.M. and Livingstone, A. (1986) The effect of alpha-two adrenergic agonist drugs and their antagonists on the respiratory blood gases in conscious sheep. *Journal of the Association of Veterinary Anaesthetists* **14**: 11–13.

Watney, G.C.G. (1986/87) Effects of xylazine/halothane anaesthesia on the pulmonary mechanics of cattle. *Journal of the Association of Veterinary Anaesthetists* **14**: 16–27.

Wilson, D.V. (1991) Pharmacologic treatment of priapism in two horses. *Journal of the American Veterinary Medical Association* **199**: 1183–1184.

Young, L.E. (1992) Clinical evaluation of romifidine/ketamine/halothane anaesthesia in horses. *Journal of Veterinary Anaesthesia* **19**: 89.

General pharmacology of the injectable agents used in anaesthesia

5

INTRODUCTION

In the past, injectable or intravenous agents were regarded as being particularly useful for either the induction of anaesthesia to be continued by an inhalation technique or for anaesthesia of short duration. They are now increasingly used as alternatives to inhalation anaesthetic agents when prolonged periods of anaesthesia are desired. For these longer periods they may be given by intermittent injection or by continuous infusion.

While it is perfectly possible to obtain satisfactory anaesthesia using manual control of infusion rates, the procedure is facilitated greatly by the use of a computer controlled continuous infusion where the anaesthetist specifies the 'target' blood concentration rather than an infusion rate and the computer is programed to determine the appropriate rate of injection to achieve this target concentration. Computer controlled infusions are not yet so widely used in veterinary anaesthesia as they are in medical practice, largely because the necessary pharmacokinetic data are not available, but their use is likely to increase as the necessary information is revealed by research.

With intravenous agents (in particular the barbiturates), the clinical level of anaesthesia is more related to the intensity of stimulation than it is with most of the inhalation agents. An undisturbed animal may be breathing quietly and have marked relaxation of the jaw and abdominal mus-

cles, giving a picture of deep unconsciousness. However, on surgical stimulation the breathing may accelerate or deepen, muscle relaxation may be lost, reflex movement of a limb occur, and blood pressure and heart rate suddenly increase. Herein lies one of the major hazards of intravenous anaesthesia because if this animal is now given sufficient of the intravenous agent to abolish these reactions to stimulation, a dangerous degree of respiratory depression may occur when the stimulation ceases. Moreover, because of the larger quantity of agent being administered more prolonged unconsciousness can be expected. Although similar considerations apply to anaesthesia with some inhalation agents it must always be borne in mind that a major difference between the intravenous anaesthetics and those given by inhalation is that the action of intravenous agents is not as quickly reversible because, unlike the inhalation agents, they cannot be recovered from the patient.

Another significant difference from the inhalation agents is that specific receptor sites for many of the intravenous agents have been identified in the central nervous system, whereas no such specific receptors have been shown to exist for the inhalation agents. The inhalation agents act on cell membranes generally and are much more prone to demonstrate undesirable side effects from their actions on cell function in the body outside the central nervous system.

Intravenous anaesthetic agents should, when given in adequate doses, produce loss of consciousness in one injection site–brain circulation time so that the dose can be titrated against the animal's requirements. Drugs with a slower onset of action, such as ketamine, are more difficult to use as induction agents. Rapidity of effect requires the drug to be lipophilic at physiological pH and they must also be non-toxic to any body organ or tissue as well as being non-allergenic. Other important characteristics include biotransformation to inactive metabolites and, even at high dose rates, non-saturability of the enzyme systems responsible for their elimination from the body

The terms 'ultra-short acting' and 'short acting' were originally used in the classification of the effects of barbiturates but they have come to be employed for a wider range of anaesthetic agents. They are both confusing and misleading and should be reserved for drugs which are indeed broken down rapidly in the body (propofol, for example). In contrast to these, return of consciousness following an intravenous barbiturate such as thiopental (which was originally classified as an 'ultra-short acting' compound) occurs with a large amount of active drug still in the body so that if left undisturbed animals tend to lapse back into a deep sleep from which they can only be aroused with difficulty.

Total intravenous anaesthesia (TIVA) avoids the use of both volatile agents and nitrous oxide during anaesthesia. An intravenous analgesic (e.g. fentanyl) ensures adequate pain relief during the perioperative and early postoperative period. In practice many prefer to use a combination of nitrous oxide with intravenous supplementation (intravenous anaesthesia; IVA). In a number of clinical situations IVA and TIVA can offer advantages over the more traditional volatile agent anaesthesia.

THE BARBITURATES

It is more correct to regard barbituric acid as a pyrimidine derivative but it is usually depicted in either the keto or enol form (Fig.5.1).From Dundee and Wyant (1988) it seems that the many occurring variations are all derived by substitutions in the 1,2 and 5,5' positions and that four distinct groups of compounds can be recognized:

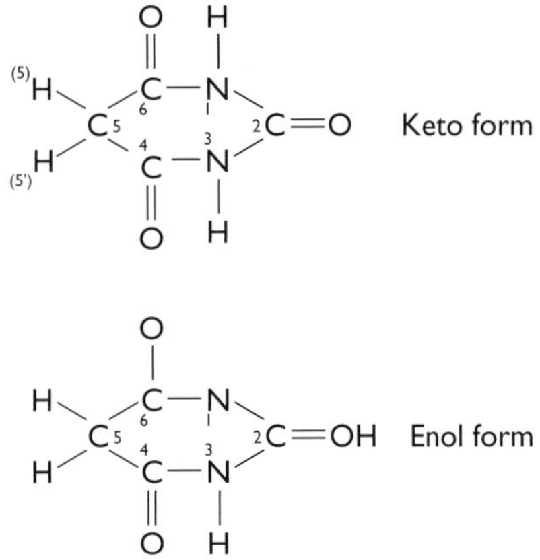

FIG. 5.1 Keto and enol forms of barbituric acid.

1. Barbiturates (or oxybarbiturates): 1 = H, 2 = O.
2. Methylated oxybarbiturates: 1 = CH_3, 2 = O.
3. Thiobarbiturates: 1 = H, 2 = S
4. Methylated thiobarbiturates: 1 = CH_3, 2 = S.

Unconsciousness cannot be produced in one injection site–brain circulation time by the intravenous injection of any of the group 1 compounds; they have a very limited use in veterinary practice as hypnotics or sedatives. Group 2 compounds frequently, but not invariably, will produce unconsciousness in one injection site–brain circulation time. The methyl group confers convulsive activity, of which tremor, involuntary muscle movement and hypertonicity are manifestations. Intravenous injection of an adequate dose of one of the Group 3 thiobarbiturates produces unconsciousness in one injection site–brain time and return to consciousness is more rapid than after the same dose of the comparable oxybarbiturate. Methylated barbiturates of Group 4 produce such severe convulsive manifestations as to preclude their use in clinical anaesthesia.

All barbiturates commonly used as anaesthetics are prepared for clinical use as sodium salts and are usually available as powders to be dissolved in water or saline before use. Commercial preparations of most barbiturate anaesthetics contain a mixture of six parts of anhydrous sodium carbonate and 100 parts (w/w) of the barbiturate to prevent precipitation of the insoluble free acid by atmospheric CO_2. Aqueous solutions are strongly alkaline and are incompatible with acids such as most solutions of analgesics, phenothiazine derivatives, adrenaline and some preparations of neuromuscular blocking drugs. Methohexital is a colourless compound and its solution is readily distinguishable from the yellow solution of sulphur-containing compounds.

The terminology applied to the barbiturates formerly varied between North America and the UK, the former using the suffix '-al' and the latter '-one', hence 'thiopental' and 'thiopentone' referred to the same compound. The use of the '-al' suffix is now universal.

THIOPENTAL SODIUM

In the UK thiopental (thiopentone) was introduced into veterinary practice in 1937 (Sheppard & Sheppard, 1937; Wright, 1937) and over the next 60 years came to be the most widely used induction agent, especially for dogs and cats. Studies of its pharmacology did not keep pace with progress in the clinical field and it was not until the 1950s that any notable contribution to an understanding of its clinical pharmacology was made when Brodie and his co-workers (Brodie, 1952; Brodie et al., 1951; 1953) followed the concentration of the drug in the urine and various body tissues both in dogs and in man. It was found that the liver and plasma concentrations of thiopental, which were high almost immediately after a single injection, soon fell rapidly. The muscle concentration, although high almost immediately after injection, continued to rise for some 20 minutes, then fell – the fall being fairly rapid during the first hour but then becoming progressively slower in the next two to three hours. In contrast to this, the concentration in the body fat, which was negligible at first, increased rapidly during the first hour and then more slowly until a maximum was reached in three to six hours. It was obvious that the concentration in the fat rose at the expense of that in the plasma and all other tissues. Although the brain concentration of thiopental was below that of the blood plasma, both showed similar changes and therefore the depth of narcosis could be related to the plasma concentration of the drug.

From these findings it is clear that the factors which govern the duration and depth of narcosis due to an injection of thiopental are:

1. The amount of the drug injected
2. The speed of injection
3. The rate of distribution of the drug in the non-fatty tissues of the body
4. The rate of uptake of thiopental by the body fat.

The speed of injection and the quantity injected are related. For example, a small amount injected rapidly may produce a high plasma concentration of undissociated drug and consequently a parallel high brain level so that deep narcosis is induced rapidly. However, the drug soon becomes distributed throughout the non-fatty tissues of the body so that the plasma concentration and the brain concentration are reduced and there is a rapid decrease in the depth of narcosis. In contrast, a slow rate of injection of a larger quantity of the drug has the effect of maintaining the plasma level as the drug is distributed to the body tissues. This means that a larger amount of thiopental will be necessary to obtain any given depth of narcosis and recovery will depend more on the uptake of the drug by the body fat and detoxication, since the concentration of thiopental in the non-fatty tissues will already be high at the end of injection.

Thiopental appears to cross the blood–brain barrier with very great speed. The factor which limits the time of response following an injection is the circulation time from the site of injection to the brain. The absence of any appreciable blood–brain barrier makes the rapid injection of the drug very useful for the production of short periods of narcosis with rapid recovery as redistribution occurs. Induction doses of the drug are usually between 5 and 10 mg/kg for most species of animal, but the anaesthetist always aims to combine the effects of injection speed and total dose in such a manner as to minimize the quantity needed by any individual for any given procedure, and takes full advantage of the reduction in dose offered by suitable premedication.

Carbon dioxide (CO_2) retention or the administration of CO_2 has the effect of reducing plasma pH. Alteration of the plasma pH has a complex effect on the distribution of thiopental in the body. The drug is partially ionized and acts as a weak organic acid; the dissociation constant is such that a small change in pH will markedly affect the degree of ionization. If the plasma pH is lowered by CO_2, the undissociated fraction is increased and since only this fraction is fat soluble, the decrease in pH results in an increase in the uptake of the drug by fatty tissues. This lowers the plasma concentration and narcosis might be expected to lighten. However, this does not occur and Brodie has suggested that although the total plasma thiopental is reduced, the concentration of the undissociated (active) fraction remains roughly the same.

A further mechanism may be implicated since thiopental becomes bound to the plasma protein and the degree of binding depends on the protein concentration and the pH of the plasma. Protein binding is reduced by a reduction in pH and because the pharmacological activity resides in the unbound fraction, narcosis might be expected to deepen when the plasma pH is reduced by CO_2. To complicate matters further, hyperventilation, which should have the opposite effect to hypercapnia, has been shown to to reduce the amount of thiopental necessary for the maintenance of anaesthesia. This, of course, is not necessarily contradictory since all three factors, the uptake by body fat, the degree of dissociaton and the degree of binding by the plasma proteins, affect the concentration of active drug. It is unlikely that all three factors will be affected to the same degree and in the same way by changes in the pH of the plasma.

Comparatively little attention has been given to the reduction of plasma thiopental concentration by detoxication. Animal experiments show prolongation of the action of large doses following liver damage caused by other agents, revealing the importance of the liver for recovery from thiopental. Mark and co-workers (1963) showed that up to 50% of thiopental is removed in its passage through the human liver and although there are known to be marked species variations, metabolism in animals is now generally agreed. In dogs, Saidman and Eger (1966) concluded that although the uptake in muscle still plays the dominant role in the early fall of arterial thiopental levels, this is rivalled by the additive effect of metabolism and uptake in fat. Decreased liver metabolism was also shown to be involved in the prolonged recovery from thiopental found in greyhounds (Ilkiw et al., 1985).

After intravenous injection thiopental rapidly reaches the central nervous system and its effects become apparent within 15–30s of injection. Concentrations of the drug in the plasma and cerebrospinal fluid run parallel so the depth of narcosis can be assumed to be dependent on, and vary with, the blood level. However, this relationship is not a simple linear one, as acute tolerance to the drug develops. The plasma concentration of the drug at which the animal wakens increases as the duration of narcosis proceeds. Moreover, the depth and duration of narcosis bear some relation to the initial dose. When a large dose has been injected for the induction of narcosis, the animal will awaken at a higher plasma level than after a small dose. This acute tolerance is probably the explanation for the clinical observation that recovery from the rapid injection of a given dose is quicker than if the same amount is given slowly. The initial concentration of the drug reaching the brain is greater when the drug is injected quickly so that consciousness returns at a higher plasma concentration than after a slower administration.

In clinical practice the intravenous injection of the drug is usually carried out at such a rate that surgical anaesthesia is reached within, at the most, 1–2 minutes. Apnoea sometimes occurs at a depth of anaesthesia sufficient to permit surgical intervention but excitement is very rarely seen during the induction of anaesthesia. The drug, like all barbiturates, has little, if any, analgesic action and reflex response to stimuli is not abolished until an appreciably greater depth of unconsciousness is reached than is required with many other anaesthetic agents. Because of the lack of analgesic properties anaesthesia is more affected by premedication with analgesic drugs than is the case with other anaesthetic agents. This applies also to supplementation during anaesthesia with analgesics whether these be of the opioid type (e.g. alfentanil) or analgesic mixtures of nitrous oxide and oxygen. They reduce or abolish reflex response to stimuli and enable operative procedures to be performed at plasma levels of thiopental which would be insufficient if the drug were given alone.

All barbiturate drugs cause respiratory depression and a short period of apnoea usually follows the intravenous injection of thiopental. This is probably due to the central nervous depression caused by the initial high plasma concentration. The sensitivity of the respiratory centre to CO_2 is reduced progressively as narcosis deepens. As a result of the central depression the alveolar ventilation is diminished, raising the CO_2 tension of the arterial blood.

As with many other agents, anaesthesia in horses is often associated with a peculiar respiratory effect – a complete arrest of respiration for 20–30 s followed by four to eight respiratory movements. These bursts of activity followed by inactivity may persist throughout anaesthesia (Longley, 1950; Waddington, 1950; Ford, 1951; Jones *et al.*, 1960; Tyagi *et al.* 1964).

There is an apparent increase in the sensitivity of the laryngeal and bronchial reflexes under light thiopental anaesthesia. This is generally attributed vaguely to parasympathetic preponderance under thiopental anaesthesia. It would be wrong, however, to assume that thiopental itself produces laryngeal and bronchial spasm for these are reflex phenomena, usually evoked by stimulation of sensory afferent nerves by small amounts of mucus, regurgitated gastric contents or by foreign bodies such as endotracheal tubes. They may also be initiated by stimuli from other parts of the body. During anaesthesia these reflexes are depressed centrally and it is probable that thiopental does not affect the afferent side of the reflex pathway as much as other agents do, so that deeper levels of unconsciousness are necessary for the suppression of these effects. Certainly, spasm is no more common in deep thiopental anaesthesia than with other anaesthetic agents.

There is considerable disagreement among research workers concerning the effects of thiopental on the cardiovascular system. This may well be due to varying methods used for determinations of such things as cardiac output, differences of premedication, depth of narcosis and the degree of CO_2 retention, as well as on the speed of injection. It appears to be generally agreed, however, that the rapid intravenous injection of the drug causes a fall in blood pressure even in normovolaemic animals and that this can be serious in hypovolaemic states. After the initial fall in normovolaemic animals the blood pressure returns to about the normal level but often with a persistent tachycardia.

The drug appears to have a direct depressant effect on the myocardium and in certain circumstances may produce cardiac arrhythmias such as ventricular extrasystoles. It is doubtful whether these have any clinical significance since they do not seem to progress to fibrillation and usually pass off spontaneously. In most instances only the ECG provides any indication of their presence. Where myocardial damage is present, it is unwise to use a very rapid rate of injection because this will submit the heart to a very high initial concentration of the drug.

In many types of anaemia the amount of thiopental necessary for any given level of narcosis is reduced, for the plasma protein concentration as well as the haemoglobin level are low and decreased protein binding is then responsible for increased sensitivity to the drug.

Thiopental modifies the vasomotor response to increase in intrathoracic pressure (Valsalva manoeuvre). In the absence of thiopental, too vigorous controlled respiration will produce a fall in arterial pressure by increasing the mean intrathoracic pressure, although a degree of recovery ensues as the result of compensatory venoconstriction. This compensatory mechanism is impaired by thiopental and persistent hypotension may result from injudicious positive pressure ventilation of the lungs.

Thiopental does not effectively block motor nerve impulses and muscular relaxation can be provided only by excessive central nervous depression. Shivering is common in all species of animal in the recovery period and may be due to persistent cutaneous vasodilatation in a cold environment. It is probably a reflection of the lack of analgesic action because it is usually readily controlled by small doses of analgesic drugs.

The incidence of hepatic damage is related to the dose administered and hepatic dysfunction always follows the use of large doses. However, the presence of liver damage does not contraindicate the drug so long as only minimal doses are employed. Uraemia increases the duration of thiopental narcosis and the drug should be used with care, and in only minimal doses, in uraemic animals. Renal blood flow varies with the arterial blood pressure and prolonged hypotension caused by thiopental can be followed by temporary oliguria. The drug is associated with a small but sometimes persistent fall in plasma potassium concentration.

Foetal respiration seems particularly sensitive to the depressant effects of thiopental. It has never been clearly established whether, in animals, a long or short induction–delivery interval is beneficial to the offspring. At Cambridge it has been used as an induction agent for obstetrical cases for over 40 years without evidence of serious harm to the offspring. Only minimal doses are administered for the induction of anaesthesia and a relatively long induction–delivery interval is allowed. Other induction agents, with the possible exception of propofol, and in horses ketamine, appear to have no remarkable advantages.

Presentation

In dogs a 2.5% solution (0.5 g in 20 ml) should be used and 1.25% solution is preferable in very small dogs and in cats. The intravenous injection of a 5% or stronger solution causes spasm of the vein and perivascular injection causes sloughing of overlying tissues. The use of a 2.5% solution does not cause venous thrombosis and ensures that accidental perivascular injection is much less likely to be followed by tissue necrosis. In small animals where the total dose is likely to be between 50 and 100 mg, further dilution of the 1.25% solution is advisable to give the injection bulk and ensure that the dose is not given too quickly. When it seems possible that more than 20 ml of the 2.5 % solution will be required for a dog or similar sized animal, thought should be given to the use of suitable premedication to reduce the thiopental dose.

It may be essential to use concentrated solutions (e.g. up to 10%) in horses and the larger farm animals but necrosis, sloughing and even aneurysms may follow their accidental perivascular injection. The likelihood of accidental perivascular injection may be reduced by always injecting the solution through a correctly placed intravenous catheter that is well secured in position in the vein.

It is a remarkable and as yet unexplained fact that the use of a 2.5% rather than a 5% solution halves the total dose of the drug which has to be administered to small animal patients. There is no completely acceptable explanation for this

but it seems likely that acute tolerance may be involved.

Thiopental is usually supplied together with the appropriate quantities of water for injection to make a 2.5 or 5% solution. When prepared as a 2.5% solution dose and stored in multidose vials at room temperature the solution will generally remain fit for use for up to four or five days but freshly prepared 10% solutions may precipitate out at lower environmental temperatures.

Contraindications

Porphyria, a disease characterized by progressive acute demyelination of nerves, with clinical signs depending on those most affected, is well documented in man. In a latent stage any barbiturate may provoke an acute exacerbation. Progressive paralysis may end in the death of the patient. During these acute excerbations porphobilinogen is usually present in the urine and can be detected by a simple test in the absence of laboratory facilities. When first voided, urine containing porphobilinogen is usually normal in colour but it darkens when left standing in daylight for a few hours. The classic case presents with colicky abdominal pain and many are subjected to unnecessary laparatomy. Porphyria has been diagnosed in cattle and pigs (Blood & Henderson, 1961) and while it is probably of little importance in these species, the anaesthetist must note that it has also been diagnosed in cats (Tobias, 1964) although the exact type of porphyria was uncertain. In the light of our present knowledge porphyria must be considered an absolute contraindication to the use of thiopental in veterinary practice. There are no other absolute contraindications.

Thiamylal sodium

Thiamylal closely resembles thiopental in chemical structure except that while the latter is the ethyl derivative of the series, the former is the allyl compound. It is no longer available.

METHOHEXITAL SODIUM

Methohexital sodium is a racemic mixture of the α-d and a-l isomers of sodium 5-allyl-1-methyl-5-

(1-methyl-2-ynyl) barbiturate, and differs from thiopental in having no sulphur in the molecule. It is stable for at least six weeks in aqueous solutions kept at room temperature.

There are important differences between this and other barbiturates. The significant features characteristic of methohexital sodium compared to thiopental are:

1. Potency is two or three times greater
2. Shorter duration of effect
3. More rapid recovery to full alertness, even after prolonged anaesthesia (it is the only barbiturate drug for which there is convincing evidence of a more rapid recovery than from the 'standard' barbiturate, thiopental).

Its action is characterized by a rapid induction, satisfactory surgical anaesthesia and a recovery which seldom exceeds 30 minutes. Unfortunately, the recovery period is often complicated by muscle tremors or even frank convulsions. Muscle tremors may also occur during the induction of anaesthesia. These undesirable features are usually suppressed by the use of an opioid or acepromazine for premedication. The short duration of action depends both on marked fat solubility and also on rapid hepatic breakdown to inactive compounds.

It is best administered to small animals as a 1% solution (10 mg/ml) but when large volumes of this solution would be required to administer a dose of 3–5 mg/kg, a 2.5% (25 mg/ml) solution may be used. In large animals more concentrated solutions of up to 6% are more convenient. Owing to differences in pH, solutions of methohexital sodium should not be mixed with acid solutions such as atropine sulphate.

Rapid injection, especially of the more concentrated solutions, usually produces apnoea of 30 to 60 s duration. Rapid injection may also produce transient hypotension but the blood pressure soon returns to normal levels. Laryngospasm is reputed to occur less frequently than with the other intravenous anaesthetics.

Undoubtedly, there is a place in veterinary anaesthesia for an agent which can safely produce rapid anaesthesia with recovery that is fast and complete. Methohexital sodium fulfills most requirements, although the occurrence of muscle tremors indicates that it is not the perfect agent. It seems to have an advantage over the thiobarbiturates in that recovery may be completed earlier as the animal is more alert and coordinated on regaining consciousness. It seems probable, however, that in the near future it will be superseded by propofol and in some countries it is no longer available.

RAPIDLY ACTING NON-BARBITURATES

SAFFAN

Research into the anaesthetic activity of steroids produced a number of hypnotic compounds. Of these alphaxalone was the most promising and, although virtually insoluble in water, when dissolved in cremophor EL the addition of another weakly hypnotic steroid, alphadolone, increased its solubility more than threefold. 'Saffan' is a mixture of the two steroids in cremophor EL and this mixture has never been given an 'official' name. In medical practice an identical formulation was known as 'Althesin'. Solution in cremophor EL being no longer acceptable for drugs to be used in man, Althesin was withdrawn from medical clinical use in 1984, although many anaesthetists considered its withdrawal unwarranted.

Each millitre of Saffan contains 9 mg of alphaxalone and 3 mg of alphadolone. The ready-to-use solution is viscid, has a pH of about 7 and is isotonic with blood. Like all solutions made up in cremophor EL it froths when drawn up into the syringe but is miscible with water. The dose of Saffan may be expressed in several ways but in veterinary anaesthesia it has been usual to record it as mg (total steroid) per kg body weight. Pharmacological studies in Glaxo laboratories (Child et al., 1971) led to the introduction of Saffan as an anaesthetic for cats, but it can be used in all domesticated animals, except dogs (in these animals it causes histamine release), without major problems (Hall, 1972; Eales et al., 1974; Eales 1976; Komar, 1984) and in monkeys (Dhiri, 1984).

The electroencephalographic pattern of cerebral depression is similar to that produced by other anaesthetics. Some evidence has been produced which suggests that Saffan selectively decreases cerebral oxygen consumption to an extent greater than can be attributed to a reduction in cerebral blood flow. Thus, it may be a useful agent for anaesthetizing animals other than dogs suffering from head injuries. When given to cats by intravenous injection induction is not as smooth as with thiopental and, in the authors' experience, retching and even vomiting may occur unless the induction dose is given rapidly. Twitching of limb and facial muscles is also seen but appears to have no clinical significance. Saffan produces similar falls in arterial blood pressure, central venous pressure and stroke volume to thiopental, but the hypotension is not dose related and is accompanied by tachycardia. It causes no significant changes in cardiac index or systemic vascular resistance (Dyson *et al.*, 1987). With moderate doses the arterial hypotension is transient but large doses have a more prolonged effect. Foex and Prys-Roberts (1972) observed a dose-related increase in pulmonary vascular resistance in goats and concluded that Saffan appeared to cause a greater fall in cardiac output than equipotent doses of other induction agents. Sheep appear to be unduly sensitive to Saffan (Clarke & Hall, 1975) for in these animals it produces a marked fall in cardiac output, pulse rate and arterial blood pressure. In dogs cremophor EL produces histamine release, thus causing a further fall in arterial blood pressure and making Saffan unsuitable for use without prior antihistamine medication; even then it cannot be recommended.

It is claimed that Saffan produces good muscle relaxation in cats without at the same time causing severe respiratory depression. Malignant hyperthermia-susceptible pigs have been safely anaesthetized with Saffan (Hall *et al.*, 1972).

The only endocrine effect of Saffan is a weak anti-oestrogenic action. The major route for excretion of steroids is via the bile and in rats 60–70% of alphaxalone and alphadolone are excreted by this route within three hours of administration. There is some evidence that, like progesterone, the anaesthetic steroids are involved in enterohepatic circulation.

Information relating to the transfer of Saffan across the placental barrier is scanty but clinical results show very minor adverse effects on kittens when induction doses of up to 6 mg/kg are given to the mother. It has been claimed that kittens breathe almost immediately after delivery when the dose of Saffan given to the mother is restricted to less than 4 mg/kg.

Cats recovering from Saffan anaesthesia often show tremor of muscles, paddle and, if stimulated, may become extremely excited or convulse. This excitement and convulsions disappear as soon as the stimulation ceases. Oedema and/or hyperaemia of the ear pinnae and paws is common under Saffan anaesthesia. Measurement of paw and ear thickness suggests that this occurs more frequently than can be recognized by simple visual inspection. Currently, it has to be accepted that these side effects result from some idiosyncrasy in some cats to some unidentified ingredient in the product. Informed opinion seems to be that this type of reaction, probably related to histamine release, is usually without clinical significance – although there have been occasional reports of ear pinna and paw necrosis.

Other reports of possible histamine release in cats cannot be dismissed so easily. These are clinical reports, only seldom supported by autopsy findings, associating the administration of Saffan with pulmonary oedema. However, in about 30 instances, lung oedema has been confirmed histologically at autopsy. Evans (1979) attributed pulmonary oedema to an administration or administrator-related problem because most reports stem from very few practitioners and he estimated that about 30 000 cats are anaesthetized with Saffan each month. There seems to be no way of preventing it occurring and because it is a potentially lethal problem others take the view that Saffan is not an acceptable alternative to thiopental. However, in at least one region of the UK from which pulmonary oedema has been reported similar trouble has followed the use of thiopental and this may indicate the operation of some factor peculiar to a geographical region. In such a region an endemic chronic infection may prime the complement systems, making them susceptible to activation by an intravenously administered compound. This would lead to histamine release in affected animals by the so-called 'alternative pathway' without involvement of immune recognition so no previous exposure to Saffan or to any other intravenous agent would be necessary for such a reaction as histamine-induced pulmonary oedema to occur. There are also reliable reports of laryngeal oedema following induction of anaesthesia with Saffan with no history of previous exposure to the steroids.

Although all the genus *Canis* show a dose-related anaphylactoid type of reaction to surface-active agents such as cremophor EL, a constituent of Saffan, the preparation has been used in dogs after premedication with acepromazine and chlorpheniramine. Attempts to follow this regimen in dogs in the UK have revealed a high incidence of skin erythema and vomiting. It is difficult to accept that the prior administration of an antihistamine merely to enable Saffan to be used is good practice, especially now that other and better agents such as propofol are available for use in dogs.

Unlike many induction agents Saffan may be given by intramuscular injection but, despite this possible use, there is no doubt that the prime role for the formulation is as an intravenous induction agent, or as a total anaesthetic (using incremental dosage or a continuous infusion technique). Metabolism is so fast that subcutaneous injection fails to produce any evidence of effect on the central nervous system, making it possible to disregard inadvertent perivascular injection as far as subsequent doses are concerned.

OTHER STEROIDS

Minaxolone

Following enthusiastic reports of its use in early clinical trials in man, minaxolone, a rapidly acting, water soluble steroid was subjected to clinical trials involving 70 dogs and six anaesthetists (Clarke & Hall, 1984). It proved to be an adequate anaesthetic, with usually smooth induction but prolonged recovery times. The commonest side effect noted was twitching, while the most serious was respiratory depression often needing oxygen supplementation coupled with intermittent positive pressure ventilation of the lungs, to maintain an adequate PaO_2. Occasionally, there was a marked delay between intravenous injection and the attainment of maximal anaesthesia. Cardiovascular effects were minimal, a slight fall in arterial

pressure occurring immediately after injection but pressure rapidly returned to normal or slightly elevated levels.

Unfortunately the drug did not live up to expectations with regard to smoothness of recovery or speed of recovery and was withdrawn from the market.

5 β Pregnanolone and other steroids

The pregnanes were first reported to possess anaesthetic activity in 1957 but it was a decade later that the anaesthetic effects of some were described. 5 β Pregnanolone is insoluble in water but it has been used as an emulsion in man. To date there are no published data on its efficacy in veterinary anaesthesia. It *may* have an impact on intravenous anaesthetic techniques.

METOMIDATE

Metomidate (Hypnodil) is a non-barbiturate intravenous hypnotic synthesized in the laboratories of Janssen Pharmaceutica in Belgium. It was the first representative of a completely new group of hypnotics, the imidazole derivatives. It is a white crystalline powder, freely soluble in water, but aqueous solutions are unstable and should be used within 24 hours of preparation. A 1% solution has a pH of 2.9 and a 5% solution a pH of 2.4. It was introduced as a hypnotic for pigs and its use has mainly been confined to these animals.

Metomidate has strong central muscle relaxant properties but little ability to suppress response to painful stimulation. However, since it has usually been used with other agents, such as fentanyl or azaperone, it is difficult to establish the effects of the agent alone. Given by intravenous injection it produces unconsciousness in one injection site–brain circulation time. In pigs, after azaperone premedication, induction of unconsciousness is smooth and side effects are rarely seen. Occasionally muscle tremors occur and although they may persist for a few hours they appear to be of little clinical significance. Metomidate has also been given by intraperitoneal injection at the same time as an intramuscular injection of azaperone but the results were unpredictable.

In pigs, injection of metomidate is followed by slight hypotension, with a decreased pulse rate and a mild decrease in cardiac output. During sedation there is remarkable stability of the cardiovascular system. Under azaperone–metomidate sedation the minute volume of respiration is equal to that of the rested, conscious pig, with a decreased frequency but an increased tidal volume. Piglets delivered by caesarean section from sows under metomidate hypnosis are sleepy but usually recover from this depressed state if they are kept warm. When high doses of metomidate are given to the sow the piglets may show tremors for several hours after birth.

Although introduced as a hypnotic for pigs it has also been used experimentally in horses (Cox, 1973; Hillidge *et al.*, 1973) and for restraint for a variety of species of birds (Cooper, 1974). In horses metomidate produces sweating, muscular tremors and involuntary head and limb movements ; it cannot be recommended for clinical use.

Role

Although possibly indicated for pigs, there is currently little call for its use in the field because of farm economics and although pigs are becoming widely used as experimental animals other agents are usually more satisfactory for laboratory purposes.

ETOMIDATE

The commercial preparation, Hypnomidate, contains 20 mg of the dextrorotatory isomer of the compound dissolved in 10 ml of a mixture of 35% propylene glycol and 65% water v/v, because injection of plain aqueous solutions causes pain. Etomidate is currently much more expensive than metomidate.

The pharmacokinetics of etomidate favour its use as an infusion and, combined with its low cardiovascular toxicity it is not surprising that this became a popular technique (usually combined with an opioid such as fentanyl) in man. In dogs it is 76% bound to albumin and like thiopental it quickly enters the brain and leaves rapidly as it becomes redistributed in the body. Of the total dose given, in rats 83% is excreted in the urine in 24 hours (2% as unchanged etomidate) and 13% is excreted in the bile. It is quickly hydrolysed by esterases in the liver and plasma to pharmacologically inert metabolites. The pharmacokinetics of etomidate in cats have been investigated (Wertz *et al.*, 1990) and are best described by a three-compartment open model similar to those determined in people and rats.

In effective doses etomidate causes loss of consciousness in one injection site–brain circulation time and in dogs doses of 1.5 to 3 mg/kg produce hypnosis, in a dose dependent manner, lasting from 10 to 20 minutes. Thus on a weight-for-weight basis it appears to be about 10 times more potent than thiopental. Side effects are no more likely to occur with the higher dose rates than with lower ones.

Intravenous injection is associated with a high incidence of involuntary muscle movement, tremor and hypertonus. The EEG changes produced by etomidate at induction are similar to those seen with barbiturates and no specific epileptogenic or convulsive activity is observed, so the muscle movements cannot be attributed to central nervous activity. Premedication with diazepam, fentanyl or pethidine reduces the incidence of these side effects so they may be related to pain on intravenous injection when the drug is administered through a small calibre vein.

Lack of cardiovascular depression is claimed to be one of the outstanding features of etomidate (Nagel *et al.*, 1979). The drug does release significant amounts of histamine and there is a very low incidence of thrombosis after injection. Injection of etomidate is frequently followed by a short bout of coughing in unpremedicated dogs but in general respiration is less depressed than after other intravenous hypnotics.

A slight rise in serum potassium occurs when marked, persistent myoclonic movements occur, but the main effect of importance is that etomidate inhibits increases in plasma cortisol and aldosterone concentrations during surgical stress, even when adrenocorticotropic hormone levels are normal or increased. In canine surgical patients adrenocortical function is suppressed for two to three hours after the administration of etomidate (Kruse-Elliott *et al.*, 1987). Suppression of the endocrine response to surgical stress has been deemed by some to be beneficial, although this suppression has resulted in etomidate no longer being used for sedation of human patients in intensive care units.

Role

It is impossible to assess whether etomidate has a place in veterinary anaesthesia. Erhardt (1984) has reported acceptable results with a mixture of etomidate and alfentanil mixed in a ratio of 1.000 mg to 0.015 mg in dogs, cats, rats, rabbits, sheep, goats and calves but etomidate has so far failed to make any impact in veterinary practice in North America or the UK.

EUGENOLS

The eugenols are related to oil of cloves and three derivatives have been subjected to clinical trials in man. The first, known as G29505 or Estil, was abandoned because of its deleterious effects on veins. Another derivative, Propinal, was abandoned very quickly because of its effects on respiration and the circulation. The third eugenol, propanidid (Epontol), became available in the UK in 1967. Doses of 5 mg/kg given to very small ponies by extremely rapid intravenous injection produced anaesthesia sufficient for castration followed by complete recovery in less than 10 minutes. Because of the extremely short duration of action it was found to be physically impossible to give the drug fast enough to produce anaesthesia in larger horses, and violent excitement followed the administration of subanaesthetic doses. In dogs, Epontol was found to produce profound hypotension, probably because propanidid was dissolved in cremophor EL.

PROPOFOL

Propofol is an intravenous anaesthetic agent unrelated to barbiturates, eugenols, or steroid anaesthetic agents. The active ingredient, 2,6 di-isopropylphenol, exists as an oil at room temperatures. Originally introduced in a preparation containing the surface-active agent cremophor EL it is now presented as a free flowing oil-in-water emulsion containing 1% w/v soya bean oil, 1.2%

w/v purified egg phosphatide and 2.25% w/v glycerol.

Like thiopental, propofol is a rapidly-acting agent producing anaesthesia of short duration without side effects. Both agents produce equivalent cardiovascular and respiratory effects but, unlike thiopental, propofol does not damage tissue when injected perivascularly or intra-arterially. Pain on injection into small veins has been reported in man and occasionally dogs seem to resent injection into the cephalic vein. The reason for pain on injection is not known but the various possible explanations have been reviewed by Tan & Onsiong (1998). Greater reflex depression and more pronounced EEG changes are associated with propofol than with thiopental.

Details of pharmacological studies performed in rabbits, cats, pigs and monkeys were published (Glen, 1980; James & Glen, 1980; Glen & Hunter, 1984), and preliminary clinical trials in 10 dogs and one cat soon followed (Hall, 1984). Propofol has been shown to be compatible with a wide range of drugs used for premedication, inhalation anaesthesia and neuromuscular block (James & Glen, 1980). It lacks any central anticholinergic effect, is not potentiated by other non-anaesthetic drugs, does not affect bronchomotor tone or gastrointestinal motility, and decreases the risk for catecholamine induced cardiac arrhythmias.

The propofol blood concentration profile following a single bolus dose can be described by the sum of three exponential functions representing;

(i) distribution from blood into tissues
(ii) metabolic clearance from blood
(iii) metabolic clearance constrained by the slow return of propofol into the blood from a poorly perfused tissue compartment.

It is highly lipophilic and rapidly metabolized primarily to inactive glucuronide conjugates, the metabolites being excreted in the urine. In man, liver disease and renal failure have little effect on pharmacokinetic parameters and it seems likely that extrahepatic mechanisms contribute to the metabolism of propofol, but this has not been investigated in any detail in other animals. In dogs premedication with 10 μg/kg of medetomidine, which might be expected to reduce hepatic blood flow, does not significantly alter the kinetic

TABLE 5.1 **Mean utilization rate of propofol (data supplied by J.B. Glen)**

Species	Mean utilization rate (mg/kg/min)
Mouse	2.22
Rabbit	1.55
Rat	0.61
Pig	0.28
Cat	0.19

TABLE 5.2 **Disposition of propofol in mongrel and laboratory beagle dogs.** V_{SS}= apparent volume of distribution at steady state. $T_{1/2}\beta$ = elimination half-life. [*] indicates a significant difference at $p > 0.05$ (data from Hall et al., 1994; 1997);

Disposition	Mongrel dogs	Laboratory beagles
	(n = 6)	(n = 6)
V_{SS} (L/kg)	6.04 (0.71)	3.27 (0.26)[*]
Systemic clearance (ml/kg/min)	34.40 (1.92)	47.46 (6.21)
$T_{1/2\beta}$ (min)	486.2 (56.4)	131.30 (12.82)[*]

variables (Hall et al., 1994). In cats considerable first pass extraction of propofol occurs in the lung (Matot et al., 1993) and it is uncertain whether all of the drug is released back into the circulation or if some is metabolized in the pulmonary tissue.

The mean 'utilization rate' of propofol varies from species to species (Table 5.1) and is probably related to differences in the rate of biotransformation and conjugation as the cat, with the smallest utilization rate of the animals studied, has a deficiency in its ability to conjugate phenols.

Propofol is now accepted as a most useful agent in all domestic animals, although its current price precludes its widespread use in adult farm animals and horses. The principal advantage of propofol over thiopental is the more rapid recovery of consciousness. As it is very lipophilic it has a very large volume of distribution. There are noticeable differences between the disposition data from mongrels and beagle dogs (Table 5.2). It is metabolized very quickly although, at least in man, concurrent administration of fentanyl reduces clearance and increases plasma concentrations (Cockshott, 1985).

The dose for induction of anaesthesia in unpremedicated dogs and cats is between 6 and 7 mg/kg. Premedication with between 0.02 and 0.04 mg/kg of acepromazine reduces this induction dose by about 30% in dogs but this effect is not so marked in cats premedicated with 0.04 mg/kg of acepromazine (Brearley et al., 1988). Premedication with 10 or 20 μg/kg of medetomidine decreases the anaesthetic induction dose in dogs to about 5 mg/kg and 3 mg/kg respectively (Hall et al., 1994; 1997). Blood systemic clearance is almost halved by premedication with medetomidine 20 μg/kg whereas 10 μg/kg produces very little effect. ·It has been demonstrated that the pharmacokinetics of propofol differ in grey-

hounds and mixed breed dogs (Zoran & Riedesel, 1993) so that breed differences must be expected.

In dogs, anaesthesia maintained by continuous infusion (Chambers, 1988; Vainio 1991; Nolan & Reid, 1993; Hammond & England, 1994) appeared to be less controllable than that maintained by halothane/nitrous oxide (Hall & Chambers, 1987; Chambers, 1988) although it is perhaps better when maintained by intermittent injections of the agent (Watkins et al., 1987). Following a single intravenous dose of 6 mg/kg recovery in dogs is complete (awake, no ataxia) after about 20 minutes and neither acepromazine nor medetomidine premedication appear to increase the recovery time. Recovery in greyhounds and other sighthounds is no longer than in other breeds. There is a suggestion that some families of boxer dogs may be more susceptible to the drug since recovery was prolonged in some related animals of this breed (Hall & Chambers, 1987). In cats recovery after a single dose is less rapid – about 30 minutes – presumably because of relative inability to conjugate phenols. In cats the incidence of postanaesthetic side effects such as vomiting/retching and sneezing or pawing at the mouth is about 15% but this can be slightly reduced by acepromazine premedication (Brearley et al., 1988). Vomiting and retching may also be seen during recovery in dogs, the incidence being about 16% following infusion at 0.4 mg/kg/min after atropine and acepromazine premedication (Chambers, 1988).

Propofol has also been used for anaesthesia in horses (Nolan, 1982; Nolan & Hall, 1985; Aguiar et al., 1993), goats (Nolan et al., 1991), macacaque monkeys (Sainsbury et al., 1991) and many other species of animal. It does not appear to trigger malignant hyperthermia in susceptible pigs (Raff & Harrison, 1989)

The great attraction for using propofol is the rapid and complete, excitement-free awakening, irrespective of the duration of anaesthesia. However, animals require careful observation during the recovery period to ensure that they come to no harm from vomiting. In dogs, excitatory phenomena associated with the use of propofol have been reported (Davies, 1991; Davies & Hall, 1991). These have been mainly muscle twitching, extensor rigidity and opisthotonus, and have not given rise to life-threatening situations.

LESS RAPIDLY ACTING INTRAVENOUS AGENTS

The less rapidly acting intravenous agents include chloral hydrate, the dissociative agents and pentobarbital sodium. In the past all have been used as anaesthetics but appropriate doses do not produce unconsciousness in one injection site–brain circulation time.

CHLORAL HYDRATE

Chloral hydrate is a white, translucent, crystalline substance which volatilizes on exposure to air, producing a penetrating smell. It is not deliquescent, but it is readily soluble in water and aqueous solutions are generally stable although the drug decomposes in the presence of alkali. Solutions may be sterilized by boiling for a few minutes. In the blood chloral hydrate is reduced to 2,2,2-trichloroethanol and its narcotic effect is generally attributed to this substance. When given by intravenous injection its effects are slow in appearing and this means that it is difficult to assess the degree of depression produced by a given dose as injection proceeds. Even following slow intravenous infusion of a dilute solution, narcosis continues to deepen for several minutes and additional doses should not be administered until it is clear that the maximum depth of depression from the initial dose has been reached. Perivascular injection causes severe tissue reaction,

often followed by sloughing of the overlying tissues. A small amount appears unchanged in the urine but most is excreted after conjugation with glycuronic acid through the kidneys as trichloroethylglycuronic acid.

Chloral hydrate is a hypnotic and not an anaesthetic. The dose needed to produce anaesthesia is very close to the minimal lethal dose. It has only very weak analgesic action. Hypnotic doses cause respiratory depression and large doses result in arterial hypotension. Death from chloral hydrate results as a result of respiratory depression.

The drug was never used as an anaesthetic in dogs and cats but formerly it was used extensively in large animals, sometimes with a barbiturate (Wright, 1957). Recovery from chloral hydrate anaesthesia in horses occupies one to four or more hours and unless tranquillizers are given is often accompanied by struggling to rise. Its action in cattle is similar to that in horses except that recovery is always quiet. It was often given, well diluted with water, by stomach tube into the rumen. More recently introduced agents are safer and more convenient to administer to both horses and cattle and there is little to recommend its continuing use.

CHLORALOSE

Chloralose is prepared by heating equal quantities of glucose and chloral hydrate under controlled conditions so that two isomers are produced. Only α-chloralose has narcotic properties; β chloralose can produce muscular pain. α-Chloralose is available commercially as a white, crystalline powder and it is used as a 1% solution in water or saline. The solution is prepared fresh immediately before use by heating to 60°C. Heating above this temperature results in decomposition and precipitation occurs on standing. Chloralose is still extensively used in physiological and pharmacological non-survival experiments. Because large volumes of solution have to be given before consciousness is lost, anaesthesia is often induced with some other agent such as methohexital or, today, propofol. An intravenous dose of 80–100 mg/kg of chloralose causes loss of consciousness but spontaneous muscular activity is common. The peak narcotic action of chloralose is seen some 15 to 20 minutes after injection. The arterial blood pressure is elevated and the activity of the autonomic nervous system is believed to be unaffected. The heart rate is often greatly increased and respiratory depression does not occur until very large doses are given. In the body chloralose is broken down to chloral and glucose and the safety margin is relatively wide.

Disadvantages are its relative insolubility, the long comparatively shallow depth of anaesthesia and the slow recovery accompanied by struggling. It has no place in veterinary practice but it is regarded by many experimentalists as a valuable drug for maintenance of unconsciousness for long, non-survival experiments.

URETHANE

Urethane is no longer commonly used as an anaesthetic for any laboratory experiments. It was often given with chloralose to suppress the muscular activity which may occur when chloralose is used alone. Urethane has little effect on respiration and arterial blood pressure. It is believed to be carcinogenic and laboratory workers still having contact with this compound should handle it with care.

PENTOBARBITAL SODIUM

Pentobarbital sodium in the form of a racemic mixture of sodium 5-ethyl-5-(1-methylbutyl) barbiturate is marketed as a sterile 6.5% solution containing propylene glycol, as a powder in gelatine capsules and, for euthanasia, in non-sterile solutions of about 20%.

The main action of pentobarbital sodium is to depress the central nervous system, and effects upon other systems of the body only become important as the toxic limitations to the use of the drug are approached. It depresses the cerebral cortex and, probably, the hypothalamus. Because it depresses the motor areas of the brain it is used to control convulsive seizures. It has only a weak analgesic action and relatively large doses must be administered before pain perception is affected; like all barbiturates, it is primarily a hypnotic drug. Pentobarbital sodium takes an appreciable time to cross the blood–brain barrier and when given by intravenous injection the rate of injection

must be slow if the full effects are to be assessed as injection proceeds. The drug markedly depresses the respiratory centre and in pregnant animals it diffuses readily across the placenta into the fetal circulation, inhibiting fetal respiratory movements. One of its isomers causes a transient period of excitement before depressing the central nervous system while the other produces smoother, progressive hypnosis.

In sheep, pentobarbital causes a marked decrease in stroke volume and in the acceleration of blood in the pulmonary artery. Pulse rate increases but this does not compensate for the fall in stroke volume so cardiac output falls to an average of 64% of the resting volume in the conscious animal (Clarke & Hall, 1975). The blood pressure may subsequently rise due to hypercapnia consequent upon respiratory depression produced by the drug. The drug alters both myocardial function and the distribution of blood flow in most laboratory animals so that although often used in the past as an anaesthetic for physiological and pharmacological studies their results require critical evaluation.

The drug has no appreciable effect on the gastrointestinal system or on liver function but large doses may cause further damage to an already damaged liver. It is destroyed primarily in the liver although other tissues may have the power of breaking it down. Some of the administered dose is excreted in the urine so that if a diuresis can be produced by intravenous infusion of fluid, awakening may be accelerated. Pentobarbital has no direct action on the kidney but may inhibit water diuresis, probably by causing a release of antidiuretic hormone from the pituitary gland (Blake, 1957).

Recovery from pentobarbital is always slow but the duration varies according to the species of animal. The drug is metabolized more rapidly in horses, sheep and goats than in pigs, dogs and cats. Convulsive movements, paddling and vocalization may occur in the recovery period but such excitatory phenomena can usually be suppressed with analgesics or tranquillizers although these will further delay complete recovery. The 'glucose effect' – a reanaesthetizing effect due to a glucose induced decreased microsomal activity – exhibits a marked species variability and is of no significance in dogs, cats, mice or rats, although it has been demonstrated to prolong recovery in rabbits and guinea pigs (Hamlin *et al.*, 1965).

Role

In horses pentobarbital may be used to prolong the duration of chloral hydrate hypnosis. Horses metabolize pentobarbital relatively quickly but unless combined with chloral hydrate recovery is usually associated with excitement. Sheep and goats also metabolize the drug rapidly. In the field it may used in cattle for anaesthesia of short duration, although the prolonged recovery period constitutes a disadvantage. In dogs and cats it can be used on its own as a hypnotic or anaesthetic but analgesics are needed to reduce distress in recovery after surgery. In the laboratory it is still a most widely used injectable anaesthetic in dogs and cats despite its disadvantages. It is becoming increasingly used to maintain hypnosis in pigs for long, non-survival experiments.

DISSOCIATIVE AGENTS

Three cyclohexylamine derivatives have been used in several species of animal to produce a state that enables a surgical operation to be carried out. These substances, phencyclidine, tiletamine and ketamine, differ markedly both in chemical and physical properties as well as in their clinical effects when compared to the non-inhalation agents already described. They have been described as having cataleptic, analgesic and anaesthetic action, but no hypnotic properties. Catalepsy is defined as a characteristic akinetic state with loss of orthostatic reflexes but without impairment of consciousness in which the extremities appear to be paralysed by motor and sensory failure.

Another definition of the state produced by these agents is 'dissociative anaesthesia' which is characterized by complete analgesia combined with only superficial sleep. In man, hallucinations and emergence delirium phenomena are known to occur. It cannot be established whether similar phenomena are experienced by animals but the state produced by these substances is clinically very different from anaesthesia produced by other agents. Spontaneous involuntary muscle movement and hypertonus are not uncommon during induction and purposeless tonic-clonic movements of the extremities may be mistaken to indicate an inadequate level of anaesthesia and the need for additional doses and unless this possibility is recognized, overdoses may be given.

Electroencephalographic studies show a functional dissociation between the thalamoneocortical and limbic systems, the former being depressed before there is a significant effect on the reticular activating and limbic systems. This differs from the effects of other non-inhalation anaesthetics and is manifested by the state of the animal. Hypertonus and muscle movement have already been mentioned; in addition animals may remain with their eyes open and have a good tone in the jaw muscles with active laryngeal and pharyngeal reflexes, whilst analgesia appears to be extremely good.

Phencyclidine

Phencyclidine was the first dissociative agent used in veterinary anaesthesia but is no longer generally available.

Tiletamine

Tiletamine hydrochloride is a cataleptic agent similar to phencyclidine hydrochloride but at least twice as potent. The lack of muscle relaxation and long recovery period together with pain on injection of the available preparation (Garmer, 1969) resulted in it not being used in the UK.

TILETAMINE-ZOLAZEPAM MIXTURE

Tiletamine is currently marketed in combination with a diazepam analogue, zolazepam ('Telazol', 'Zoletil') in the USA, Australia, Europe and elsewhere, but not in the UK. This preparation is a 1:1 dry powder with a long shelf-life. It can be made into highly concentrated solutions convenient for administration to wild animals by dart gun.

In domestic cats the drug combination causes tachycardia with slight rises in blood pressure and cardiac output coupled with initial respiratory stimulation followed by mild depression of breathing. Its use in non-domesticated cats has been well described by Lewis (1994). In dogs, the tranquillizing effects of zolazepam seem to wane before those of tiletamine so that recovery is often violent. Muscle rigidity is common and some seizure-like manifestations may be seen. In the UK the mixture has yet to be subjected to clinical trials but initial reports indicate that the combination is unlikely to find favour.

KETAMINE

The ketamine molecule exists as two optical isomers and the racemic mixture is currently used clinically. It is available in 10, 50 and 100 mg/ml strengths suitable for i.m. or i.v. injection. The 10 mg/ml solution is made isotonic with sodium chloride. In all species of animal ketamine appears to have a much shorter duration of action than phencyclidine or tiletamine.

The effects of the two enantiomers of ketamine differ. The potency ratio between the two isomers appears to be greater for ketamine's analgesic action than for its anaesthetic effect. White et al. (1980) have suggested that d-ketamine (about four times as potent than the l form) would be more useful than either the racemic mixture or the l isomer, retaining the desirable but lacking the undesirable properties of the drug. It is unlikely that this will be followed up because it would involve considerable pharmaceutical outlay, which might have been very much more worthwhile if it had preceded the introduction of propofol.

The effects of ketamine on the central nervous system become apparent rapidly for the brain/plasma ratio becomes constant in less than one minute. It also rapidly crosses the placental barrier. Liver metabolism produces at least four metabolites which are excreted in the urine; they may have some slight additive effect to the action of the parent drug. Ketamine produces profound analgesia without muscle relaxtion, and tonic-clonic spasms of limb muscles may occur even in the absence of surgical or other stimulation. Salivation is increased and saliva can obstruct the airway even though laryngeal and pharyngeal reflexes are retained. To eliminate side effects a variety of other compounds such as atropine, diazepam, midazolam, xylazine, detomidine, medetomidine and even the thiobarbiturates or an inhalation agent are commonly given concurrently with ketamine.

Mild respiratory depression has been reported and in clinical practice this is usually manifested by an increased rate which does not compensate for a decreased tidal volume. Although laryngeal reflexes may be present it is still necessary for the airway to be kept under close observation because the degree of protection of the upper airway is less than was once thought.

In contrast with the action of other i.v. induction agents ketamine causes a rise in arterial blood pressure. The rate of injection is not an important factor in the production of hypertension and i.m. injection results in no less a rise in blood pressure than the i.v. route. The picture is one of stimulation by an agent which has a direct depressant action on the isolated heart preparation. This is probably due to an increase in circulating catecholamines caused by ketamine blocking the reuptake of noradrenaline by adrenergic nerve terminals. Cardiac arrhythmias are uncommon in animals under ketamine anaesthesia and the minimal arterial blood pressure is always similar to and rarely less than the preoperative level.

Ketamine produces little, if any, muscle relaxation. There is generally an increase in skeletal muscle tonus and tendon reflexes are brisk. Athetoid limb movements occur without external stimuli and are not dose-related.

There is no evidence of tolerance developing after repeated injections of ketamine and no significant cumulative effects have been reported in the veterinary literature, although a case of tolerance has been noted in a young child (Stevens & Hain, 1981). Daily injections of ketamine in rats, dogs and monkeys caused no alterations in haematological, urine or bone marrow values or in blood chemistry. According to the manufacturers there were no adverse effects on the dam or the pups when pregnant bitches were given 25 mg/kg ketamine twice a week over a three-week period during each third of pregnancy and pregnant rabbits given ketamine daily during the period of organogenesis produced normal litters.

There is little published information regarding the use of ketamine for caesarian section in any species of animal. In the authors' experience lambs delivered from ewes that have had anaesthesia induced with ketamine behave as though they are unaware of their surroundings for up to 12 hours after delivery. Extreme difficulty was experienced in getting them to suckle in the first six hours of life. The behaviour of young of other animal species born to mothers after ketamine has apparently not been studied but for caesarian section in mares, induction of anaesthesia with ketamine after xylazine premedication seems to have little effect on the survival of the foal.

The difficulty in assessing the depth of unconsciousness coupled with the poor muscle relaxation produced by the drug make it doubtful whether ketamine should ever be used alone for surgical operations, although its ease of administration makes its use superficially attractive in animals such as sheep and cats. Ketamine alone in sheep, or in any other animals, in the authors' experience and that of others (Taylor *et al.*, 1972; Thurmon *et al.*, 1973) fails to produce satisfactory anaesthesia. In cats it is doubtful if ketamine alone should be used, except possibly to subdue a particularly wild individual. However, there is general agreement that if injectables have to be used, ketamine is the agent of choice for the sedation of reptiles (Bree & Gross, 1969; Borzio,1973; Harding, 1977). Similarly, ketamine has proved to be of value in many species of birds (Gerlach, 1969; Kittle, 1971; Mattingly, 1972; Klide, 1973; Mandelker, 1973; Boever & Wright, 1975) when inhalation agents are unavailable.

REFERENCES

Aguiar, A.J.A., Hussni, C.A., Luna, S.P.L., Castro, G.B., Massone, F. and Alves, A.L.G. (1993) Propofol compared with propofol/guaiphenesin after detomidine premedication for equine surgery. *Journal of Veterinary Anaesthesia* **20**: 26–28.

Blake, W.D. (1957) Some effects of pentobarbital and anesthesia on renal hemodynamics. *American Journal of Physiology* **191**: 393–398.

Blood, D.C. and Henderson, J.A. (1961). In: *Veterinary Medicine*. London: Baillière, Tindall and Cox.

Boever, W.J. and Wright, W. (1975). Use of ketamine for restraint and anaesthesia of birds. *Veterinary Medicine – Small Animal Clinician* **70**: 86–88.

Borzio, F. (1973) Ketamine hydrochloride as an anesthetic for wild fowl. *Veterinary Medicine – Small Animal Clinician* **68**: 1364–1367.

Brearley, J.C., Kellagher, R.E.B. and Hall, L.W. (1988)

Propofol anaesthesia in cats. *Journal of Small Animal Practice* **29**: 315–322.

Bree, M.M. and Gross, N.B. (1969). Anesthesia of pigeons with CI581 (ketamine) and pentobarbital. *Laboratory Animal Care* **19**: 500–502.

Brodie, B.B. (1952). Physiological disposition and chemical fate of thiobarbiturates in the body. *Federal Proceedings* **11**: 632–639.

Brodie, B.B., Mark, L. C., Papper, E.M., Lief, P.A., Bernstein, E. and Papper, E.M. (1951). Acute tolerance to thiopentone. *Journal of Pharmacology and Experimental Therapeutics* **102**: 215–218.

Brodie, B.B, Burns, J.J., Mark, L.C., Lief, P.A., Bernstein,E. and Papper, E.M. (1953). Fate of pentobarbital in man and dog, and method for its estimation in biological material. *Journal of Pharmacology and Experimental Therapeutics* **109**: 26–34.

Chambers, J.P. (1988). Propofol infusion anaesthesia in dogs. *Journal of the Association of Veterinary Anaesthetists* **15**: 135.

Child, K.J., Currie, J.P., Davis, B., Dodds, M.G., Pearce, D.R. and Twissell, D.J. (1971). The pharmacological properties in animals of CT1341 – a new steroid anaesthetic agent. *British Journal of Anaesthesia* **43**: 2–13.

Clarke, K.W. and Hall, L.W. (1975). The effect of some intravenous anaesthetics on cardiac output. *Proceedings of the 20th. World Veterinary Congress,Thessaloniki.* **2**: 1688–1692 (published in 1976).

Clarke, K.W. and Hall, L.W. (1984). Minaxolone : a clinical trial in the dog. *Journal of the Association of Veterinary Anaesthetists* **12**: 83–92.

Cockshott, I.D. (1985). Propofol ('Diprivan') pharmacokinetics and metabolism – an overview. *Postgraduate Medical Journal.*, **61** (Suppl 13): 45–50.

Cooper, J.E. (1974). Metomidate anaesthesia of some birds of prey for laparotomy and sexing. *Veterinary Record* **94**: 437–440.

Cox, J.E. (1973). Immobilization and anaesthesia of the pig. *Veterinary Record* **92**: 143–147.

Davies, C. (1991). Excitatory phenomena following the use of propofol in dogs. *Journal of Veterinary Anaesthesia* **18**: 48–51.

Davies, C. and Hall, L.W. (1991). Propofol and excitatory sequelae in dogs. *Anaesthesia* **46**: 797–798.

Dhiri, A.K. (1984). Continuous intravenous infusion using Saffan (CT1341) in the Patas monkey. *Journal of the Association of Veterinary Anaesthetists of Great Britain and Ireland* **12**: 68–77.

Dundee, J.W. and Wyant, G.M. (1988) In: *Intravenous Anaesthesia* 2nd Edition, Edinburgh. Churchill Livingstone.

Dyson, D.H., Allen, D.A., Ingwersen, W., Pascoe, P.J. and O'Grady, M. (1987). Efects of Saffan on cardiopulmonary functions in healthy cats. *Canadian Journal of Veterinary Research* **51**: 236–239.

Eales, F.A., Hall, L.W. and Massey G.M. (1974) 'Saffan' a new steroid anaesthetic in veterinary anaesthesia. *Proceedings of the Association of Veterinary Anaesthetists of Great Britain and Ireland.* **No. 5**: 1–5.

Eales, F.A. (1976). Effects of Saffan administered intravenously in the horse. *Veterinary Record* **99**: 270–272.

Erhardt, W. (1984). Anaesthesia with alfentanil and etomidate in several animal species. *Journal of the Association of Veterinary Anaesthetists of Great Britain and Ireland* **12**: 196–196.

Evans, J.M. (1979). Steroid anaesthesia five years on. *Proceedings of the Association of Veterinary Anaesthetists of Great Britain and Ireland* **8**: 73–84.

Foex, P. and Prys-Roberts, C. (1972). Pulmonary haemodynamics and myocardial effects of Althesin (CT1341) in goat. *Postgraduate Medical Journal. (Suppl 2).* 48–24.

Ford, E.J.H. (1951) Some observations on the use of thiopentone in large animals. *Veterinary Record* **63**: 636–638.

Garmer, L.N. (1969). Effects of 2-ethylamino- 2'-(2'phenyl) cyclohexanone HCl (CI-634) in cats. *Research in Veterinary Science* **10**: 382–388.

Gerlach, H. (1969). Surgical conditions in wild and pet birds. *Veterinary Record* **84**: 342.

Glen, J.B. (1980). Pharmacokinetics in laboratory animals of ICI 35868: a new i.v. anaesthetic agent. *British Journal of Anaesthesia* **52**: 743–746.

Glen, J.B. and Hunter, S.C. (1984) Pharmacology of an emulsion formulation of ICI 35868. *British Journal of Anaesthesia* **56**: 617–626.

Hall, L.W. (1972). Althesin in the larger animal. *Postgraduate Medical Journal.* **48** *(Suppl2).* 55–58.

Hall, L.W. (1984). A clinical study of a new intravenous agent in dogs and cats. *Journal of the Association of Veterinary Anaesthetists of Great Britain and Ireland* **12**: 115–121.

Hall, L.W. and Chambers, J.P. (1987). A clinical trial of propofol infusion anaesthesia in dogs. *Journal of Small Animal Practice* **28**: 623–637.

Hall, L.W., Trim, C.M. and Woolf, N. (1972). Further studies of porcine malignant hyperthermia. *British Medical Journal* **ii**: 1145–1148.

Hall, L.W., Lagerweij, E., Nolan, A.M. and Sear, J.W. (1994). Effect of medetomidine on the pharmacokinetics of propofol in dogs. *American Journal of Veterinary Research* **55**: 116–120.

Hall. L. W., Lagerweij, E., Nolan, A.M. and Sear, J.W. (1997). Disposition of propofol after medetomidine premedication in beagle dogs. *Journal of Veterinary Anaesthesia* **24**: 23–29.

Hamlin, R.L., Redding, R.W., Rieger, J.E., Smith, R.C. and Prynn, B. (1965). Insignificance of the 'glucose effect' in dogs anesthetized with pentobarbital. *Journal of the American Veterinary Medical Association* **146**: 238–241.

Hammond, R.A. and England, G.C.W. (1994). The effect of medetomidine premedication upon propofol induction and infusion anaesthesia in the dog. *Journal of Veterinary Anaesthesia* **21**: 24–28.

Harding, K.A. (1977). The use of ketamine anaesthesia to milk tropical rattlesnakes (*Crotalus durissus terrificus*). *Veterinary Record* **100**: 289–290.

Hillidge, C.J., Lees, P. and Serrano, L. (1973) Investigations of azaperone-metomidate anaesthesia in the horse. *Veterinary Record* **93**: 307–311.

Ilkiw, J.E., Sampson, D. and Cutler, D. (1985) Thiopentone sodium in the Greyhound. *Proceedings of the 2nd. International Congress of Veterinary Anesthesia* Oct. pp 118–119.

James, R. and Glen, J.B. (1980) Synthesis, biological evaluation and preliminary structure-activity considerations of a series of alkylphenols as intravenous anaesthetic agents. *Journal of Medicinal Chemistry*, **23**: 1350.

Jones, E.W., Johnson, L. and Heinze, C.D. (1960). Anesthesia in the horse. *Journal of the American Veterinary Medical Association* **137**: 19–122.

Klide, A.M. (1973). Avian anesthesia (cage birds).*Veterinary Clinics of North America* **3**: p. 175–186.

Komar, E. (1984). Steroid anaesthesia in horses. *Journal of the Association of Veterinary Anaesthetists of Great Britain and Ireland* **12**: 127–131.

Kruse-Elliott, K.T., Swanson, C.R. and Aucoin, D.P. (1987). Effects of metomidate function on canine surgical patients. *American Journal of Veterinary Research* **48**: 1098–1100.

Lewis, J.C.M. (1994). Anaesthesia of non-domestic cats. In: Hall, L.W. and Taylor, P.M. (eds) *Anaesthesia of the Cat.* London: Baillière Tindall, pp. 329–330.

Longley, E.O. (1950). Thiopentone (pentothal sodium) as a general anaesthetic in the horse. *Veterinary Record* **62**: 17–20.

Mandelker, L. (1973). A toxicity study of ketamine HCl in parakeets.*Veterinary Medicine – Small Animal Clinician* **68**: 487–488.

Mark, L.C. (1963). Thiobarbiturates. In: Papper, E.M., Kitz, R.J. (eds) *Uptake and Distribution of Anesthetic Agents.* New York, McGraw-Hill, ch 23.

Matot, I., Neely, C.F., Ray, M.D., Katz, R.Y. and Neufield, G.R. (1993). Pulmonary uptake of propofol in cats, effect of fentanyl and halothane. *Anesthesiology* **78**: 1157–1165.

Mattingly, B.E. (1972) Injectable anesthetic for raptors. *Raptor Research* **6**: 51–52.

Nagel, M.L., Muir, W.W. and Nguyen, K (1979). Comparison of the cardiopulmonary effects of etomidate and thiamylal in dogs. *American Journal of Veterinary Research* **40**: 193–196.

Nolan, A.M. (1982). Disoprofol anaesthesia in horses – a preliminary report. *Proceedings of the Association of Veterinary Anaesthetists of Great Britain and Ireland* **10**: 204–207.

Nolan, A.M. and Hall, L.W. (1985). Total intravenous anaesthesia in the horse with propofol. *Equine Veterinary Journal* **17**: 394–398.

Nolan, A.M. and Reid, J. (1993). Pharmacokinetics of propofol administered by infusion in dogs undergoing surgery. *British Journal of Anaesthesia* **70**: 546–551.

Nolan, A.M., Reid, J. and Welsh, E. (1991). Use of propofol as an induction agent in goats. *Journal of Veterinary Anaesthesia* **18**: 53–54.

Raff, M. and Harrison, G.G. (1989). The screening of propofol in MH swine. *Canadian Journal of Anaesthesia* **36**: 186–197.

Saidman, L.J. and Egger, E.I. (1966) The effect of thiopental metabolism on duration of anaesthesia. *Anesthesiology*, **27**: 118–126.

Sheppard, M. and Sheppard, D.H. (1937). The use of pentothal sodium as a short-duration anaesthetic in small animals. *Veterinary Record* **49**: 424–425.

Stevens, R.W. and Hain, W.R. (1981) Tolerance to rectal ketamine in paediatric anaesthesia. *Anaesthesia* **36**: 1089–1093.

Tan, C.H. and Onsiong, M.K. (1998) Pain on injection of propofol. *Anaesthesia* **53**: 468–476.

Taylor, P.M., Hopkins, L., Young, M. and McFadyen, I.R. (1972). Ketamine anaesthesia in the pregnant sheep. *Veterinary Record* **90**: 35–36.

Thurman, J.C., Kumar, A. and Link, R.P. (1973) Evaluation of ketamine hydrochloride as an anesthetic in sheep. *Journal of the American Veterinary Medical Association* **162**: 293–297.

Tobias, G. (1964). Congenital porphyria in a cat. *Journal of the American Veterinary Medical Association* **145**: 462–463.

Tyagi, R.P.S., Arnold, J.P., Usenik, E.A. and Fletcher, T.F. (1964) Effects of thiopental sodium (pentothal sodium) anesthesia in the horse. *Cornell Veterinarian* **54**: 584–692.

Vanio, O. (1991) Propofol infusion anaesthesia in dogs pre-medicated with medetomidine. *Journal of Veterinary Anaesthesia* **18**: 35–37.

Waddington, F.G. (1950). Thiopentone as an anaesthetic in the horse. *Veterinary Record* **62**: 100–101.

Watkins, S.M., Hall, L.W. and Clarke, K.W. (1987). Propofol as an intravenous anaesthetic agent in dogs. *Veterinary Record* **120**: 326–329.

Wertz, E.M., Benson, G.J., Thurmon, J.C. and Tranquilli, W.J. (1990). Pharmacokinetics of etomidate in cats. *American Journal of Veterinary Research* **51**(2): 281–285.

White, P.F., Ham, J., Way, W.L. and Trevor, A.J. (1980). Pharmacology of ketamine isomers in surgical patients. *Anesthesiology* **52**: 231–239 .

Wright, J.G. (1937). The use of a new short-acting barbiturate – pentothal sodium – as a general anaesthetic in canine surgery. *Veterinary Record* **49**: 27–29.

Wright, J.G. (1957). *Veterinary Anaesthesia*, 4th edn. London: Baillière, Tindall & Cox.

Zoran, D.L. and Riedesel, D.H. (1993). Pharmacokinetics of propofol in mixed breed dogs and greyhounds. *American Journal of Veterinary Research* **54**: 755–760.

General pharmacology of the inhalation anaesthetics

6

An inhalation anaesthetic cannot be introduced into the brain without at the same time being distributed through the entire body, and this distribution exerts a controlling influence over the rate of uptake or elimination of the anaesthetic by brain tissue. So far, no specific receptors mediating the actions of used inhalation anaesthetics have been identified. It seems that they act via a non-specific (? physical) mechanism on the lipid bilayer of cell membranes and thus it is not unexpected that profound effects on other organ systems besides the central nervous system have been readily identified.

The influence of the physical characteristics shown in Table 6.1 on the pharmacokinetics of the volatile anaesthetic agents (and therefore on the speed on induction of and recovery from anaesthesia) have been described in detail in Chapter 3. The anaesthetist needs to know these and other physical and pharmacodynamic properties of the currently used inhalation agents in order to use these agents in the safest possible manner.

NON-INFLAMMABILITY

Modern anaesthetics must be non-inflammable in the range of concentrations and in the range of gas mixtures (usually of O_2 and N_2O) used in clinical practice. In the past, quenching gases such as helium were used to make otherwise explosive mixtures of agents such as cyclopropane safe for

TABLE 6.1 **Physical characteristics for some anaesthetic agents. Values taken from various sources in the literature but mainly from Halsey (1981), Steward et al. (1900), Eger (1987), Rhône Mèrieux data sheets and Ohio Medical Products**

Compound	Water/gas part. coeff.	Blood/gas part. coeff.	Oil/gas part. coeff.	Boiling Point (°C)	Vapour Pressure at 20°C. (mmHG)
Cyclopropane	0.21	0.55	11.50	−34.0	Gas at 20 °C
Desflurane	0.23	0.42	18.70	23.5	664
Enflurane	0.78	1.90	98.00	56.5	172
Ether	13.00	12.00	65.00	34.6	442
Halothane	0.80	1.94	220.00	50.2	240
Isoflurane	0.62	1.40	97.00	48.5	236
Methoxyflurane		12.00	970.00	104.8	23
Nitrous oxide	0.47	0.47	1.40	−89.0	Gas at 20 °C
Sevoflurane	0.36	0.60	53.00	58.5	157

clinical purposes but today non-inflammability is usually achieved by halogenation – in particular fluorination – of the agent. In most cases this does not greatly change inflammability limits but it does greatly increase the energy necessary to ignite the agents and it is this which renders these agents non-inflammable in clinical use. They require a spark having an energy of 10–30 joules to ignite them and a static spark released within an anaesthetic system has an energy of only a few hundred millijoules. Thus, the halothane/oxygen mixture within the vaporizing chamber of a plenum type vaporizer (see p.67) may contain about 33% of halothane at 20 °C, well within the flammable range for halothane, but it could only be ignited by a powerful energy source which cannot be present during normal use.

Promising anaesthetic agents have often been rejected on grounds of inflammability and it is worth noting that N_2O increases the flammability of organic vapours because it is an endothermic compound whose decomposition results in the evolution of heat together with the production of an oxygen-rich mixture (33% O_2). Thus, although the lowest concentration of halothane in oxygen which can be ignited is around 14% it can be shown that in pure N_2O, 2% of halothane vapour is ignitable by an ignition energy as low as 0.3 joules.

CHEMICAL STABILITY

The use of completely closed breathing systems (see p.68) imposes a severe test on the chemical stability of an agent because of its continuing passage over hot, moist CO_2 absorbents (soda lime or Barolyme). A compound which is toxic to mice in the concentration range of 100–5000 ppm has been detected after one hour of closed circuit halothane anaesthesia (Sharp et al., 1979) but halothane has now been used very extensively with soda lime carbon dioxide absorption during prolonged anaesthesia in all species of domestic animal without any reports of harmful effects. Halothane is, however, broken down by ultraviolet light and samples removed from an anaesthetic system for analysis by an ultraviolet absorption meter should not be returned to the breathing circuit, and indeed it is for this reason that the economical

ultraviolet method of anaesthetic gas analysis is no longer used.

Sevoflurane when used in closed systems, produces a number of breakdown products of which 'Compound A' (CF_3=C(CF_3)-O-CH_2F) is nephrotoxic in rats. Although toxic values (in rats) usually need to exceed 1000 ppm, under certain circumstances levels as low as 50 ppm may cause medullary tubular necrosis (Callan et al., 1994). The concentrations of Compound A which occur are greatest at higher temperatures, with dry absorbents, with low flow or closed systems and, not surprisingly, with high concentrations of sevoflurane (Baum & Aitenhead, 1995). Levels in man and the dog using closed systems are usually about 20 ppm, but in certain circumstamces reach over 50 ppm in individuals (Smith et al., 1996). Nevertheless, in man there is no evidence that renal failure has resulted from sevoflurane anaesthesia (Malan, 1995).

The passage of some volatile anaesthetic agents over very dry CO_2 absorbents results in accumulation of carbon monoxide (CO) within a closed anaesthetic system. Of the volatile agents in common use, desflurane produces the greatest amount of CO, and halothane probably the least (Fang et al., 1995). The problem can be avoided by turning off the O_2 flow of 'fail-safe' machines when they are not in use to avoid the drying effect of continuous gas flow through the system.

BIOTRANSFORMATION OF ANAESTHETIC GASES AND VAPOURS AND ORGAN TOXICITY

Damage to organs as a result of inhalation anaesthetic agents may be due to direct toxic effects of the agent, to effects mediated by metabolites, or to hypoxic changes, usually from poor organ blood flow. Except in sensitivity reactions the toxicity of the unchanged compound is normally directly related to the concentration present and decreasing the concentration present and/or the duration of exposure to it will decrease toxicity. Metabolite formation is more complicated and may be faster when the concentration of the parent compound is low. The mechanism of this concentration/time dependence is unknown but it seems that biotransformation reaches a maximum at relatively low concentrations of anaesthetic and later as its concentration in the liver increases the efficiency of the enzyme system decreases. The plateau in biotransformation rate could be because the amount of enzyme available becomes the rate limiting factor or its activity is depressed either by inhibition due to the anaesthetic substrate or the metabolites produced. The important implication for toxicity caused by metabolism of anaesthetics is that greater quantities of metabolites may be produced by subanaesthetic concentrations than by exposure to an anaesthetizing concentration when each is administered for the same number of MAC hours. Furthermore, increasing the duration of anaesthesia does not proportionally increase the quantity of metabolites produced in the body. Finally, while a large reduction in the concentration of an administered anaesthetic might reduce direct toxicity to below threshold for harm this might not be the case for indirect toxicity due to metabolites.

Toxic effects of anaesthetic drugs are most commonly seen in the liver and kidneys. The most commonly cited example is that of halothane, which is extensively metabolized, catalysed by enzymes such as cytochrome P450. Breakdown products include trifluoroacetyl halides, which can link to liver proteins. In some cases antibodies are formed against the halothane-induced antigen, resulting in immune mediated liver damage (the so-called 'halothane hepatitis'). However, isoflurane and enflurane produce similar breakdown products to halothane, but to a lesser extent, so similar autoimmune mediated hepatitis may occur (Frink, 1995; Kenna & Jones, 1995), but more uncommonly. The renal damage which was reported following the prolonged use of methoxyflurane was thought to be due to the action of free fluoride ions formed from hepatic metabolism. The threshold for plasma fluoride to cause nephrotoxicity is approximately 50 mmol/l. However, levels close to this occur after prolonged enflurane or sevoflurane anaesthesia, but appear to have only transient effects and serious renal damage is rare (Kenna & Jones, 1955).

DEPRESSION OF VITAL BODY FUNCTIONS

In experiments on isolated organs all anaesthetics have a depressant effect but in an intact animal these depressant effects may be modified or even controlled by various mechanisms. With the exception of N_2O, all the inhalation anaesthetics produce a concentration dependent depression of respiration although there is some difference of degree between the agents currently used in their tendency to produce this effect. In clinical practice this is offset by surgical stimulation so that all the standard agents can be used in spontaneously breathing animals without undue accumulation of carbon dioxide provided excessively deep levels of central nervous depression are avoided.

On the cardiovascular system all the inhalational agents have a directly depressant action and the differences in their overall effects can be attributed to their action on baroreceptor activity and on the activity of the sympathoadrenal system as reflected in plasma adrenaline and noradrenaline. The direct effects on the cardiovascular system are opposed by sympathetic activity resulting from surgical stimulation and the changes in cardiovascular function seen will depend on the balance between inhibitory and excitatory influences.

INTERACTION WITH OTHER DRUGS

All neuromuscular blocking drugs are potentiated by inhalational anaesthetics in a dose-dependent manner and since muscle relaxation quite adequate for most operations can be produced by inhalation agents alone it is reasonable to assume that at least part of this potentiation is due to the central nervous depression produced by the anaesthetic agent. In addition, it has been shown that inhalational agents decrease the sensitivity of the postjunctional membrane of the neuromuscular junction and possibly act at a more distal site such as the muscle membrane itself. The different anaesthetic agents differ in the extent they potentiate relaxants. For example, enflurane and isoflurane are considerably more potent in potentiating d-tubocurarine in man than are halothane or N_2O (Ali & Savarese, 1976). The reason for this is quite unknown but, clearly, it may be considered advantageous for an inhalational agent to contribute to neuromuscular block since this component can be removed by ventilation of the lungs, so increasing the flexibility of control because there are then at least two methods of reducing or abolishing the block – use of an anticholinesterase and augmented ventilation.

The sensitization of the myocardium to both endogenous and exogenous adrenaline by the inhalational agents has been the subject of much investigation and it can be concluded that while straight-chain hydrocarbons tend to sensitize the heart to catecholamines, the ethers, especially if fluorinated, do not have this effect. Indeed, fluorinated ethers such as enflurane and isoflurane, have the desirable attribute of conferring good stability to adrenaline.

ANALGESIA

For as yet unknown reasons subanaesthetic concentrations of agents such as nitrous oxide produce marked analgesia, whereas others such as halothane do not. It may be speculated that this effect depends on the release of endorphins (encephalins) but, except for N_2O evidence for this is lacking. If an agent having good analgesic properties has a high solubility (e.g methoxyflurane) then elimination of it will be slow and analgesia will be present during recovery. Unfortunately, less desirable effects such as respiratory depression and arterial hypotension are also prolonged so that it is usually better to rely on specific analgesic drugs in the postoperative period rather than the retention of the anaesthetic agent.

INDIVIDUAL INHALATION ANAESTHETICS

NITROUS OXIDE (N_2O)

N_2O is a colourless gas with a faint, rather pleasant smell; it is not flammable or explosive but it will support combustion, even in the absence of free O_2. Compressed into cylinders ('tanks' in North America) at 40 atmospheres pressure it liquifies so that the amount in a cylinder can only be determined by weighing since the pressure of the gaseous N_2O above the liquid level remains constant as long as any liquid remains. Thus a pressure gauge screwed into the cylinder outlet will register a constant pressure until all the N_2O has vaporized and after this the reading drops rapidly

as gas leaves the cylinder. Some type of 'regulator' or pressure-reducing valve must be attached to the cylinder before the rate of flow of the gas can be accurately adjusted or measured.

It is not irritant to the respiratory mucosa and because short periods of inhalation do not cause toxicity it was given for prolonged periods in intensive care units. However, exposure to it for several days caused bone marrow depression in humans due to interference with methionine synthase giving rise to disturbances of folate metabolism and megablastosis (Armstrong & Spence, 1993). N_2O has little or no effect on the liver and kidneys and although it has a direct depressant effect on the myocardium this is offset by its sympathetic stimulating properties.

The results of several studies suggest that N_2O may increase pulmonary ventilation (Eckenhoff & Helrich, 1958; Hornbein *et al.*, 1982; Hall, 1988). The tachypnoea produced by N_2O may result from direct central stimulation similar to that postulated for potent inhalation agents but the impact of N_2O appears to be greater than that of other inhalation anaesthetics. The greater increase in respiratory rate and minute ventilation associated with its use is also found when it is combined with some of the inhaled anaesthetics but not with opioid analgesics. Respiratory rate and minute ventilation are greater at a given MAC level when N_2O and isoflurane are combined than when isoflurane is given alone (Dolan *et al.*, 1974). This is also true for halothane but not enflurane. Adding N_2O to a stable level of alfentanil narcosis appears to have no effect (Andrews *et al.*, 1982).

As already discussed N_2O tends to enter gas-filled spaces in the body at a greater rate than nitrogen can diffuse out. This is of considerable importance in herbivores and in the presence of a closed pneumothorax.

During the induction of anaesthesia a large gradient exists between the tension of N_2O in the inspired gas and the arterial blood so that in the early moments of induction the blood takes up large volumes of gas. Its rapid removal from the alveoli by the blood elevates the tension of any remaining (second) gas or vapour such as oxygen, or a volatile anaesthetic agent, and augments alveolar ventilation. Thus, during the first few minutes of N_2O administration anaesthetic uptake is facilitated because the enhanced tension of the second gas ensures a steeper tension gradient for its passage into the blood. This is known as 'the second gas effect'.

The phenomenon known as 'diffusion hypoxia' occurs immediately following anaesthesia when the gas is being rapidly eliminated from the lungs; N_2O may form 10% or more of the volume of expired gas, and the outward diffusion of N_2O into the alveoli lowers the the partial pressure of O_2 in the lungs (PaO_2). This effect appears to have little clinical significance in healthy animals but any hypoxia may be dangerous in elderly animals or in those suffering from cardiovascular or pulmonary disease and such animals should have an O_2 enriched mixture to inhale for some 10 minutes after the termination of N_2O administration. Many anaesthetists consider that even healthy animals benefit from 5–10 minutes of O_2 inhalation when N_2O is discontinued at the end of a lengthy procedure. When the insoluble agent desflurane is used with N_2O, it is imperative that O_2 is given for some minutes after termination of the anaesthetic administration.

Being only a very weak anaesthetic, with a MAC of over 100%, N_2O cannot, on its own, be used to produce anaesthesia because it must be given with sufficient O_2 (>25%) to prevent hypoxia. Its strong analgesic properties make it most useful to provide additional analgesia for both intravenous and inhalation anaesthetic agents, i.e. it is best regarded as an anaesthetic adjuvant.

DIETHYL ETHER

Diethyl ether, commonly known simply as 'ether', was one of the earliest inhalation anaesthetics introduced into clinical practice but its use is currently declining rapidly. The chief reason for this is its inflammability and also its great water and blood solubility which, together with its irritant smell, make for a slow induction and recovery. Nevertheless, ether has always had the justification of being a very safe anaesthetic agent.

It is a transparent, colourless liquid with a vapour twice as heavy as air, which is highly inflammable in air and explosive in O_2 rich atmospheres. Ether is decomposed by air, light and heat;

the liquid is, therefore, stored in amber-coloured bottles kept in a cool dark place. Its heavy vapour tends to pool on the floor and unless ventilation is good the possibility of fires is very great. Sparks of static electricity from faulty connections in electrical switches and apparatus can easily ignite ether/air mixtures and ether/oxygen mixtures are explosive. Fires have resulted from the vapour rolling into an adjoining room and being ignited there. Ether should not be administered in locations where equipment such as radiographic apparatus or diathermy is to be used.

Ether is safe in the presence of adrenaline. Indeed, its administration is associated with sympathoadrenal stimulation which opposes its negative inotropic effect and the concurrent use of β-adrenergic blocking drugs allows this effect to become dangerous. Normally, cardiac output is well maintained even at deep levels of unconsciousness. During light levels of unconsciousness, ether does not depress respiration. The spleen contracts while the intestines become dilated and atonic. The blood sugar level rises due to the mobilization of liver glycogen under the influence of the increased secretion of adrenaline. Liver and kidney function is depressed but these organs usually recover their normal function within 24 hours. The inhalation of ether causes metabolic acidosis and ketone bodies may appear in the urine. Although ether does undergo some metabolism it contains no halogens so that its intermediate metabolites are such relatively non-toxic substances as ethyl alcohol, acetic acid and acetaldehyde.

Ether possesses many disadvantages in addition to its inflammability. Its inhalation provokes the secretion of saliva and of mucus within the respiratory tract (although this problem can be counteracted by premedication with an anticholinergic agent). In man, postanaesthetic nausea appears to be pronounced and it is a fact that animals are reluctant to eat for several hours following ether anaesthesia, possibly indicating they too experience nausea.

Ether has now been in continuous use for well over 100 years and millions of operations must have been performed on animals under ether anaesthesia. The number of deaths directly attributable to ether, apart from accidents (e.g.

explosions and fires) and errors of technique, must be very small indeed or its use would have been discontinued long ago. It must still be considered a safe agent for the inexperienced anaesthetist to use because, in addition to being slow in action, it produces a graded series of signs useful in indicating the depth of central nervous depression.

CHLOROFORM

Chloroform is a most powerful anaesthetic which is no longer used. It has a toxic effect on the liver and kidneys, causing cloudy swelling and even acute fatty change in the cells. When severe these changes give rise to delayed poisoning, the symptoms of which develop some 24–48 hours after administration. Delayed poisoning is characterized by acute acidosis, severe vomiting (in dogs and cats), acetonuria, albuminuria, mild pyrexia and icterus, and frequently terminates fatally with severe hyperpyrexia. In addition, chloroform sensitizes the myocardium to the effects of catecholamines and sudden death has occurred from ventricular fibrillation during anaesthesia or recovery from chloroform.

CYCLOPROPANE

Cyclopropane is as inflammable as ether and mixtures with both air and oxygen are explosive. It has solubility characteristics which commend it as an anaesthetic agent for induction and recovery but it produces marked respiratory depression. In the 1950s it was extensively employed in veterinary hospitals in the UK and was noted for causing vomiting in the recovery period in pigs and dogs. The explosion risk associated with its use is a very real one and it is no longer available.

HALOTHANE

Halothane was introduced into veterinary anaesthesia in 1956 (Hall, 1957) and was so greatly superior to existing agents that it soon became used throughout the world. It is probable that halothane has been subjected to more investigational studies than any other anaesthetic agent and in the veterinary field alone there is now an extremely large number of references to this agent.

Vapour concentrations from 2 to 4% in the inspired air produce smooth and rapid induction of anaesthesia in all species of domestic animal. Anaesthesia can then be maintained with inspired concentrations of 0.8 to 2%, the MAC being about 0.85% in all mammals. Recovery from short-duration halothane anaesthesia is also reasonably rapid and free from excitement although unrelieved pain can give rise to restlessness during recovery. When no other agents are administered most animals are able to walk without ataxia in 15 to 30 minutes, depending on the duration of anaesthesia and the degree of obesity of the animal. Blood concentrations are around 14 mg/dl during maintenance of anaesthesia and fall rapidly during recovery so that levels of 4–6 mg/dl have been recorded 15 minutes after the discontinuation of administration.

The mucosa of the respiratory tract is not irritated and and it is for this reason that halothane has (until the advent of sevoflurane), remained the agent of choice in man for mask induction of anaesthesia. Halothane has been shown to produce bronchodilatation with an increase in expiratory reserve volume in ponies (Watney et al., 1987). The $PaCO_2$ is directly related to the alveolar concentration of halothane when this is above 0.7% (Merkel & Eger, 1963).

Halothane causes a dose-dependent depression of cardiac output and arterial blood pressure due mainly to a negative inotropic effect although it does cause some block of transmission at sympathetic ganglia. Evidence for the mode of action of halothane on the peripheral vasculature is still both controversial and more than a little confusing. In dogs Perry et al. (1974) showed that halothane decreases plasma catecholamine levels and this may explain the reduction of arterial pressure and decreased myocardial contractility and cardiac output.

Dose-dependent respiratory depression occurs, both the depth and rate being decreased so that the minute volume of respiration is greatly reduced leading to a progressive rise in $PaCO_2$ until equilibrium between production and elimination of this gas is reached. In small dogs and in cats tachypnoea has been related to a central action of the anaesthetic (Mazzarelli et al., 1979; Berkenbosch et al., 1982). Except in horses, respiratory failure from overdose precedes cardiac failure by a considerable margin. Adaptation of both cardiovascular and respiratory function occurs with time (Steffey *et al.*, 1987) After about four hours cardiac output in horses increases by about 40% from that at 30 minutes and the values for $PaCO_2$ and the ratio of inspired to expired gas flow become significantly higher than those at 30 minutes of anaesthesia.

Bradycardia is common during halothane anaesthesia due apparently to activity in the vagus nerves. Usually a perfectly normal electrocardiogram persists throughout anaesthesia although ventricular extrasystoles and bigeminal rhythm have been reported as occurring in dogs; these can largely be prevented by premedication with acepromazine (Wiersig *et al.*, 1974). In cats A-V dissociation with interference and extrasystoles may occur (Muir *et al.*, 1959). Arrhythmias are usually associated with CO_2 accumulation from respiratory depression, hypoxia, catecholamine release and overdosage. Changes in heart rate and rhythm should not be treated with atropine as a routine since the abolition of vagal tone may accentuate their severity and even induce ventricular fibrillation. Catecholamine-induced tachyarrhythmias may be treated with propranolol or by switching to another inhalation agent.

Halothane has minimal neuromuscular blocking effect and the muscle relaxation seen during halothane anaesthesia (which is only moderate at deep levels of central nervous depression) does, however, potentiate the effects of non-depolarizing muscle relaxants and antagonize those of depolarizing agents (Graham, 1958). Shivering is often seen in all species of domestic animals during recovery but the reason for it is not completely understood. It does not seem to be related to whole body or environmental temperature and its only importance is that it may be harmful by increasing oxygen demands in animals suffering from respiratory and/or cardiovascular diseases which limit oxygen uptake when they are breathing air.

Because of its lack of analgesic properties halothane anaesthesia is more affected by premedication with analgesic drugs than is the case for many other agents. This also applies to supplementation during anaesthesia with analgesics, whether these be of the opioid type or analgesic mixtures of N_2O and O_2. Postoperative analgesia during recovery is not a feature of unsupplemented halothane anaesthesia.

Minimal pathological changes have been found in the liver and kidneys of dogs, horses and sheep anaesthetized for long periods with halothane (Stephen *et al.*, 1958; Wolff *et al.*, 1967). Susceptibility to hepatic damage varies from species to species. For example, rat liver microsomes, which contain the cytochrome P450, will bind to reductive metabolites of halothane and if these microsomal enzymes are pre-induced hepatoxicity results. Mice have the same isoenzyme P450 as rats but even when this is induced, hepatotoxicity cannot be provoked by halothane (Gorsky & Cascorbi, 1979). The guinea pig does not metabolize halothane well under reductive conditions, yet develops hepatotoxicity (Lunam *et al.*, 1985).

The question of hepatotoxicity in man has been much discussed but its actual incidence seems small because the estimated incidence of fatal fulminant hepatic failure is less than 1:35000 (National Halothane Study, Washington DC, 1969) and is associated with repeated exposure to the drug, often at short intervals (Elliott & Strunin, 1993). A second, more common syndrome, characterized by moderately increased concentrations of liver transaminases and sometimes transient jaundice, carries a low morbidity. These conditions, however, only relate to people given halothane anaesthetics and the veterinary anaesthetist is more concerned by the risk of adverse effects from exposure of anaesthetic personnel to the low concentrations of halothane in operating rooms. After a detailed and extensive review, Armstrong and Spence (1993) concluded that evidence for a severe problem with pollution from anaesthetic waste gases, including halothane, is small but nevertheless they *may* cause adverse effects in pregnant women and have an effect on the immune system (although this is probably of no clinical relevance).

Halothane and ether form an azeotropic mixture (31.7% diethyl ether and 68.3% halothane, v/v) with a boiling point of 51.5 °C. This mixture has been employed in veterinary anaesthesia (Hime, 1963) but it is an illogical one and is no longer used.

METHOXYFLURANE

Methoxyflurane is a clear, colourless liquid which boils at 104.65 °C. at 760 mmHg (101 kPa) pressure and freezes at –35 °C. Although the boiling point is slightly higher than that of water it volatilizes more readily as a result of low latent heat of vaporization (49 cal/g). It is non-explosive and non-inflammable in air or oxygen and conditions encountered in anaesthesia.

It is chemically stable and is not decomposed by air, light, moisture or alkali such as soda lime. It may, however, slowly form a brownish discoloration due to the antioxidant used in its formulation. Chenworth *et al.* (1962) have shown that the urine contains only minute traces of methoxyflurane, but polyuric renal dysfunction (high output renal failure) has been reported in people and laboratory animals. It follows the prolonged administration of high concentrations and is said to be due to the release of free fluoride by metabolism in the body: this resulted in the withdrawal of methoxyflurane from medical practice. High output renal failure, except when flunixin was given concurrently, has not been reported in veterinary anaesthesia where methoxyflurane was used extensively for small animals. The agent has now been completely withdrawn from clinical use by the manufacturers, although it can still be obtained from them for research purposes and is apparently still available in Australia.

ISOFLURANE

Isoflurane is similar to enflurane in general, physical and chemical properties. A great deal of experimental work has been carried out in evaluating isoflurane and comprehensive reviews of its pharmacological properties are those of Eger (1981), Wade & Stevens (1981) and Forrest (1983). Isoflurane does not decompose in the presence of moist soda lime but has been reported to interact with dry carbon dioxide absorbents to form carbon monoxide (Rhône Mérieux Ltd, Data Sheet).

It may be administered with oxygen or nitrous oxide/oxygen mixtures and because it is a potent anaesthetic an accurately calibrated vaporizer should be used. Isoflurane has a pungent odour but animals breathe it without breath holding or coughing. Clinical signs of anaesthesia resemble those seen with halothane.

Like most inhalation agents it undergoes some biotransformation (approximately 1%), the main metabolites being trifluroacetic acid and inorganic fluoride, but the possibility of fluoride nephrotoxicity is very remote. Respiratory and cardiovascular depression are dose-dependent. Respiratory depression in the unstimulated subject is greater than with halothane but surgical stimulation counteracts this and tends to equalize respiratory rates under anaesthesia with the two agents. Arterial blood pressure is as depressed as it is under halothane anaesthesia. However, heart rate is increased and cardiac output and stroke volume are reduced less than they are with halothane; a greater fall in peripheral resistance must be responsible for the similarity of the blood pressure response, for at clinical concentrations halothane has little effect on total peripheral resistance. There is evidence that at 1.5 and 2.0 × MAC isoflurane lowers peripheral resistance and maintains or increases blood flow to organs and muscle. Arrhythmias have not been reported and because it is an ether irregularities following the injection of catecholamines are less likely to occur than under halothane anaesthesia.

In horses a limited number of tests have shown minimal or no toxicity (Davidcova *et al.*, 1988) and recovery is usually quiet although problems with the quality of recovery have been reported, particulary after the use of ketamine as an induction agent. The quick elimination of isoflurane allows mares to nurse shortly after completion of surgery.

The high volatility, coupled with low blood solubility, provide for relatively rapid induction and recovery and easy control of the depth of anaesthesia. Its low solubility in fatty tissues avoids accumulation in obese subjects. Isoflurane increases splanchnic blood flow and thus enhances hepatic oxygenation. Renal blood flow is well maintained during isoflurane anaesthesia and because there is very little production of fluoride ions, coupled with less than 1% elimination via the kidneys, it can generally be administered quite safely to animals with renal dysfunction. Isoflurane should not be used in animals with a known susceptibility to malignant hyperthermia. Fully comprehensive data concern-

TABLE 6.2 **Inspired concentrations for the induction and maintenance of anaesthesia with isoflurane for different species of animal. The precise concentration depends on the other drugs administered and the type of anaesthetic delivery system. The concentrations shown here refer to situations where the induction of anaesthesia has been with isoflurane alone and could represent gross overdoses when anaesthesia is induced with other drugs (data from Mallinckrodt Veterinary, 1996)**

SPECIES	MAC (%)	Induction (%)	Maintenance
Horse	1.31	3.0–5.0 (foals)	1.5–2.5
Dog	1.28	Up to 5.0	1.5–2.5
Cat	1.63	Up to 4.0	1.5–3.0
Ornamental birds	About 1.45	3.0–5.0	0.6–5.0
Reptiles	?	2.0–4.0	1.0–3.0
Mouse	1.34	2.0–3.0	0.25–2.0
Rat	1.38–2.40	2.0–3.0	0.25–2.0
Rabbits	2.05	2.0–3.0	0.25–2.0

TABLE 6.3 **Median recovery times to swallowing, response to voice, spontaneous head lift and walking without ataxia in 12 dogs after anaesthesia induced with propofol and maintained for a median time of 18 minutes with halothane, enflurane and isoflurane in N_2O / O_2. None of the dogs received premedication or underwent surgical procedures (data from Peshin & Hall, 1996)**

Agent	Time to swallowing (min)	Time response to voice (min)	Time to head lift (min)	Time to walking (min)
Halothane	3	5	8	12.5
Enflurane	2.2	4.5	8	12
Isoflurane	4.5	8	10	12.5

ing its use in pregnant, breeding or lactating domestic animals are not yet available, although Funkquist *et al.* (1993) have reported its use for caesarian section in bitches. The use of isoflurane in reptiles has been reported by Hochleithner (1995).

Despite the popularity isoflurane has gained, especially in North America, it is doubtful whether it will replace halothane in veterinary anaesthesia except possibly in certain indications such as in obese animals or those suffering from cardiac disease. The much publicized rapid recovery has not been substantiated in dogs (Zbinden *et al.*, 1988). Moreover, after propofol induced anaesthesia maintained with isoflurane/N_2O/O_2 (Peshin & Hall, 1996) significant differences in recovery times from halothane, enflurane and isoflurane were not observed (Table 6.3).

ENFLURANE

Enflurane was first synthesized in 1963 and was released for general clinical use in people in North America in 1972. Fears about possible epileptogenic properties have not been realized although some anaesthetists have reported muscle twitching in enflurane anaesthetized dogs. Like halothane it depresses cardiovascular function in a

dose-dependent manner, and the effects of the two agents are comparable. It has a negative inotropic effect on the canine heart, which is accompanied by a decrease in myocardial oxygen demand. In equipotent concentrations enflurane causes slightly greater impairment of left ventricular function than does halothane (Horan *et al.*, 1977). Heart rate and rhythm are stable with enflurane and it only mildly sensitizes the heart muscle to catecholamines. Thus, subcutaneous injection of adrenaline by the surgeon is unlikely to cause serious cardiac irregularities. Arterial hypotension is often a conspicuous feature (Wolff *et al.*, 1967; Steffey *et al.*, 1975). Comparative studies of equipotent concentrations of enflurane, isoflurane, sevoflurane and halothane in dogs showed that enflurane produced the greatest falls in cardiac output and arterial blood pressure (Mutoh *et al.*, 1997). Under light anaesthesia surgical stimulation produces an immediate increase in arterial blood pressure, possibly due to increased sympathetic activity. All the commonly used neuromuscular blocking drugs are compatible with this agent but the actions of the non-depolarizing relaxants may be markedly enhanced so that smaller doses become adequate.

The degree of metabolic biotransformation is approximately 2–8% (Elliot & Strunin, 1993). The production of inorganic fluoride is probably not great enough to pose a threat to the health of normal kidneys so any potential hazard from renal fluoride toxicity is unlikely to occur but 'enflurane hepatitis' has been reported. The ability to produce rapid changes in the depth of anaesthesia coupled with apparent absence of adverse side effects suggested that this agent might be useful in veterinary practice, particularly for horses and small animals undergoing surgery on a day case basis. In horses recovery not covered by xylazine administration is unpleasant (Taylor & Hall, 1985) but in dogs enflurane has been used very satisfactorily for radiotherapy treatment (Peshin & Hall, 1996).

DESFLURANE

Desflurane is a fluorinated methyl ethyl ether, differing from isoflurane only in the substitution of fluorine for chlorine at the α-ethyl carbon atom (Fig.6.1). It is a clear, colourless and virtually odourless fluid, with a boiling point of 23.5 °C and a saturated vapour pressure of 88.53 kPa (664 mmHg) at 20 °C. Substitution of fluorine for chlorine on the α-ethyl carbon atom confers a high degree of chemical stability so that desflurane can be stored at room temperature for up to one year without the need for added preservatives. It is not degraded by artificial light and is inflammable at a concentration of 17%.

Although decomposing when in contact with dry soda lime it is not significantly decomposed by warm, moist soda lime, thus it can be used in the minimal flow systems so important in the current awareness of the need for cost containment in veterinary anaesthesia. Desflurane has a very low solubility in blood (0.42; N_2O is 0.46 – Eger (1987)) and might, therefore, be expected to induce anaesthesia very rapidly, as well as permitting rapid changes in depth of anaesthesia when the inspired concentration is altered (Eger, 1992; Smiley 1992; White, 1992; Jones & Nay, 1994). Similarly, recovery should be rapid. Problems have arisen in man where the quality of induction of anaesthesia is complicated by breath holding, coughing, laryngeal spasm and increased airway secretions from irritation of the airways (White, 1992; Smiley, 1992; Whitton et al., 1993). No similar problems have been reported when desflurane has been used to induce anaesthesia in the dog and cat and dogs recovered within 3–9 minutes following 5–9 hours of desflurane anaesthesia (Hammond et al., 1994; McMurphy & Hodgson, 1994).

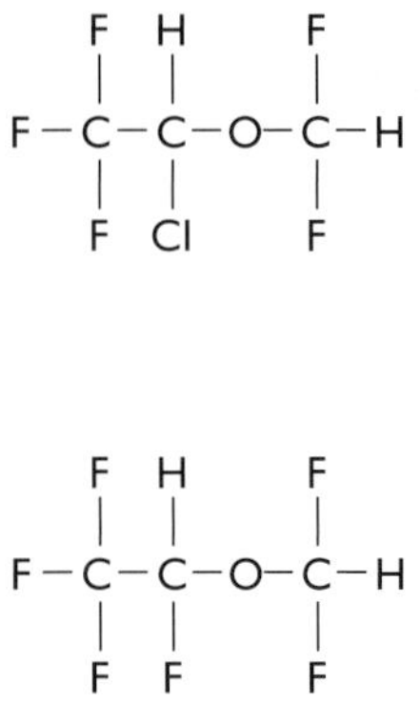

FIG. 6.1 Formulae of isoflurane and desflurane.

The minimum alveolar concentration (MAC) of desflurane varies between species and between individuals within that species. For example, the measured MAC of desflurane in human surgical patients has been reported as 7.25% in the age group 18–30 years and 6% in those aged 31–65 years (Rampil et al., 1991), while in neonates it is about 9.16% (Taylor & Lerman, 1991). In non-human primates MAC varies between 5.7 and 10.3% (Eger, 1992). After induction of anaesthesia with xylazine and ketamine, Clarke et al. (1996, 1996a) reported the MAC in ponies aged 1 or 2 years to be 7.0% (SD 0.85) with a range of 5.8 to 8.3%.

In an individual the MAC of an inhalation agent does not usually vary by more than 10% (Quasha et al., 1980) and sudden large increases of MAC during the period of measurement as reported by Eger et al. (1988) or Clarke et al. (1996), have not been reported for other inhalation agents.

Desflurane boils at close to room temperature, and a special vaporizer, such as the Tec 6 vaporizer produced by Ohmeda, is essential. Any volume of gas flowing through the vaporizing chamber of a traditional vaporizer will contain several volumes of desflurane because of the high volatility of the agent. The resulting volume expansion will produce uncontrollable efflux of gas from the chamber. Moreover, the low potency of desflurane necessitates the vaporization of large quantities of liquid during the course of an anaesthetic and in the absence of any heat source this will cause excessive cooling of the vaporizer. In the special vaporizer desflurane is contained in a sump which is electrically heated and thermostatically controlled to maintain a constant temperature of 37 °C, while an electronically controlled pressure regulating valve ensures a precise, controllable output from the vaporizer which is not affected by the rate of gas flow through the sump but is reduced by up to 2% by the concurrent use of N_2O in the carrier gas flow (Johnston *et al.*, 1994).

Desflurane undergoes minimal metabolism (0.2%) and therefore the potential for toxicity is low (Koblin, 1992). It does not prevent the development of malignant hyperthermia in susceptible pigs (Wedal *et al.*, 1993) and in experimental circumstances the effects of desflurane on vital organ function are similar to those of isoflurane (Merin *et al.*, 1991; Hartman *et al.*, 1992; Warltier and Pagel, 1992) in that it causes dose-related vasodilatation, moderate impairment of myocardial function and a similar degree of respiratory depression. The heart is not sensitized to adrenaline-induced arrhythmias. However, experimentally Weiskoptf *et al.* reported 'sympathetic storms' in man whereby an increase in inhaled concentration was followed by tachycardia and an increase in arterial blood pressure (Ebert & Muzi, 1993; Weiskopft *et al.*, 1994). Such sympathetic storms have not been reported in animals but the variations in reported MAC may be due to a similar occurrence.

The major potential advantages of desflurane in comparison with isoflurane result from its low solubilities in blood and fat. However, in most veterinary species it is probable that the advantages are minimal. The exception is in the horse (p.298), where desflurane renders it exceptionally easy to maintain stable anaesthesia and is possible to run in a totally closed system, making it very economical in use. Clarke *et al.* (1996) reported that in ponies recovery after desflurane, when coupled with low dose xylazine (0.2 mg/kg i.v. given after extubation), proved to be extremely rapid, quiet and uneventful; without xylazine, animals tended to fall at their first attempt to stand.

The availability of desflurane for use in animals will probably depend on its fate in the medical anaesthetic market where it does not seem to be proving popular because of its irritant nature (preventing mask inductions of anaesthesia) and the occurrence of sympathetic storms.

SEVOFLURANE

Sevoflurane is a fluorinated ether (Fig. 6.2) which has been licenced for medical use in Japan since 1990 and is now approved for clinical use in medical practice in the USA, the UK and Continental Europe. Although the blood/gas partition coefficient of sevoflurane is quite low (0.62), dictating rapidity of uptake and elimination, the tissue/blood partition coefficients are greater than those of isoflurane (Table 6.4)

The data in Table 6.4 do not prevent sevoflurane being a rapidly acting general anaesthetic with faster induction and emergence than isoflurane, but not as fast as desflurane. Both induction and emergence phases are smooth although there have been reports of emergence excitement in man and unsedated recoveries in horses may be violent (Clarke, 1999). The vapour pressure of sevoflurane is such that a conventional vaporizer can be employed rather than the special, and expensive, vaporizer required for desflurane.

The respiratory and cardiovascular (Ebert *et al.*, 1995) actions of sevoflurane are similar to those of the other halogenated agents. No seizure-like activity has been noted for sevoflurane. Sevoflurane depresses myocardial contractility and decreases peripheral blood flow but it is non-irritant to the respiratory passages so that induction of anaesthesia is not complicated by coughing or breath-holding.

Sevoflurane undergoes biotransformation to free fluoride ions and hexafluoroisopropanol which is rapidly glucuronidated. Its potential for hepatotoxicity is low as its metabolic pathway is not via trifluroacetic acid, but the release of free fluoride ions has given rise to some concern. Investigations into this issue demonstrate no evidence of renal toxicity and extensive clinical experience in man has brought to light no cases of renal failure following its use.

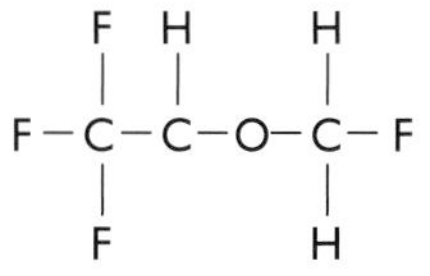

FIG. 6.2 Chemical structure of sevoflurane.

TABLE 6.4 **Physiochemical and partition data for isoflurane and sevoflurane in human subjects (part. coeff. = partition coefficient)**

	Sevoflurane	Isoflurane
Boiling point (°C)	58.5	48.5
Vapour pressure (20°C)	157	236
Blood/gas partit. coeff.	0.62	1.36
Oil/Gas part. coeff.	47	98
MAC in O_2 (%)	2.05	1.20
Tissue/fat part. coeff.	47.5	44.9
Tissue/brain part. coeff.	1.70	1.57
Tissue/muscle part. coeff.	3.13	2.92
Tissue/liver part. coeff.	1.85	1.75

Another question which has been raised concerns the stability of sevoflurane in the presence of strongly alkaline carbon dioxide absorbers since the molecule is more susceptible to spontaneous base degradation than are other anaesthetic molecules, such as those of isoflurane and desflurane. Two of the decomposition compounds generated in carbon dioxide absorbers during medical clinical use are known as compounds A and B. In clinical practice the maximum concentration of the degradation product, compound A, was far below the toxic concentration found experimentally.

The MAC of sevoflurane in horses has been determined by Aida *et al.* (1994) as 2.31 and Aida *et al.* (1966) have described its cardiovascular and pulmonary effects in these animals. Its use following atropine/xylazine/guaifenesin/thiopental induction of anaesthesia in horses was recorded by Hikasa *et al.* (1994a).

In adult spontaneously breathing cattle its use following atropine/guaifenesin/thiopental induction of anaesthesia was reported by Hikasa *et al.* (1994b), while Yasuda *et al.* (1990) compared its pharmacokinetics with those of desflurane, isoflurane and halothane in pigs. Hikasa *et al.* studied the effects of these same agents in spontaneously breathing cats and compared their ventricular arrhythmogenic activities (Hikasa *et al.*, 1996). Sevoflurane has also been used in dogs (Mutoh *et al.*, 1995, 1995a) and cats (Hikasa *et al.*, 1994c). Its cardipulmonary effects were compared with those of halothane, enflurane and isoflurane in healthy Beagles by Mutoh *et al.* (1997).

OCCUPATIONAL EXPOSURE TO INHALATION ANAESTHETIC AGENTS

Personnel are often exposed to trace concentrations of inhalation anaesthetics in the atmosphere. Contamination of ambient air occurs during the filling of vaporizers, via known or unsuspected leaks in breathing systems, and accidental spillage of liquid agent. Personnel inhale and apparently retain these agents in their bodies for some hours or even days and slow elimination of anaesthetics such as halothane allows accumulation of retained quantities from one day to the next and the persistent low concentration of the agent may encourage the formation of toxic metabolites.

The Control of Substance Hazardous to Human Health (COSHH) regulations in the UK require employers to evaluate and control the risks to health for all their employees from exposure to hazardous substances at work. Occupational Exposure Standards (OES) on an eight hour time weighted average (TWA) have been set by the Health and Safety Commision and are shown in Table 6.5.

The critical health effect was considered to be toxicity to reproduction but reproductive effects have not been proven following occupational exposures. In the USA levels of exposure which should not be exceeded are, for example, by government recommendation 2.0 ppm for volatile agents and 25 ppm for N_2O.

There seems to be no good evidence on which to base any recommendations such as those above but there is now a legal obligation in the UK for employers to meet these conditions. Anaesthetists throughout the UK were united in opposing (unsuccessfully) the imposition of COSHH regulations to anaesthetic practice. Monitoring of levels of these supposedly hazardous substances in the

TABLE 6.5 **Occupational exposure standards (Health and Safety Commission of the UK). The standard for isoflurane is five times that for halothane**

Halothane	10	ppm
Isoflurane	50	ppm
Nitrous Oxide	100	ppm

environment will, of course, entail expense for the purchase of suitable equipment. It must also be noted that work using better controlled groups and improved methods of data collection indicate that pollution of theatre atmosphere with anaesthetic gases is not as great a hazard as was thought some 20 years ago (Armstrong & Spence, 1993). However, even now there is still sufficient doubt about the safety of trace concentrations of anaesthetic gases for further research to be needed.

REFERENCES

Aida, H., Mizuno, Y., Hobo, S., Yoshida, K. and Fujinaga, T. (1994) Determination of the minimum alveolar concentration (MAC) and physical response to sevoflurane inhalation in horses. *Journal of Veterinary Medical Science* **56**: 1161–1165.

Aida, H., Mizuno, Y., Hobo, S., Yoshida, K. and Fujinaga, T. (1996) Cardiovascular and pulmonary effects of sevoflurane in horses. *Veterinary Surgery* **25**: 164–170.

Andrews, C.J.H., Sinclair, M., Dye, A., Dye, J., Harvey, J. and Prys-Roberts, C. (1982) The additive effect of nitrous oxide on respiratory depression in patients having fentanyl or alfentanil infusions. *British Journal of Anaesthesia* **54**.

Armstrong, P.J. and Spence, A.A. (1993) Toxicity of inhalational anaesthesia: long-term exposure of anaesthetic personnel – environmental pollution. *Baillière's Clinical Anaesthesiology* **7**(4): 915–935.

Baum, J.A., Aikenhead, A.R. (1995) Low flow anaesthesia. *Anaesthesia* **50**: S37.

Berkenbosch, A., de Goede, J., Olievier, C.N. and Quanjer, M.D. (1982) Sites of action of halothane on respiratory pattern and ventilatory response to CO_2 in cats. *Anesthesiology* **57**: 389–398.

Callan, C., Prokocimer, P., Delado-Herrer, L. *et al* (1994) Effect of compound A on the kidney of Spragu-Dawley rats. *Anesthesiology* **81**(3A): A1284.

Chenworth, M.B., Robertson, D.N., Erley, D.S. and Golhke, M.S. (1962) Blood and tissue levels of ether, chloroform, halothane and methyflurane in dogs. *Anesthesiology* **23**: 101–106.

Clarke, K.W. (1999) Desflurane and sevoflurane. *Clinical Anaesthesia. Veterinary Clinics of North America: Small Animal Practice* **29**(3): 793–810.

Clarke, K.W., Song, D.Y., Alibhai, H.I.K. and Lee, Y.H. (1996) Cardiopulmonary effects of desflurane in ponies after induction of anaesthesia with xylazine and ketamine. *Veterinary Record* **139**: 180–185.

Clarke, K.W., Song, D.Y., Lee, Y.H. and Alibhai, H.I.K. (1996a) Desflurane anaesthesia in the horse; minimum alveolar concentration following induction of anaesthesia with xylazine and ketamine. *Journal of Veterinary Anaesthesia* **23**: 56–59.

Davidkova, T., Kikucchi, H., Fujii, K., Mukaida, K., Sato, N., Kawachi, S. and Motio, M. (1988) Biotransformation of isoflurane: urinary and serum fluoride ion and organic fluorine. *Anesthesiology* **69**: 218–222.

Dolan, W.M., Stevens, W.C., Eger, E.I. *et al.* (1974) The cardiovascular and respiratory effects of isoflurane-nitrous oxide anaesthesia. *Canadian Anaesthetists Society Journal* **21**: 557–568.

Ebert, T.J., Harkin, C.P. and Muzi, M. (1995) Cardiovascular responses to sevoflurane: a review. *Anesthesia and Analgesia* **81** (Suppl): 11–22.

Ebert, T.J. and Muzi, M. (1993) Sympathetic hyperactivity during desflurane anaesthesia in healthy volunteers: a comparison with isoflurane. *Anesthesiology* **79**(3): 444–453.

Eckenhoff, J.E. and Helrich, M. (1958) The effect of narcotics, thiopental and nitrous oxide upon respiration and respiratory responses to hypercapina. *Anesthesiology* **19**(2): 240–243.

Eger, E.I. II (1981) Isoflurane; a review. *Anesthesiology* **55**: 559–576.

Eger, E.I. II (1987) *Anesthesia and Analgesia* **66**: 971.

Eger, E.I. II (1992) Desflurane – animal and human pharmacology: aspects kinetics, safety and MAC. *Anesthesia and Analgesia* **75**(4): 3–9.

Elliott, R.H. and Strunin, L. (1993) Hepatotoxicity of volatile anaesthetics. *British Journal of Anaesthesia* **70**: 339–348.

Fang, Z.X., Eger E.I. II, Laster M.J., Chortkoff, B.S., Kandel, L. and Lonescu, P. (1995) Carbon monoxide production from degradation of desflurane, enflurane, isoflurane, halothane and sevoflurane by soda-lime and Baralyme. *Anesthesia and Analgesia* **80**(6): 1187–1193.

Fink, B.R. (1955) Diffusion anoxia. *Anesthesiology* **16**: 511–519.

Forrest, J.B. (1983) *Clinics in Anaesthesiology* **1**(2): 251.

Frink, E.J. Jr (1995) The hepatic effects of sevoflurane. *Anesthesia and Analgesia* **81** (Suppl): S46.

Funkquist, P., Lofgren, A.M. and Nyman, G. (1993) Propofol-isoflurane anaesthesia for caesarian section in bitches. *Svensk Veterinartidning* **45**: 675–680.

Gorsky, B.H. and Cascorbi, H.F. (1979) Halothane toxicity and fluoride production in mice and rats. *Anesthesiology* **50**: 123–125.

Graham, J.D.P. (1958) The myoneural blocking action of anaesthetic drugs. *British Medical Bulletin* **14**: 15–17.

Hall, L. W. (1957) Bromochlorotrifluroethane (fluothane); a new volatile anaesthetic agent. *Veterinary Record* **69**: 615–618.

Hall, L.W. (1988) Effects of nitrous oxide on respiration during halothane anaesthesia in the dog. *British Journal of Anaesthesia* **60**: 207–215.

Halsey, M.L. (1981) *British Journal of Anesthesia* **53**: 4S.

Hammond, R.A., Alibhai, H.I.K., Walsh, K.P., Clarke, K.W., Holden, D.J. and White, R.N. (1994) Desflurane in the dog: minimum alveolar concentration alone and in combination with nitrous oxide. *Journal of Veterinary Anaesthesia* **21**: 21–23.

Hartman, J.C., Pagel, P.S., Proctor, L.T., Kampine, J.P., Schmeling, W.T. and Warltier, D.C. (1992) Influence of desflurane, isoflurane and halothane on regional tissue perfusion in dogs. *Canadian Journal of Anaesthesia* **39**: 877–887.

Hikasa, Y., Takase, K., Kondou, K. and Ogasawara, S. (1994) Sevoflurane and oxygen anaesthesia following administration of atropine-xylazine-guaifenesin-thiopental in spontaneously breathing horses. *Zentralblat Veterinarmedizin - A* **41**: 700–708.

Hikasa, Y., Takase, K., Kondou, K. and Ogasawara, S. (1994a) Sevoflurane and oxygen anaesthesia following administration of atropine-xylazine-guaifenesin-thiopental in spontaneously breathing adult cattle. *Journal of Veterinary Medical Science* **56**(3): 613–616.

Hikasa, Y., Kawanabe, H., Takase, K. and Ogasawara, S. (1994b) Comparison of sevoflurane, isoflurane and halothane anaesthesia in spontaneously breathing cats. *Veterinary Surgery* **25**: 234–243.

Hikasa, Y., Okabe, C., Takase, K. and Ogasawara, S. (1996) Ventricular arrhythmogenic dose of adrenaline during sevoflurane, isoflurane and halothane anaesthesia either with or without ketamine or thiopentone in cats. *Research in Veterinary Science* **60**(2): 134–137.

Hime, J.M. (1963) Observations on the use of halothane and ether in constant boiling (azeotropic) mixture in general anaesthesia in a small series of dogs. *Veterinary Record* **75**: 426–427.

Hochleithner, K. (1995) Isoflurane anaesthesia in birds and reptiles. *European Journal of Companion Animal Medicine* **1**: 37–41.

Horan, B.F., Prys-Roberts, C., Bennett, M.J. and Foex, P. (1977) Haemodynamic responses to isoflurane anaesthesia and hypovolaemia in the dog and their modification by propranolol. *British Journal of Anaesthesia* **49**(12): 1189–1197.

Hornbein, T.F., Eger. E.I., Winter, P.M., Smith, G., Wetstone, D. and Smith, K.H. (1982) The minimum alveolar concentration of nitrous oxide in man. *Anesthesia and Analgesia* **61**: 553–556.

Johnston, R.V. Jr, Andrews, J.J., Deyo, D.J. *et al.* (1994). *Anesthesia and Analgesia* **79**: 548.

Jones, R.M. and Nay, P.G. (1994) Desflurane. *Anesthetic Pharmacology Review* **2**: 51–60.

Kenna, J.G. and Jones, R.M. (1995) The organ toxicity of inhaled anesthetics. *Anesthesia and Analgesia* **81**(6) (Suppl): S51–S56.

Koblin, D.D. (1992) Characteristics and implications of desflurane metabolism and toxicity. *Anesthesia and Analgesia* **75** (Suppl): S10–S16.

Lunam, C.A., Cousins, M.J. and Hall, P. (1985) Guinea pig model of halothane associated heptotoxicity in the absence of enzyme induction and hypoxia.

Journal of Pharmacology and Experimental Therapeutics **232**(3): 802–809.

Malan, T.P. Jr (1995) Sevoflurane and renal function. *Anesthesia and Analgesia* **81**: S39–S45.

Mazzarelli, M., Haberer, J.P., Jaspar, N. and Miserocchi, M.D. (1979) Mechanism of halothane induced tachypnea in cats. *Anesthesiology* **51**(6): 522–527.

McMurphy, R.M. and Hodgson, D.S. (1994) Cardiopulmonary effects of desflurane in cats. *Proceedings of the 5th International Congress of Veterinary Anaesthesia, Guelph, Canada* p. 191.

McMurphy, R.M. and Hodgson, D.S. (1995) The minimum alveolar concentration of desflurane in cats. *Veterinary Surgery* **24**: 435.

Merin, R.G., Benard, J.M., Doursout, M.F., Cohen, M. and Chelly, J.E. (1991) Comparison of the effects of isoflurane and desflurane on cardiovascular dynamics and regional blood flow in the chronically instrumented dog. *Anesthesiology* **74**(3): 568–574.

Merkel, G and Eger, E.I. II (1963) A comparative study of halothane and halopropane anaesthesia. *Anesthesiology* **24**: 346–357.

Muir, B.J., Hall, L.W. and Littlewort, M.C.G. (1959) Cardiac irregularities in cats under halothane anaesthesia. *British Journal of Anaesthesia* **31**: 488–489.

Mutoh, T., Nishimura, R., Kim, H.Y. *et al.* (1995) Clinical application of rapid induction of anesthesia using isoflurane and sevoflurane with nitrous oxide in dogs. *Journal of Veterinary Medical Science* **57**(6): 1007–1013.

Mutoh, T., Nishimura, R., Kim, H.Y. *et al.* (1995a) Rapid inhalation induction of anesthesia by halothane, enflurane, isoflurane and sevoflurane and their cardiopulmonary effects in dogs. *Journal of Veterinary Medical Science* **57**: 1007–1013.

Mutoh, T., Nishimura, R., Kim, H.Y., matsunaga, S. and Sasaki, N. (1997) Cardiopulmonary effects of sevoflurane, compared with halothane, enflurane and isoflurane, in dogs. *American Journal of Veterinary Research* **58**: 885–890.

National Halothane Study (1969) Bunker, J.P., Forrest, W.H., Mosteller, F. and Vandam, L.D. (eds) A study of the possible association between halothane anesthesia and post operative hepatic necrosis. Washington DC: US Government Printing Office.

Peshin, P.K. and Hall, L.W. (1996) Short duration anaesthesia for minor procedures in dogs. *Journal of Veterinary Anaesthesiatar* **23**: 70–74.

Quasha, A.L., Eger E.I.II, and Tinker, J.H. (1980) Determination and applications of MAC. *Anesthesiology* **53**: 315–334.

Rampil, I.J., Lockhart, S.H., Zwass, M.S. *et al.*, (1991) Clinical characteristics of desflurane in surgical patients: minimum alveolar concentration. *Anesthesiology* **74**(3): 429–433.

Smiley, R.M. (1992) An overview of induction and emergence characteristics of desflurane in pediatric, adult and geriatric patients. *Anesthesia and Analgesia* **74** (Suppl 4): 38–46; discussion S44–S46.

Smith. I., Nathanson, M. and White, P.F. (1996) Sevoflurane – a long awaited volatile anaesthetic. *British Journal of Anaesthesia* **76**: 435–445.

Steffey, E.P., Gillespie, J.R., Berry, J.D., Eger, E.I.II and Rhode, E.A. (1975) Circulatory effects of halothane and halothane-nitrous oxide anaesthesia in the dog: spontaneous ventilation. *American Journal of Veterinary Research* **36**(2): 197–200.

Steffey, E.P. Kelly, A.B. and Woliner, M.J. (1987) Time related responses of spontaneously breathing, laterally recumbent horses to prolonged anesthesia with halothane. *American Journal of Veterinary Research* **48**(6): 952–957.

Stephen, C.R., Margolisd, G., Fabian, L.W. and Bourgeois- Garvardin, M. (1958) Laboratory observations with fluothane. *Anesthesiology* **19**: 770–781.

Steward, A. *et al.* (1900) *British Journal of Anaesthesia* **45**: 282.

Taylor, P.M. and Hall, L.W. (1985) Clinical anaesthesia in the horse: comparison of enflurane and halothane. *Equine Veterinary Journal* **17**: 51–57.

Taylor, R.H. and Lerman, J. (1991) Minimum alveolar concentration of desflurane and hemodynamic responses in neonates, infants and children. *Anesthesiology* **75**: 975–979.

Wade, J.G. and Stevens, W.C. (1981) Isoflurane: an anesthetic for the eighties? *Anesthesia and Analgesia* **60**: 666–682.

Warltier, D.C. and Pagel, P.S. (1992) Cardiovascular and respiratory actions of desflurane: is desflurane diferent from isoflurane? *Anesthesia and Analgesia* **75** (Suppl 4): S17–29; discussion S29–S31.

Watney, G.C.G., Jordan, C. and Hall, L.W. (1987) Effect of halothane, enflurane and isoflurane on bronchomotor tone in anaesthetized ponies. *British Journal of Anaesthesia* **59**(8): 1022–1026.

Wedal, D.J., Gammel, S.A., Milde, J.H. and Iaizzo, P.A. (1993) Delayed onset of malignant hyperthermia induced by isoflurane and desflurane compared with halothane in susceptible swine. *Anesthesiology* **78**: 1138–1144.

Weiskopf, R.B., Moore, M.A., Eger, E.I. II, Noorani, M., McKay, L., Chortkoff, B., Hart, P.S. and Damask, M. (1994) Rapid increase in desflurane concentration is associated with greater transient cardiovascular stimulation than with rapid increase in isoflurane concentration in humans. *Anesthesiology* **80**(5): 1035–1045.

White, P.F. (1992) Studies of desflurane for outpatient anesthesia. *Anesthesia and Analgesia* **74** (Suppl 4): S47–S53; discussion S53–S54.

Whitton, C.W., Elmore, J.C. and Latson, T.W. (1993) Desflurane; a review. *Progress in Anesthesiology* **78**: 46–58.

Wiersig, D.O., Davis, R.H. and Szabiniewicvz, M. (1974) Prevention of induced ventricular fibrillation in dogs anesthetized with ultra-short acting barbiturates and halothane. *Journal of the American Veterinary Medical Association* **165**(4): 341–345.

Wolff, W.A., Lumb, W.V. and Ramsaya, K. (1967) Effects of halothane and chloroform anesthesia on the equine liver. *American Journal of Veterinary Research* **28**(126): 1363–1372.

Yasuda, N., Targ, A.G., Eger, E.I.II, Johnson, B.H. and Weiskopf, R.B. (1990) Pharmacokinetics of desflurane, sevoflurane, isoflurane and halothane in pigs. *Anesthesia and Analgesia* **71**(4): 340–348.

Relaxation of the skeletal muscles

7

INTRODUCTION

To relax skeletal muscles it is necessary to abolish voluntary muscle contractions and modify the slight tension which is the normal state (the 'tone' or 'tonus' of the muscle). Tone is maintained by many complex mechanisms but, briefly, it can be said that all result in the slow asynchronous discharge of impulses from cells in the ventral horn region of the spinal cord. This discharge gives rise to impulses in the α motor neurones which cause the muscle fibres to contract. Activity of these ventral horn cells is controlled by impulses from the higher centres (cerebrum, cerebellum, or medulla oblongata) exciting the α motor neurone direct, or by impulses through the small motor nerve fibre system (the γ efferents) which activate them indirectly via the stretch reflex arc. Movements controlled by the γ fibre system are essentially directed towards governing the length of the muscle. Voluntary movement, on the other hand, involving direct activity in the γ fibres, results in muscle tension of a given magnitude.

The relevance to anaesthesia lies in the fact that the small motor nerve fibre system is, like the motor fibres to the skeletal muscles themselves, a cholinergic one. Any drug which can affect the neuromuscular junction may, therefore, also interfere with the effect of the γ-fibres on the muscle spindles. A paralysis of the γ fibre/muscle spindle junction will have, as a major consequence, a reduction in the afferent inflow from the muscle spindles and the mere reduction of such a flow to the brainstem may have subtle effects. For example, there is a possibility that a drug which paralyses the γ fibres and so reduces muscle spindle proprioceptive inflow to the higher centres actually contributes to a sleep-like state.

METHODS OF ABOLISHING MUSCLE TONE AND ABILITY TO CONTRACT

During anaesthesia abolition of muscle tone and ability to contract can be brought about in three ways:

1. *By the use of anaesthetic agents which act centrally.*

The anaesthetic agents cause decreased activity of ventral horn cells in the spinal cord and, thus, muscle relaxation. A profound degree of muscle relaxation can be obtained when a potent drug is administered in doses which produce a deep generalized depression of the whole central nervous system. However, the consequences are widespread for these agents produce dose-dependent depression of the cardiovascular and respiratory systems. Also, deep depression and immobility in the recovery period can predispose to complications such as pneumonia in horses and aspiration of regurgitated ingesta in ruminants or of stomach acid in other animals.

Other centrally acting drugs, such as guaiphenesin, which produce muscle relaxation by selectively depressing the transmission of impulses at the internuncial neurones of the spinal cord, brain stem and subcortical regions of the brain, may be more acceptable but the relaxation produced by them is seldom profound. Muscle relaxation can also be produced by the benzodiazepines and α_2 adrenoceptor agonists but this is weak and no substitute for the complete relaxation produced by neuromuscular blocking agents.

2. Utilizing drugs which have a peripheral action.

Local analgesics injected directly into a muscle mass, or around nerve fibres or nerve endings, block the transmission of impulses and muscle fibres are effectively isolated from nervous influences. This is strikingly demonstrated by paravertebral nerve block in cattle. At the same time this method also has its disadvantages. The temperament of some animals renders them unsuitable subjects for the use of local analgesics alone, especially when limb muscles are involved, and even in docile animals immobility of the whole body can only be assured when local analgesia is combined with general anaesthesia or very deep sedation. The injection of local analgesics is a time-consuming procedure and even after simple techniques there is a delay before the full degree of relaxation is obtained. In addition, techniques such as neuraxial blocks can cause loss of control of much of the circulatory system as a result of paralysis of sympathetic nerves.

In spite of the disadvantages it is probable that combinations of local analgesia and general anaesthesia are used much less than they should be in veterinary anaesthesia. Peripheral nerve blocks such as brachial plexus block, or epidural blocks with low dose bupivacaine and opioids, are the only reliable methods of preventing wind-up in the dorsal horn cells of the spinal cord and can thus make a marked contribution to postoperative pain control.

3. Using specific neuromuscular blocking agents.

Modern neuromuscular blocking agents have little or no significant action in the body other than at the neuromuscular junction, and by their use it is possible to produce quickly, and with certainty, any degree of muscle relaxation without influencing the excitability and functioning of the central nervous and cardiovascular systems. They are commonly called 'muscle relaxants' or simply 'relaxants'.

In order that their mode of action be understood it is essential that the phenomena which occur at the neuromuscular junction upon the arrival of an impulse in the motor nerve should be appreciated. The following brief review of neuromuscular transmission is concerned with those aspects that are of importance in anaesthesia. For a detailed study of these phenomena reference should be made to the standard texts of physiology.

THEORY OF NEUROMUSCULAR TRANSMISSION

The neuromuscular junction is the most accessible of the synapses in the body to study and over the last 100 years very much has been revealed about it. Even so, there are many processes involved in synaptic transmission which still await explanation. It is now well established that acetylcholine is synthesized and stored in the motor nerve in vesicles, each of which contains one packet or 'quantum' of acetylcholine. This is the transmitter substance released as a result of a propagated impulse in the nerve fibre. After release, the acetylcholine diffuses across the synaptic gap (cleft) and interacts with nicotinic acetylcholine receptors embedded in the postjunctional membrane directly opposite the sites of its release. This interaction causes the receptor–ion channel complex to undergo a conformational change from a closed to an open state. The channnel is relatively nonspecific and in the open state it can conduct sodium and potassium ions, together with other less important cations, down their respective chemical and electrical gradients resulting in a localized fall in membrane potential measured by physiologists as the 'end-plate potential'. The end-plate potential causes local circuit currents which lower the membrane potential in the electrically excitable adjacent muscle membrane and, if this lowering is of great enough amplitude, sodium channels open to initiate the muscle action potential which results in muscle contraction.

Release of acetylcholine from the nerve terminal occurs in discrete quanta and it is now believed that transmitter release is an exocytotic process whereby each quantum of acetylcholine released represents the exocytotic liberation of the contents of a single synaptic vesicle found in the terminal region of the nerve. Acetylcholine is synthesized in the nerve cytoplasm by choline acetyl-O-transferase and must be pumped into these vesicles against its concentration gradient, but the mechanism by which this occurs is poorly understood. There must also be mechanisms which link the initiation of exocytosis and promote the fusion of the synaptic vesicle membrane with the nerve terminal membrane together with the formation of a 'pore' linking the inside of the vesicle to the extracellular space of the synaptic cleft. There is still much controversy and uncertainty with respect to vesicular exocytotic processes.

The release of acetylcholine can only occur at active or 'critical' zones, meaning that there is a limited compartment of acetylcholine which can be regarded as available for release. In simple terms, 'mobilization' must occur, bringing reserve supplies of either acetylcholine itself or acetylcholine-containing vesicles into the available compartment as depletion occurs from vesicular exocytosis. One proposal which has gained ground is that prejunctional nicotinic acetylcholine receptors exist on nerve terminals allowing a positive feedback control mechanism such that acetylcholine can enhance its own release. The importance of effective mobilization becomes critical at high rates of nerve stimulation when the acetylcholine output of the nerve terminal is greatest. The phenomenon known as 'tetanic fade', i.e. the inability of the muscle to maintain a constant tension in reponse to high frequency stimulation of its motor nerve, is used by some anaesthetists to monitor the degree of neuromuscular block (Klide, 1973). A rate of stimulation of 50 Hz is considered to be the maximum physiological rate as the evoked muscle tension is similar to that developed during maximum voluntary effort.

All nicotinic receptors so far isolated and characterized, function as cation channels, the activation of which causes a change in postjunctional membrane potential. Thus they behave in a similar manner to receptors for other known chemical transmitters and belong to a family of closely related receptors (5-HT$_3$ receptor, GABA$_A$ receptor,

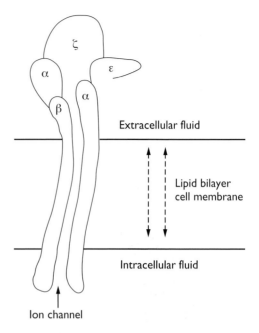

FIG. 7.1 Diagram of the nicotinic receptor at the neuromuscular junction. There are thought to be five subunits, two of which, the α receptors, are similar. The other subunits are called β, δ and ε. Another type of nicotinic receptor has a γ subunit instead of ε, the so-called extrajunctional or foetal receptor, because it occurs in relatively low numbers outside the neuromuscular junction in skeletal muscle. The five units are arranged as a cylinder around a central funnel-shaped pore.

glycine receptor and kainate-type glutamate receptor). The common element in this receptor family is that the receptors consist of five glycosylated protein subunits of varying molecular type. In mature skeletal muscle these have been designated α, β, γ, δ and ε (Fig. 7.1) having changed from embryonic types during the neonatal period when the size and number of end plates and the number of receptors increases. Each of the subunits traverses the muscle membrane at the end plate region and they are arranged to form the walls of an aqueous pore representing the ion channel through which mainly sodium and potassium ions flow to produce the single channel current measurable by the physiologists' patch-clamping technique.

Neurotransmitter acetylcholine must bind to sites on two α subunits for the ion channel to open and produce the single channel current. Competitive neuromuscular blocking agents bind on these sites so that acetylcholine has a reduced chance of binding and opening the channel. It is known that tubocurarine has different binding affinities for α subunits and it is possible that differential binding of other chemical classes of neuromuscular blocking agents may explain some of the interactions that can be observed clinically with such agents (Pedersen & Cohen, 1990).

General anaesthetics, local analgesics and antibiotics are all potential causes of end plate ion channel block. The most widely documented form of channel block is the 'open channel block' (Lambert *et al.*, 1983). After the channel is opened by acetylcholine this type of block is produced by drugs which themselves have no affinity for the binding sites on the α subunits but which, once the channel is open, enter it and bind to amino acids in the transmembrane domains. The result is that the active or open form of the receptor becomes blocked in a non-competitive way and increasing the agonist concentration (acetylcholine) leads to more open channels and hence more opportunity for the blocking compound to act. This type of block is, consequently, not reversible by anticholinesterase agents such as neostigmine.

Calcium is recognized as an essential intermediary linking depolarization of the presynaptic terminals to transmitter release. Release of acetylcholine is triggered by an increase in the concentration of intracellular calcium ions (Ca^{++}). Depolarization opens channels in the membrane that allow calcium to pass into the cell, possibly through the cyclic adenosine monophosphate (cAMP) mechanism. Thus, it is generally believed that depolarization activates membrane-bound adenyl cyclase which converts ATP to cAMP and that the latter acts on a protein kinase which causes opening of the Ca^{++} channel. Calcium itself does not cause transmitter mobilization and release – an essential intermediary is calmodulin, a Ca^{++} binding protein which regulates its action. Binding of four Ca^{++} to calmodulin changes its shape and activates it. Activated calmodulin combines with an inactive receptor protein, activating it by changing its shape, and this activated form is known to be associated with the aggregation of acetylcholine vesicles and their subsequent interaction with the presynaptic membrane. It seems probable that release of transmitter (exocytosis) is dependent on calcium ions and calmodulin.

Drugs may interfere with this complex Ca^{++} mechanism in many ways. For example, Ca^{++} antagonists such as verapamil may act by inhibiting calmodulin combination. One molecule of this drug may be sufficient to block the uptake of several thousand Ca^{++}. There is evidence that the change in quantal release of acetylcholine is proportional to the fourth power of the change in Ca^{++} concentration. In dogs, a dose of 1 mg/kg of verapamil has been shown to produce a significant interaction with the non-depolarizing agent, pancuronium, which persists long beyond the period of the calcium antagonist's cardiac effects (Jones, 1984). Volatile anaesthetics may be considered to be non-specific calcium antagonists and so potentiate neuromuscular blockade (Pollard & Millar, 1973).

In recent years there has been an increasing awareness that in addition to nicotinic cholinergic receptors at the end plate there are prejunctional receptors which have an influence on normal neuromuscular transmission. It is thought that there are at least two populations of presynaptic cholinergic receptors, each subserving different physiological functions. One group is the presynaptic nicotinic receptor which acts as a positive feedback and responds to low concentrations of acetylcholine by facilitating its release at the end plate. This is believed to be mediated at least partly by its action on synapsin I causing an increase in the immediately available store of the transmitter. The second group are presynaptic muscarinic receptors which respond to a high concentration of acetylcholine and act in a negative feedback mechanism. Stimulation of these receptors causes reduced release of transmitter in response to motor nerve activity. There are also adrenoreceptors on motor nerve endings which may modulate synaptic function, and noradrenaline is known to increase transmitter output in skeletal muscle. The catecholamine effect on the motor nerve endings is thought to be an α effect in the presynaptic region contributing to an anticurare action; it contrasts with the β effect on the postsynaptic membrane which leads to hyperpolarization and a deepening of non-depolarising neuromuscular block.

A remarkable property known as 'desensitization' is displayed by the acetylcholine receptor of striated muscle and its associated systems. This appears as the waning of a stimulant effect or development of repolarization (usually partial but under some circumstances complete) despite the continued presence of acetylcholine or some other depolarizing substance at the end plate. The rate of this repolarization increases with the concentration of the drug and is faster when the extracellular concentration of Ca^{++} is high. The extent of desensitization appears to vary between individuals of any one species. Acetylcholine has been shown to change the affinity of the receptor for certain blocking agents in a way which may be connected with the desensitization process.

NEUROMUSCULAR BLOCK

Consideration of the mechanisms of neuromuscular transmission outlined above suggests many ways in which the process may be modified to produce failure or block of transmission.

Non-depolarizing, antagonist, curare-like or competitive block results when the drug reduces the degree of depolarization of the postsynaptic membrane caused by acetylcholine following motor nerve stimulation. When the reduction in the degree of depolarization is such that a threshold depolarization of the membrane adjacent to the end plate is not achieved, a neuromuscular block is present. As the effect is 'all or none' for each motor end plate, what is seen in any particular muscle during this type of block represents a spectrum of these thresholds. For complete suppression of the motor response to occur even the most resistant synapses must be blocked.

In normal neuromuscular transmission an excess of acetylcholine is produced by motor nerve stimulation. There also exist many more receptors than necessary for the production of a total increase in cation conductance required to trigger an action potential. This results in a substantial 'safety factor' (Jones, 1984). It has been shown that under certain conditions in cat tibialis muscle four to five times as much acetylcholine is released as is needed for threshold action. Expressed in terms of receptors this means that 75–80% of the receptors must be occluded before the threshold is reached (Cookson & Paton, 1969).

The existence of a safety factor has obvious practical significance. It means, for example, that the action of the drug is far from terminated at the time when transmission is apparently normal. There is likely to be considerable 'subthreshold action' which is only detectable when a tetanic stimulus is applied to the motor nerve or when some other drug is potentiated. It also explains the properties of muscles partially blocked by competitive drugs, such as the fall of tension during a tetanus, the sensitivity of the depth of block to anticholinesterases, catecholamines, previous tetanization, anaesthesia and a wide range of drugs.

Depolarizing drugs will increase the variation of the safety factor. Slightly depolarized fibres become more excitable, i.e. their safety factor becomes greater than normal conversely, deeply depolarized fibres become less excitable. If the depolarization is sufficient, the propagation threshold may rise above the maximum depolarization which can be achieved by acetylcholine and the safety factor becomes zero. It is likely that this underlies the general insensitivity of partial depolarization block.

Drugs which produce depolarization and then prevent the passage of excitation from motor nerves have been termed 'depolarizing agents' and the analysis of their actions brought to light a variety of stimulant effects analogous to those of acetylcholine itself, and attributable to end plate depolarization. In themselves, however, these effects do not explain how synaptic block is produced, nor why the overt signs of stimulation (such as fasciculations and limb movements) are quite transient although the depolarization persists. During the block produced by a depolarizing agent there is a decrease of electrical excitability of the postsynaptic membrane as a result of the persisting depolarization (Burns & Paton, 1951).

Depolarizing block may be followed by an alteration of the threshold of the end plate region to depolarization by acetylcholine. This 'raised threshold block' was originally described as 'dual block' but now the commonly used term is 'phase II block', indicating that it follows 'phase I' which is the depolarizing activity of the drug. Phase II block following prolonged suxamethonium depolarization may be due to 'channel block', the molecule of the drug being small enough to actually penetrate the open ion channels.

In the past, neuromuscular block was classified as 'depolarizing' or 'non-depolarizing' ('competitive') solely on characteristics such as the response to an anticholinesterase, behaviour during and after the application of a tetanic stimulus, and interaction with other drugs. This now seems a dangerous outlook. Erosion of the safety factor makes it possible for a block to develop from quite a small rise in propagation threshold produced by a depolarizing drug without greatly increasing the variation in safety factor; such a block would show many of the characteristics of a competitive block. When it is realized that some neuromuscular blocking agents may be 'partial agonists' (i.e. possessing limited ability themselves to depolarize as well as to compete) and that drugs may act presynaptically as well as postsynaptically, it becomes clear that under clinical conditions many situations will arise where the underlying mechanisms can only be guessed. To interpret the effect of neuromuscular blocking drugs clinically it is necessary to assess contributions due to depolarization, competitive antagonism and presynaptic action produced by the various drugs used.

PATTERN OF NEUROMUSCULAR BLOCK

Attempts have been made to take advantage of the different susceptibilities of the body muscle to paralysis by neuromuscular blocking drugs by giving doses which were just enough to paralyse the abdominal muscles without paralysis of the intercostal muscles and diaphragm. However, useful relaxation of the abdominal muscles is invariably associated with a marked diminution in the tidal volume of respiration. When it is of a minor degree the animal may compensate for this respiratory impairment by an increase in respiratory rate. The breathing which results is characterized by a pause between inspiration and expiration, producing a rectangular pattern when recorded spirometrically. The increased respiratory rate is accompanied by over-activity of the diaphragm resulting in very turbulent conditions for intra-abdominal surgery. Larger doses of the neuromuscular blocking agent result in depression which cannot be compensated for by an increase in respiratory rate. Because of the oxygen-rich mixtures commonly used in breathing circuits hypoxia may not occur but, nevertheless, the decreased minute volume of respiration will lead to an inefficient elimination of carbon dioxide. The results are likely to be a rising blood pressure, an increased oozing from cut cutaneous vessels and distressed respiratory efforts. Thus, it is now generally recognized that if a neuromuscular blocking drug is administered for any purpose some form of artificial respiration (IPPV) will be required.

Sensitivity of muscles to neuromuscular block

The concept of sensitivity refers to the concentration of drug at the neuromuscular junction needed to produce a specific degree of blockade. From the earliest attempts to use these drugs it has been recognised that the neuromuscular junctions of various muscles differ in response with regard to intensity and duration of blockade. The recent progress in monitoring and assessing the relationship between the response of different muscles has not, unfortunately, been equalled by an understanding of the mechanisms underlying the different responses of muscles to neuromuscular blocking agents. If it were available it might allow objective predictions of the sensitivities of muscles that are inaccessible to easy monitoring under a wide range of pathological states.

Among the mechanisms suggested as being responsible for differing responses are:

1. Perfusion.
This is important since neuromuscular block can only be produced when the drug binds with acetylcholine receptors at the neuromuscular junction. Therefore, after i.v. injection the onset time for the block in any particular muscle depends on circulatory factors such as cardiac output and circulation time from injection site to the muscle, muscle blood flow and proximity to the central arterial circulation (Donati, 1988). This explains the more rapid onset of paralysis at the diaphragm, laryngeal, masseter, abdominal and facial muscles which are nearer to the aorta and probably better perfused than muscles of the distal limbs. For the onset phase concentration gradients

between the plasma and the receptors are large and thus perfusion plays a major part in the development of neuromuscular block. Perfusion, however, does not appear to contribute to unequal durations of paralysis of different muscles, at least for longer acting paralysing drugs (Goat *et al.*, 1976). During recovery from block plasma concentration changes slowly with time, so that the concentration gradient between plasma and receptors on the different muscles is likely to be small as a result perfusion plays only a minor role, duration of blockade being determined mainly by plasma concentration and sensitivity of each muscle.

2. *Acetylcholine receptor numbers, distribution and type.*

The motor innervation pattern of muscles, acetylcholinesterase activity and number and density of receptors at end plate regions may all play a part but it is not known exactly how these may contribute to muscle sensitivity to neuromuscular blocking drugs.

3. *Fibre size in the muscle.*

In goats there is a direct association between time to spontaneous recovery from vecuronium or suxamethonium blockade and size of fibres in the diaphragm, posterior cricoarytenoideus, thyroary-tenoideus and ulnaris lateralis muscles (Ibebunjo & Hall, 1993). This evidence for influence of fibre size is supported by the fact that laryngeal and facial muscles contain very small fibres while larger fibres are found in the diaphragm and still larger ones in peripheral muscles, a rank order identical to the relative sensitivities of these muscles to neuromuscular block (Donati *et al.*, 1990).

The respiratory muscles

The anaesthetist is interested in the sensitivity of the respiratory muscles to neuromuscular blocking drugs but there is a paucity of information relating to the response of intercostal, abdominal and accessory respiratory muscles to these agents. The upper airway is kept patent and protected by the laryngeal adductors, laryngeal abductors, the masseter muscle and the muscles of the tongue and pharynx, but again little is known about their sensitivity to neuromuscular blockade.

The diaphragm requires more neuromuscular blocker than a peripheral limb muscle for an identical degree of blockade. Monitoring of neuromuscular blockade during recovery is, because of their relative sensitivity, clearly best carried out by observing the responses of peripheral muscles to stimulation of their motor nerves.

MONITORING OF NEUROMUSCULAR BLOCK

The large variability in onset times, duration and depth of neuromuscular blockade following a given dose of a neuromuscular blocking agent makes it impossible to predict its effect in any individual animal. It is desirable to monitor blockade to allow drug dosage to be titrated against response of the individual. Monitoring assesses response of a muscle following electrical stimulation of its motor nerve somewhere in the nerve's peripheral course. This does not mean that neuromuscular blocking drugs should not be used in the absence of monitoring apparatus – they were used quite safely for very many years before these devices became available in clinical practice, but their use does, undeniably, add to the ease with which the degree of muscle relaxation can be controlled.

PERIPHERAL NERVE STIMULATION

A peripheral motor nerve is stimulated to produce a propagated action potential when the electrical potential inside the fibre is decreased from the normal resting value of –90 mV to a threshold of around –50 mV. A peripheral nerve stimulator achieves this when a sufficient current density is produced to decrease the potential in the tissue surrounding the nerve whereby the effective membrane potential is decreased to the threshold value. This is most easily achieved when the negative electrode of the stimulator is placed closest to the nerve, for a smaller current is then required than if the positive electrode is nearest. After a nerve has been depolarized to produce an action potential, it is resistant to further stimulation for its refractory period of some 0.5 to 1.0 ms. The observed muscle response following stimulation

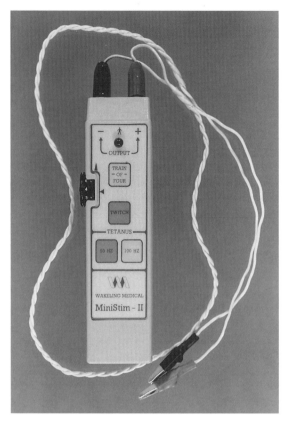

FIG. 7.2 MiniStim nerve stimulator. This is typical of the small, hand-held inexpensive nerve stimulators used for monitoring neuromuscular block.

of a peripheral nerve is only reliable when the nerve is depolarized once in response to the electrical stimulus, the same number of nerve fibres are stimulated each time and the direct stimulation of muscle fibres is avoided. The duration and shape of the stimulus pulse is important for if the duration of the impulse exceeds the refractory period of the nerve, or a non-square wave impulse is delivered, repetitive nerve stimulation may occur. A long stimulus duration is also likely to result in direct muscle stimulation (Fig. 7.2).

The single twitch

Single twitch stimulation at slow frequencies has been used extensively to investigate effects of neuromuscular blocking agents in human subjects. At a stimulus frequency greater than about 0.15 Hz the response becomes progressively smaller owing

to presynaptic effects of non-depolarizing agents impairing release of acetylcholine. Its usefulness in veterinary anaesthesia is limited as the size of the response must be quantified against a control response obtained before the administration of any drug and simple visual inspection of the twitch is insufficiently accurate for this.

Train-of-four (TOF)

Since its description by Ali *et al.*, (1970) the train-of- four (four pulses at 2.0 Hz) has become the most popular of the methods available to the clinical anaesthetist to monitor competitive neuromuscular blockade. The method as developed by these workers involves recording four twitch responses evoked in a muscle by supramaximal stimulation of its motor nerve at a rate of 2 Hz. The frequency of 2 Hz was adopted to allow maximum separation of individual twitch responses; to avoid fade between successive train-of-four (TOF) stimuli, the stimulation should not be repeated at intervals of less than 12 s. The great advantage of the TOF is that it is not necessary to establish a control response before the administration of the neuromuscular blocking agent (Cullen & Jones, 1984). The technique is simple and evaluation of the evoked response requires no special equipment. Response of the muscle can be assessed either as the number of palpable twitches (TOF count) or ratio of the fourth and the first response (TOF ratio). Fig. 7.3 illustrates the relationship during recovery from non-depolarizing blockade.

The relationship shown in Fig. 7.4 is relatively constant for all the different non-depolarizing

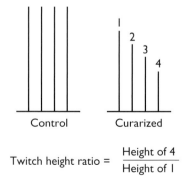

$$\text{Twitch height ratio} = \frac{\text{Height of 4}}{\text{Height of 1}}$$

FIG. 7.3 'Train-of-four' (TOF) stimulation of a motor nerve.

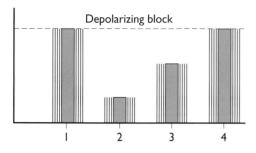

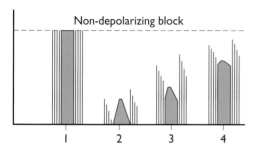

FIG. 7.4 Pattern of responses to TOF stimulation during recovery from non-depolarizing neuromuscular block. Twitch height calculated as percentage inhibition of first response to TOF stimulation.

agents (O'Hara *et al.*, 1986). A TOF ratio of > 0.5 is generally accepted as being compatible with clinically safe recovery but a TOF ratio of 0.6 to 0.7 can still be associated with fade (Drenck *et al.*, 1989). As the consequences of missing residual curarization are more serious than failing to recogzise full recovery, the prudent anaesthetist is only satisfied with a TOF ratio of 0.8 to 0.9. The fourth twitch is said to be as strong as the first when 25–30% of the receptors are free of the blocking drug. During depolarizing neuromuscular blockade, the responses to TOF stimulation are all of approximately equal height. The detection of fade is associated with the appearance of a phase II block.

The TOF has been used to study suxamethonium (Cullen & Jones, 1980), atracurium (Jones & Brearley, 1985), gallamine and pancuronium (Gleed & Jones, 1982), vecuronium (Jones & Seymour, 1985), pipecuronium (Jones, 1987) and rocuronium (Martinez *et al.*, 1996) in dogs, but its value in other animals has been questioned. According to Klein *et al.*(1988) in halothane anaesthetized horses there may be very obvious 'fade' during 50 Hz stimulation when no fade exists at

2 Hz, and thus stimulation at the higher rate is a much more sensitive method to indicate a slight blockade. However, tetanic stimulation induces recovery in the muscles stimulated so that all subsequent events are shifted towards normality (Ali & Salvarese, 1976). Moreover, stimulation of the nerve at 50 Hz results in sustained tension when only 20–25% of receptors are free, less than the 25–30% as indicated by TOF restoration of the fourth twitch. Conflicting views may result from observations in different species of animal and stimulation of different muscles.

Tetanus

Repetitive high frequency stimulation of the motor nerve where the responses to individual stimuli fuse and summate to produce a sustained muscle contraction causes what is known as 'tetany'. The absence or presence of fade due to presynaptic effect of non-depolarizing blockade has been used to assess adequacy of recovery in order to judge whether any clinically significant blockade persists to endanger the life of the animal. A tetanic stimulation of 50 Hz for 5 s stresses neuromuscular function to much the same extent as does maximal voluntary effort and it may be possible to decide, by visual or tactile means, whether there is any fade in response to tetanic stimulation.

A sustained tetanus correlates with a TOF ratio of 0.7 or greater. It seems certain that fade represents interaction of neuromuscular blocking agents with different sites within the neuromuscular junction. A site of action at presynaptic nicotinic receptors or ion channels could impede the mobilization and/or release of the transmitter in response to repeated stimulation of the motor nerve; ion channel block might also be involved.

Increased mobilization and release of transmitter substance occuring following tetanic stimulation in the presence of a neuromuscular blocking agent can cause the magnitude of response to a subsequent stimulus to be enhanced. This is termed post-tetanic facilitation or potentiation. The effect increases with the duration and frequency of tetanic stimulus and can persist for up to 30 minutes. It can lead to underestimation of neuromuscular block and to avoid it is necessary to delay further tetanic stimlation for at least two minutes (Brul *et al.*, 1991; Silverman & Brul, 1993).

During profound neuromuscular blockade when all responses to single twitch, TOF and tetanic stimulation have been abolished, post-tetanic facilitation following a tetanic burst may allow responses to occur with single twitch stimulation. Post tetanic count (PTC) is the number of responses to 1 Hz stimulation 3 s after a 5 s 50 Hz tetanus (Viby-Mogensen *et al.*, 1981). The number of post-tetanic responses is inversely related to depth of blockade: the smaller the PTC the deeper the neuromuscular block.

Double burst stimulation (DBS)

The DBS consists of two short lasting bursts of tetanus (2 to 4 pulses at 50 Hz) separated by 0.75 s. The interval of 0.75 s allows the muscle to relax completely between tetanic bursts, so that response to this pattern of stimulation is two single separated muscle contractions perceived as two twitches. The tetanic bursts fatigue the neuromuscular synapse more than two single twitches so that fade is exaggerated. Several diferent combinations of tetanic stimulation have been used but the pattern known as DBS$_{3,3}$ seems the most satisfactory. This consists of three bursts at 50 Hz followed by a further three at 50 Hz after a 0.75 s delay (Fig. 7.5). The stimulus pattern is of limited use during operations; the larger response to DBS means that the first response reappears just before that from

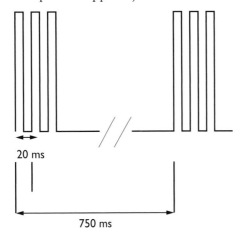

FIG. 7.5 Preferred pattern of double-burst stimulation. In each burst three impulses are given at a frequency of 50 Hz and the two bursts are separated by 750 ms (= 0.75 s).

TOF stimulation and the second response occurs slightly before the fourth response to TOF (Gill *et al.*, 1990) DBS was designed to improve clinical detection of residual curarization because it is easier to compare the strength of the two contractions to DBS than to compare the strength of the first and fourth contractions with TOF ratio.

When any nerve stimulator is used, supramaximal stimulation must be employed (e.g. 200 to 300 V for 0.3 ms) and results of stimulation should be observed before neuromuscular block is induced to ascertain that the placing of the electrodes is correct and that twitches can be obtained. Supramaximal stimulation can be achieved using surface or needle electrodes. Paediatric ECG silver/silver chloride gel electrodes are excellent provided the underlying skin is properly prepared by shaving but needle electrodes may be necessary in obese animals or those having very thick skins.

Recognition of twitches in clinical practice

In clinical practice the most convenient way of assessing the response to stimulation of the motor nerve is to observe or feel for contraction of muscles. This obviously means that the accurate evaluation of the strength of muscle activity obtained by mechanical recording with a force transducer as employed in the laboratory, cannot be expected. However, even under laboratory conditions stability of recording with time tends to be poor so perhaps the limitations imposed in the clinical situation are not a major drawback. Visual appraisal of the relevant muscle twitch is probably the simplest way of recognizing the response to nerve stimulation but other means exist.

When the ulnar nerve is stimulated accelerography may be used to measure the acceleration of the distal limb. The mass of the limb is taken to be constant and by Newton's law (force = mass × acceleration) changes in force are directly proportional to changes in acceleration. Fixation of the limb is not critical and small hand-held accelerograph monitors are available but these devices are not very reliable. Slight alteration in the position of the limb may alter the measured response.

Another method of monitoring involves recording of the electromyogram (EMG) from the stimulated muscle. This involves insertion of three needle electrodes – the active electrode from the belly of the muscle, a reference electrode on the point of origin of the muscle and a ground electrode positioned between the recording and stimulating electrodes. The recording signal is gated and usually delayed for 3 to 4 ms following nerve stimulation to avoid stimulus artefact. The equipment is expensive and the technique is usually reserved for experimental studies.

Recognition of paralysis when a nerve stimulator is not used

There can be little doubt that the reliance on simple clinical evaluations of the degree of neuromuscular blockade (using such criteria as the respiratory efforts in the anaesthetized animal) is inadequate. There is a remarkably wide variation in the sensitivity of individuals to neuromuscular blocking drugs but after spontaneous or evoked recovery from neuromuscular blockade routine clinical monitoring may allow the prediction of which individuals are likely to be able to maintain and clear their airways.

Abolition of diaphragmatic activity can be taken to indicate complete muscle paralysis. If an animal can move its limbs in such a way as to be able to maintain itself in sternal recumbency it usually means that at the most only partial neuromuscular block is present. Short, jerky respiratory efforts are often seen in animals where diaphragmatic activity is not in evidence and marked blockade exists. To assess the ability of a partially paralysed animal to breathe, the endotracheal tube may be occluded and the negative pressure generated in the tracheal tube during an attempt at inspiration measured with a simple anaeroid manometer. Depending on depth of anaesthesia and the prevailing $PaCO_2$, a pressure of -10 to $-20\,cm\,H_2O$ can usually be taken to indicate that the block is insufficient to produce respiratory inadequacy. However, although in these circumstances gas exchange may be adequate in an animal whose airway is safeguarded by an endotracheal tube, the degree of neuromuscular block may not leave enough margin of safety after extubation because of residual paralysis of the muscles of the pharynx and larynx causing upper airway obstruction.

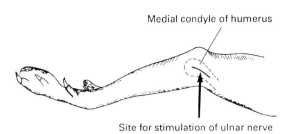

Medial condyle of humerus

Site for stimulation of ulnar nerve

FIG. 7.6 Site for stimulation of the ulnar nerve in the dog and cat.

Sites for electrical stimulation of motor nerves

In theory, neuromuscular block can be monitored by stimulation of any superficially placed peripheral motor nerve and evaluation of the response of any muscle supplied by that nerve. Monitoring is usually performed at some site where there is an accessible peripheral nerve and a readily available muscle for assessment of the results of the nerve stimulation.

The dog and cat

In dogs muscle responses to electrical stimulation of the ulnar (Heckman et al., 1977; Cullen et al., 1980), tibial (Curtis & Eiker, 1991), peroneal (Bowen, 1969) and facial (Cullen et al., 1980a) nerves have been reported. Probably the best of these, which should be used when accessible during an operation, is the ulnar nerve. It is stimulated at its most superficial location on the medial aspect of the elbow and contraction involving the forepaw is assessed visually or by palpation. The peroneal nerve is stimulated on the lateral aspect of the stifle and muscle twitch of the hindfoot assessed; this site is particularly useful when the head end of the animal is covered, for example during ocular surgery. Accurate recording of muscle twitches is not possible with facial nerve stimulation (Cullen and Jones, 1980a).

The horse

The most commonly stimulated nerve is the facial nerve (Fig. 7.7) where it can be palpated on the masseter muscle ventral to the lateral canthus of the eye. This produces easily visible contractions of the muscles of the lip and nostrils (Bowen, 1969;

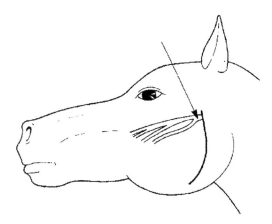

FIG. 7.7 Site for stimulation of the facial nerve in the horse.

Jones & Prentice, 1976). The peroneal nerve (Fig. 7.8) can be stimulated as it crosses the head of the fibula (Klein *et al.*, 1988) to produce contractions of the digital extensor muscles. It is advisable to restrain the hind leg when this nerve is stimulated even if no mechanical recording of the response is proposed. In horses and ponies stimulation of the peroneal nerve shows greater sensitivity to neuro-

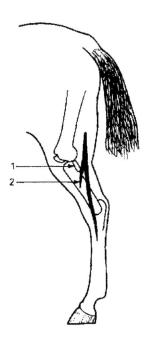

FIG. 7.8 Site for stimulation of the peroneal nerve in the horse. The nerve crosses the shaft of the tibia just distal to the head of the fibula and is often palpable at this site in thin-skinned horses.

muscular blocking agents than the facial muscle twitch (Manley *et al.*, 1983 ; Hildebrand & Arpin, 1988; Hildebrand *et al.*, 1989).

Other animals

Peroneal nerve stimulation has been used in the assessment of neuromuscular block in cows (Bowen, 1969), calves (Hildebrand & Howitt, 1984) and llamas (Hildebrand & Hill, 1991).

Factors affecting monitoring

Some patient conditions and errors in monitoring techniques can affect the muscle response observed following stimulation of a motor nerve and can lead to erroneous conclusions being drawn.

Hypothermia

Hypothermia is a common finding during general anaesthesia and may cause the degree of neuromuscular block to be overestimated. It is generally accepted that there is a 10% decrease in twitch height per °C, although the TOF ratio shows only a minimal effect. Hypothermia seems to have a smaller and more consistent effect on the EMG compared to mechanical recording (Engbaek *et al.*, 1992).

Reduction in body temperature decreases renal, hepatic and biliary elimination of non-depolarizing drugs and during hypothermia reduced doses may be needed to produce any given degree of blockade. Below a body core temperature of 34.5 °C monitoring may become increasingly inaccurate as thermoregulatory vasoconstriction occurs. Reduction of muscle blood flow in hypothermic animals may lead to delay in the onset of the block and unless allowance is made for this unduly deep block can result when assessment is carried out too soon after the injection of the drug because the anaesthetist is persuaded to administer further, unnecessary, doses.

Overstimulation

Overstimulation caused by an excessive current directly stimulating muscle or by inducing repetitive firing leads to the degree of blockade being underestimated. Overstimulation is most likely to follow when the nerve stimulator is applied after the administration of the first dose of neuromuscular blocking agent.

AGENTS WHICH PRODUCE NON-DEPOLARIZING (COMPETITIVE) BLOCK

d-TUBOCURARINE CHLORIDE

A purified, biologically standardized preparation of curare (Intocostrin) was used in dogs in 1951. Intocostrin was, however, a relatively crude substance, and the pure quaternary alkaloid, d-tubocurarine, which had become available in 1944, was used in the UK and elsewhere. After intravenous injection maximum activity is apparent within 2–3 minutes and lasts for 35–40 minutes in most species of animal. Some 30–40% of the dose is excreted unchanged in the urine within 3–4 hours. Plasma proteins have the power of binding d-tubocurarine chloride and full discussion of the fate of tubocurarine in the body has been given by Kalow (1959).

Use of an effective dose, i.e. dose that corresponds to 90% depression of twitch response under light general anaesthesia, showed that in dogs d-tubocurarine chloride has actions other than at the neuromuscular junction for although even large doses of the drug do not affect the canine myocardium it causes a severe fall in blood pressure and an increase in heart rate. The fall in arterial blood pressure appears to be due to block of impulse transmission across autonomic ganglia – hence tachycardia from vagal block – and/or release of histamine. A similar fall in arterial blood pressure occurs when the drug is administered intravenously to cats. In pigs, doses of the order of 0.3 mg/kg cause complete relaxation with respiratory paralysis without at the same time causing any marked fall in arterial blood pressure. Although unlikely to be of any use in clinical porcine anaesthesia, d-tubocurarine chloride has proved to be a useful agent for the production of relaxation required for experimental surgery.

Relatively little is known about the action of d-tubocurarine chloride in ruminant animals. Young lambs and calves appear very sensitive to the paralysing action of the drug but doses of up to 0.06 mg/kg have been given without harmful effects being noted. Intocostrin, the crude curare preparation, was used in horses during chloral hydrate narcosis and Booth and Rankin (1953) came to the conclusion that this combination of drugs had no value in equine anaesthesia. However, the dose of curare used (about 0.12 mg/kg when expressed in terms of the pure d-tubocurarine was much less than what is today regarded as the minimal effective dose. Doses of 0.22 to 0.25 mg/kg produce good relaxation with respiratory arrest in anaesthetized horses breathing 0.8 to 1.0% halothane and no significant hypotension is encountered.

DIMETHYL ETHER OF d-TUBOCURARINE

The dimethyl ether of d-tubocurarine has been used as a relaxant during anaesthesia in dogs, cats, pigs and horses. It appeared to be two to three times as potent as d-tubocurarine chloride but the duration of neuromuscular blockade was slightly shorter. It never gained a wide popularity and has not been available a in the UK since about 1965 but it is available in the USA under the name of 'Metocurine'.

GALLAMINE TRIETHIODIDE

Gallamine block of cardiac muscarinic activity can be useful during halothane anaesthesia since halothane tends to produce bradycardia via the vagus nerve. Tachycardia occurs within 1.0 to 1.5 min after i.v. injection and in dogs and pigs the heart rate increases by 10–20%. The rise in heart rate is sometimes accompanied by a rise in arterial blood pressure. It is not detoxicated and is excreted unchanged in the urine. Gallamine does not give rise to histamine release so that it is a useful non-depolarizing relaxant in dogs.

In dogs doses of 1.0 mg/kg by i.v. injection usually cause complete relaxation for 15 to 20 minutes. Apart from a slight tachycardia, the drug appears to produce few side effects, but occasionally hypertension follows its administration. In cats 1.0 mg/kg produces apnoea of 10 to 20 min duration. Pigs are very resistant to gallamine and doses of 4 mg/kg are needed to produce complete relaxation with apnoea. In horses, doses of 0.5 to 1.0 mg/kg result in complete paralysis with apnoea of 10 to 20 min duration. Young lambs and calves have been given doses of 0.5–1.0 mg/kg without harmful effect but in these animals apnoea may be prolonged.

ALCURONIUM CHLORIDE

Alcuronium is not available in the USA. It is diallylnortoxiferine, a derivative of the alkaloid toxiferine obtained from calabash curare. It has been used quite extensively in dogs and horses and seems to have no significant histamine liberating or ganglionic blocking effects. During light halothane anaesthesia the dose required to produce complete relaxation with respiratory arrest is 0.1 mg/kg. Intravenous injection produces no change in heart rate, arterial blood pressure or central venous pressure. The return of spontaneous breathing is apparently followed by a prolonged period of partial paresis; because of this, reversal of the myoneural block is obligatory. If only one dose of alcuronium chloride has been given during the course of an operation, the block is very readily reversed with neostigmine or other anticholinesterases, but when more than one dose of alcuronium has been administered some difficulty may be experienced in antagonizing its effects. It is, therefore, probably advisable to limit the use of alcuronium for operations which can be completed in the 70 ± 18 minute period of relaxation which follows one injection of the drug (Jones *et al.*, 1978).

PANCURONIUM BROMIDE

Pancuronium bromide, an amino steroid free from any hormonal action, is a rapidly acting, nondepolarizing neuromuscular blocker with a medium duration of activity. It has no major undesirable side effects but its administration may be followed by a slight, short lived, rise in arterial blood pressure. A study in 1970 of the effects of pancuronium in dogs, cats and horses (G.M. Thompson, personal communication) showed that the i.v. injection of the drug causes minimal change in heart rate or central venous pressure and no alteration of the ECG. During light anaesthesia doses of 0.06 mg/kg have been found to produce

complete relaxation with apnoea in dogs and horses of about 40 min duration together with a short-lived rise in arterial blood pressure. A similar period of apnoea follows a second dose of 0.03 mg/kg. The delay in achieving maximum effect after i.v. administration is much less than is found with d-tubocurarine or alcuronium. Complete antagonism with neostigmine (always given with an anticholinergic) is readily obtained and no cases of relapse into neuromuscular block have been encountered. Care should be taken in dogs suffering from chronic nephritis and other conditions which impair kidney function, because it is, in part, excreted unchanged in the urine and its action is also prolonged in cases of biliary obstruction.

VECURONIUM

Vecuronium is a monoquarternary analogue of pancuronium, the only difference in structure being that in this compound the nitrogen in the piperidine group attached to the steroid nucleus is not quarternary and positively charged whereas in pancuronium it is. Due to the instability of the 3-acetyl group in high concentrations in solution the drug is marketed as a freeze-dried buffered powder with water in a separate ampoule. The powder can be kept on the shelf at room temperature without deterioration. Vecuronium is currently the most specific neuromuscular blocking drug in clinical use and is more potent and shorter acting than pancuronium. It shows a low propensity to liberate histamine and possesses a negligible ganglionic blocking action, hence cardiovascular side effects are unlikely to be seen during clinical use.

Although the mechanism and exact pathway of inactivation in the body is not fully understood, by analogy with pancuronium there are likely to be three main metabolites that could arise by deacetylation to the corresponding alcohol. The principal metabolite appears to be the 3-hydroxyl derivative for up to 10% of an injected dose may appear in this form in the urine.

In dogs doses of 0.06 mg/kg produce an initial block of about 20 min and in horses this dose appears to produce apnoea of 20 to 30 min duration. Although the ED_{50} of vecuronium is about 0.04 mg/kg compared with 0.05 mg/kg for pancuronium, at this dose the recovery from neuromuscular block to 50% twitch depression is less than 10 min and this period is less than adequate for most surgical procedures, whereas that produced by pancuronium is much longer lasting. As a result, if longer lasting relaxation is to be obtained it is necessary to use a larger bolus dose of vecuronium to produce a rather greater initial block than with pancuronium.

Vecuronium has both hepatic and renal pathways for excretion but renal failure has little effect on its clearance. Biliary excretion accounts for about 50% of the injected dose so that clearance is much reduced in severe hepatic disease. In the absence of renal and hepatic disease it is not markedly cumulative and, indeed, in healthy dogs up to six incremental doses of 0.4 mg/kg have been shown to be non-cumulative (Jones & Seymour, 1985). It has also been used as an infusion in dogs (Clutton, 1992).

PIPECURONIUM

Pipecuronium bromide, a long acting non-depolarizing neuromuscular blocking agent, is an analogue of pancuronium. It was originally used in 1980 in Hungary but it is now approved for clinical use in man in both the UK and the USA. In dogs about 77% of the injected drug is said to be eliminated in the urine with less than 5% being excreted in the bile. One potential advantage of pipecuronium is that it is apparently free from cardiovascular side effects. Its neuromuscular blocking effects in the dog have been investigated (Jones 1987;1987a).

ROCURONIUM

Rocuronium, formerly known as Org 9426, a steroidal non-depolarizing neuromuscular blocker, is a derivative of vecuronium. Initial animal studies (Muir *et al.*, 1989 ; Cason *et al.*, 1990) demonstrated that compared with vecuronium the onset of block was more rapid, its duration of action very similar and its potency about one-fifth. It has no or minimal cardiovascular effects but in anaesthetized cats it has been shown to possess a vagal/neuromuscular blocking ratio of 7 compared to 3 for pancuronium (Marshall *et al.*, 1994), so that compared to vecuronium it may be consid-

ered to have some mild vagolytic activity. In cats more than 50% of the injected dose is eliminated unchanged in the bile and only 9% in the urine (Khuenl-Brady *et al.*, 1990). No signs of histamine release or anaphylactoid responses have been reported after its administration but it has been reported that in man the injection of rocuronium is painful and, therefore, the drug should only be injected after the deeper stages of anaesthesia have been achieved (Borgeat & Kwiatkowski, 1997).

ATRACURIUM

Atracurium besylate is a bisquaternary isoquinoline compound and is available as a mixture of 10 sterioisomers (Amaki *et al.*, 1985). It is eliminated by pH and temperature-dependent Hofmann degradation, giving rise to laudanosine and a monoquaternary ester which is further degraded to a second laudanosine molecule and an acrylate ester (Stenlake *et al.*, 1981). None of these degraduation products is active at the neuromuscular junction. The half-life of this process in cats is about 19 minutes (Payne & Hughes, 1981). Coupled with uptake by the liver, kidney and other tissues, this produces a rapid plasma clearance and an apparent large distribution volume. The Hofmann degradation process does not need an enzyme system and attains a linear relationship between the dose of drug and the rate of metabolism irrespective of the substrate load. Obviously, the reason why the duration of block is unaffected by hepatic disease or anuria is because neither process involves liver metabolism or renal excretion.

Because of its propensity to release histamine, atracurium cannot be administered in multiples of its ED_{50} to give the same sort of flexibility of duration of action associated with vecuronium where a large single bolus dose can be used to provide relaxation for a moderately prolonged operation. It is in short procedures that its relatively rapid onset, medium duration of action and rapid recovery are most useful.

The paralysing dose for the dog is from 0.3 to 0.5 mg/kg (Jones & Clutton, 1984) and recovery from these doses occurs in about 40 min (Jones *et al.*, 1983) although there is a very wide range in the duration of effect. The reason for this wide variability in duration is unknown. The drug has also been administered to dogs by continuous infusion of 0.5 mg/kg/hour after a loading dose of 0.5 mg/kg (Jones & Brearley, 1985).

A single injection of 0.11 mg/kg of atracuronium produces paralysis of about 20 to 30 min duration in halothane anaesthetized horses (Hildebrand et al., 1986). It has also been administered by infusion to horses under halothane anaesthesia (Klein et al., 1988). After a loading dose of 0.05 mg/kg in another investigation a 95 to 99 % reduction in TOF hoof-twitch response was produced by an infusion of 0.17 ± 0.01 mg/kg/hour (Hildebrand & Hill, 1989).

Some anxiety has been expressed about a possible central nervous system effect of the tertiary metabolite of atracurium. This compound, laudanosine, does penetrate the blood–brain barrier and, in higher concentrations than are likely to be produced with clinical doses in normal animals, it can cause analeptic or convulsant effects. To date, no reports of these effects have been described in the veterinary literature.

MIVACURIUM

Savarese and colleagues in Massachusetts investigated a series of compounds which are non-depolarizing and metabolized by plasma cholinesterase. One of these, mivacurium, is a benzylisoquinoline diester compound with a potency approximately one third to one half that of atracurium. It consists of three sterioisomers of which one is active. Unlike atracurium, its breakdown products are pharmacologically inactive. Breakdown is by plasma cholinesterase and both acetylcholinesterase and spontaneous hydrolysis appear to have only minimal effects. Low plasma cholinesterase levels are associated with a longer duration of action and a decreased plasma cholinesterase due to hepatic failure results in prolonged activity, although alternative pathways for clearance are available (Saverese et al., 1988).

Re-establishment of paralysis using very small doses of mivacurium following apparent full recovery from mivacurium-induced neuromuscular block has been reported in man (Kopman et al., 1996). Even at a TOF of 0.95 the neuromuscular junction's margin of safety remains considerably reduced.

PHARMACOKINETICS OF THE NON-DEPOLARIZING AGENTS

All neuromuscular blocking agents contain quaternary ammonium groups making them positively charged at body temperature. Because of this ionization they are highly water soluble and relatively insoluble in fat. Their pharmacokinetics can be described by a two or three compartment model, with a rapid distribution phase in which they distribute from a central into a peripheral compartment. This is followed by one or two slower elimination phases, consisting of biotransformation and excretion. For most drugs a two compartment model is suitable and thus two half-lives can be determined: the half-life of distribution ($t_{1/2\alpha}$) and the half-life of elimination ($t_{1/2\beta}$). The mean residence time (MRT) has been introduced for statistical purposes – the time for 63.2 % of the administered dose to be excreted. The value known as C_{SS95} is the plasma concentration at which a 95% decrease in muscle contraction occurs. This is particularly important to the anaesthetist because it represents the surgically optimal level of neuromuscular block.

All pharmacokinetic data are relevant to the full understanding of the pharmacological profile of a drug under particular circumstances, but only a few are of immediate clinical importance to the anaesthetist who principally wishes to utilize them for calculation of the appropriate infusion rate for any particular drug. These clinically important data are summarized in Table 7.1 which shows mean figures culled from the literature. The published data show a marked variability resulting from differences in the doses administered, the anaesthetic technique employed, the time of sampling, the extraction and assay methods for measuring the concentrations, the species of animal and in the pharmacokinetic model used for the calculations.

Vd_c governs the peak plasma concentration following injection of a bolus dose. Because drug distribution depends on tissue perfusion, cardiac output is an important factor in pharmacokinetics. Reduction in cardiac output leads to slow and lesser distribution with lengthening of $t_{1/2\alpha}$, a slower onset of action and eventually, a stronger effect. With increased cardiac output tissue perfusion is

TABLE 7.1 **Pharmacokinetic data (rounded figures).** Vd_c = initial volume of distribution; Vd_{ss} = volume of distribution, central and peripheral compartment; Clp = plasma clearance; $t_{1/2\,\beta}$ = half-life of elimination; MRT = mean residence time; C_{ss95} = plasma concentration for 95 % decrease in first twitch of TOF

Drug	C_{ss95} (mg/kg)	Vd_c (l/kg)	Cd_{ss} (l/kg)	Cl_p (ml/kg/min)	$t_{1/2}\,\beta$ (min)	MRT (min)
Alcuronium	0.08	0.15	0.33	1.34	143	
Atracurium	1.30	0.05	0.20	6.60	21	
Doxacurium			0.22	2.76	99	91.9
Gallamine	10.00	0.10	0.20	1.20	134	
Metocurine	0.60	0.05	0.57	1.20	360	
Mivacurium			0.11	70.00	18	1.5
Pancuronium	0.35	0.10	0.26	1.80	132	134.0
Pipecuronium		0.11	0.31	2.30	137	140.0
Rocuronium		0.04	0.21	3.70	97	58.3
Vecuronium	0.23	0.07	0.27	5.20	71	52.0

greater than normal which means a more extensive and faster distribution and thus a higher dose is needed to cause the same effect. When the plasma concentration of a drug to produce a given level of neuromuscular block (e.g. C_{ss95}) is known, the single bolus dose or the rate of a continuous infusion needed for it to be achieved can be calculated:

$$\text{Bolus dose} = C_{ss95} \times Vd_{ss},$$
$$\text{and infusion rate} = C_{ss95} \times Clp$$

It must be remembered, however, that a wide biological variability in response to neuromuscular blocking drugs exists between individual animals.

Another important factor in pharmacokinetic behaviour is protein binding which influences the volume of distribution, metabolism and excretion of neuromuscular blocking agents. Changes in plasma protein concentration in diseased states and binding of concurrently administered drugs will both influence the protein binding of these agents.

AGENTS WHICH PRODUCE DEPOLARIZING BLOCK

Muscle paralysis due to depolarization differs from that caused by non-depolarizing drugs in the following respects:

1. The paralysis is preceded by the transient stimulation of muscle fibres, probably caused by the initial depolarization. The muscle twitching which results from this is visible in animal subjects.

2. Substances which antagonize the non-depolarizing agents tend to potentiate the depolarizing ones and thus in clinical practice it is important to note that anticholinestrases such as neostigmine may prolong the action of depolarizing relaxants.

3. In a nerve–muscle preparation it can be demonstrated that after partial paralysis with a non-depolarizing drug there is a rapid decay of an induced tetanus, whereas after a corresponding degree of paralysis caused by a depolarizing agent an induced tetanus is sustained.

4. It is unlikely that depolarizing agents ever produce a pure type of neuromuscular block. For example, in dogs they cause both depolarization and desensitization.

5. In the cat, rat and mouse, the depolarizing agents affect the red muscles more than the white, whereas non-depolarizers have the opposite effect.

In certain animal species esters of choline, notably the succinyl derivatives, cause neuromuscular block of short duration by depolarization. Two of these compounds are dimethylsuccinylcholine and diethylsuccinylcholine. The former substance is known as suxamethonium and the latter as suxethonium. They resemble each other pharmacologically, with the sole difference that the paralysis caused by suxethonium is rather more rapid in onset and of slightly shorter duration. The first two of the compounds to be used clinically in veterinary anaesthesia was suxethonium bromide (Hall, 1952) but the suxamethonium compound is the one generally employed today.

SUXAMETHONIUM

Suxamethonium consists of two acetylcholine molecules coupled back to back. Like acetylcholine, it is hydrolysed by cholinesterases and this hydrolysis is believed to be responsible for recovery from its effects. It has been shown in dogs that the injection of a purified cholinesterase preparation produces a marked increase in resistance to the effect of the drug (Hall *et al.*, 1953). Because of this, attempts have been made to correlate the sensitivity of an animal to suxamethonium with the levels of cholinesterase present in its blood (Stowe *et al.*, 1958).

The ability of plasma cholinesterase to hydrolyse butyrylthiocholine can be used to predict sensitivity to suxamethonium in man but has not been of value in animals. Faye (1988) has made an extensive study of the role of cholinesterase in the explanation of differing species sensitivity to suxamethonium. In her opinion the affinities of cholinesterase for different substrates are different between species (Tables 7.2 and 7.3) and, furthermore, although the hydrolysis of some assay substrates parallel that of suxamethonium in man they do not in other species of animal. Therefore, the substrates used to study cholinesterase activity in man cannot be used to draw conclusions regarding suxamethonium sensitivity in other animals; for this to be done, Faye considers it is most important that the substrate used for assay is suxamethonium itself.

In birds, suxamethonium produces spastic paralysis of the whole body. An initial enhancement of the twitch produced by stimulation of the motor nerve is quickly followed by a tonic contraction and depression of neuromuscular transmission. Spasm does not require neural impulses, usually prevents muscle fasciculation and persists as long as the block lasts. In mammals, this myotonic response persists in the extraocular muscles, in partially denervated and degenerating limb muscles and to a minor degree in the jaw muscles. Animals susceptible to malignant hyperthermia also respond to suxamethonium with a spastic paralysis.

In domestic animals there is some slight variation in response of the various muscle groups but the diaphragmatic muscle is usually the last to be affected. Suxamethonium causes marked muscle fasciculation and in man these contractions frequently lead to muscle pains obvious the next day to the patient. Conscious volunteers given suxamethonium for experimental purposes have reported that the muscle fasciculations are extremely painful. Suxamethonium produces actual muscle injury; serum creatine kinase levels are raised and myoglobinuria has been seen after intermittent administration of the drug during halothane anaesthesia in horses.

Because cholinesterase is formed in the liver, the existence of severe liver damage, cachexia, or malnutrition may prolong the duration of action of suxamethonium. In man, atypical forms of cholinesterase are recognized. They have been found in animals but their significance and mode of inheritance have not been determined (Trucchi *et al*, 1988). Low cholinesterase levels are also

TABLE 7.2 **Mean values for plasma cholinesterases as determined by the use of different assay substrates (courtesy of Dr Sherry Faye, Senior Biochemist, Bristol Royal Infirmary)**				
Species	**Propionyl thiocholine**	**Benzoyl choline**	**Butyryl thiocholine**	**Succinylcholine**
Sacred baboon	4.20	0.85	7.01	89.70
Chimpanzee	5.65	0.93	6.15	76.50
Bottle-nosed dolphin	0.04	None	0.02	47.90
Pig	0.34	0.03	0.32	43.13
Horse	4.18	0.27	4.46	33.10
Dog	2.13	0.36	3.33	8.01
Cat	1.36	–	–	7.24
Indian elephant	0.01	None	0.05	7.00
Goat	0.14	0.04	0.02	6.70
Sheep	0.05	None	None	1.47
Cow	0.06	–	–	0.95

TABLE 7.3 **Plasma cholinesterase activities determined using different substrates expressed as a percentage of appropriate mean human reference range. Mean cholinesterase activity for human Elu homozygotes taken as: propionylthiocholine activity 4.58 units/ml, benzoylcholine activity 0.88 units/ml, butyryl thiocholine activity 5.04 units/ml and succinylcholine activity 58.6 units/ml (courtesy of Dr Sherry Faye, Senior Biochemist, Bristol Royal Infirmary)**

Species	Propionyl thiocholine activity	Benzoyl choline activity	Butyryl thiocholine actvity	Succinylcholine activity
Red deer	1.3	4.5	0.5	6.8
Goat	2.9	4.5	0.5	6.7
Fallow deer	1.0	–	1.3	12.4
Bottle-nosed dolphin	0.9	–	0.4	81.7
Indian elephant	0.2	–	0.9	11.9
Sacred baboon	91.7	96.6	139.1	153.1
Patas monkey	9.2	5.7	13.5	45.9
White rhino	29.7	12.5	34.3	26.4
Donkey	99.3	62.5	124.4	61.6
Muscovy duck	8.5	7.9	6.9	18.9

encountered after exposure to organophosphorus compounds.

Suxamethonium, containing two acetylcholine molecules, might be expected to have actions in the body in addition to its effects at the neuromuscular junction and this is indeed the case. Injection of suxamethonium causes a rise in blood pressure in all animals, although in some species the rise may be preceded by a fall. In cats there is an immediate marked fall in arterial blood pressure, followed by a slower rise to above the resting level. The fall in blood pressure can be prevented by the prior administration of atropine, and the rise by hexamethonium so that the prior administration of both these drugs prevents any blood pressure change. Blood pressure changes are seen after each successive dose of suxamethonium but with progressively diminishing severity. Pulse rate changes are variable, both bradycardia and tachycardia being observed, sometimes in the same animal, and often the heart rate does not change. In horses and dogs the nicotinic response predominates (Adams & Hall, 1962, 1962a) – very occasionally a fall in blood pressure with bradycardia is seen, but an increase in both blood pressure and heart rate is the usual response.

Cardiac arrhythmias are frequently seen after i.v. injection and usually take the form of atrioventricular nodal rhythm. One injection of suxamethonium causes a rise in serum potassium which is not abolished by adrenalectomy, ganglionic blockade,

adrenolytic drugs or high epidural block so it is likely to be due to release of potassium ions from muscle. This rise in serum potassium may also be associated with cardiac irregularities. Prolonged administration of suxamethonium, on the other hand, causes a large decrease in serum potassium in dogs, but the reason for this is unknown (Stevenson, 1960).

There are wide species differences in sensitivity to the neuromuscular blocking action of suxamethonium. Horses, pigs and cats are relatively resistant, but dogs, sheep and cattle are paralysed by small doses. In horses 0.12–0.15 mg/kg usually cause paralysis of the limb, head and neck muscles without producing diaphragmatic paralysis. In most horses double this dose will cause total paralysis but the exact effect produced in any individual will depend on the depth of anaesthesia at the time when the relaxant is administered. After a single dose paralysis generally lasts for about 4–5 min although limb weakness may persist for some time longer. In cattle, one-sixth of this quantity (0.02 mg/kg) produces paralysis of the body muscles without diaphragmatic paralysis and this relaxation lasts 6–8 min. Once again, double this dose will cause complete paralysis in most animals. In sheep, doses similar to those used in cattle are employed. Pigs require much larger doses; to facilitate endotracheal intubation the dose required is about 2 mg/kg, which produces complete paralysis for only 2–3 min. In cats, 3–5 mg of suxamethonium chloride (total dose) produces 5–6 min of paralysis. The dog is comparatively sensitive and doses of 0.3 mg/kg produce total paralysis of 15–20 minutes' duration. A single dose may produce phase II block in dogs and phase II block may also be produced when more than one dose is given to other animals. It is believed that the response of the motor end plate gradually alters with each successive dose but the precise time and dose relationship is not yet known.

Apart from its use to facilitate endotracheal intubation in pigs and cats, it seems that there are today no good indications for suxamethonium in veterinary anaesthesia.

FACTORS AFFECTING THE ACTION OF NEUROMUSCULAR BLOCKING DRUGS

Factors such as age, concurrent administration of other drugs, body temperature, extracellular pH, neuromuscular disease and genetic abnormalities may influence response to muscle relaxant drugs.

Age

The response of young animals to neuromuscular blocking drugs is different from that of adults. The muscles of a 7-day-old kitten are less sensitive to depolarizing drugs than those of a normal adult cat but very sensitive to tubocurarine. The anaesthetic drugs themselves have an age-dependent effect upon neuromuscular transmission so that complementary relaxation provided by some anaesthetics is variable and important.

Body temperature

The effect of muscle and body temperature on the potency and duration of action of muscle relaxants is difficult to assess because any effect of change in body temperature on neuromuscular block may be complicated by changes in regional blood flow. Reduction in body temperature decreases renal, hepatic and biliary elimination of non-depolarizing neuromuscular blocking agents and during hypothermia reduced doses may be needed to produce a given degree of neuromuscular block. In clinical practice it certainly seems that the requirements of non-depolarizing agents are decreased during moderate hypothermia. Reduction of muscle blood flow in hypothermic animals may lead to delay in onset time of block and unless allowance is made for this, gives rise to the risk of serious overdosing if the drug is being given in incremental doses to assess its effects as administration proceeds.

Administration of other drugs

Any drug which has anticholinesterase properties will prolong the action of suxamethonium and tend to antagonize non-depolarizing neuromuscular blockade. Several antibiotics, especially the aminoglycosides, may produce or enhance non-depolarizing block, possibly by binding calcium to produce hypocalcaemia, or by influencing binding of calcium at presynaptic sites. However, antibiotic induced or enhanced competitive block is not invariably antagonized by anticholinesterase drugs or by administration of calcium. Care should, therefore, be taken over the administration of antibiotics such as gentamycin during the immediate recovery period following antagonism of non-depolarizing neuromuscular blockers because refractory paralysis may occur.

General anaesthetics may have a marked effect on neuromuscular block. Halothane, methoxyflurane and isoflurane potentiate non-depolarizing relaxants such as pancuronium. Rocuronium block is potentiated by isoflurane and enflurane but only to a lesser degree by halothane.

Extracellular pH

Hypercapnia augments tubocurarine block and opposes its reversal by neostigmine. Alcuronium and pancuronium block are apparently unaffected by PCO_2, but block due to suxamethonium may be potentiated by acidosis. A number of explanations have been advanced to account for these findings and it seems likely that factors such as protein binding, ionization of the relaxant and ionization of the receptor sites may be important.

Neuromuscular disease

Animals suffering from myasthenia gravis are resistant to depolarizing neuromuscular blockers and are more than normally sensitive to competitive blocking agents. A myopathy has been described in a horse (Jones & Richie, 1965) where a generalized muscle spasm was produced by the administration of an extremely small dose of suxamethonium.

Genetic factors

Genetic factors in relation to response to suxamethonium have been described in humans. Trucchi *et al.* (1988) have demonstrated some effects on cholinesterase activity which seem to have a genetic basis in dogs.

Blood pressure and flow

Recovery from the effects of relaxant drugs is likely to be more rapid if blood flow through the muscle is high and thus maintains a steep concentration gradient between tissues and blood by removing molecules of the agent as soon as they are freed from receptors.

Electrolyte imbalance

A deficiency of calcium, potassium or sodium retards the depolarization of motor end plates and by thus inhibiting neuromuscular transmission will increase the blocking effects of the non-depolarizing muscle relaxants. On the other hand, hyperkalaemia and hypernatraemia render muscles more resistant to them.

EVOKED RECOVERY FROM NEUROMUSCULAR BLOCK

While it is possible for non-depolarizing agents to be eliminated from the body with or without significant metabolism, thus resulting in termination of action, this can never be reliably predicted. There is great individual variation in response of animals to neuromuscular blocking drugs and, in addition, with many drugs spontaneous recovery takes a very long time. Thus, antagonism of non-depolarizing neuromuscular block is usually indicated in routine clinical practice – especially in horses, for these animals appear to have a psycho-

logical need to stand immediately on recovery from anaesthesia. The presence of even a small degree of neuromuscular block can result in violent excitement and floundering about as the horse tries, unsuccessfully because of muscle weakness, to get to its feet.

The principle underlying use of antagonists to neuromuscular blocking drugs is tilting of the balance between the concentration of acetylcholine and the concentration of the drug at the neuromuscular junction in favour of the former. To do this, it is necessary to reduce breakdown of acetylcholine by cholinesterase or to facilitate greater release of it. The drugs that are in common use as antagonists of neuromuscular block are those that reduce breakdown of the transmitter, i.e. they are anticholinesterases. The anticholinesterases allow the accumulation of acetylcholine at the end plate region but acetylcholine does not actively displace the neuromuscular blocking drugs molecules from the receptor sites. There is constant attachment and reattachment of the molecules of the muscle relaxant and acetylcholine to the receptor, and with the greater numbers of acetylcholine molecules from inhibition of acetylcholinesterase there is a greater chance of one of the acetylcholine molecules occupying a temporarily 'unblocked' receptor (Bowman, 1990).

There are no effective antidotes to those agents which act by depolarization, but certain anticholinesterases are effective antidotes to the phase II block following the use of suxamethonium. It is essential to observe clear fade of TOF because, when phase II block is not present, prolonged paralysis requiring several hours of ventilatory support may result from anticholinesterase administration. The commonly used anticholinesterase agents are neostigmine, edrophonium and pyridostigmine and of these neostigmine is by far the most popular. The use of these agents in the reversal of neuromuscular blockade in veterinary anaesthesia was well reviewed by Jones (1988).

Acetylcholinesterase has two sites of action, one ionic and and the other esteratic, and its inhibitors are usually classified as acid-transferring or prosthetic. Neostigmine and pyridostigmine are acid-transferring drugs, containing a carbamate group and combining with cholinesterase in almost the same way as acetylcholine.The bond of the carbamate–enzyme is much longer lasting than that of the bond of the enzyme with acetylcholine and they are, therefore, more slowly hydrolysed than acetylcholine, thus preventing the access of the enzyme to acetylcholine. Their breakdown products also have weak anticholinesterase activity. Prosthetic inhibitors such as edrophonium have a dissociation half-life which is much shorter than that of the neostigmine–enzyme bond but, unlike neostigmine, edrophonium is not metabolized when combined with cholinesterase and is therefore free to recombine repeatedly with the enzyme (Wilson, 1955). The inhibition of acetylcholinesterase, although it is the main one, is not the only action of these drugs. Their other actions include a direct stimulation of the receptor as well as a presynaptic effect involving enhancement of acetylcholine release (Riker & Wescoe, 1946; Deana & Scuka, 1990).

Neostigmine and pyridostigmine differ from edrophonium in their effects on presynaptic receptors. Presynaptic effects of edrophonium are much greater in terms of acetylcholine liberation. This is shown by greater anti-fade effect (higher TOF ratio) when administered for reversal of neuromuscular block, fade being a presynaptic phenomenon related to liberation of more acetylcholine (Donati et al., 1983). Edrophonium may also differ from neostigmine and pyridostigmine because its inconsistent effect in deep neuromuscular block may result, at least in part, from a direct depression of the end plate channel leading to muscle weakness from accumulation of acetylcholine produced in excess due to a presynaptic effect of edrophonium (Wachtel, 1990).

If the anticholinerestases are administered in the absence of non-depolarizing neuromuscular blocking drug they produce muscle fibrillation or fasciculations and, given in large enough doses, they will produce a depolarization type of neuromuscular block.

NEOSTIGMINE

Neostigmine is probably the most widely used anticholinesterase antagonist of non-depolarizing neuromuscular block. The time course of the antagonising effect of neostigmine is roughly halfway between that of edrophonium and pyridostigmine, being about 7 to 10 minutes. Unless neuromuscular block is being monitored by a motor nerve stimulation technique, neostigmine should never be given until there is some sign of spontaneous respiratory activity, otherwise there is no way of assessing its effects and the possibility of passing from a non-depolarization to a depolarization block exists. An anticholinergic should always be given to counteract the more serious muscarinic effects of neostigmine (bradycardia, salivation, defaecation and urination). Atropine sulphate may be mixed in the syringe with neostigmine and the mixture given in small repeated doses until full respiratory activity is established or monitoring reveals a satisfactory TOF ratio. It is customary to mix atropine and neostigmine in the ratio of approximately 1 : 2 (e.g. 1.2 mg of atropine with 2.5 mg of neostigmine). This practice is quite safe because anticholinergics exert their effects before the onset of neostigmine activity.

Neostigmine, even if given with full doses of atropine, may cause serious cardiac arrhythmias if there has been gross underventilation during anaesthesia or if CO_2 has been allowed to accumulate at the end of operation with a view to ensuring return of spontaneous respiration. Hypercapnia also increases the neuromuscular block of nondepolarizing agents and so antagonism is likely to be less effective under these conditions. It has been shown that after anaesthesia in which IPPV has been used to lower the $PaCO_2$, spontaneous breathing returns at low $PaCO_2$s, provided that no depressant drugs have been used. This is probably due to the effect of stimuli arising in the trachea and bronchi, skin and, perhaps, to the effect of a sudden increase of afferent nerve impulses resulting from the return of proprioceptive activity as muscle tone is restored following the administration of neostigmine.

In the absence of facilities for monitoring of neuromuscular block reliance must be placed on clinical signs to assess when reversal is adequate. Signs of residual neuromuscular block include tracheal tug, paradoxical indrawing of intercostal muscles during inspiration similar to that seen in cases of respiratory obstruction, and a 'rectangular' breathing pattern in which the inspiratory position is held for some time before expiration begins. The atropine-neostigmine mixture should be given in small doses, with a pause between each, until these signs disappear.

EDROPHONIUM

Edrophonium is an effective and reliable anatagonist to the non-depolarizing agents. Earlier impressions that its effects were too short lasting were probably due to use of inadequate doses and, with the use of higher doses, the drug is now becoming popular. Doses of edrophonium in excess of 0.5 mg/kg appear similar in effect to that of neostigmine but the onset of action is considerably shorter (about 1 to 3 minutes) making it easier to titrate more accurately its administration to full reversal of blockade. It is usual to administer it in conjunction with atropine or glycopyrrolate although it may have fewer and more transient muscarinic effects than neostigmine.

PYRIDOSTIGMINE

In the USA pyridostigmine has found favour in some centres. It has a longer duration of action than neostigmine but its long onset time of around 10 – 15 minutes means that assessment of reversal is difficult if it is administered by a titration method. In veterinary practice, it appears to have no significant advantages over neostigmine.

4-AMINOPYRIDINE

This has not been used to increase the output of acetylcholine at nerve endings since the early 1980s. The main problems with 4-aminopyridine are its occasional inability to antagonize non-depolarizing neuromuscular block, and its effects on the central and peripheral nervous systems. Its central effects may be useful as an analeptic and respiratory stimulant but other and more satisfactory drugs exist for these purposes.

USE OF NEUROMUSCULAR BLOCKING DRUGS IN VETERINARY ANAESTHESIA

INDICATIONS

The general indications for the use of these drugs in veterinary clinical practice are:

1. To relax skeletal muscles for easier surgical access.

2. To facilitate control of respiration during intrathoracic surgery.

3. To assist in reduction of dislocated joints. Clinical experience shows that not only are dislocations more easily reduced if the muscles are paralysed but also that reluxation of the joint is facilitated by the absence of muscle tone. The reduction of fractures, on the other hand, is seldom eased by administration of relaxants since the difficulties of reduction are due to spasm of muscles around the fracture site provoked by haematomata and broken bone fragments.

4. To limit the amount of general anaesthetic used when muscle relaxation itself is not the prime requisite. For example, in dogs no muscle relaxation is needed for operations on the ear canal but surgical stimulation can be intense, resulting in head shaking unless the animal is very deeply anaesthetized. The judicious use of neuromuscular block prevents head shaking by weakening neck muscles so very much smaller quantities of anaesthetic or analgesic can be employed. In these circumstances all that is required is a light degree of unconsciousness coupled with analgesia, and thus the detrimental effects of deep depression of the central nervous system are avoided.

5. To ease the induction of full anaesthesia in animals already unconscious from intravenous narcotic drugs. For example, when thiopentone is used to induce loss of consciousness in horses before administration of an inhalant such as halothane or isoflurane, there is a period when the effect of the thiopentone is waning and the uptake of the inhalation agent is not yet sufficient to prevent movement of the limbs. The careful use of small doses of relaxant can do much to 'smooth out' this transitional period by paralysing the limb muscles.

6. To facilitate the performance of endotracheal intubation and endoscopy. Although animals can be intubated without the use of these drugs, they may make endotracheal intubation very much easier, especially in cats and pigs.

7. To reduce the need for postoperative analgesics. By making surgical access easier without forcible retraction of muscles by the surgeon they minimize bruising of muscle caused

by retractors. Much postoperative pain is due to muscle damage and minimizing this by use of neuromuscular blocking drugs contributes greatly to postoperative comfort of the animal and to wound healing.

8. To facilitate eye surgery by ensuring immobility of the eyeball.

CONTRAINDICATIONS

It must be very clearly understood that a relaxant should never be administered unless facilities are available for immediate and sustained artificial respiration to be applied. The administration of even small doses of these drugs may, on occasion, be followed by respiratory paralysis. An animal cannot be ventilated efficiently for very long by application of intermittent pressure to the chest wall and artificial respiration must be carried out by application of intermittent positive pressure to the airway through an endotracheal tube – the use of a face mask, except in an emergency when intubation attempts fail, is not really satisfactory because it is all too easy to inflate the stomach as well as the lungs.

In addition it must be clearly recognized that neuromuscular blocking drugs have no narcotic or analgesic properties. During any surgical operation an animal must be incapable of appreciating pain or fear throughout the whole period of action of any neuromuscular blocking drug which may be employed. Fortunately, provided due care is taken, it is a relatively simple matter to ensure this, but any doubt about the maintenance of unconsciousness must constitute an absolute contraindication to the use of neuromuscular blockers. When an inhalation anaesthetic such as halothane, isoflurane or sevoflurane is being used, with or without nitrous oxide, administration of $1.2 \times$ MAC should always ensure unconsciousness without producing an undesirable depth of unconsciousness.

TECHNIQUE OF USE

Induction of anaesthesia by intravenous medication is simple and pleasant for the animal so that heavy sedation with large doses of sedative/analgesic drugs is neither necessary nor desirable. When, however, the use of an intravenous in-

duction agent is deemed contraindicated and anaesthesia is induced with an inhalation agent, somewhat heavier sedation is required. The neuromuscular blocker may be given at induction or later, at the start of, or during surgery, depending on the reason for its use. Atropine or glycopyrrolate should always be given to avoid troublesome salivation and increased bronchial secretion which may otherwise follow administration of suxamethonium.

Induction of anaesthesia with an i.v. drug has very few contraindications provided that only minimal doses are employed. The dose used should only be just sufficient to induce loss of consciousness and relaxation of the jaw muscles. Dogs, horses and ruminants may then be intubated. In cats and pigs injection of the induction agent may be followed immediately unconsciousness supervenes by i.v. injection of a neuromuscular blocking agent and the animal allowed to breathe O_2 through a close-fitting face mask until respiration ceases and atraumatic endotracheal intubation can be performed. These animals are perhaps best intubated under suxamethonium-induced relaxation but pigs may be intubated under vecuronium paralysis (Richards *et al.*, 1988).

Endotracheal intubation is most desirable when relaxant drugs are used because a perfectly clear airway is required at all times (but it must never be assumed that the presence of an endotracheal tube necessarily guarantees an unobstructed airway). Owing to relaxation of pharyngeal and oesophageal muscles stomach contents may be regurgitated and aspirated into the lungs. This need not imply that a cuffed endotracheal tube is essential. In cats and other small animals, reasonably close-fitting plain tubes confer a considerable protection for with IPPV escape of gas around the tube during the inspiratory phase discourages the passage of regurgitated stomach contents down the trachea and the presence of stomach content in the pharynx, from where it can be removed by suction, will become obvious to the observant anaesthetist.

If an endotracheal tube is not used the stomach and even the intestines may be inflated by gas forced down the oesophagus when positive pressure is applied to the airway at the mouth and nostrils. This may be dangerous and is always a nuisance in abdominal surgery. Laryngeal masks

(Colgate Medical, Windsor, Berkshire), now widely used in man instead of endotracheal intubation, may not provide total airway protection in animals. Although tried in pigs they have not been extensively tested in animals and, currently, the wider exploration of their use in veterinary anaesthesia is precluded by their cost.

Maintenance of anaesthesia involves the administration of further doses of the neuromuscular blocker whenever these are indicated, and ensuring beyond all reasonable doubt that the animal remains lightly anaesthetized throughout the operation. Indications for supplementary doses of relaxant are relatively easy to state. The drugs are always best given by i.v. injection of repeated small doses, or by continuous infusion, until the desired degree of relaxation is obtained. One exception to this rule is that a dose given prior to endotracheal intubation must be large enough to abolish respiratory movements so that the tube may be introduced through a completely relaxed larynx.

Neuromuscular blockade is probably best maintained during prolonged surgical procedures by an infusion of the agent after an initial bolus dose. Infusion is commenced when the desired level of block returns after this dose and its rate is adjusted to to maintain this level, with initial adjustments of ± 20%, but adjustments are not made more frequently than every 5 minutes. Atracurium, vecuronium or mivacurium may be given in this way and infusion is stopped when relaxation is no longer needed. The desired level of block is easily established when TOF monitoring is employed because maintenance of one twitch will provide good operating conditions; desired block level is more difficult to recognize when TOF monitoring is unavailable. Most anaesthetists consider that the dose of relaxant drug used should be such that if IPPV is temporarily suspended, the animal is just capable of making feeble respiratory efforts. Resistance to lung inflation, in the absence of other obvious causes (e.g. airway obstruction) indicates that forcible respiratory efforts are imminent and a further dose of neuromuscular blocker is required. When an intermittent injection technique is used supplementary doses of neuromuscular blockers should not, in general, exceed half the initial dose.

The maintenance of a light plane of anaesthesia throughout the operation is of very great importance. Allowing the animal to awaken to consciousness during the course of an operation clearly cannot be tolerated but deep central nervous depression must be avoided or the full benefit derived from the use of neuromuscular blocking drugs will not be obtained. Once anaesthesia has been induced light anaesthesia may be ensured in one or more of several ways but it is important to note that if it becomes dangerously light, contractions of limb or facial muscles will occur either spontaneously or in response to surgical stimulation. These movements can always be seen, even when clinically paralysing doses of neuromuscular blockers have been given. The reason for this is unknown, but it is tempting to speculate that the γ fibre system nerve endings are more sensitive to the action of relaxant drugs than are the α fibre endings, for if this is so the neuromuscular blockers might abolish muscle tonus and produce relaxation without entirely preventing contraction of the muscles due to impulses in the α motor neurones.

Theoretically, it is unwise to use drugs of differing actions at the myoneural junction in the same animal at any one time. There is some clinical evidence to support this view yet with a proper appreciation of the risks involved and the avoidance of certain sequences, drugs such as suxamethonium and pancuronium can be given with safety to the animal during one operation. Jones and Gleed (1984) demonstrated that in dogs prior administration of suxamethonium reduced the duration of action of alcuronium, gallamine and pancuronium. In pigs it is often desirable to produce total paralysis rapidly with suxamethonium so as to obtain the best possible conditions for intubation of the trachea and yet to obtain relaxation throughout the subsequent operation with a nondepolarizing drug. Provided the effects of suxamethonium have worn off (as judged by the respiratory activity) few, if any, harmful effects are seen when the non-depolarizing neuromuscular blocker is given. In dogs, the use of suxamethonium at the end of a long operation when a nondepolarizing drug has provided the relaxation up to the last few minutes, seems to involve reduction in the duration of action of the depolarizing agent (Jones & Gleed, 1984a).

Cumulative effects should not be forgotten – if, when bolus administration is being employed, it is necessary to administer subsequent doses, the quantity of each dose given should not, in general, exceed half the total dose used initially to secure the desired degree of relaxation. As noted previously the aminoglycoside variety of antibiotics may cause difficulty in antagonism of neuromuscular block produced by non-depolarizing agents.

POSTOPERATIVE COMPLICATIONS OF NEUROMUSCULAR BLOCKING AGENTS

The most important complication is prolonged apnoea. The best prevention of this complication is the avoidance of excessive doses. Potentially troublesome desensitization of the postjunctional membrane can be avoided if the anaesthetist does not persist with administration of increasingly larger doses of depolarizing agents in the face of obvious tachyphylaxis to their blocking effect. In postoperative apnoea the animal should be ventilated until the cause of the apnoea can be ascertained and treated. If non-depolarizing agents were used during the operation and the cause of apnoea seems to be due to paralysis of the respiratory muscles, it may be treated by i.v. atropine and an anticholinesterase. There is no antidote to the phase I block of depolarizing drugs and the only treatment is IPPV until the return of adequate spontaneous breathing.

When an anticholinesterase agent is ineffective but the apnoea appears to be due to neuromuscular block caused by non-depolarizing agents, or is due to a phase 2 block of the depolarizing agents, the effects of the i.v. administration of potassium and/or calcium may be tried. In the absence of a urinary output potassium should be given cautiously and if possible myocardial activity should be continuously monitored for incipient electrocardiographic evidence of hyperkalaemia (e.g. high spiking T-waves, shortening of the S–T segment). If the administration of potassium is not effective and there is reason to believe that the plasma level of ionized calcium has been diminished (e.g. after transfusion of large quantities of citrated blood), calcium gluconate or calcium chloride solutions may be given.

The commonest cause of prolonged apnoea following the use of non-depolarizing agents appears to be hypothermia. Unless precautions are taken to maintain the body temperature it falls, especially during laparotomy and thoracotomy. This fall is particularly great in small animal patients and there is often difficulty in antagonizing the effects of non-depolarizing drugs in these animals until they are rewarmed. Animals should not be left in the postoperative period with any residual neuromuscular block. If dogs are returned to their cages with any residual curarization, pulmonary atelectasis may develop. Estimation of the tone of the masseter muscle, by gentle traction on the mandible, has proved to be a useful test for detecting slight degrees of muscular weakness. If the masseter tone is good there is unlikely to be trouble with respiration.

CENTRALLY ACTING MUSCLE RELAXANTS

MEPHENESIN

Mephenesin is a colourless, odourless, crystalline solid soluble in ethyl alchohol and propylene glycol. Intravenous injection of a 10% solution leads to a high incidence of venous thrombosis and also to haemolysis which may cause haemoglobinuria, oliguria, uraemia and death. The drug is partly detoxicated in the liver and partly excreted unchanged in the urine. Mephenesin mixed with pentobarbitone was introduced for canine and feline anaesthesia but the mixture did not prove to have any significant advantage over pentobarbitone alone. Mephenesin has many side effects and it is no longer used in anaesthesia.

GUAIPHENESIN

Guaiphenesin (Guaifenesin in North America), formerly known as guaicol glycerine ether, GGE or GG, is a mephenesin-like compound which has been used in Germany for many years (Westhues & Fritsch, 1961) and is now used widely throughout the world. Concentrated solutions (over 10%)

in water or 5% glucose have been associated with haemolysis, haemoglobinuria and venous thrombosis and although the recently introduced 15% stabilized solutions are said to be be free from these effects there is evidence that they cause thrombosis. Solutions of 10% in water have minimal haemolytic effect – they have an osmolality of 242 mOsm/kg which is closer to the osmolality of equine plasma than the formerly recommended 5% aqueous or dextrose solutions (Grandy & McDonell, 1980) but 10% aqueous solutions give rise to thrombus formation in the equine jugular vein (Herschl *et al.*, 1992). Injection into tissues causes pain, abscesses and necrosis so that accurate intravenous injection is essential. Venous thrombosis is potentially very serious; it is a delayed complication and may be related to speed of injection since it has been reported to occur with all formulations of guiaphenesin, particularly when they were infused under pressure (Schatzmann, 1980). However, the incidence of venous thrombosis was greatly reduced when 15 % stabilized solutions were administered to 2000 horses (Schatzmann, 1988).

Cardiovascular depression is dose dependent. In healthy horses heart rate is increased and arterial blood pressure decreased when guaiphenesin is administered with minimal doses of thiobarbiturates (Heath & Gabel, 1970; Wright *et al.*, 1979). Respiration is also depressed by guaiphenesin, and the $PaCO_2$ rises (Muir *et al.*, 1977; Muir *et al.*, 1978), an increase in frequency being insufficient to compensate for decreased tidal volume. Its effects on the cardiopulmonary system have been studied in detail by Hubbell *et al.* (1980). The duration of action in male horses is 1.5 times that in mares but there is apparently no sex difference in the doses required to produce relaxation (Davis & Wolff, 1970). In contrast to neuromuscular blocking agents significant amounts of guaiphenesin cross the placental barrier.

Following premedication with acepromazine (0.04 mg/kg i.v.) or xylazine (0.6 mg/kg i.v.) a mixture of guaiphenesin and thiobarbiturate given to effect will produce about 20 min of immobilization in horses. The usual dose requirement is about 4 mg/kg of thiobarbiturate and 100 mg/kg of guaiphenesin. Completing the induction of anaesthesia with halothane often produces marked arterial hypotension but the pressure recovers slowly over the next 20 to 30 min. Abdominal relaxation obtained with doses of guaiphenesin which do not interfere with respiratory activity is never as good as can be produced by the proper use of neuromuscular blocking drugs, but may be useful in situations where inhalation anaesthesia cannot be used or where the services of a specialist anaesthetist are not available. For short operations, doses in excess of 50 mg/kg may be associated with marked ataxia in the recovery period and this can give rise to excitement unless a small dose of a sedative such as xylazine is given at the end of operation.

Guaiphenesin is now used as an ingredient of the 'Triple drip' for total intravenous anaesthesia in horses with xylazine and ketamine (Greene *et al.*, 1986; Young *et al.*, 1993) or detomidine and ketamine (Taylor & Watkins, 1992).

The drug may be used to cast cattle. If these animals are premedicated with tranquillizers and analgesics the necessary dose for casting purposes is 4–5 g/kg, i.e. about 1 l of the 5% solution in any animal weighing 500 kg. Towards the end, or after the completion of this i.v. injection, the animal starts to sway and then falls relaxed. Barbiturates may be mixed with the solution (e.g. 0.25 g thiobarbital per 50 kg body weight) but as the two drugs potentiate each other most animals fall during the infusion, which is completed in the cast position.

Guaiphenesin has been used in other species of animal but its administration is rendered difficult by the large volumes of solution which must be infused. Even in horses and cattle this is a considerable disadvantage associated with its use, for ataxia develops as the solution is run into the vein and care has to be exercised to avoid the type of injury to the animal resulting from stumbling when the hind legs are crossed.

REFERENCES

Adams, A.K. and Hall, L.W. (1962) An experimental study of the action of suxamethonium on the circulatory system. *British Journal of Anaesthesia* **34:** 445–450.

Adams, A.K. and Hall, L.W. (1962a) The action of suxamethonium on the circulatory system. *Proceedings of the 1st European Congress of Anaesthesia, Vienna.*

Ali, H.H. and Savarese, J.J. (1976) Monitoring of neuromuscular function *Anesthesiology* **45**: 216–249.

Ali, H.H., Utting, J.E. and Gray, T.C. (1970) Stimulus frequency in the detection of neuromuscular block in humans. *British Journal of Anaesthesia* **42**: 967–978.

Amaki, Y. , Waud, B.E. and Waud, D.R. (1985) Atracurium-receptor kinetics: sample behaviour from a mixture. *Anesthesia and Analgesia* **64**: 777–780.

Booth, N.H. and Rankin, A.D. (1953) Studies on the pharmacodynamics of curare in the horse. I. Dosage and physiological activity of d-tubocurarine chloride. *American Journal of Veterinary Research* **14**: 51–59.

Borgeat, A. and Kwiatkowski, D. (19997) Spontaneous movements associate with rocuronium; is pain on injection the cause? *British Journal of Anaesthesia* **79**: 382–383.

Bowen, J.M. (1969) Monitoring neuromuscular function in intact animals. *American Journal of Veterinary Research* **30**: 857–859.

Bowman, W.C. (1990) Reversal agents. In: *Pharmacology of Neuromuscular Function*, 2nd edn. London: Wright, pp 196–202.

Brul, S.J., Connelly, N.R., O'Connor, T.Z., and Silverman, D.G. (1991) Effect of tetanus on subsequent neuromuscular monitoring in patients receiving vecuronium. *Anesthesiology* **74**: 64–70.

Burns, B.D. and Paton, W.D.M. (1951) depolarization of the motor end plate by decamethonium and acetylcholine. *Journal of Applied Physiology*. **115**: 41–73.

Cason, B., Baker, D.G.,Hickey, R.F. *et al.* (1990) Cardiovascular and neuromuscular effects of three steroidal neuromuscular blocking drugs in dogs (ORG 9616, ORG 9426, ORG 9991). *Anesthesia and Analgesia* **70**: 382–388.

Clutton, R.E. (1992) Combined bolus and infusion of vecuronium in dogs. *Journal of Veterinary Anaesthesia* **19**: 74–77.

Cookson, J.C. and Paton, W.D.M. (1969) Mechanisms of neuromuscular block. *Anaesthesia* **24**: 395–416.

Cullen, L.K. and Jones, R.S. (1980) The nature of suxamethonium neuromuscular block in the dog assessed by train-of-four stimulation. *Research in Veterinary Science*. **29**: 266–268.

Cullen, L.K. and Jones, R.S. (1980a) Recording of train-of-four evoked muscle responses from the nose and foreleg in the intact dog. *Research in Veterinary Science* **29**: 277–280.

Cullen, L.K. and Jones, R.S. (1984) Residual non-depolarizing neuromuscular block assessed by train-of-four stimulation in the dog. *Research in Veterinary Science* **32**: 121–123.

Cullen, L.K., Jones, R.S. and Snowdon, S.L. (1980) Neuromuscular activity in the intact dog: techniques for recording evoked mechanical responses. *British Veterinary Journal* **136**: 154–159.

Curtis, M.B. and Eicker, S.E. (1991) Pharmacodynamic properties of succinylcholine in greyhounds. *American Journal of Veterinary Research* **52**: 898–902.

Davis, L.E. and Wolff, W. A. (1970) Pharmacokinetics and metabolism of glyceryl guaiacolate in ponies. *American Journal of Veterinary Research* **31**: 469–473.

Deana, A. and Scuka, N. (1990) Time course of neostigmine; action on the end plate response. *Neurosciences* **118**: 82–84.

Donati, F. (1988) Onset of action of relaxants. *Canadian Journal of Anaesthesia* **35**: S52–S58.

Donati, F., Ferguson, A. and Bevan, D.R. (1983) Twitch depression and train-of-four ratio after antagonism of pancuronium with edrophonium, neostigmine or pyridostigmine. *Anesthesia and Analgesia* **62**: 314–316.

Donati, F., Meistelman, C. and Plaud, B. (1990) Vecuronium neuromuscular blockade at the diaphragm, the orbicularis oculi and the adductor pollicis muscles. *Anesthesiology* **74**: 833–837.

Drenck, N.W., Ueda, N., Olsen, N.V. *et al.* (1989) Manual evaluation of residual curarization using double burst stimulation: a comparison with train-of-four. *Anesthesiology* **70**: 578–581.

Engbaek, J., Skovgaard, L.T., Friis, B. *et al.* (1992) Monitoring of the neuromuscular transmission by electromyography (I). Stability and temperature dependence of evoked EMG response compared to mechanical twitch recordings in the cat. *Acta Anaesthesiologica Scandinavica* **36**: 495–504.

Faye, S. (1988) PhD thesis. Leeds: University of Leeds.

Gill, S.S., Donati, F. and Bevan, D.R. (1990) Clinical evaluation of double-burst stimulation. *Anaesthesia* **45**: 543–548.

Gleed, R.D. and Jones, R.S. (1982) Observations on the neuromuscular blocking action of gallamine and pancuronium and their reversal by neostigmine. *Research in Veterinary Science* **32**: 324–326.

Goat, V.A., Yeung, M.L., Blakeney, C. and Feldman, S.A. (1976) The effect of blood flow upon the activity of gallamine triethiodide. *British Journal of Anaesthesia* **48**: 69–72.

Grandy, J.L. and McDonell, W.N. (1980) Evaluation of concentrated solutions of guaifenesin for equine anesthesia. *Journal of the American Veterinary Medical Association* **176**: 619–622.

Greene, S.A., Thurmaon, J.C., Tranquilli, W.J. and Benson, G.J. (1986) Cardiopulmonary effects of continuous intravenous infusion of guaifenesin, ketamine and xylazine in ponies. *American Journal of Veterinary Research* **47**: 2364–2367.

Hall, L.W. (1952) A report on the clinical use of bis-(β-dimethylaminoethyl)–succinate bisethiodide (Brevidil E, M & B 2210) in the dog. *Veterinary Record* **64**: 491–492.

Hall, L.W., Lehmann, H. and Silk, E. (1953) Responses in dogs to relaxants derived from succinic acid and choline. *British Medical Journal* **i**, 134–136.

Heath, R.B. and Gabel, A.A. (1970) Evaluation of thiamylal sodium, succinylcholine, and glyceryl guaiacolate prior to inhalation anesthesia in horses. *Journal of the American Veterinary Medical Association* **157**: 1486–1494.

Heckmann, R., Jones, R.S. and Wuersch, W.A. (1977) A method for recording electrical and mechanical activity of muscle in the intact dog. *Research in Veterinary Science* 23: 1–6.

Herschl, M.A., Trim, C.M. and Mahaffey, E.A. (1992) Effects of 5% and 10% guaifenesin infusion on equine vascular endothelium. *Veterinary Surgery* 21: 494–497.

Hildebrand, S.V. and Arpin, D. (1988) Neuromuscular and cardiovascular effects of atracurium administered to healthy horses anesthetized with halothane. *American Journal of Veterinary Research* 49: 1066–1071.

Hildebrand, S.V. and Hill, T. (1989) Effects of atracurium administered by continuous intravenous infusion in halothane-anesthetized horses. *American Journal of Veterinary Research* 50: 2124–2126.

Hildebrand, S.V. and Hill, T. (1991) Neuromuscular blockade by atracurium in llamas. *Veterinary Surgery* 20: 153–154.

Hildebrand, S.V., Hill, T. and Holland, M. (1989) The effect of the neuromuscular blocking activity of atracurium in halothane anesthetized horses. *Journal of Veterinary Pharmacology and Therapeutics* 12: 277–282.

Hildebrand, S.V. and Howitt, G.A. (1984) Neuromuscular and cardiovascular effects of pancuronium bromide in calves anesthetized with halothane. *American Journal of Veterinary Research* 45: 1549–1552.

Hildebrand, S.V., Howitt, G.A. and Arpin, D. (1986) Neuromuscular and cardiovascular effects of atracuronium in ponies anesthetized with halothane. *American Journal of Veterinary Research* 47: 1096–1100.

Hubbell, J.A.E., Muir, W.W. and Sams, R.A. (1980) Guaifenesin: cardiopulmonary effects and plasma concentrations in horses. *American Journal of Veterinary Research* 41: 1751–1755.

Ibebunjo, C. and Hall, L.W. (1993) Muscle fibre diameter and and sensitivity to muscle relaxant drugs. *British Journal of Anaesthesia* 71: 732–733.

Jones, R.M. (1984) Calcium antagonists. *Anaesthesia* 39: 747–749.

Jones, R.S. (1987) Observations on the neuromuscular blocking action of pipecuronium in the dog. *Research in Veterinary Science* 43: 101–103.

Jones, R.S. (1987a) Interactions between pipecuronium and suxamethonium in the dog. *Research in Veterinary Science* 43: 308–312.

Jones, R.S. (1988) Reversal of neuromuscular blockade – a review. *Journal of the Association of Veterinary Anaesthetists* 15: 80–88.

Jones, R.S. and Brearley, J.C. (1985) Atracurium infusion in the dog. *Proceedings of the 2nd International Congress of Veterinary Anesthesia, Sacramento,* pp 172–173.

Jones, R.S. and Clutton, R.E. (1984) Clinical observations on the use of the muscle relaxant atracurium in the dog. *Journal of Small Animal Practice* 25: 473–477.

Jones, R.S. and Gleed, R.D. (1984) Effects of prior administration of suxamethonium on non-depolarizing muscle relaxants in dogs. *Research in Veterinary Science* 36: 43–47.

Jones, R.S. and Gleed, R.D. (1984a) Effects of prior administration of a non-depolarizing muscle relaxant on the action of suxamethonium in the dog. *Research in Veterinary Science* 36: 348–353.

Jones, R.S., Heckmann, R. and Wuersch, W. (1978) Observations on the neuromuscular blocking action of alcuronium in the dog and its reversal by neostigmine. *Research in Veterinary Science* 25: 101–102.

Jones, R.S., Hunter, J.M. and Utting, J.E. (1983) Neuromuscular blocking action of atracurium and its reversal by neostigmine. *Research in Veterinary Science* 34: 173–176.

Jones, R.S. and Prentice, D.E. (1976) A technique for investigation of the action of drugs on the neuromuscular junction in the intact horse. *British Veterinary Journal* 132: 226–230.

Jones, R. S and Richie, H.E. (1965) The effects of suxamethonium in a case of myotonia in the horse. *British Journal of Anaesthesia* 37: 142.

Jones, R.S. and Seymour, C.J. (1985) Clinical observations on the use of vecuronium as a muscle relaxant in the dog. *Journal of Small Animal Practice* 26: 213–218.

Kalow, W. (1959) The distribution, destruction and elimination of muscle relaxants. *Anesthesiology* 20: 505–518.

Khuenl-Brady, K., Castagnoli, K.P., Canfell, P.C. *et al.* (1990) The neuromuscular blocking effects and pharmacokinetics of ORG 9426 and ORG 9616 in the cat. *Anesthesiology* 72: 669–674.

Klide, A.M. (1973) *Veterinary Clinics of North America.* Philadelphia: W.B. Saunders., 3: 152.

Klein, L.V., Nann, L. and Brophy, M.A. (1988) Potency and duration of atracurium in anesthetized horses. *Advances in Anaesthesia 1988. Proceedings of the 3rd International Congress of Veterinary Anaesthesia, Brisbane,* pp 35–36.

Kopman, A.F., Mallhi, M.N., Newman, G.G. and Justo, M.D. (1996) Reestablishment of paralysis using miracurium following apparent full recovery from miracurium-induced neuromuscular block. *Anaesthesia* 51: 41–44.

Lambert, J.J., Durant, N.N. and Henderson, E.G. (1983) Characterization of end plate conductance at the neuromuscular junction. *Annual Review of Pharmacology and Toxicology* 23: 505–539.

Manley, S.V., Steffey, E.P., Howitt, G.A. and Woliner, M. (1983) Cardiovascular and neuromuscular effects of pancuronium in the pony. *American Journal of Veterinary Research* 44: 1349–1353.

Marshall, R.J., Muir, A.W., Sleigh, T. and Savage, D.S. (1994) An overview of the pharmacology of rocuronium bromide in experimental animals. *European Journal of Anaesthesia* 11: 9–15.

Martinez, E.A., Wooldridge, A.A., Mercer, D.R., Slater, M.R. and Hartsfield, S.M. (1996) Cardiovascular and neuromuscular effects of rocuronium in anesthetized dogs. *Proceedings of the Annual Meeting of the American*

College of Veterinary Anesthesiologists, New Orleans, p 32.

Muir, A.W., Houston, J., Green, K.L. *et al.* (1989) Effects of a new neuromuscular blocking agent, ORG 9426 in anaesthetized cats and pigs and in isolated nerve-muscle preparations. *British Journal of Anaesthesia* **63**: 400–410.

Muir, W.W., Skarda, R.T. and Milne, D.W. (1977) Evaluation of xylazine and ketamine hydrochloride for anesthesia *American Journal of Veterinary Research* **38**: 195–201.

Muir, W.W., Skarda, R.T. and Sheenan, W. (1978) Evaluation of xylazine, guaifenesin and ketamine hydrochloride for restraint in horses. *American Journal of Veterinary Research* **39**: 1274–1278.

O'Hara, D.A., Fragen, R.J. and Shanks, C.A. (1986) Reappearance of train-of-four after neuromuscular blockade induced with tubocurarine, vecuronium or atracurium. *British Journal of Anaesthesia* **58**: 1296–1299.

Payne, J.P. and Hughes, R. (1981) Evaluation of atracuronium in anaesthetized man. *British Journal of Anaesthesia*, **53**: 45–54.

Pedersen, S.E. and Cohen, J.B. (1990) D-tubocuraine binding sites are located at alpha-gamma and alpha-delta subunit interfaces of the nicotinic acetylcholine receptor. *Proceedings of the National Academy of Sciences of the USA* **87**: 2785–2789.

Pollard, B.J. and Millar, R.A. (1973) Potentiating and depressant effects of inhalation anaesthetics on the rat phrenic nerve – diaphragm preparation. *British Journal of Anaesthesia* **45**: 404–415.

Riker, W.F. and Wescoe, W.C. (1946) The direct action of prostigmin on skeletal muscle; its relationship to the choline esters. *Journal of Pharmacology and Experimental Therapeutics* **88**: 58–66.

Richards, D.L.S., Clutton, R.E., Boyd, C., Shipley, C. and McGrath, C.J. (1988) Conditions for tracheal intubation in pigs using vecuronium–a comparison with succinylcholine. *Journal of the Association of Veterinary Anaesthetists of GB Great Britain and Ireland* **15**: 89–90.

Savarese, J.J., Ali, H.H., Basta, S.J. *et al.* (1988) The clinical pharmacology of mivacurium (BW B1090U). *Anesthesiology* **68**: 723–732.

Schatzmann, U. (1980/81) Advantages and disadvantages of glycerol guaiacolate (Guaifenesin) in the equine species. *Proceedings of the Association of Veterinary Anaesthetists of Great Britain and Ireland.* **9**: 153–159.

Schatzmann, U. (1988) Discussion on the use of glyceryl guiacolate ether (G.G.E.). *Journal of the Association of Veterinary Anaesthetists of Great Britain and Ireland* **15**: 14–16.

Silverman, D.G. and Brul, S.J. (1993) The effect of a tetanic stimulus on the response to subsequent tetanic stimulation. *Anesthesia and Analgesia* **76**: 1284–1287.

Stenlake, J.B., Waigh, R.D. and Dewar, G.H. (1981) Biodegradable neuromuscular blocking agents part 4: atracurium besylate and related polyalkylene di-esters. *European Journal of Medical Chemistry* **16**: 515–524.

Stevenson, D.E. (1960) Changes in the blood electrolytes of anaesthetized dogs caused by suxamethonium. *British Journal of Anaesthesia* **32**: 364–371.

Stowe, C.M., Bieter, R.N. and Roepke, M.H. (1958) The relationship between cholinesterase activity and the effects of succinylcholine in the horse and cow. *Cornell Veterinarian* **48**: 241–259.

Taylor, P.M. and Watkins, S.B. (1992) Stress responses during total intravenous anaesthesia in ponies with detomidine–guaiphenesin–ketamine. *Journal of Veterinary Anaesthesia* **19**: 13–17.

Trucchi, G., Buracco, P., Mangione, M., Quaranta, G. and Berra, G.P. (1988) Correlation between the duration of action of suxamethonium, serum levels of pseudocholinesterases and dibucaine number in the dog. *Journal of the Association of Veterinary Anaesthetists of Great Britain and Ireland* **15**: 96–113.

Viby-Mogensen, J., Howard-Hansen, P., Chraemmer-Jorgensen, B. *et al.* (1981) Posttetanic count (PTC): A method of evaluating an intense nondepolarizing neuromuscular blockade. *Anesthesiology* **55**: 458–461.

Wachtel, R.E. (1990) Comparison of anticholinesterases and their effects on acetylcholine-activated ion channels. *Anesthesiology* **72**: 496–503.

Westhues, M. and Fritsch, R. (1961) In: Weaver, A.D. (trans) *Animal Anaesthesia*, volume 2. Berlin: Paul Parey Translated in 1965.

Wilson, I.B. (1955) The interaction of tensilon and neostigmine with acetylcholinesterase. *Archives Internationales de Pharmacodynamie et de Therapie* **54**: 204–213.

Wright, M., McGrath, C.J. and Raffe, M. (1979) Indirect blood pressure readings in horses before and after induction of general anesthesia with acepromazine, glyceryl guaiacolate and sodium thiamylal. *Veterinary Anesthesia* **VI**: 41–44.

Young, L.E., Bartram, D.H., Diamond, M.J. Gregg, A.S. and Jones, R.S. (1993) Clinical evaluation of xylazine, guaifenesin and ketamine for maintenance of anaesthesia in horses. *Equine Veterinary Journal* **25**: 115–119.

Pulmonary gas exchange: artifical ventilation of the lungs

8

INTRODUCTION

Special techniques to ventilate the lungs when the respiratory muscles are paralysed by neuromuscular blocking drugs or rendered inactive by central nervous depression have evolved gradually over a number of years. Today, they usually involve endotracheal intubation together with periodic inflation of the lungs and the commonest method used is known as 'intermittent positive pressure ventilation' of the lungs or IPPV. It was first employed during intrathoracic surgery but it is now much more widely used in anaesthesia. It is also a routine technique in intensive care whenever respiratory failure occurs. There are differences between spontaneous breathing and IPPV, and IPPV when the thoracic cage is opened widely at thoracotomy from when it is intact. The anaesthetist must appreciate what these differences are if IPPV is to be correctly managed under all circumstances.

SPONTANEOUS RESPIRATION

In a spontaneously breathing animal active contraction of the inspiratory muscles lowers the normally subatmospheric intrapleural pressure still further by enlarging the relatively rigid thoracic cavity. The decrease in intrapleural pressure lowers the alveolar pressure (Fig. 8.1) so that a pressure gradient or driving force is set up between the

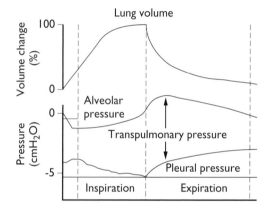

FIG. 8.1 Changes in lung volume, pleural and transpulmonary pressures during normal spontaneous breathing (diagramatic only).

exterior and the alveoli. This overcomes the airway resistance and air flows into the alveoli until at the end of inspiration the alveolar pressure becomes equal to the atmospheric pressure. During expiration the pressure gradient is reversed and air flows out of the alveoli.

The transpulmonary pressure is a measure of the elastic forces which tend to collapse the lungs and there is no one intrapleural pressure. In the ventral parts of the chest it is just sufficient to keep the lungs expanded. Because of the influence of gravity acting on the lungs, the intrapleural pressure in the dorsal parts of the chest should be much more below atmospheric, but it is not at all certain how uniform the pressure on the pleural

Spontaneous breathing

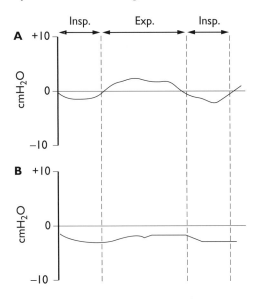

IPPV

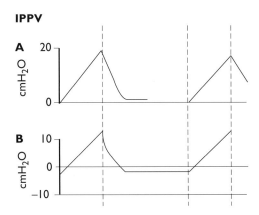

FIG. 8.2 Pressure changes (**A**) at the mouth end of endotracheal tube, (**B**) in the thoracic oesophagus during spontaneous breathing and IPPV with closed chest (diagramatic only).

surface ot the lung really is. The hilar forces, the buoyancy of the lung in the pleural cavity and the different shapes of the lung and chest wall are all possible sources of local pressure differences. Thus, it is customary to measure the intra-oesophageal pressure as being representative of the mean intrapleural pressure (Fig. 8.2)

The alveolar pressure changes generate airflow into and out of the lungs against a resistance in a way analagous to that stated by Ohm's Law for

electricity, where:

$$R = \frac{E}{R}$$

So that:

$$\text{Resistance} = \frac{\text{alveolar pressure change}}{\text{air flow}}$$

Airway resistance is largely influenced by the lung volume because the elastic recoil of lung parenchyma exerts traction on the pleural surfaces and walls of airways (holding them patent) when the lungs are inflated above residual volume. As the lungs are further inflated, elastic recoil pressure increases, thus further dilating the airways and decreasing resistance to air flow. This relationship between airway resistance and lung volume is hyperbolic in nature, as shown in Fig. 8. 3. Airway resistance also depends on the nature of airflow through the airway. With a clear airway and a low gas flow rate, intrapulmonary flow is largely laminar (streamlined) and airway resistance is also low, but obstruction or a high flow velocity will give rise to turbulence and a greatly increased resistance. Measurement of airway resistance must be made when gas is flowing. During IPPV when the chest wall is intact, resistance to expansion of the lungs is also offered by the chest wall which then contributes to the total respiratory resistance.

Total respiratory resistance (Rr_s) may be estimated by the application of an oscillating airflow to the airways with measurement of the resultant

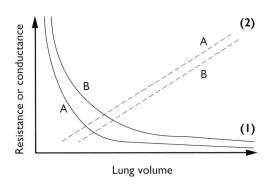

FIG. 8.3 Resistance and volume curves together with lower airways conductance curves (G_{law}). (1): Resistance curves; (2): (G_{law}); A: normal airway B: obstructed airway (Lehane et al., 1980).

pressure and airflow changes. A technique was developed by Lehane *et al.* (1980) to measure airway resistance as a function of lung volume during a vital capacity manoeuvre and so to derive specific lower airways conductance, $s.G_{law}$, (conductance being the reciprocal of resistance) and the expiratory reserve volume (ERV). The method was modified by Watney for use in anaesthetized and paralysed horses and dogs (Watney *et al.*, 1987; 1988) and it was demonstrated that in ponies xylazine, acepromazine, halothane and enflurane produce bronchodilatation and a decrease in ERV while isoflurane appears to increase ERV. In dogs, it was concluded that both bronchoconstriction and changes in lung volume may be responsible for changes in airway resistance seen during hypoxia. During spontaneous breathing changes in resistance may necessitate a great increase in the work of breathing. The effect of inhalation anaesthetics on total respiratory resistance in conscious horses was studied by Hall and Young (1992) who showed that halothane appeared to have no effect while enflurane and isoflurane seemed to increase it.

Resistance is not the only factor opposing movement of air in and out of the chest; a full analysis includes the effects of compliance and inertance. Adding the compliance and inertance forms the reactance and this can be combined with the resistance in one complex term called the 'impedance'. If the impedance of the respiratory system is known then the resistance and reactance can be determined. A completely non-invasive method suggested by Michaelson *et al.* (1975) has, since the introduction of computers, been used quite extensively to determine the frequency dependence of resistance in man. Because it does not require patient cooperation it is relatively simple to use in conscious animals as described by Young and Hall (1989) for horses but it is difficult to use in anaesthetized, intubated animals because the impedance of the tube alone is much greater than that of a non-intubated animal. Commercially available apparatus is expensive but, nevertheless, it can provide a useful diagnostic tool for the identification of horses suffering from chronic obstructive pulmonary disease (COPD) which can pose problems during anaesthesia with IPPV because of a sudden increase airway resistance at the end of

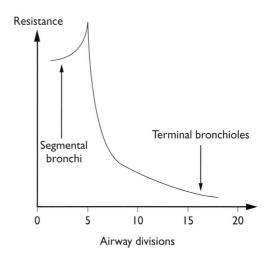

FIG. 8.4 Contribution of the major and minor airways to total respiratory resistance. The resistance offered by the small airways, each of which has a high resistance, is small because they are in parallel (by analogy with electrical resistance: $1/R_{total} = 1/R_1 + 1/R_2 + 1/R_{33} \ldots 1/R_n$).

expiration (Gillespie *et al.*, 1966). This increase does not usually present problems during anaesthesia with spontaneous breathing but may necessitate a prolonged expiratory period during IPPV. Unfortunately, small airways contribute little to the total lung resistance; although each one has a large individual resistance, there are large numbers in parallel so that the overall effect is small (Fig. 8.4). This is important because small airway disease (which increases local resistance) is not detected by measurement of total airway resistance until the condition is well advanced.

Anaesthetic apparatus may afford resistance that is considerably higher than that offered by the animal's respiratory tract. It is difficult to say at what value this apparatus resistance becomes intolerable because a healthy anaesthetized animal seems able to compensate for increases in resistance to airflow. Anaesthetized human subjects breathe at 80 % of control tidal volume against an inspiratory load of 10 cm H_2O (Nunn & Ezi-Ashi, 1961). It is unlikely that moderate expiratory resistance will cause serious problems in spontaneously breathing animals provided the $PaCO_2$ remains within acceptable limits. In halothane anaesthetized horses, Hall and Trim (1975) found that 10 and 20 cm H_2O of expiratory resistance did not affect the PaO_2 but was associated with increases in $PaCO_2$ of about 1.2 mmHg (0.16 kPa) per min. However, common sense would seem to suggest that apparatus resistance should be kept to a minimum. Purchase (1965; 1965a) studied the resistance afforded by four closed breathing systems used in horses and cattle and in three, all of which had internal bores of 5 cm, found it to be of the order of 1 cm H_2O (0.1 kPa) per 100 l/min at flow rates of 600 l/min, which he judged to be quite acceptable. He also found that the resistance of endotracheal tube connectors was relatively high in comparison with that of the remainder of the apparatus.

During a breathing cycle mean intrathoracic pressure may be above or below atmospheric pressure as a result of apparatus resistance. For example, if the expiratory flow through a piece of apparatus with a high resistance is great enough to induce turbulence, whilst the inspiratory rate is lower (as it often is in horses) so that during inspiration the flow is laminar, the mean intrathoracic pressure will be above atmospheric. Conversely, if the inspiratory flow rate is greater there may be a subatmospheric mean intrathoracic pressure. Mean intrathoracic pressures above atmospheric may cause cardiovascular failure in hypovolaemic states by reducing the effect of the thoraco-abdominal pump for venous return. Large subatmospheric mean intrathoracic pressures may be equally dangerous, perhaps by producing pulmonary oedema, but probably more importantly by reducing lung volume. Trapping of gas in the lungs occurs more readily at low lung volumes and gas trapping produces widespread airway obstruction with serious impairment of respiratory function.

IPPV WHEN THE CHEST WALL IS INTACT

IPPV is easily applied during anaesthesia by rhythmical compression of the reservoir bag of a breathing circuit. This is most simply achieved by manual squeezing, but machines have been designed and built to relieve the anaesthetist of the bag-squeezing duty. If the bag is squeezed as the animal breathes in, the tidal volume may be augmented ('*assisted ventilation*'). The increased ventilation produced results in 'washout' of CO_2 and

the $PaCO_2$ falls below the threshold for stimulating the respiratory centre so that spontaneous breathing movements cease and the anaesthetist can impose whatever respiratory rhythm is required – 'controlled respiration'.

A properly used machine undoubtedly provides the most efficient means of ventilating the lungs for prolonged periods, but to use a machine properly or even to squeeze a bag correctly, it is essential to understand the principles underlying IPPV and to know under what circumstances any possible harmful effects may arise.

Compliance has been defined in many ways but the simplest definition is that it is the volume change produced by unit pressure change ($\delta V / \delta P$). Compliance shows hysteresis (Fig.8.5) and it is changes in surfactant which seem to be responsible; airway resistance and tissue viscosity play only a small part. Ideally, measurements needed for the calculation necessary to obtain this value should be made when no air is flowing into or out of the lungs (i.e. at the end of inspiration). Compliance measures cannot be compared unless related to a lung volume such as the functional

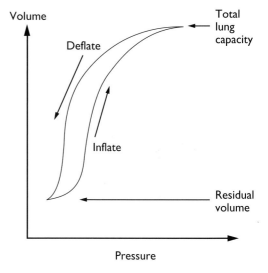

FIG. 8.5 Total thoracic compliance curves showing hysteresis. The compliance can be altered by a number of factors: (a) the lung compliance is reduced by lack of surfactant (respiratory distress syndrome), reduction of elastic tissue in the lungs (as in emphysema), and fibrosis or scar tissue; (b) the chest wall compliance is altered by obesity and splinting of the diaphragm by abdominal disorders.

residual capacity (FRC). Unfortunately, measurement of FRC is not a simple procedure and such measurements of compliance as have been made in animals have often omitted this refinement.

As commonly measured, compliance has two components and compliance values can be found for both the lungs themselves and the thoracic cage but, of course, when the chest wall is not intact the total compliance measured approaches that of the lungs alone. It might seem that methods using high airway pressures to inflate the lungs might be safe if, when compliance is reduced, it is the thoracic cage itself which is uncompliant because alveoli only rupture when overdistended. On the other hand, decreased compliance of the lungs themselves is apt to be non-uniform, an airway pressure which produces little ventilation of some regions may overdistend and even rupture alveoli in other regions. During anaesthesia compliance may be altered by assistants resting their weight on the chest, by the use of retractors and by the degree of muscle relaxation.

Airway resistance has to be overcome to deliver gas to the alveoli at inspiration and to expel it during expiration. Resistance during anaesthesia is increased by the resistance of apparatus used, such as endotracheal tubes. Animals with pulmonary disease may also have increased airway resistance so that it is necessary to allow a more prolonged expiratory period if the lungs are to deflate to FRC. If this is not done lung volume will be greater at the start of the next inspiration and there will be a steady increase in FRC until the retractive forces of the lung, which increase with increase in lung volume, become sufficient to empty the lungs to a new FRC in the time available and the inspiratory and expiratory tidal volumes become normally related. While conscious, the animal with expiratory obstruction empties its lungs by active expiratory movements but, when anaesthetized and paralysed or made otherwise apnoeic, expiration may become passive and, consequently, of longer duration. The pattern of IPPV used must make allowance for this, and large tidal volumes should be delivered with long expiratory pauses between each inspiration to allow the chest to return to its original resting position.

The induction of general anaesthesia is usually associated with an increase in resistance due to

a decrease in lung volume but this may be countered to some extent by bronchodilation due to the agents given, e.g. xylazine, acepromazine, halothane and enflurane.

Perhaps the most obvious effect of IPPV when the chest is closed is on the circulatory system. During spontaneous breathing, by lowering intrathoracic pressure inspiration augments the venous return to the heart; in many animals, as can often be seen on a tracing of continuously recorded blood pressure, there are indications that a increased stroke volume is produced. During IPPV, however, intrathoracic pressure rises during inspiration, blood is dammed back from the thorax, venous return and stroke volume decrease; blood flows freely into the thoracic vessels during the expiratory period. Fortunately, by causing distension of veins this damming back of blood during inspiration produces a reflex increase in venous tone which in normal animals appears to compensate for the changed intrathoracic conditions during the inspiratory period and restores the venous return towards normality. Obviously the extent to which an increase in venous tone can compensate will depend on the degree of venomotor integrity (which can be affected by drugs), the blood volume, the magnitude of the intrathoracic pressure rise and its duration.

The magnitude and duration of the increased pressure within the thorax during the inspiratory phase of IPPV are, therefore, critical and are reflected in the '*mean intrathoracic pressure*'. This mean pressure, like the mean arterial blood pressure, is not the simple arithmetical mean between the highest and lowest pressures reached in the system and its calculation is not always easy for the non-mathematician. It is clearly important to keep this mean pressure as low as possible during the respiratory cycle and this can be accomplished in a variety of ways:

1. *Short application of positive pressure.*
The shorter the inspiratory period during IPPV the lower the mean intrathoracic pressure will be for any given applied pressure. Theoretically, it might seem that the peak pressure should never be maintained – expiration should commence as soon as the peak pressure is achieved – or the circulation

will suffer. However, the short application of a positive pressure may not result in very good distribution of fresh gas within the lungs. In man very short inspiratory periods have the effect of increasing the physiological dead space, while Hall *et al.* (1968) found a decrease in the physiological dead space/tidal volume ratio in horses ventilated with a ventilator which had a relatively long inspiratory phase. A compromise seems to be necessary here, but exactly what it is likely to be for any one animal of any one species remains pure speculation. It is usually taught that in small animals (dogs, cats, foals, calves, sheep) the inspiratory time should be 10–1.5 s and in adult horses and cattle 2–3 s provided the lungs are healthy.

2. *Rapid gas flow rate.*

If the necessary tidal volume of gas is to be delivered to the lungs in a short inspiratory period it is clear that the flow rate will need to be high. The rate at which gas can flow into the lungs, however, is largely dictated by the resistance offered by the apparatus used and the airway resistance. The airway resistance to the various lung regions may not be uniform. For example, a bleb of mucus may partially obstruct a small bronchus and greatly increase the resistance to gas flow through it. A high gas flow rate through a neighbouring, unobstructed bronchus may result in overdistension of the alveoli supplied by it in an interval of time so short that the alveoli supplied by the partially obstructed bronchus will not have time for more than minimal expansion. Theoretically, it would seem that under these circumstances alveolar rupture might occur, but in practice this complication seems rare.

3. *Low expiratory resistance.*

Because any resistance to the airflow created by the passive phase of IPPV will delay the fall in intrathoracic pressure, it will result in an increase in mean intrathoracic pressure and possibly in circulatory embarrassment. However, expiratory resistance can result in more orderly emptying of alveoli and an increase in FRC with consequent widening of the airways (Comroe *et al.*, 1962). Thus, at least in some cases (e.g. in animals with obstructive emphysema) a higher expiratory resistance may be advantageous to the animal.

4. *Subatmospheric pressure during the expiratory phase.*

If a subatmospheric pressure is applied to the airway during the expiratory phase of IPPV the inspiratory pressure will be applied from a lower baseline. Hence the pressure gradient necessary to produce the required volume change in the lungs can be achieved with a lower peak pressure. This might be expected to help maintain cardiac output, but changes in arterial blood pressure and cardiac output are proportional to the duration of the increased airway pressure and not necessarily to the peak pressures reached. Consequently, merely decreasing the peak airway pressure may have but little effect if the inspiratory phase is long. Clinical experience in dogs suggests that any beneficial effects resulting from a subatmospheric expiratory phase are difficult to appreciate. In animals suffering from emphysema where air trapping occurs, its use will result in further impairment of the expiratory gas flow. During thoracotomy its application will cause such marked lung collapse that re-expansion may be difficult.

IPPV AFTER OPENING OF THE PLEURAL CAVITY

COLLAPSE OF THE LUNG

Normally, distension of the lungs to fill the thoracic cavity is due to the existence of a pressure gradient between the airway and the pleural cavity. The airway pressure is usually atmospheric and the intrapleural pressure subatmospheric due to the outward recoil forces of the chest wall, the lymphatic removal of fluid from the pleural cavity and the limited expansibility of the lungs. This distending force is opposed by what has been termed the 'elasticity' of the lung tissue, although the term 'elasticity' is not strictly applicable because surface tension in the alveoli contributes in a most important manner to the lung retractive force. When the chest is opened and atmospheric pressure allowed to act directly in the pleural cavity, the normal pressure gradient is abolished and the retractive forces cause the lung to collapse (Fig.8.6).

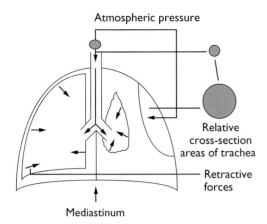

FIG. 8.6 Forces responsible for collapse of the lung following unilateral opening of the chest wall during spontaneous breathing. The volume of air entering the pleural cavity at each breath will depend on the relative cross-sectional area of the trachea and the defect in the chest wall.

Paradoxical respiration

The paradox is that during spontaneous breathing following unilateral large openings into the pleural cavity the lung on the damaged side of the chest becomes smaller on inspiration and larger on expiration. Normally, when the thorax enlarges due to activity of the inspiratory muscles its increased volume comes to be occupied by air which enters via the trachea and blood which enters the right atrium and thin-walled great veins. In the presence of a unilateral open pneumothorax air enters not only into the lungs via the trachea but also through the chest wall defect into the pleural cavity. The proportion of air entering by each route is largely governed by the relative size of the the chest wall defect to the tracheal lumen. When the opening to the hemithorax is large, or when there is any degree of airway obstruction, the greater volume of air will enter through the hole in the chest wall and the mediastinum will be pushed towards the intact side of the chest. During inspiration pressure in the bronchi on the open side of the chest will be greater than in the trachea because of the addition of the normal retractive forces of the lung to the atmospheric pressure acting on the pleural surface of the exposed lung (Fig. 8.7). Thus, on inspiration the increased volume on the intact side of the chest is occupied by air from the collapsed lung as well

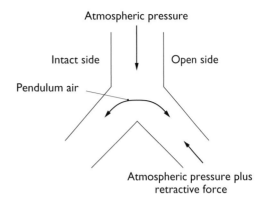

FIG. 8.7 Effect of unilateral pneumothorax on intrabronchial pressure.

as from the atmosphere. The exposed lung, therefore, becomes smaller. On expiration the lung on the intact side is discharged partly into the collapsed lung, which becomes larger. In this way an animal with a unilateral open pneumothorax breathing spontaneously shuttles air from one lung to the other. This 'pendulum air' produces, in effect, an increase in respiratory dead space, and the animal's respiratory efforts are less effective in producing overall ventilation. It is not seen after bilateral opening of the pleural cavity through a sternotomy. Applying positive pressure to the airway during inspiration abolishes paradoxical respiration.

MEDIASTINAL MOVEMENT

In any normal animal the mediastinum is not a rigid partition between the two halves of the chest. Veterinary anatomists have made much of the presence or absence of fenestration in the mediastinum but in practice this seems unimportant and the behaviour of each half of the chest during respiration is always dependent on the conditions prevailing in the other half. Unilateral pneumothorax can occur in all domestic animals and its presence causes the mediastinum to move towards the intact side during inspiration and the opposite way during expiration. This movement of the mediastinum results in obstruction of the thin-walled great veins and thus impedes the venous return to the heart. However, this impediment poses little problem and death is usually due to hypoxia rather than circulatory failure. Rigidity of the mediastinum may be encountered in chronic inflammatory pleuritis.

EFFECTS ON THE CIRCULATION

It might be expected that most of the potentially harmful effects of IPPV on the circulatory system would be absent when the pleura is opened widely because an opening in the chest wall should prevent compression of intrathoracic vessels when positive pressure is applied to the airway. Nevertheless, in dogs it has been found that thoracotomy reduces the cardiac output to below levels that might be expected to result from the application of IPPV alone, apparently by causing a further reduction in venous return to the heart. It may be that the airway pressure results in compression of pulmonary capillaries leading to a diminished return to the left atrium.

POSSIBLE HARMFUL EFFECTS OF IPPV

The effects of IPPV on pulmonary ventilation are, of course, in the main clearly beneficial, or the procedure would not have found such extensive use in the treatment of respiratory failure. Rupture of lung tissue is no more likely to occur during properly conducted IPPV than during the ordinary activities of life. Very high intrapulmonary pressures develop during activities such as coughing, or straining at defaecation or parturition. In dogs, pressures above 100 mmHg (13.3 kPa) will produce fatal air embolism, while during thoracotomy pressures above 70 mmHg (9.3 kPa) can produce mediastinal emphysema but pressures of this order are most unlikely to be encountered during normal IPPV where it is seldom possible to create pressure above 60 cm H_2O (6 kPa) by compression of the reservoir bag. Care is needed when ventilators are used for, in some, sticking of valves may expose the patient's airway directly to the high pressures at which gases are delivered from the anaesthetic machine to the ventilator. As already mentioned, uneven inflation of alveoli is a distinct possibility during IPPV but the surrounding tissues seem to provide sufficient support to prevent rupture of the relatively overinflated alveoli.

Any uneven distribution of gas must have the effect of disturbing the normal ventilation/perfusion relationships within the lungs. It appears that these are often upset by anaesthesia itself and if IPPV produces more uneven gas distribution it will probably fail to affect any improvement in the alveolar–arterial oxygen tension gradient found during anaesthesia in spite of any improvement in tidal exchange which it may produce. For example, in laterally recumbent horses it is possible that the gravitational force gradient from the top to the bottom of the lungs acting on the low pressure pulmonary circulation may, by reducing the circulation to the upper lung, cause this lung to be overventilated in relation to its perfusion. Due to the weight of the horse's abdominal viscera acting on the lower cone of the diaphragm, IPPV is more successful in inflating the upper than the lower lung and hence the upper lung receives an even more disproportionally large part of the ventilation to the further detriment of its ventilation/perfusion relationships. Certainly, in the laterally recumbent horse IPPV appears to produce very little improvement in the alveolar–arterial oxygen tension gradient found during general anaesthesia. Other situations in which the normal relationships between ventilation may be upset occur in all animals where the expansion of one lung or part of a lung is limited by surgical procedures such as 'packing off' and retraction of lung lobes during intrathoracic surgery.

IPPV should remove CO_2 from the animal's lungs and it is possible, over a period of time, to remove either too much or too little causing the animal to suffer from either respiratory alkalosis or acidosis. Respiratory acidosis (hypercapnia) is characterized by sympathetic overactivity, cutaneous vasodilatation, a rise in arterial blood pressure and a bounding pulse. Respiratory alkalosis (hypocapnia) may, it has been claimed, lead to cerebral damage from cerebral vasoconstriction because the calibre of the cerebral blood vessels depends on the $PaCO_2$. However, convincing evidence of cerebral damage due to hypocapnia has yet to be produced. Moreover, although it has been demonstrated that hypocapnia reduces cardiac output in horses (Hall *et al.*, 1968), at least in normovolaemic states no disaster appears to result.

IPPV carried out with a face mask instead of through an endotracheal tube can be harmful unless care is taken to avoid forcing gases down the oesophagus into the stomach. This entails careful limiting of the pressure applied at the mouth and nostrils and observations of the epigastric region to detect any inflation of the stomach. An inflated stomach not only hinders intra-abdominal surgery – if it becomes sufficiently distended with gas, regurgitation of gastric fluid is a distinct possibility. Gas accidentally forced into the stomach should be removed as soon as possible by passing a stomach tube.

MANAGEMENT OF IPPV

Before IPPV can be applied all spontaneous breathing movements have to be abolished if the animal is not to 'fight' the imposed ventilation. This is usually accomplished by:

1. Depressing the respiratory centres by relative overdose of anaesthetics or agents such as morphine or fentanyl.

2. Paralysis of the respiratory muscles by neuromuscular block.

3. Lowering the PCO_2 by hyperventilation. This may be done by forcing a little more gas into the lungs at the end of a normal inspiration, or by ventilating between spontaneous breaths.

4. Reflexly inhibiting the respiratory centres by regular rhythmical lung inflation. This inhibition does not depend on changes in blood pH and $PaCO_2$. For example, in the cat subjected to IPPV it is known that respiratory neuronal activity usually synchronizes with the ventilator cycle within two to three respiratory cycles; this is too rapid for significant changes in the arterial blood gases to occur. It is believed that if the lungs are slightly overdistended at each inspiration afferent impulses from pulmonary receptors inhibit the medullary centres.

MANUAL VENTILATION

When IPPV is carried out by manual squeezing of the reservoir bag (a procedure often known in North America as 'bagging the animal') this should be done gently and rhythmically. Once the desired degree of lung inflation has been produced the bag should be released and the lungs allowed to empty freely. The rate of lung ventilation should be faster than the normal respiratory rate of the animal and the chest wall movement produced should be more obvious than in normal breathing. During thoracotomy, expansion of the lung beyond the limits of the wound indicates that excessive inflation on the lungs is being produced. Simple observations such as these ensure that ventilation is being carried out in a manner which will result in no harm to the animal.

Because the rhythmical squeezing of a reservoir bag for long periods is both tedious and monotonous, mechanical devices ('ventilators') are commonly used to perform this duty. The use of a ventilator frees the anaesthetist to set up intravenous infusions, keep records, suck out the tracheobronchial tree, and otherwise attend to the welfare of the patient. Nevertheless, it should be noted that the manual squeezing of a reservoir bag is not to be despised. Observation of the bag between compressions shows volume changes due to the heart beat; the anaesthetist can alter the rate, rhythm and character of lung inflation to suit the convenience of the surgeon at any particularly critical stage of an operation, and the presence of respiratory obstruction is immediately obvious. Theoretically, the effort necessary to produce the desired degree of lung inflation should give the anaesthetist information about the level of anaesthesia or degree of relaxation of the respiratory muscles, more difficult inflation meaning waning relaxation or lighter anaesthesia. As relaxation wears off it is undoubtedly necessary to exert a greater pressure to maintain the tidal exchange as may be observed by anyone using suitably calibrated apparatus, but the authors have seldom been able to appreciate this while actually squeezing a reservoir bag. There may be such a thing as an 'educated hand' which recognizes every flicker of the diaphragm, or attempted cough, or waning relaxation, but it does not seem to be all that easily acquired.

LUNG VENTILATORS

A description of every commercially available ventilator is quite outside the scope of this book and the principles that underlie their operation can only be outlined. In general, the respiratory cycle of a ventilator can be divided into four parts :

1. The inspiratory phase provided by either flow generators or pressure generators. With flow generators the tidal volume delivered to the patient is independent of factors outside the ventilator – if, for example, the patient's airway resistance rises then the inflation pressure increases. The flow is not necessarily constant and can be generated by a bellows compressed by a cam mechanism or by pneumatic compression of the anaesthetic reservoir bag situated in a gas-tight chamber. Pressure generators maintain a constant pressure during the inspiratory phase of the respiratory cycle, often by a weight acting on a concertina bag. The volume delivered by a pressure ventilator will depend on such factors as the airway resistance (Mushin *et al.*, 1969).

2. The changeover from inspiratory to expiratory phase, i.e. the manner in which the ventilator cycles, may be (a) time cycled, in which inspiration is terminated after a set time, (b) volume cycled, where inspiration is terminated after a preset volume has been delivered, or (c) pressure cycled, in which case inspiration ceases as soon as a preset pressure is reached. Not all machines conform to this classification in that some show mixed cycling with hybrid cycling mechanisms. Each type of apparatus has its own advantages and disadvantages and discussion of their relative merits is, again, outside the scope of this book.

3. In the expiratory phase a machine may act as a flow generator (e.g. an injector) or a pressure generator and the commonest arrangement is to expose the patient's airway to atmospheric pressure.

4. The changeover from the expiratory to the inspiratory phase may be time cycled or patient triggered. In the patient triggered ventilator a slight inspiratory effort by the patient triggers the changeover to the inspiratory phase.

Ventilator performance in the presence of changed parameters in the patient is extremely complex and anyone contemplating the use of an unfamiliar ventilator is well advised to read any instructions provided by the manufacturer and become thoroughly conversant with its mode of operation before attempting to employ it. As a guide, provided a machine meets the following requirements it should be adequate in most circumstances no matter what its mode of operation or mechanism of cycling may be.

Essential characteristics

For use in cats, dogs, sheep, goats, small calves and small pigs, a ventilator needs to provide tidal volumes up to 1000 ml at a cycling rate of from 8 to about 40 cycles/minute. The duration of the inspiratory phase should be variable, independent of the other settings and range from about 0.5 to 3.0 s duration. Whenever possible the expired volume should be monitored since due to leaks the 'stroke volume' of the ventilator may not represent the tidal volume delivered to the animal.

Difficulty is experienced in using many commercially available ventilators in cats and small dogs. The problems involve the provision of high respiratory rates, and low tidal volumes. Adaptation of ventilators designed for adult humans can be accomplished by employing a controlled leak or a parallel resistance and compliance used in conjunction with an Ayre's T-piece. However, such systems are complicated and the ventilators designed specifically for veterinary purposes offer a better solution to the problem (Fig 8.8).

Since there is nothing more tiresome than having to adjust all the controls of a ventilator when only one setting needs correction, control of the length of expiratory period should, like that of the inspiratory period, be independent of the other settings. It should be possible to obtain inspiratory: expiratory ratios of at least 1:3, the expiratory period beginning immediately the desired tidal volume has been delivered to the lungs. Resistance to expiration should be low although it may sometimes be to an animal's advantage if the expiratory resistance can be increased (e.g. in emphysematous animals).

A high peak gas flow rate during the inspiratory phase is always desirable if the lungs are to be inflated in a short inspiratory period. It is comparatively easy to adapt a ventilator which gives a high peak flow rate to give a lower flow rate but it is impossible to obtain a high peak flow rate from a machine which is not designed to achieve this.

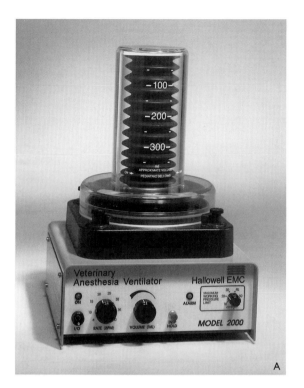

A

Provided a ventilator satisfies these general criteria, its method of cycling is unimportant. There are, however, several points which should be taken into account before buying a machine. First, for safety, it is essential that provision is made for a change to manual squeezing of a reservoir bag should any mechanical fault develop during the course of an operation. Secondly, if electrically driven, the machine must be electrically safe and explosion proof. Possibly less important, the machinery should not be noisy and if free standing it should occupy the minimum of floor space. In practice, the choice of ventilator is largely one of personal preference, convenience of operation for the particular circumstances in which it is to be used and the financial resources available.

The basic clinical criteria for ventilators for adult horses, cattle and large pigs are similar to those for the other animals described above (Fig. 8.9). A useful ventilator has a tidal volume of between 2 and 20 l with a cycling rate of between 4 and 15/min and an inspiratory phase of 2 to 3 s duration. It should be capable of sustaining pressures

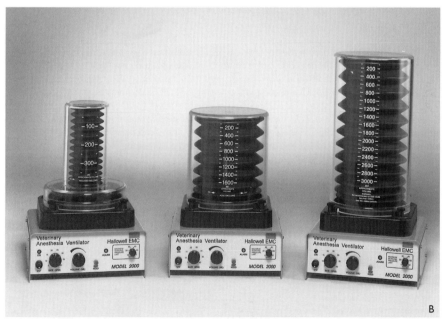

B

FIG. 8.8 A, B One example of a ventilator specially designed for veterinary use is the Hallowell ventilator, which is widely used in North America and elsewhere. It is electronically controlled, time-cycled and pressure-limited. Interchangeable bellows and housings enable it to deliver accurate tidal volumes of from 20 ml to 3000 ml at safe working pressures of 10–60 cm H_2O with respiratory rates of 6–40 breaths per minute. It can be fitted to all anaesthesia systems with out-of-circuit vaporizers (photographs courtesy of Hallowell EMC, 63 Eagle Street, Pittsfield, Massachusetts 01201, USA).

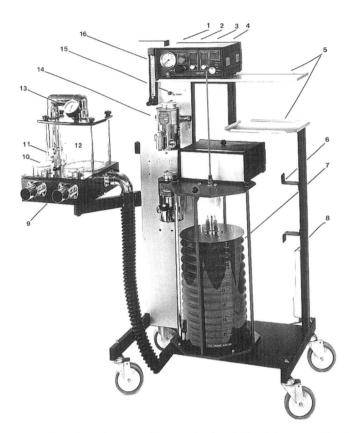

FIG. 8.9 On the Mallard Medical ventilator the controls are easily identified and the setting clearly displayed, making this ventilator very easy to set up. Rachel Model 2800 Large animal anaesthesia ventilator with model 2850 large animal absorber circuit. **1**: Microprocessor based ventilator; **2**: expanded flow rate control for paediatric through to large adult application 0–600 litres per minute; **3**: positive end-expiratory pressure (PEEP) control to enhance oxygenation of the patient; **4**: LED display of respiratory values and IE ratio; **5**: convenient shelves for monitors and accessories; **6**: mounting wraps on frame and backboard for hoses; **7**: 21 litre ascending bellows with resolution of less than 1 litre; **8**: surge and noise suppresser to protect all electronic instruments and provide multiple electrical outlets; **9**: model 2850 large animal absorber circuit; **10**: visible directional valves to observe inhalation and exhalation; **11**: new advanced design gas balance valve from human medicine. Allows for visual indication of setting and instant breathing circuit pressure relief; **12**: ultra capacity soda lime canister for removal of carbon dioxide; **13**: patient airway pressure gauge; **14**: vaporizer (not part of model 2800) backboard has holes located for either two Ohmeda or two Drager vaporizers, or a combination; **15**: oxygen flush, delivers 100% oxygen to absorber circuit; **16**: anaesthesia flowmeter (1–10 litres per minute) to vaporizer; **Note**: not shown is an optional paediatric bellows assembly, providing tidal volumes of 200 ml to 2.20 litres (photograph courtesy of Mallard Medical, Inc., 20268 Skypark Drive, Redding, California 96002, USA).

of up to 60 cmH$_2$O (6 kPa) in the upper airway during inspiration, although it must be noted that Schatzmann (1988) reported that peak inspiratory pressures above 20 cmH$_2$O lead to overdistension of lung tissue in the apical regions of the horse's lungs and to discharge of unidentified fluid out of the lungs during recovery from anaesthesia. The inspiratory: expiratory ratio should be at least 1:2. To achieve sufficiently high gas flows and tidal volumes special machines were developed for use

with large animals and often constructed to local specifications. Commercially made ventilators for adult horses and cattle are now available but proper data on their performance is scarce.

Ventilator settings

A survey of the literature reveals wide variations in the recommendations for tidal and minute volumes of respiration when IPPV is used. There are no generally agreed values for the production of adequate levels of ventilation in horses and even in dogs, where more studies have been done, published figures range from 20 to 30 ml/kg (tidal volume) and from 400 to 600 ml/kg (minute volume), so it is clear that numbers such as these can only be regarded as a very rough guide. In horses and cattle it is suggested that a tidal volume of 10 ml/kg at a rate of 8 to 12 breaths per minute, with an inspiratory: expiratory time ratio of 1:2 and a peak airway pressure not exceeding 30 cm H_2O should provide suitable initial settings for IPPV, although these may need to be modified as anaesthesia proceeds. Ideally, the end tidal concentration of carbon dioxide may be monitored continuously and, once the end tidal to arterial tension difference has been derived from blood gas analysis, the ventilation may be adjusted to yield a normal $PaCO_2$; it is important to note, however, that the end tidal to arterial carbon dioxide gradient may change during the course of anaesthesia. In practice, facilities for rapid gas and blood analysis are limited by financial and other constraints and it is often necessary to perform IPPV without such assistance.

For small animal patients, where non-rebreathing systems can be employed, it is relatively easy to ensure the maintenance of satisfactory $PaCO_2$ by deliberately hyperventilating at large tidal volumes with a gas mixture containing 4% CO_2 and at least 30% O_2. Using such a gas mixture in this way it is only necessary to ensure that large tidal and minute volumes are being imposed and this can be done from observation of the frequency of lung inflation and the amplitude of the chest wall excursions.

In large animals, where for reasons of economy in the use of gases it is essential to employ rebreathing systems, it is much less easy to ensure satisfactory blood gas levels and, in the absence of monitoring facilities, the anaesthetist has to rely on experience and aim to err, if at all, on the side of providing a mild degree of hyperventilation. In general, it is better to ventilate at slower rates with large tidal volumes than to achieve the same minute volumes by faster rates and smaller tidal volumes because low tidal volumes predispose to the lung collapse which necessitated the 'obligatory sigh' incorporated into the mechanism of earlier ventilators.

WEANING FROM IPPV

It is important to note that while in most animals apnoea may be established with the aid of neuromuscular blocking or centrally depressant drugs, in all cases at the end of operation apnoea should be mainly due to reflex inhibition of respiration by the rhythmical slight overinflation of the lungs and, possibly, hypocapnia. Thus, prompt resumption of spontaneous breathing usually follows if:

1. The rhythm of lung inflation is broken.
2. Some accumulation of CO_2 is allowed by either by slowing the ventilation rate, removing the soda lime canister or, in non-rebreathing systems, by adding more CO_2 to the inspired gases.

Residual neuromuscular block should be counteracted where appropriate by the i.v. administration of anticholinergic and anticholinesterase drugs. This should be done before any CO_2 accumulation is encouraged because anticholinesterases appear less likely to produce cardiac irregularities when the $PaCO_2$ is low. When inhalation anaesthetics have been used the inspired anaesthetic concentration should be decreased. Provided only minimal central depression by anaesthetic agents is present animals will resume spontaneous breathing at very low $PaCO_2$. Dogs have been observed to start breathing with $PaCO_2$ as low as 18–20 mmHg (approx. 2.2 kPa).

In cases where apnoea is established by the use of centrally acting drugs, antagonists such as naloxone may be given at the end of operation to overcome the respiratory depressant effects, but the relatively short action of the drugs commonly used today (e.g. fentanyl) usually makes this unnecessary.

PEEP and CPAP

In many conditions of advanced lung disease the imposition of an expiratory threshold has been shown to have beneficial effects on the PaO_2. According to Nunn (1977), use of an expiratory resistor during IPPV is known as PEEP (positive end-expiratory pressure) and during spontaneous breathing as CPAP (continuous positive airway pressure).

The respiratory benefits of an expiratory resistor include an overall reduction in airway resistance due to an increase in FRC, movement of the tidal volume above the airway closing volume, a tendency towards re-expansion of any collapsed lung and, possibly, a reduction in total lung water. The net result is that ventilation/perfusion relationships are improved. However, these advantages are, in some circumstances, counterbalanced by circulatory disadvantages due to the inevitable rise in mean intrathoracic pressure. Although the venous return can be restored by an α adrenergic stimulator such as dobutamine, or by over-transfusion, in clinical practice the situation is more complicated.

Both disease and drugs have profound effects on the circulatory response to a rise in mean intrathoracic pressure due to PEEP (or CPAP). Certain conditions may aggravate the reduction in cardiac output but others actually oppose it and it is in these latter conditions that PEEP or CPAP is likely to be of benefit. In animals with poor lung compliance much of the applied end-expiratory pressure will be opposed by the excessive pulmonary transmural pressure, thus minimizing the increase in intrathoracic pressure. Thus, the stiffer the lungs, the safer is the application of PEEP or CPAP likely to be.

To summarize, PEEP and CPAP may confer respiratory advantages and circulatory disadvantages which interact in a complicated manner rendering it necessary to make direct measurements of the relevant physiological functions to ensure that overall benefit results.

The results of PEEP and CPAP during routine anaesthesia are disappointing. Colgan *et al.* (1971) showed that PEEP produced no change in the alveolar–arterial gradient in anaesthetized dogs. Hall and Trim (1975) failed to demonstrate any benefit from CPAP in anaesthetized horses, and broadly similar results were obtained by Beadle *et al.* (1975). These results all probably indicate that anaesthesia produces no reduction in lung compliance in veterinary patients free from pulmonary disease. There would, therefore, seem to be no indication for the use of PEEP or CPAP in routine anaesthesia in healthy animals. Use of PEEP or CPAP in animals suffering from respiratory disease does not appear to have been documented.

HIGH FREQUENCY LUNG VENTILATION

Ventilation with tidal volumes of less than the anatomical dead space volume can provide adequate gas exchange in the lungs. The means of achieving this are not immediately obvious. Effective gas exchange in the lungs requires fresh gas to be presented to the animal's alveoli and the removal of used gas from the alveoli. The amount of gas required per minute to accomplish this is determined by the size and metabolic rate of the animal. Conventional artificial ventilation described in this chapter uses rates and tidal volumes within the physiological range but using small tidal volumes and higher respiratory frequencies is associated with lower peak inspiratory airway pressures and less fluctuation in intrathoracic pressure.

The transition from the conducting airways, with no gas exchanging function, to the alveolar sacs where gas exchange takes place, is not sharply demarcated anatomically. The respiratory bronchioles are predominently conducting passages but do have alveolar sacs opening off them. The alveolar ducts have gas exchanging epithelium throughout and in addition conduct gas to the alveoli. Thus any gas which penetrates to the respiratory bronchioles by bulk convection from the mouth and nose will take part in gas exchange.

Within the lung differing regions have different time constants (product of compliance and airway resistance). Some areas of the lung are fast fillers with short time constants, whereas other areas are slow fillers with long time constants. During early inspiration the fast filling regions become full and during late inspiration are actually emptying into the slow fillers. This is known as 'Pendelluft', and the sum of gas movement within the lung is greater than the gas flow down the trachea; there is gas movement between regions of the lung without gas movement in the trachea. It is, therefore, apparent that when small tidal volumes are delivered at high frequency, a slow filler could still be filling from a fast filler which at the same time is providing gas for expiration up the trachea.

Even with high ventilation frequencies fresh gas presented to the alveoli has ample time to diffuse across the alveolar zone (for this is complete within 10 ms.) and thus there is an enhanced potential for molecular diffusion to take a considerably greater role in the movement of gas across the alveoli.

High ventilation frequency

In the conventional model of ventilation a mass of gas under pressure (potential energy) is presented at the airway opening. This potential energy is converted to kinetic energy to allow the gas to flow down the airway. By the end of inspiration this kinetic energy has become zero for the gas is then static and the energy is stored as potential energy in the distended lungs. The time course for this change is determined by the time constant for the lung and it is known that 95% of change occurs within three time constants. It is obvious that with higher frequencies of ventilation there will be insufficient time for inspiration to go to completion, i.e. with static gas distending the lung alveoli. It therefore follows that with higher ventilatory frequencies either a reduced tidal volume is delivered to the lung periphery or a higher peak pressure is required to force the gas into the lung periphery within the time available.

With high frequencies of ventilation the kinetic energy of the molecules of gas undergoing bulk convection as ventilation cycles from inspiration to expiration becomes increasingly important. As ventilation changes from inspiration to expiration the gas retains its forward kinetic energy and will continue to progress peripherally until this kinetic energy is dissipated. This inertia of gas molecules is not present with conventional IPPV since end-inspiration is a static state.

The pressure–flow relationships at conventional breathing rates are adequately expressed by airways resistance but with higher frequencies airways resistance can no longer be assumed to be constant and inertia makes an increasing contribution. Thus, at higher frequencies airway impedance, which takes inertia into account, must be used to express pressure–flow relationships. By far the largest component of impedance to high frequency ventilation lies in the endotracheal tube. This impedance is greatest with a wide bore endo-

tracheal tube and high gas flow rates (large tidal volumes at high frequency).

At normal breathing rates gas distribution within the lung is determined by regional compliance. However, with higher respiratory rates airway resistance and gas inertia have an increasing effect on the distribution of ventilation. Potentially, this will result in a change of ventilation from areas of high compliance to areas of low impedance. Since there is no evidence to suggest that regional lung perfusion is altered, high frequency ventilation must, therefore, result in changes in lung ventilation–perfusion ratios.

Another aspect of high frequency ventilation is that it involves less time for the bulk convection of gas during inspiration and expiration so that the gas path length becomes increasingly important. Thus, in animals such as horses with long tracheas, pressures at the airway distend the major conducting passages, then the nearby fast filling lung units and finally the peripheral slow filling units. With a progressive shortening of the inspiratory time a situation will arise when there is insufficient time for the tidal volume to get beyond the major conducting passages which will then act in a way analogous to that of an electrical capacitor. The implication of this is that pressure at the airway opening is not transmitted to the lung periphery and hence the pleural space. However, the reverse will also occure in that there will not be enough time for the intra-alveolar pressure to empty the alveoli so that there will be a continuous positive pressure in the peripheral lung units. This should, in theory, be beneficial in elderly animals or in those with a reduced FRC since small airway closure is most likely to occur in these patients.

Methods for achieving high frequency ventilation of the lungs

Conventional ventilators deliver a volume of gas during inspiration by occlusion of a relatively wide bore orifice through which expiration takes place and the device to occlude the expiratory orifice must function rapidly. The more rapidly this device is made to operate the more likely valve bounce is to occur so that conventional ventilators cannot, in general, operate at frequencies above

2 Hz. Because of this limitation high frequency ventilation is normally provided by either high frequency jet ventilation (HFJV) or high frequency oscillation (HFO).

High frequency jet ventilators

These ventilators allow a high pressure gas source to flow into the airway during part of the respiratory cycle, usually 20–35% of the cycle time, through a narrow diameter tube usually at tracheal level. They require no expiratory seal and hence the airway is open to atmospheric pressure throughout the cycle. This potentially results in entrainment of an unknown quantity of ambient gas and thus the volume and composition of the tidal volume is unknown. The system has the inherent safety advantage that the animal can take a spontaneous breath at any time during the respiratory cycle.

High frequency oscillators

Oscillator type ventilators tend to be used for higher frequencies (6 to 40 Hz). A piston driven by a motor or an electronically driven diaphragm at the airway opening generates a to-and-fro motion of gas within the airway. The tidal volume results from displacement of the piston or diaphragm and a subatmospheric airway pressure is generated during the expiratory half of the respiratory cycle. Fresh gas is fed in at the airway opening and a low-pass filter exhaust port allows gas to exit the system. The low-pass filter offers a high impedance to high frequencies which are thus able to direct the tidal volume down the airway, which has a lower impedance, rather than be lost through the exhaust port.

Carbon dioxide elimination and oxygen delivery

On theoretical grounds it might be expected that with a constant tidal volume there should be a linear relationship between CO_2 removal and ventilatory frequency until such a time as the duration of inspiration is insufficient to permit the gas to penetrate the conducting airways to the gas exchanging regions of the lung. In practice this seems to be the case and there is a critical frequency at which CO_2 elimination reaches a peak. Above this frequency CO_2 elimination becomes a function of tidal volume and independent of ventilatory frequency. The critical frequency is dependent on the anatomy of the lung and is certainly higher in dogs than in horses.

One of the original hopes for high frequency ventilation was that the change from compliance/airway resistance distribution of ventilation to one determined by airway resistance/gas inertia would result in improved distribution of gas within the lung and an improvement in ventilation. However, it is now generally accepted that, at equivalent tidal volumes, neither HFJV nor HFO produce improvement in PaO_2, over that which can be attained by conventional ventilation techniques. Reports to date of high frequency lung ventilation in veterinary patients (Wilson *et al.*, 1985; Dunlop *et al.*, 1985; Dodman *et al*, 1985) are not encouraging.

LUNG VENTILATION IN INTENSIVE CARE

Long term IPPV over several days may be necessary after cardiopulmonary resuscitation, prolonged recovery from anaesthesia, or in animals presently unable to maintain an adequate PaO_2 when breathing 60% O_2 but which are expected to recover after appropriate treatment. IPPV is usually carried out with an air/oxygen mixture, the inspired O_2 concentration being adjusted to yield an arterial O_2 saturation of over 90% as shown by pulse oximetry.

Animals which are restless may require sedation or even light general anaesthesia for tolerance of the endotracheal tube (which is obligatory for the performance of IPPV). In dogs, cats and small ruminants an oral endotracheal tube is usual but in foals it is customary to employ a nasotracheal tube. Humidification of the inspired gases is necessary if high gas flows are employed but at low flows sufficient water vapour appears to condense on the inside of a rebreathing circuit to provide the water necessary for humidification. With high gas flows a disposable condenser-humidifier between the endotracheal tube and and delivery circuit is a convenient method of ensuring proper humidification of the inspired gas.

REFERENCES

Beadle, R.E., Robinson, N.E. and Sorensen, P.R. (1975) Cardiopulmonary effects of positive end-expiratory pressure in anesthetized horses. *American Journal of Veterinary Research.* **36**: 1435– 1438.

Colgan, F.J., Barrow, R.E and Fanning, G. (1971) Constant positive pressure breathing and cardiorespiratory function. *Anesthesiology* **34**: 145–151.

Comroe, J.H., Forster, R.E., Dubois, A.B., Briscoe, W.A. and Carlsen, E. (1962) *The Lung*, 2nd edn. Chicago: Year Book Medical.

Dodman, N.H., Lehr, J.L. and Spaulding, G.L. (1985) High frequency ventilation in large animals. *Proceedings of the 2nd International Congress of Veterinary Anaesthesia, Sacramento*, pp 186–187.

Dunlop, C., Steffey, E.P., Daunt, D., Kock, N. and Hodgson, D. (1985) Experiences with high frequency jet ventilation in conscious horses. *Proceedings of the 2nd International Congress of Veterinary Anaesthesia, Sacramento*, pp 190–191.

Gillespie, J.R., Tyler, W.S. and Eberly, V.E. (1966) Pulmonary ventilation and resistance in emphysematous and control horses. *Journal of Applied Physiology.* **21**: 416–422.

Hall, L.W., Gillespie, J.R. and Tyler, W.S. (1968) Alveolar–arterial oxygen tension differences in anaesthetized horses. *British Journal of Anaesthesia* **40**: 560–568.

Hall, L. W. and Trim, C.M. (1975) Positive end-expiratory pressure in anaesthetized spontaneously breathing horses. *British Journal of Anaesthesia* **47**: 819–824.

Hall, L.W. and Young, S.S. (1992) Effect of inhalation anaesthetics on total respiratory resistance in conscious ponies. *Journal of Veterinary Pharmacology and Therapeutics* **15**: 174–179.

Lehane, J.R. Jordan, C. and Jones, J.G. (1980) Influence of halothane and enflurane on respiratory airflow resistance and specific conductance in anaesthetized man. *British Journal of Anaesthesia* **52**: 773–781.

Michaelson, E.D., Grassman, E.D. and Peters, W.R. (1975) Pulmonary mechanics by spectral analysis of forced random noise. *Journal of Clinical Investigation* **56**: 1210–1230.

Mushin, W.W., Rendell-Baker, L., Thompson, P. and Mapleson, W.W. (1969) *Automatic Ventilation of the Lungs*. Oxford: Blackwell Scientific.

Nunn, J.F. (1977) *Applied Respiratory Physiology*. London: Butterworths, p 128.

Nunn, J.F. and Azi-Ashi, T.I. (1961) Respiratory effects of resistance to breathing in anaesthetized man. *Anesthesiology* **22**: 174–175.

Purchase I.F.H. (1965) Function tests on four large animal anaesthetic circuits. *Veterinary Record* **77**: 913–919.

Purchase I.F.H. (1965a) Some respiratory parameters in horses and cattle. *Veterinary Record* **77**: 859–860.

Schatzmann, U. (1988) Artificial ventilation in the horse. *Advances in Veterinary Anaesthesia: Proceedings of the 3rd International Congress of Veterinary Anaesthesia, Brisbane*, pp 29–34.

Watney, G.C.G., Jordan, C. and Hall, L.W. (1987) Effect of halothane, enflurane and isoflurane on bronchomotor tone in anaesthetized ponies. *British Journal of Anaesthesia* **59**: 1022–1026.

Watney, G.C.G., Jordan, C., Hall, L.W. and Nolan, A.M. (1988) Effects of xylazine and acepromazine on bronchomotor tone of anaesthetized ponies. *Equine Veterinary Journal.* **20**: 185–188.

Wilson, D.V., Soma, L.R. and Klein, L.V. (1985) High frequency positive pressure ventilation in the equine. *Proceedings of the 2nd International Congress of Veterinary Anaesthesia, Sacramento*, pp 188–189.

Young, S.S. and Hall, L.W. (1989) A rapid, non-invasive method for measuring total respiratory impedance in the horse. *Equine Veterinary Journal* **21**: 99–105.

Apparatus for the administration of anaesthetics

9

ADMINISTRATION OF INTRAVENOUS AGENTS

For agents which are intended to reach the central nervous system and produce narcosis or anaesthesia the intravenous route is obviously more direct than one through the respiratory tract. But it must always be borne in mind that unlike the respiratory pathway the intravenous one does not provide an exit as well as an entrance and, for this reason, apparatus used for the administration of intravenous agents must be designed to allow accurate control of the amount given, for once injected it cannot be recovered from the animal's body.

Although any superficial vein may be used, the choice of vein does not influence the apparatus which may be employed and detailed descriptions of the techniques of venepuncture will be found in the chapters concerned with anaesthesia of the various species of animal.

SYRINGES, NEEDLES AND CATHETERS

The largest syringe which can be handled conveniently is one of 50 to 60 ml capacity and for easy percutaneous venepuncture all those of greater capacity than 2 ml should have eccentrically placed nozzles. All-glass syringes are easy to sterilize but have plungers which tend to stick during injection and, although theoretically the best in which to collect samples of blood for blood gas

analysis (see Chapter 2) even for this purpose they have been replaced by the disposable plastic variety when no delay between collection of the sample and its analysis is anticipated.

Needles must be sharp and their points should, preferably, have a short bevel to reduce the risk of transfixing the vein: good quality disposable needles are always sharp. In small animals insertion of a needle or catheter through the skin may be rendered painless by the prior application of a local analgesic cream to the skin after suitable hair clipping. EMLA cream, a eutectic mixture of lignocaine base 2.5% with prilocaine base 2.5% applied under an occlusive dressing for 60 min prior to venepuncture, has been reported to be effective, but amethocaine 4% gel also applied under an occlusive dressing needs only 30 min to produce similar analgesia. In horses and cattle it is customary to desensitize the skin by the intradermal or s.c. injection of a small bleb of 2% lignocaine hydrochloride through a 25 gauge needle or via an air powered intradermal injector, prior to the insertion of a large bore catheter.

The administration of intermittent small doses of a drug, or its constant infusion, normally requires that a catheter be kept in the vein and free from blood clot. Methods in which a needle is left in the vein and an attached, loaded, syringe strapped to the patient are rarely satisfactory because movement between the skin and the vein, or of the patient, results in displacement of the needle. Unless this mishap is noticed it may lead to

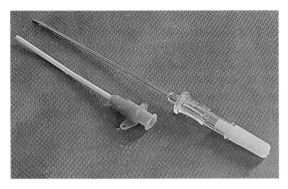

FIG. 9.1 Disposable plastic 'catheter over-needle'. Many patterns are available.

haematoma formation and/or the extravascular injection of drugs, some of which (e.g. guaiphenesin, thiopentone) may be highly irritant to the surrounding tissues.

Where anaesthesia is to be supervised by nursing staff or a technician it is particularly important to ensure there is a secure open venous line before commencing surgery. Venous access is usually ensured with a plastic catheter (Fig. 9.1). Proprietary catheters for this purpose are supplied sterile: they consist of a nylon, polythene or teflon catheter around a hollow metal needle or trocar, the point of which projects just beyond the tapered end of the catheter. The catheter is inserted into the vein with the trocar needle in position and the needle is withdrawn when blood flows from its proximal end or is seen to enter the catheter hub. The needle hub is then held firmly while the catheter is advanced well up the vein and secured in position with adhesive tape or a stitch. Because the catheter is blunt ended it does not transfix the vein and a long length can be threaded into the vein. Once the catheter is in position the needle is completely withdrawn. To prevent unwelcome spilling of blood from a peripheral vein it is customary, as soon as the catheter has been sited, to occlude the vein by exerting digital pressure over the catheter tip (usually easily located by palpation) until an obturator or tap is affixed or an infusion connected.

An attempt to insert one of these catheters directly through the skin may result in the tip of the catheter opening out into a bell-mouth shape which is almost impossible to introduce into the vein, so they should be inserted through a small skin incision. Often, a small skin incision for this

purpose can be made with the cutting edge of a needle. Should venepuncture be found to be unsuccessful, even if the needle has only been partially withdrawn from the catheter, it must not be reinserted unless the catheter is completely removed from the tissues because it may penetrate the side wall of the catheter and sheer off the distal portion.

More than than 25 different patterns of 'catheter over needle' are commercially available in the United Kingdom alone. There is some variation on their general shape and some have small handles to aid insertion. Most have plastic needle hubs through which which blood can be seen when the needle enters the vein. Three important factors govern the choice of catheter. First, it should be no longer than strictly necessary. The length of most catheters (up to 7 cm) is always adequate and there is no need for the larger diameters to be longer. However, exceptions to this rule may be made in circumstances when the need to ensure that the catheter remains in the vein at all costs (e.g. when administering guaiphenesin to a horse) outweigh the effect of the increased length on resistance to flow. The second important feature is the wall thickness. It is the external diameter which largely determines the size chosen in any given situation and catheters with thinner walls obviously permit more rapid infusions. The third factor is that the external shape should be as smooth as possible, for catheters with smooth contours are the easiest to introduce.

Longer catheters are available for special purposes such as measurement of the central venous pressure (see Chapter 2). Although it is possible to obtain some of the catheters described above up to 5.25 inches (13.3 cm) in length (which may be adequate for central venous pressure measurement in cats and small dogs), the longer catheters are generally not provided with introducing needles. Whenever possible, they are introduced into the vein through a previously placed large bore catheter. Some long catheters (e.g. Abbotts Drum Reel) are supplied with an additional short, wider bore catheter of the 'over needle pattern' that is introduced into the vein so that the longer one can be threaded through it.

Veins (and arteries) can be catheterized over a guidewire. Originally described as the 'Seldinger'

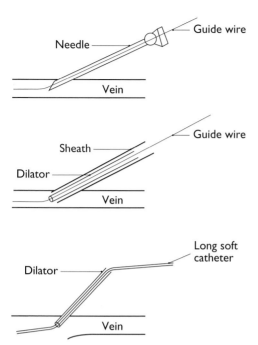

FIG. 9.2 Technique for the insertion of a long, soft catheter (e.g. Swan–Ganz) into a vein by the modified Seldinger technique. The vein is first penetrated with a needle through which the guide wire is threaded as soon as the needle is placed in the vein. After withdrawing the needle, a sheathed vein dilator is introduced over the guide wire and the dilator and guide wire are removed to leave the dilator sheath patent for the introduction of the catheter.

technique for arterial cannulation, this method is now used to introduce catheters which are too flexible, blunt ended or too large to be inserted directly percutaneously. It is commonly used for arterial catheters, right atrial feeding catheters, catheters for injecting radiological contrast media, cardiac pacing catheters and pulmonary artery flow directed catheters, but it may be used for any intravenous catheter placement. A relatively small needle or catheter is introduced into the vessel, a guidewire is inserted through it and the catheter is withdrawn. A large bore vein dilator is threaded over the guidewire. Most vein dilators are fragile and a scalpel incision must be made to clear a track to the vessel. Dilators usually consist of an inner section and a sheath; the inner section is removed with the guidewire. The catheter proper is inserted through the vein dilator sheath (Fig. 9.2). There are several designs of guidewire; most have flexible

tips followed by a stiffer section. The tip may be preformed into a J-shape to facilitate its passage through angles in the vessels. Some catheters (e.g. radiographic catheters) are stiff enough to be threaded over the guidewire and passed into the vessel but softer catheters need to be passed through the vein dilator. For asepsis it is safer to 'gown-up' completely and towel up a large disinfected area of skin to avoid contamination of a very expensive catheter which may not be re-sterilizable.

The number of proprietary catheters of various lengths now available is bewilderingly large and choice is difficult. Because the wrong choice is made intravenous infusions which appear to run smoothly when originally set up with electrolyte solutions may prove infuriatingly slow when blood or a colloid solution has to be given. Such a disadvantage may cost an animal's life. Consideration of some of the factors influencing the flow makes the choice of catheter more rational and less dependent on the information given on the packet by the manufacturers of any particular product.

The flow through a tube is proportional to the driving pressure, which is equal to the pressure difference between the two ends of the tube, multiplied by a constant, $\pi/8$. Flow is also inversely proportional to the viscosity of the fluid, since the more viscous it is the harder it will be to force it through the tube. The final factor governing the flow is the internal diameter of the tube, flow being directly proportional to the fourth power of the radius, and inversely proportional to the length of the bore. Thus, for maximum flow of any given fluid at any given pressure, the tube should be short, and the diameter large. It must be noted that a small change in diameter has a great effect on flow velocity.

At very high flow rates it may be found that the resistance to flow is disproportionately high. There is a critical flow velocity at which flow changes from streamline to turbulent. During turbulence the driving pressure is largely used up in creating the kinetic energy of the turbulent eddies. The flow no longer depends on the viscosity of the fluid but on its density. However, the critical velocity at which turbulence occurs depends mainly on the viscosity and density of the fluid as well as the radius of the bore of the tube through which it is

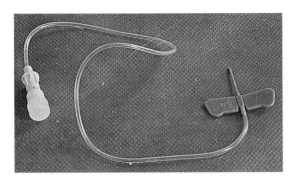

FIG. 9.3 'Butterfly' or 'small vein set' or 'infant scalp vein set'. Many types are available but all have lengths of plastic tubing attached and most have winged needles to aid insertion and subsequent fixation to the patient.

flowing. In an intravenous infusion system the critical velocity is likely to be exceeded at very high flow rates and also at local points in the apparatus at which, because of sudden change in internal configuration, the velocity of flow momentarily rises. Thus, at points at which the internal diameter changes suddenly, turbulence will occur.

The viscosity of blood is considerably greater than that of water, mainly because of the presence of erythrocytes. It increases with the haematocrit and above about 60% packed cell volume blood hardly behaves as a fluid. Viscosity is also increased by a drop in temperature, and the viscosity of blood at 0 °C is about 2.5 times as great as at 37 °C. Blood warming coils are, therefore, justified on grounds of increasing the speed of transfusion as well as of preventing the development of hypothermia in the recipient.

An alternative to a catheter for very small veins is a needle attached to a hub by a length of plastic tubing. There are at least nine types of 'small vein' needles currently available (Fig. 9.3). Some have winged handles to aid insertion and subsquent fixation to the patient. Flow performance of most of the 'small vein sets' (often called 'scalp vein sets' or 'butterflies') is surprisingly poor, and it is usually best to choose one with the shortest length of tubing attached.

INFUSION APPARATUS

Where, as in larger farm animals and horses, large volume infusions are to be given rapidly, simple apparatus may be used. However, if a fairly accurate control of flow rate is needed, or the infusion is to be given slowly as may be necessary in small animal patients or when potent drugs are to be administered, a system giving a greater degree of control is essential. Proprietary disposable plastic 'giving sets' or 'administration sets' are convenient for these purposes and can be obtained in a variety of patterns.

Essentially, a 'giving set' consists of an outlet tube which may or may not incorporate a filter depending on whether the set is for blood and blood products or crystalloids alone, a drip chamber and a long length of plastic delivery tubing which can be occluded by some form of adjustable clamp. If it is intended for use with *bottles* of fluid an air inlet with a filter is incorporated. All plastic sets include a short piece of rubber tubing towards the needle mount end of the delivery tube, or a rubber capped short side arm so that injections can be made through a fine bore needle whilst the tubing is pinched between the finger and thumb on the drip chamber side of the injection site to prevent the pressure damming back fluid in the drip chamber. The flow rate is controlled by means of the clamp and can be estimated from number of drops which pass through the drip chamber in one minute. For example, with most sets 40 drops/minute means the administration of approximately 500 ml in 4 hours. Much more accurate control of infusion rate can be obtained by the use of a drip rate controller between the fluid container and the patient. These are electronic devices which monitor the drip chamber and, by changing the effective cross-section area of a section of the standard administration set tubing, maintain a constant infusion rate. The automatic control eliminates the need for frequent adjustment of the drip rate. However, drip rate controllers are expensive and cannot compensate for variations in drip size so that the actual delivery rate depends on the drop size.

Drip rate pumps are similar in cost and appearance to drop rate controllers and most operate satisfactorily with standard administration sets. They generate a pressure by peristaltic fingers or rollers acting on deformable tubing to give a constant infusion rate.

Volumetric pumps are designed to avoid problems associated with variations in drop size. Very

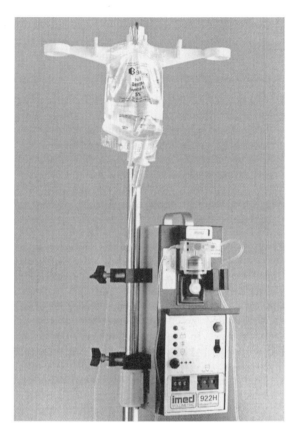

FIG. 9.4 Volumetric or constant infusion pump. Types such as this drive a disposable piston pump and the need to refill the barrel of the pump means that the infusion rate is not actually constant. They will, however, maintain a reliable infusion rate. Most have devices which warn of the presence of air in the infusion line or occlusion of the line.

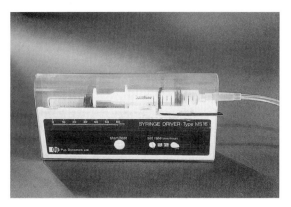

FIG. 9.5 Syringe driver. Many types of electrically driven syringe drivers are available. Some must be used with one specified size of syringe, others can be used with a variety of syringes.

good volumetric accuracy is obtained with either a reciprocating piston type pump or by peristaltic pumping on an accurately made tube which forms part of the administration set. With the piston type pump (Fig. 9.4) no fluid is delivered to the patient during the refilling stage of the cycle so that at low flow rates significant fluctuations in delivery rate occur. The need for a dedicated infusion set adds to the cost of each infusion and the volume of fluid needed to prime these sets can also be in the region of 20 ml which may give rise to significant wastage of expensive solutions. These pumps are, however, particularly valuable for longer procedures where the solution can be withdrawn from a large container such as a 3 l plastic bag.

Electrically driven syringe drivers (Fig. 9.5) overcome many of the problems associated with the administration of relatively small volumes of fluid (e.g. to cats or for the continuous administration of small volumes of drug solutions during anaesthesia). They are usually calibrated for a particular type and size of syringe. The delivery rate control alters the rate of plunger travel and hence the cross-sectional area of the barrel is critical in ensuring that the delivery rate is correct. The syringe can be filled from a large container of fluid and connected to the intravenous catheter with a simple administration extension set so that priming volume is minimal. Syringe drivers are generally less expensive than volumetric pumps or drip rate pumps or controllers as well as being more portable. Further developments include the use of programmed microprocessor control with an ability (if the pharmacokinetics of the infused substance are known) to deliver a changing infusion rate such that a steady state of blood concentrations can be achieved and maintained.

Most infusion pumps monitor line pressure by detecting changes in the motor current needed for driving and to avoid frequent false alarms the pressure at which an occlusion is indicated is usually set well above the anticipated line pressure. This means that occlusion alarms on infusion pumps have little value in indicating that the fluid is being injected into the tissues rather than into a vein. With low flow rates, the time required for a significant increase in interstitial, and subsequently line pressure, will be long and substantial amounts of fluid may be injected before any warning is given.

Pharmaceutical companies now provide intravenous fluids in plastic disposable bag containers and some provide bags with an integral giving set. Because such bags are collapsible, no air inlet is necessary, air embolism cannot occur and infusions can be left running unattended, which may be an advantage for veterinary use. When bottles of fluid are used, there is a possibility of air embolism should the bottle empty unobserved, as air has to enter the bottle before fluid can leave.

When fluids are administered under the influence of gravity the speed of infusion depends more on the bore of the needle or catheter than on the pressure applied (i.e. the height above the needle or catheter at which the container is held). Doubling the diameter of the needle or catheter gives a 16-fold increase in the rate of flow, whereas a four-fold increase in the pressure is required to double the rate. However, in the case of the 'flutter valve' apparatus traditional and formerly so popular in veterinary practice, the vertical distance between the needle and the air inlet opening determines the rate at which air enters the system; increasing this distance increases the rate of air entry and hence the speed of infusion. The 'flutter valve' is unreliable and there is little justification for its continued use in veterinary anaesthetic practice except, perhaps, when short duration fast infusion needs to be given.

In circumstances where the maximum size of the needle or catheter is limited, the maximum rate of flow of fluid can be increased by pressurizing the system. Where bottles are in use, they can be pressurized by pumping air under pressure through the air inlet. This procedure carries a high risk of producing air embolism if the supply of fluid runs out, so it should be used with caution and the infusion should never be left unattended. Pressure can be applied to plastic bags of fluid by placing them in a second bag or container pressurized by pumping in air; there is then no danger of air embolism.

ADMINISTRATION OF INHALATION AGENTS

The administration of an inhalation anaesthetic requires:

1. A source of oxygen (which may be air)
2. A vaporizer or a source of anaesthetic gas
3. A 'patient' or 'breathing' system.

In its simplest form modern anaesthetic apparatus consists of an oxygen cylinder, with pressure gauge, pressure regulator and flowmeter, delivering oxygen to a suitable patient breathing system. A vaporizer for an inhalation anaesthetic agent may be included inside or outside the patient breathing system.

DELIVERY AND REGULATION OF ANAESTHETIC GASES

Oxygen cylinders ('tanks' in North America)

For medical use oxygen is obtained compressed at high pressure (138 atmospheres or $2000 \, lb/in^2$) into metal cylinders or as liquid oxygen in special containers. For veterinary purposes cylinders are usually used. In the United Kingdom they are colour coded black with a white top but in other countries there is no adherence to what was intended to be a universal code. In the USA they are coloured all green and in Canada all white. When delivered, all cylinders have a plastic seal over their outlet to exclude dust and this seal should be removed only immediately before use. There are two types of cylinder outlet. Some cylinders fit into a yoke over pins which are indexed for different gases so as to make it impossible to attach an incorrect cylinder. A small washer termed a 'Bodcock seal' is needed around the inlet on the yoke of these pin-indexed fittings. Larger cylinders utilize 'bull-nose' fittings which screw into place and require no sealing washer.

Pressure gauge

It is essential for the anaesthetist to know that there is an adequate supply of oxygen in the cylinder so when in use they are coupled to a pressure gauge to register the pressure inside and, therefore, the quantity of oxygen available. Pressure gauges are most commonly of the Bourdon type (see Fig. 9.6), consisting of a metal tube, the end of which is attached to a pointer. The application of pressure to the inside of the tube causes it to straighten and moves the pointer over a scale.

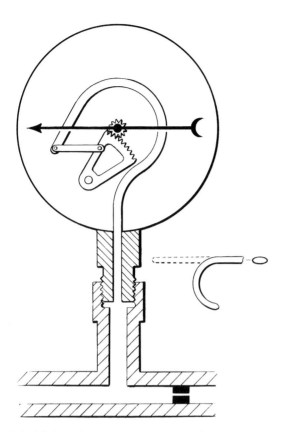

FIG. 9.6 Bourdon gauge. These are used for measuring gas pressure and, placed before an orifice, for gas flow measurement.

Reducing valves or regulators

A pressure reducing valve at the cylinder outlet or on a pipeline supply is necessary for three reasons:

1. For cylinder supplies, once the flow has been set for any particular level, frequent readjustment of the flowmeter control, which would be necessary as the pressure in the cylinder fell off, is obviated. Because the reducing valve exerts this automatic control it is often referred to as a 'regulator'.

2. By supplying a low gas pressure to the control valve spindle small variations in the gas flow can be made easily. Where a high pressure cylinder is controlled directly by a simple needle-type valve large changes in flow result from very small movements of the control valve spindle.

3. The regulator limits the pressure within the connecting tubing to a low level and the likelihood of bursting the connecting tube when the flow is

shut off by the flowmeter control is very much reduced.

The regulators in common use in anaesthesia usually reduce the pressure at which oxygen is delivered to below 200 lb/in^2 (13.8 atm) and many modern anaesthetic machines incorporate the valve into the block featuring the cylinder pin index so that on superficial inspection of the machine they may be difficult to identify. Further details of these regulators can be obtained from such texts as *Ward's Anaesthetic Equipment* by Moyle and Davey (4th edn. (1997) W. B. Saunders) and will not be considered here.

Flowmeters

Today most of the flowmeters used in anaesthesia in the UK are known as 'rotameters' (Fig. 9.7). They make use of the interdependence of flow rate, size of an orifice and the pressure difference on either side of the orifice. The rotameter consists

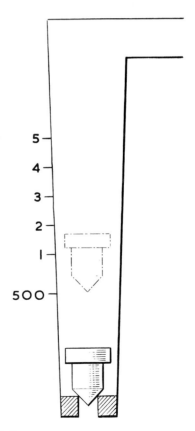

FIG. 9.7 Rotameter.

of a glass tube inside which a rotating bobbin is free to move. The bore of the tube gradually increases from below upwards. The bobbin floats up and down the tube, allowing gas to flow around it. The higher the bobbin in the tube the wider the annular space between the tube and bobbin (orifice) and the greater the flow rate through it. The bobbin, usually made of aluminium, has an upper rim which is of a diameter slightly greater than that of the body, and in which specially shaped channels are cut. As the gas enters the rotameter tube it impinges on the bobbin and causes it to rise and to spin because the rim with its set of channels acts like a set of vanes. The result is that the bobbin rides on a cushion of gas thereby eliminating errors due to friction between the tube and bobbin. The gas flow rate is read from the top of the bobbin against a scale etched on the outside of the glass tube. If the tube is mounted in a truly upright position these meters are capable of readings of an accuracy of ± 2% but only for the gas for which they have been calibrated.

The Heidbrink flowmeter, commonly used in the USA, has a metal tube, the inside of which is tapered in the same way as a rotameter tube. The bobbin is replaced by a rod, the tip of which is visible through a glass tube fitted at the top of the metal tube. A scale is fitted to the side of the glass tube and the gas flow rate can be read off from the position of the tip of the metal rod against this scale. In the UK this type of meter is most commonly found on oxygen therapy apparatus.

Ball float meters, like the rotameter and Heidbrink, have a tapering bore and are, therefore, variable orifice meters. The bobbin or rod is replaced by a special ball and if the tube is mounted on an inclined plane one ball is sufficient, but if the tube is vertical the ball tends to oscillate; this is overcome by using two ball floats. The reading is taken from the centre of the ball or, in two ball types, the point of contact between the balls. The Connell flowmeter has two balls in contact in an inclined tube. With all inclined tube meters it is important that they are set at the correct angle or inaccuracies will occur.

A much more crude flowmeter utilizes a Bourdon pressure gauge (Fig. 9.8). The gas flowing from the cylinder issues from the reducing valve

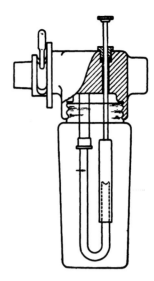

FIG. 9.8 Boyle-type vaporizer. This relatively crude type of vaporizer is not temperature or flow compensated and is mostly used in developing countries for the volatilization of ether in a stream of O_2 or air.

and is made to pass through a small orifice. A pressure builds up proximal to the constriction and this pressure is transmitted to the flexible, metal, oval cross-section, Bourdon tube. The tube tends to straighten, the degree of straightening depending on the pressure within it which, in turn, depends on the gas flow through the orifice. The tip of the Bourdon tube is linked by a simple mechanism to an indicator needle which moves over a scale calibrated in terms of rate of gas flow. In fact, in this meter the gauge indicates the pressure difference between the proximal side of the orifice and the atmosphere. This is virtually equivalent to measuring the pressure gradient across the orifice since in anaesthetic practice the pressure on the distal side of the orifice approximates very closely to atmospheric.

The Bourdon type of flowmeter is not satisfactory for measuring small rates of gas flow. Owing to the pressure necessary to cause the Bourdon tube to straighten out, a very small orifice must be used to provide the resistance to gas flow. If this orifice becomes partially blocked by dirt the meter reading increases whereas the actual flow of gas is decreased; if the orifice becomes completely blocked the meter reading suggests that the flow is being maintained. On the other hand, if the orifice is enlarged due to wear, the gas flow will be increased while the decreased resistance to gas flow will lead to a low meter reading.

Pipeline systems

Where large quantities of oxygen (or other gases) are used, it is more convenient and more economical to utilize larger cylinders. As these are awkward to handle they are kept outside the operating area and the gas is supplied to the anaesthetic machine through a pipeline. The central depot has a number of large cylinders connected to a manifold so that gas is taken from all the cylinders in the bank. Warning devices are included so that the manifold can be changed to a second bank of cylinders when the supply pressure drops, or, with more complex apparatus where there are two or more manifolds, the change to the bank of fresh cylinders takes place automatically. If extremely large quantities of oxygen are used daily, as they may be in a large hospital, the cylinder bank may be replaced by liquid oxygen containers but this is most unlikely to be necessary for veterinary practice.

In the UK the outlets from the pipelines in the theatre are colour coded and indexed so that at least in theory, pipes from the anaesthetic machine cannot be connected to the wrong outlet. In practice, it is not unknown for force to be used to circumvent this precautionary system. Oxygen and other gases are delivered at a low pressure to the anaesthetic machine and are fed directly from the piped supply to the flowmeter. However, most pipeline machines also carry a small oxygen cylinder and an associated pressure regulator for emergency use in the event of a failure in the pipeline supply.

Oxygen failure warning devices

Devices which warn the anaesthetist that the pressure of the oxygen supply is low have been largely neglected in veterinary anaesthesia, yet it is in this field, when often in general practice there is minimal assistance available to monitor the oxygen delivery, where they should be considered an essential feature of anaesthetic machines. Some types depend on a second source of gas, usually nitrous oxide, for their operation. When the oxy-

gen pressure falls a diaphragm moves to allow the second gas to pass through a whistle and an easily audible warning note is emitted. In other types a valve opens as the oxygen pressure drops and the remaining oxygen passes through the whistle; the whistling noise ceases as the oxygen pressure falls to atmospheric pressure.

Gases other than oxygen

Gases other than oxygen which are commonly found on anaesthetic machines include nitrous oxide (in the UK cylinders are colour coded blue) and carbon dioxide (grey cylinders). These gases are compressed in cylinders under a pressure which liquifies them at ordinary room temperatures. The amount of gas present in the cylinder can only be found by weighing (all have full and empty weights stamped on them) since the pressure of the gas above the liquid remains almost constant as long as any liquid remains. Thus, a pressure gauge at the cylinder outlet will register only a small fall as the gas is being drawn off due to cooling causing a fall in the saturated vapour pressure, but this will rise again as the cylinder warms and the pressure registered will not drop rapidly until all the liquid has been vaporized and the residual gas is being drawn off.

The saturation pressure of 20 °C of N_2O and CO_2 is sufficiently high that the cylinders need to be fitted with reducing valves ('pressure regulators'). It is now possible to mix two gases using a monitored dial mixer unit before delivery into a final common pathway. This type of system (Quantiflex) has been used for nitrous oxide/oxygen mixtures in any proportions from 21 to 100% oxygen at flow rates of 1–20 l/min. The system is costly, but it has the advantage that it can be more convenient and mistakes are less likely. It is inherently safe because hypoxic gas mixtures cannot be delivered.

When an oxygen flow is being mixed with a nitrous oxide without the aid of a Quantiflex mixer, failure of the oxygen supply is disastrous because the machine will then deliver 100% N_2O. Oxygen warning devices such as those described above reduce the chance of this happening without the knowledge of the anaesthetist, but many modern machines incorporate a cut-off device so that should O_2 flow cease the N_2O flow is also cut off. This cut-off device may prevent the machine from being fitted with some types of oxygen failure alarm.

VAPORIZERS

The ideal vaporizer would be one that delivered a suitable and accurately known quantity of a volatile anaesthetic agent at all times and under all conditions of use. However, many factors which vary during the course of administration influence vaporization and only the most modern of expensive, sophisticated pieces of apparatus approach anywhere near this ideal.

Factors which have most influence include temperature, gas flow rate through the vaporizer, and back pressure transmitted during IPPV. A low resistance to gas flow may also be important if the vaporizer is to be used in the breathing circuit (p. 000).

Uncalibrated vaporizers

If a liquid volatile anaesthetic is contained in a bottle it is possible to bubble gas through it or to allow the gas to flow over its surface. This arrangement is sometimes known as a 'plenum vaporizer' because gas is being forced into a chamber, and 'plenum' is a chamber or container in which the pressure inside is greater than that outside it.

In the UK Boyle pattern vaporizers are still occasionally encountered and they are common in some developing countries. In these vaporizers the method of varying the concentration of anaesthetic vapour delivered utilizes a permanent partition to prevent the direct passage of gases from the flowmeters to the patient. When the control lever is in the OFF position all gases are diverted around the partition but away from the bottle. With the tap in the ON position all gases pass through the bottle containing the liquid. The control can be placed in any intermediate position and this determines how much of the total gas flow passes through the bottle.

A further means of controlling the vapour concentration is also provided. The gases are made to pass through a J-shaped tube before emerging into the space above the liquid anaesthetic in the bottle.

The open end of the J-tube is covered by a metal hood which can be positioned as required by moving the rod attached to it up or down. As the hood is pushed downwards the gas is deflected nearer and nearer to the surface of the liquid and finally, when the open end of the hood is pushed below the surface of the liquid gases are made to bubble through the liquid anaesthetic. When the tap is in the ON position and the hood, or cowl, fully depressed, the whole of the gas flow is made to bubble through the liquid and a maximum concentration of the anaesthetic vapour is picked up. Boyle pattern vaporizers for potent agents such as halothane have a single, straight inlet tube with a side port and no cowl arrangement.

When air or other gas flows over the surface of a liquid, the vapour of the liquid is carried away, and is replaced by fresh vapour. This continuous process of vaporization is accompanied by a corresponding loss of heat, the magnitude of which is determined by the rate at which the vapour is removed and by the latent heat of vaporization of the liquid. The loss of heat results in a fall in the temperature of the liquid unless heat is conducted to the liquid from some outside source. With a fall in the temperature of the liquid there is a corresponding decrease in the speed of vaporization and, if the gas flow remains constant, the concentration of anaesthetic vapour in the gas stream from a Boyle pattern vaporizer decreases with time until the heat loss due to vaporization is balanced by the conduction of heat through the glass bottle from the surrounding atmosphere. When ether was used in this type of vaporizer it was not uncommon to see ice crystals forming on the outside of the bottle as its temperature fell due to volatilization of the ether.

Calibrated vaporizers

There are today many precision vaporizers on the market, all designed to deliver an accurately known concentration of specific volatile anaesthetics over a wide range of gas flow rates. They consist of a vaporizing chamber and a bypass. The fresh gas stream flowing into the vaporizer is divided into two portions, the larger of which passes straight through the bypass. The smaller portion is ducted through the vaporizing chamber where it becomes saturated with the vapour, and this ensures that:

1. There is no sudden burst of high vapour concentration when the vaporizer is first switched on.
2. The output of the vaporizer is unaffected by shaking.

As already pointed out, vaporization of the liquid anaesthetic results in the removal of heat from the liquid with a resultant fall in its temperature. Modern calibrated vaporizers are constructed from metal (mainly copper) which ensure the ready conduction of heat from the room to the contained liquid, the high thermal conductivity of the metal container together with the high thermal capacity of its mass, ensure a sufficient supply of heat for vaporization, holding the liquid temperature constant. In these modern vaporizers the only control to set is the output concentration.

A major problem in vaporizer design lies in the design of the splitting valves. In the earlier types it proved impossible to ensure that the flow division of this valve remained constant over a wide range of flow rates, and the vaporizers were supplied with graphs which needed to be consulted to determine the concentration of volatile agent being delivered when they were used with gas flow rates below 4 l/min. In current models this problem has been overcome and it is generally accepted that most deliver accurately indicated concentrations at flow rates above 500 ml/min.

Pressure fluctuations produced by IPPV have a pumping effect and this may have a considerable effect on the output, even doubling the output concentration at low gas flow rates. Modern vaporizers incorporate a non-return valve to overcome this.

The volatile anaesthetic agent, desflurane, requires a special vaporizer as its boiling point is too close to room temperature for it to be used in the conventional systems.

The 'Selectatec' and similar systems enable the easy removal or placement of the vaporizer on the 'back bar' of the anaesthetic machine for filling in another environment, or for exchange for a vaporizer containing a different anaesthetic agent or for service. Calibrated vaporizers need regular service at intervals as recommended by the manufacturers if they are to retain their accuracy.

All the vaporizers described so far have a high resistance to gas flow, which is unimportant when the carrier gas is pushed through them by the power of the compressed gases in the cylinders or pipelines. However, if the vaporizer is to be used where the gas flow is powered by the respiratory efforts of the animal, then a low resistance vaporizer is essential and vaporizers of this type are necessary for use in 'in-circle' systems.

Low resistance vaporizers

Vaporizers offering a low resistance to gas flow are usually of a simple type with wide-bore entry and exit ports and no wicks to impede the flow of gases. A simple low resistance, low efficiency vaporizer of this type often used in dental surgery is the Goldman (Fig. 9.9).

The EMO vaporizer (Epstein-Macintosh-Oxford) (Fig. 9.10) was specifically designed for the volatilization of ether and is generally recognized as the best of this type of vaporizer. It is

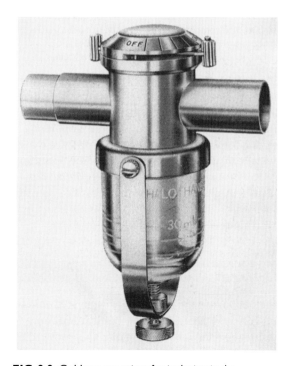

FIG. 9.9 Goldman vaporizer for inclusion in the breathing system. Commonly used for halothane.

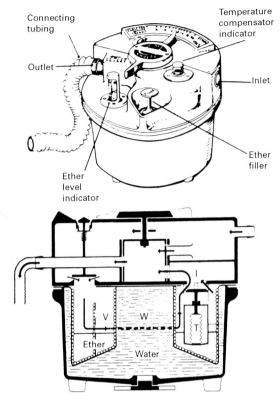

Connecting tubing

Outlet

Temperature compensator indicator

Inlet

Ether filler

Ether level indicator

V   W

Ether   Water

FIG. 9.10 The EMO vaporizer for ether. This draw-over, temperature compensated unit may be used in situations where supplies of O_2 are not readily available and, consequently, it is very popular in some developing countries.

portable, has a temperature compensating device and is employed in a non-rebreathing system. Ether/air anaesthesia administered from it meets criteria for acceptability in general practice where the veterinarian may be assisted in the operating theatre by a nurse or may be entirely alone. It may be used in situations where supplies of oxygen are not readily available and, consequently, it is popular in many developing countries.

BREATHING SYSTEMS

The purpose of the breathing system is to convey oxygen and anaesthetic to the patient, and to ensure the removal of carbon dioxide produced by the patient. It does not seem possible to classify all the ways in which this can be done in a completely logical manner and as yet there is no universally agreed system. A system of classification formerly in common use in the UK was:

1. The open method
2. The semi-open method
3. (a) The closed method with carbon dioxide absorption (b) The semi-closed method with carbon dioxide absorption
4. The semi-closed method without carbon dioxide absorption.

This classification has been criticised on the grounds that it is impractical and does not fit all systems. A more clinically useful definition of systems is based on the two methods by which carbon dioxide is removed from the inspired gases:

1. *Non-rebreathing*
The system is designed so that the expired gases are vented to the atmosphere and cannot be rebreathed.
2. *Rebreathing*
The expired gases are passed through an absorber which contains soda lime or another absorbent (e.g. Baralyme) to remove the carbon dioxide.

The open and semi-open methods were used to volatilize agents such as chloroform and ether. The methods are often referred to as 'rag and bottle anaesthesia' and they survived through over a hundred years of anaesthetic history. In the semi-open or 'perhalation' method all the inspired air was made to pass through a mask on which the vaporization of the agent occurred. In horse and cattle special masks were often used for the semi-open administration of chloroform. These masks were cylinders of leather and canvas applied over either the upper or both jaws. Chloroform was applied to a sponge inserted in the open end of the cylinder. In the cruder types of mask the sponge was actually in contact with the nostrils, but in more refined patterns a wire mesh partition prevented this direct contact.

Today, the open and semi-open methods of administration are seldom used. In them, the anaesthetic agents are diluted to an unknown extent by air and this dilution is greatest when the minute volume of breathing is large so the inspiratory gas flow rate is high. The greater the ventilation (and hence, the dilution of the anaesthetic inhaled), the closer the alveolar concentration of the anaesthetic will approach zero, and anaesthesia lightens as ventilation increases. On the other hand, depression of breathing decreases the air dilution and thereby increases the concentration of anaesthetic inspired. Under these circumstances unless there is an increase in the uptake of the anaesthetic by the body, the alveolar concentration of the anaesthetic must rise. A rise in the alveolar concentration produces deeper unconsciousness and further respiratory depression. In addition, deepening anaesthesia reduces the cardiac output and hence the uptake of anaesthetic by the body, thus adding still further to the rise in the alveolar concentration. If this process is allowed to proceed unchecked, unconsciousness deepens until the ventilation becomes inadequate. In other words, with the open and semi-open methods of administration, animals which become more lightly anaesthetized tend to continue awakening and animals which become more deeply anaesthetized tend to continue becoming more depressed and nearer to death.

NON-REBREATHING SYSTEMS

The general principle behind non-rebreathing systems is that the fresh gases flow from the anaesthetic machine into a reservoir from which the patient inhales and the exhaled gases are spilled, usually through an expiratory valve, to the atmosphere. Carbon dioxide removal depends on the fresh gas flow rate, and on the tidal and minute volumes of respiration of the patient. Many systems have been devised but, in general, they are all variations of those classified by Mapleson (1954). The performance of many of these systems has been reviewed by Sykes (1968). Strictly speaking, they often cannot be regarded as non-rebreathing systems because some rebreathing of exhaled gases takes place, but they are operated to ensure that this rebreathed gas constitutes no more than the gas coming from the deadspace of the animals' respiratory tract, i.e. fresh gas in so far as the inhaled concentration of anaesthetic gases is concerned. In veterinary anaesthesia the most commonly used non-rebreathing systems are the Magill (Mapleson A), the T-piece (Mapleson E) and coaxial circuits (variations of Mapleson A and D) (Fig. 9.11).

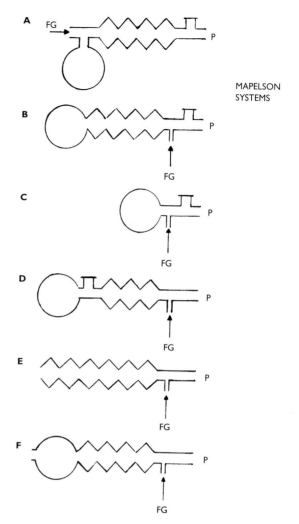

FIG. 9.11 The Mapleson classification of patient breathing systems. **A**: Magill and Lack circuits; **E**: T-piece system; FG: fresh gas flow; P: patient.

The Magill system

The Magill attachment, which incorporates a reservoir bag, wide bore corrugated tubing and a spring loaded expiratory valve is probably the most generally useful of all the non-rebreathing systems. With this system rebreathing is prevented by maintaining the total gas flow rate slightly in excess of the patient's respiratory minute volume. The animal inhales from the bag and wide bore tubing; the exhaled mixture passes back up the tubing displacing the gas in it back into the bag

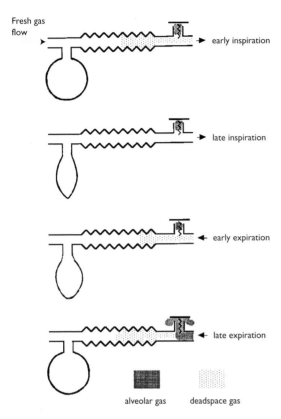

Fresh gas flow

→ early inspiration

→ late inspiration

← early expiration

← late expiration

alveolar gas   deadspace gas

FIG. 9.12 The Magill system (spontaneous breathing) showing the mode of operation to prevent rebreathing of exhaled gas.

until it is full. The exhaled gases never reach the bag because the capacity of the tube is too great and once the bag is distended the build up of pressure inside the system causes the expiratory valve to open so that the terminal part of expiration (rich in carbon dioxide – the alveolar gas) passes out of the valve into the atmosphere. During the pause which follows expiration and before the next inspiration fresh gas from the anaesthetic apparatus sweeps the first part of the exhaled gases from the corrugated tube out through the expiratory valve (Fig. 9.12).

To ensure minimal rebreathing of the expired gases the fresh gas flow rate should be equal to, or greater than, the minute volume of respiration of the patient. However, as the system leads to the preferential removal of alveolar gas, a lower fresh gas flow rate (equal to the alveolar ventilation) may be adequate and, in man, Kain and Nunn

(1968) have shown that in spontaneously breathing patients significant rebreathing does not occur until the fresh gas flow rate falls below 70% of the patient's minute volume. If, however, IPPV is applied by compression of the reservoir bag, then very much higher fresh gas flows are needed to prevent rebreathing because under these circumstances the fresh gas is spilled through the expiratory valve at the end of inspiration.

Various non-return valves have been incorporated in the Magill system in place of the simple spring loaded expiratory valve. All these valves prevent any rebreathing of the exhaled gases other than those contained in the valve itself and its connections. Where they are used the gas flow rates from the apparatus require frequent adjustment, for any alteration in the rate or depth of the patient's breathing affects the degree of distension of the reservoir bag. If the gas flow rate is kept constant, deep or rapid breathing empties the bag quickly, while slow or shallow breathing allows the bag to become over distended. These non-return valves can be used to measure the minute volume of respiration for if the flow rates are adjusted to maintain the bag at a constant average size at the end of expiration the total flow rate as read from the flowmeters will equal the respiratory minute volume. In practice because of the necessity for repeated adjustments of the total gas flow rate, an excessive flow is employed and a spill valve is incorporated between the reservoir bag and the non-return valve.

The T-piece system

The low resistance and small deadspace make the T-piece system, first described by Ayre in 1937, very suitable for small dogs and cats. As shown in Fig. 9.13 an open tube acts as a reservoir and there are no valves. The exhaled gases are swept out of the open end of the reservoir tube by fresh gases flowing in from the anaesthetic apparatus during the expiratory phase. Unless the capacity of the reservoir tube is at least equal to the tidal volume of the animal the terminal part of inspiration will be air, but unless its capacity is very small this is unimportant for the air will only enter the respiratory dead-space and no dilution of the anaesthetic gases will take place.

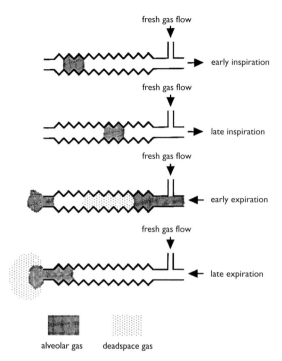

fresh gas flow

early inspiration

fresh gas flow

late inspiration

fresh gas flow

early expiration

fresh gas flow

late expiration

alveolar gas   deadspace gas

FIG. 9.13 Mode of operation of the T-piece system in preventing rebreathing provided the fresh gas flow exceeds about twice the patient's minute volume.

The resistance and fresh gas requirements are obviously related to the expiratory flow rate and flow patterns which occur in animals of any particular size. The minimum fresh gas flow rate required to prevent rebreathing and air dilution during both spontaneous and controlled ventilation is generally recommended to be 2.5 – 3.0 times the minute volume of respiration, provided the expiratory limb has a capacity greater than the tidal volume.

Using the basic T-piece system IPPV may be applied by intermittently blocking the open end of the reservoir tube thus directing the fresh gas into the animal's lungs. However, the inflation pressure, being that supplied by the anaesthetic machine, may be so high as to cause massive pulmonary damage if over inflation is allowed to occur. Ventilation may be controlled more safely by squeezing an open-tailed bag attached to the end of the expiratory limb – the Jackson–Rees modification. The orifice of the open tail can be controlled between the finger and thumb of the anaesthetist and the inflation pressure adjusted to

suit the circumstances. Scavenging of waste gases from the T-piece system presents some difficulties if the overall resistance of the apparatus is not to be increased.

Coaxial systems

The desirability of controlling atmospheric pollution in operating theatres has led to an interest in the use of coaxial circuits because it is relatively easy to duct the waste gases from them to the atmosphere by valves placed at the anaesthetic machine and well away from the patient. The Bain (Fig 9.14) and the Lack (Fig. 9.15) systems are two types of coaxial circuits.

In the Bain system fresh gas passes up the central tube and expired gas through the outer sleeve. It can be seen that this arrangement is basically that of the T-piece system and, therefore, in general, the same gas flow considerations will apply. However, higher gas flow rates are needed to prevent rebreathing of expired gases during spontaneous respiration and the pattern of respiration is important. These high flows directed via a narrow pipe to the animal's airway themselves cause quite marked expiratory respiratory resistance through a venturi effect. An animal which breathes slowly with a long expiratory pause will make more efficient use of the fresh gas inflow than an animal with a rapid, shallow respiratory pattern.

The Lack circuit uses the alternative arrangement in which the fresh gas flows in the outer sleeve and expiration through the inner tube. This arrangement was designed to aid scavenging of expired gas and is more satisfactory than the conventional Mapleson A system in this respect. The Lack system cannot be used with controlled ventilation in the same way as the Bain system without excessive rebreathing so its use is restricted to spontaneously breathing animals.

The modified Bain system collects the expired gas in a reservoir bag connected to a blow-off valve at the end of the expiratory tube and has proved reasonably satisfactory for use in dogs over 10 kg body weight. Compression of this reservoir bag or the introduction of air during the inspiratory cycle of a ventilator connected to the bag mount gives very good results for IPPV in dogs over 20 kg body weight.

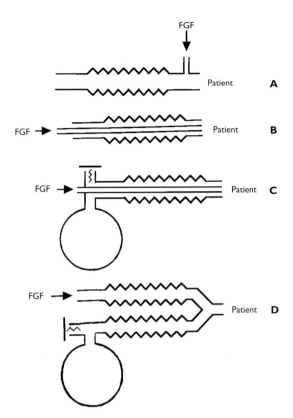

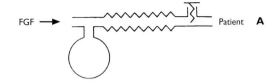

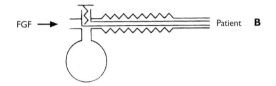

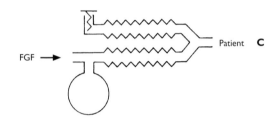

FIG. 9.14 The T-piece system (**A**) compared to the original Bain coaxial system (**B**), the modified Bain system (**C**) and the modified, parallel Bain system (**D**). It is important to note that in the modified systems the bag is on the *expiratory* limb (FGF: fresh gas flow).

FIG. 9.15 The Lack coaxial system (**B**) compared to the standard Magill system (**A**) and the parallel Lack system (**C**). In all these systems the bag is on the *inspiratory* limb of the system (FGF: fresh gas flow)

Use of these coaxial systems in veterinary anaesthesia has revealed a number of problems. In some cases the internal or external tubing has been of such a small bore that excessive demands were made on the animal's inspiratory or expiratory efforts. More serious, perhaps, the inner tube may become detached from the anaesthetic machine or the patient resulting in a very large deadspace.

The potential for a large increase in deadspace if the inner tube of a coaxial system becomes detached at the end nearest the anaesthetic machine has been appreciated in respect of the Bain system for some considerable time and it is most important that the system is tested immediately before use. Testing may be done by connecting it to the common gas outlet of the anaesthetic machine and passing a flow of at least 6 l/min of oxygen through the inner tube of the system. The distal (patient) end of this inner tube is then occluded (with the finger or the plunger of a 5 ml syringe) and the oxygen flowmeter bobbin should be seen to dip and the machine pressure relief valve heard blowing off, indicating that all is well.

Parallel systems which operate in the same manner as the Bain and Lack systems have two tubes running alongside one another rather than one inside the other (Figs 9.14 & 9.15). Although perhaps slightly more cumbersome, faults in the systems are more easily recognized.

Modifications of non-rebreathing systems

The Humphrey ADE system is designed to facilitate changing from a Mapleson A configuration during spontaneous ventilation to a Mapleson D or E mode during controlled ventilation. Recently the system has been adapted to include the optional use of a carbon dioxide absorber. Resistance in the system is reduced by the use of a flat (non-corrugated) lining to the tubing, which reduces turbulence. In man, the system has proved suitable for use in adults and children. To have one system adaptable for rebreathing, non-rebreathing, spontaneous and controlled ventilation for all sizes of cats and dogs would be of great convenience in veterinary practice. The Humphrey system has proved suitable for dogs weighing from 5.4–89.0 Kg (Lilja *et al.*, 1999), but its use in smaller dogs or cats has yet to be investigated.

The Maxima breathing system (Miller 1995) also can be used for both controlled and spontaneous ventilation. It is a lightweight valveless non-absorber system that allows selective elimination of alveolar gas in both spontaneous and controlled ventilation modes. In spontaneous ventilation mode it behaves as a Mapleson A system.

Flow rates required in non-rebreathing systems

Non-rebreathing systems have major advantages in that they may have low deadspace and resistance, and the anaesthetist knows the concentration of gases which the animal is breathing. Their disadvantage is the wastefulness of using high flow rates of gases. Although most textbooks advocate the need for administering the minute volume (for Mapleson A systems) or more (Mapleson E), a survey of existing literature demonstrates that there are few recommendations as to what is the minute volume of a particular type of animal. Most studies have suggested that tidal volume ranges from 10–20 ml/kg in dogs (Clutton 1995), and respiratory rate may be counted in order to obtain minute volume (this is not accurate if the dog is panting). A second approach is to set flow rates based on ml/kg/minute. With a Mapleson A circuit the flow rates recommended to prevent rebreathing are approximately 130 ml/kg/minute for dogs weighing less than 10 Kg, and 95 ml/kg/min for those weighing more (Holden, personal communication; Waterman 1986; Lilja *et al.*, 1999). The higher metabolic rate of the smaller animal provides an explanation for the differences in requirement in relation to weight, and it has been suggested that it should be possible to find a single suitable flow rate for a moderately wide range of weights. Lilja

et al. (1999) has demonstrated that with a Mapleson A circuit, a flow rate of 4 l/min. was sufficient to prevent rebreathing in all but one of 49 dogs, weights ranging from 5.4 – 89.0 kg, but one dog (not the heaviest but with a weight of 59 kg) required a flow of 5 l/min. The disadvantage of using any of the set 'formulae' discussed above is that in order to ensure that flow rates are adequate for every single animal, they will be excessive for many, leading to waste and expense. Ideally, where there is the ability to monitor end tidal carbon dioxide, gas flows can be reduced to those just sufficient to prevent rebreathing, and where this is practicable, it will be found that for small animals non-rebreathing circuits can be used with minimal expense.

REBREATHING SYSTEMS

Anaesthetic gases and vapours are said to be more or less physiologically 'indifferent', in that they are largely exhaled from the body unchanged, but when exhaled they are mixed with carbon dioxide. The exhaled gas can be directed into a closed bag and if the carbon dioxide is removed, and sufficient oxygen added to satisfy the metabolic requirements of the animal, the same gas or vapour can be rebreathed continuously from the bag. This is the principle of closed system anaesthetic administration. The same apparatus may also be employed as a 'low flow' system if slightly higher gas flow rates are fed in and the excess gases allowed to escape through an overflow valve.

In anaesthesia, the carbon dioxide is usually removed by directing the exhaled mixture over the surface of soda lime. This is a mixture of 90% calcium hydroxide and 5% sodium hydroxide together with 5% of silicate and water to prevent powdering. It is used in a granular form, the granules being 4–8 mesh in size, and ideally packed in a container so that the space between the granules is at least equal to the tidal volume of the animal. Some brands of soda lime contain an indicator dye that changes colour (e.g. from white to violet) when the carbon dioxide absorbing capacity is exhausted. Absence of visible colour change is no guarantee that the soda line is capable of absorbing more carbon dioxide – a small quantity should be wrapped in gauze and a brisk flow of carbon dioxide directed through it. When this is done active soda lime becomes very hot but exhausted absorbent remains cool. Unfortunately, the modern practice of removing carbon dioxide supplies from anaesthetic machines means that this simple test may be impossible to carry out although simply breathing out over a small quantity is effective, albeit taking a longer time, for the heat change to become palpable. When a capnograph is available the inspired gases should not contain more than 0.1 to 1% of carbon dioxide and thus any rise in the inspired concentration of this gas in a circle system may be the only indication that the soda lime is exhausted. Due to the exothermic nature of the reaction between soda lime and carbon dioxide, the soda lime container should become warm as anaesthesia proceeds and this should be detectable if absorption is efficient.

Theoretically, during closed circuit administration, once anaesthesia has been induced and a state of equilibrium established, all that the animal requires from the apparatus is a continuous stream of oxygen just sufficient to satisfy its metabolic needs, and efficient absorption of carbon dioxide. In practice, however, most periods of anaesthesia are too short to allow a state of equilibrium to be reached and the body continues to take up the anaesthetic agent throughout the administration, so that the agent has to be given all the time in order to maintain the alveolar concentration.

The closed method of administration is simple, and much less anaesthetic is used than in non-rebreathing methods because there is no wastage to the atmosphere. The chief disadvantage of closed system anaesthesia was assumed to be the resistance due to the packed soda lime and this resistance was considered sufficiently great to render the method unsuitable for cats, puppies and very small adult dogs. These reservations were applied to the use of systems designed for use in human adults for these small veterinary patients. Although the mechanical deadspace imposed by some of the Y-piece connectors was excessive, physiological factors such as muscle fatigue, inefficient ventilation and a tendency to lung collapse were probably responsible for some of the respiratory problems observed in small animals breathing spontaneously from systems designed for use with adult

humans. Another disadvantage is that the conservation of heat and water vapour afforded by the method may give rise to heat stroke in dogs and sheep if the ambient temperature is high.

There are two systems in use for carbon dioxide absorption in anaesthesia:

1. The 'to-and-fro' system
2. The 'circle' system.

The 'to-and-fro' system

A canister full of CO_2 absorbent is interposed between animal and the rebreathing bag, fresh gases being fed into the system as close to the animal as possible to effect changes in the mixture rapidly (Fig 9.16A). This system is simple but has several drawbacks. It is difficult to maintain the heavy, awkward apparatus in a gas-tight condition and the inspired gases become undesirably hot due to the chemical action between the soda lime and the carbon dioxide. Furthermore, irritating dust may be inhaled from the soda lime and give rise to a bronchitis. Nevertheless, the system has been most commonly used in veterinary anaesthesia for the necessary apparatus is relatively inexpensive and may be improvized.

For small animal anaesthesia (dogs, sheep and goats, young calves, young foals and small pigs) the standard soda lime canisters used in man, which are known as Water's canisters after their designer, are quite satisfactory. They are available in various sizes: one containing 1 lb (approx 0.5 kg) and a second one containing 10 oz (approx 0.3 kg) of soda lime are adequate for most veterinary purposes. These canisters are used horizontally and unless the soda lime is tightly packed when the canister is filled it tends the settle, leaving a channel along the top through which gases may pass following the path of least resistance without being subjected to the action of the soda lime. In the larger canisters a domestic nylon pot-scrub may be used so as to leave about half of it to be compressed by the wire gauze in the lid of the canister when the cap is screwed on.

Adult horses, cattle and large pigs need much larger soda lime canisters. They are designed on the principle that the animal's tidal volume should be accommodated in the spaces between the soda lime granules. Because of the difficulty of packing

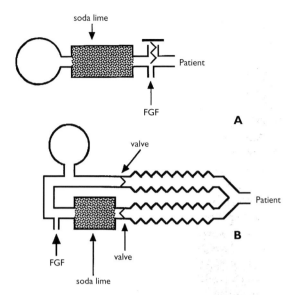

FIG. 9.16 To-and-fro (**A**) and circle absorber (**B**) systems (FGF: fresh gas flow).

these canister sufficiently tightly with soda lime, special to-and-fro canisters have been designed and developed for large animals. The vertical position of these soda lime canisters means that tight packing is not necessary and their cross-sectional area is large to ensure than the respired gases pass through the absorbent slowly. For adult horses and cattle a rebreathing bag having a capacity of about 15 l is used.

The to-and-fro systems can never be really efficient absorbers of carbon dioxide. The exhaled gases all come into contact with the soda lime at the end of the canister nearest to the patient and the absorbent in this region is quickly exhausted. Thus, as this occurs, the gases have to travel further and further into the canister before carbon dioxide is absorbed or, in other words, the apparatus deadspace steadily increases during anaesthesia. Thus, ideally the absorbent in these circuits should be changed between every case.

The 'circle' system

The circle system for carbon dioxide absorption incorporates an inspiratory and an expiratory tube with unidirectional valves to ensure a one-way flow of gases; the rebreathing bag and soda lime

canister are placed between these tubes. The valves and tubing offer an appreciable resistance to breathing and unless the apparatus is carefully designed with regard to the diameter of airways in relation to flow rates, breathing through the apparatus can impose a considerable strain on the animal, and the inevitable degree of rebreathing which occurs at the T-piece connexion to the patient limits the removal of CO_2 from the exhaled gas. This rebreathing can be prevented by placing the unidirectional valves at the face-piece or endotracheal tube connection, but it is difficult to design robust, competent valves for use at these situations. In the majority of modern circle type units the unidirectional valves are of the turret type; they are robust and competent but must be kept upright and of necessity, therefore, have to be mounted on the apparatus at some distance away from the animal.

Circle absorber units (Fig. 9.16B) are more efficient absorbers of carbon dioxide than are to-and-fro units because their dead space is constant since all the charge of soda lime is available to the respired gases. Exhaustion of soda lime is noticed more suddenly than in to-and-fro absorbers and once it occurs the inspired carbon dioxide concentration may soon become excessive.

To avoid this sudden exhaustion of soda lime and for economy in its use, canisters are now often made with two compartments. The compartment of the canister which first receives the expired gases and, therefore, whose soda lime is first used, can be refilled and the position of the canister reversed so that expired gases pass through the remaining partially used soda lime, using this to complete exhaustion before reaching the newly filled compartment.

Standard circle absorbers designed for man are satisfactory for spontaneously breathing young foals, young calves, sheep, goats, most pigs, and dogs over 15 kg body weight. Circle absorbers for large animal patients are now readily available from commercial sources but there are few reports of their efficiency in terms of carbon dioxide absorbing capacity or resistance to breathing. In North America human paediatric circle absorbers are often used for small dogs (and even cats) but they have never found favour in the UK for patients of this size. In adapting circle systems for use in small animals, it was originally assumed that all components of the standard adult human systems should be reduced in proportion to the size of animal in order to minimize deadspace and resistance to breathing. Several minaturized circle systems were manufactured, of which the Bloomquist and Ohio Infant Circle Systems are probably the best known (Dorsch & Dorsch, 1975). However, it was an error to assume that smaller valves would result in less resistance to breathing because resistance is inversely proportional to the diameter of the valve (Hunt, 1955). Moreover, being non-standard apparatus, all these small animal circle systems involve a considerable nuisance factor for the anaesthetist, requiring a complete changeover from standard adult human systems. The general practice in medical anaesthesia today is to anaesthetize paediatric patients using standard adult size apparatus but with IPPV overcome the physiological factors such as muscle fatigue and inefficient ventilation involved.

Practical problems involved in the use of closed rebreathing systems

All anaesthetists using closed rebreathing systems must fully understand how the concentrations of gases which the animal breathes from the reservoir bag are altered by the uptake, utilization, and elimination of gases and vapours by the patient.

When anaesthesia is first induced with an inhalation anaesthetic the animal takes up the anaesthetic and the expired gases contain a lower concentration of the anaesthetic than in the inspired gases. Thus, the concentration of anaesthetic in a completely closed circuit will be diluted. The speed of uptake of the anaesthetic depends on many factors (Chapter 6) but the larger the animal, the greater the dilution, and the longer the time before equilibrium is attained. Also, during induction, nitrogen from the patient accumulates in the anaesthetic circuit and decreases the concentration of O_2 therein.

The problems of denitrogenation and of maintaining an adequate concentration of anaesthetic for the induction of anaesthesia are best overcome by increasing the fresh gas flow rate, opening overspill valves, frequently emptying the rebreathing bag ('dumping') and thus converting the system into a semi-closed system for the duration of the induction period. Rapidly decreasing the depth of

anaesthesia presents problems similar to those encountered in induction of anaesthesia but the gases exhaled by the patient will contain anaesthetic in higher concentrations than the inspired gas, so that the concentration in the breathing circuit will tend to increase, and the depth of anaesthesia will only lighten very slowly. Again, this can be overcome by increasing the gas inflow rates and emptying the rebreathing bag at frequent intervals.

When a completely closed rebreathing system is employed maintenance of a stable depth of anaesthesia also poses problems. Theoretically, all that is required is a fresh gas inflow containing exactly the oxygen requirements of the animal together with low concentrations of the anaesthetic just sufficient to replenish that being absorbed by the patient or lost from the wound surfaces etc. In large animals where the oxygen need exceeds 1 l/min., the completely closed system works well and can be used throughout the anaesthetic maintenance period. In small animals, however, it is often difficult to maintain smooth stable anaesthesia without extreme care being paid by the anaesthetist to every aspect of administration. This is because these small animals have very low basal metabolic requirements of oxygen and the vaporizers used to deliver volatile anaesthetics are often very inefficient at low gas flow rates. Even modern vaporizers only deliver accurately known concentrations of the volatile agents with carrier gas flow rates of more than 0.5 l/min. and stable anaesthesia can only be achieved by increasing the fresh gas flow rate to a level at which the vaporizer will deliver an accurately known concentrations of anaesthetic, and allowing the excess to escape from an overflow valve. Some veterinarians attempt to overcome these problems by filling the circuit intermittently with high fresh gas flow rates but this results in fluctuating levels of anaesthesia.

A second method of overcoming the problem of vaporization of the anaesthetic at low fresh gas flow rates is to place the vaporizer inside the breathing system. If the vaporizer is placed in the fresh gas supply line outside the breathing system the system receives a steady supply of anaesthetic. When the vaporizer is placed in the breathing circuit (vic), however, the flow through it depends on the respiratory efforts of the patient so that vaporization of the anaesthetic depends on this rather than the fresh gas flow rate.

All anaesthetists using vaporizers inside the breathing circuit must understand clearly the way in which the alveolar concentration and hence the depth of anaesthesia, is dependent on the factors of ventilation, fresh gas inflow and vaporizer characteristics. In general, when the vaporizer is in the breathing circuit:

1. If anaesthesia is too light surgical stimulation will lead to increased ventilation and a deepening of unconsciousness. A sudden increase in ventilation and, therefore, of inspired concentration may be dangerous.

2. If the vaporizer setting is too high, deepening anaesthesia depresses ventilation and reduces vaporization. This acts to some extent as a built-in safety factor.

3. If the animal stops breathing no fresh vapour enters the circuit.

4. The smaller the fresh gas inflow the greater the economy in the use of the volatile agent.

5. A simple, low efficiency vaporizer is all that is required (e.g. The Goldman vaporizer for halothane which limits the concentration delivered to less than 3% by volume whatever the gas flow through it).

6. The safety of the circuit will depend on the anaesthetic agent. The concentration achieved will depend on the volatility of the agent, and the safety of that concentration on the MAC of the agent. For example, the boiling points and thus the concentration achieved at any setting of the vaporizer for halothane and isoflurane are similar, but as the MAC of isoflurane is higher, theoretically its use should be safer in this system than halothane (Laredo *et al.*, 1998). The boiling point of sevoflurane is higher, its MAC is 2.5%, and it has proved necessary to increase the efficacy of the standard vaporizer by adding a wick in order to use sevoflurane efficiently in a VIC (Muir & Gadawski, 1998). The low boiling point of desflurane means that it would be impossible to use in such a vaporizer.

7. The fact that respired gases pass through the vaporizer introduces problems of resistance to breathing.

There is wide concern among anaesthetists that inadvertent high flows through the vaporizer may lead to undesirably high concentrations of the volatile agent accumulating in the circuit during assisted lung ventilation with consequent danger from overdose. However, used cautiously with, if possible, monitoring of the circuit concentrations of the volatile agent the method can be very satisfactory.

When the vaporizer is outside the breathing system:

1. Ventilation has no effect on vaporization. Assisted or controlled respiration by IPPV has little effect on the depth of anaesthesia and is therefore much safer than is the case when the vaporizer is in the breathing system.

2. In most instances for any particular setting of the vaporizer control the smaller the fresh gas flow, the lower is the inspired concentration.

3. Too deep anaesthesia with respiratory depression does not have the built in safety factor found when the vaporizer is in the breathing system and the animal is in the breathing spontaneously.

Because of the difficulties with both in-circuit and out-of-circuit vaporizer positions many workers are adopting a simple system of injecting the liquid volatile agents directly into the closed breathing system. Vaporization takes place inside the tubing of the system and a metal sleeve with or without some gauze may be used to aid vaporization. Drip feeds of liquid anaesthetics into anaesthetic systems were common in the past but current interest is in the injection of liquid anaesthetic into the system using an electrically driven syringe pump which greatly facilitates automatic, computer control. Using a monitoring device in the inspiratory limb it is possible to set up a computer assisted system to maintain a constant inspired concentration of the anaesthetic agent. The closed circuit system also lends itself to various methods of automatically controlling gas flow into the system. One sophisticated approach uses a concertina bellows in the circuit as a volume transducer which is attached to a linear transducer to control the inflow of oxygen and nitrous oxide. In this system the gas flows can be electrically controlled to produce any desired flow rate from 50 to 1000 ml/min with an accuracy of ±1%, an oxygen sensor controlling oxygen flow to maintain a predetermined concentration and the nitrous oxide to maintain the volume. Work with such systems for veterinary use has been reported by Moens (1985).

The influence of the location of the vaporizer on the inspired tension of the anaesthetic agent must always be taken into account. Each placement has its own advantages and disadvantages, but in the hands of an experienced anaesthetist either arrangement is equally safe (or unsafe). The inexperienced anaesthetist is advised, especially with potent anaesthetics such as halothane or isoflurane, to use a calibrated and preferably thermostatically controlled vaporizer placed outside the breathing system.

DEFINITION OF ANAESTHETIC SYSTEMS

There have been many multiple and inconsistent definitions in British and North American literature and, as yet, there is no universal nomenclature. The systems of terminology consist of 'closed' and 'open' themes with variations, but this terminology is now of very little value. Moreover, these systems attempt to use rebreathing as the distinguishing factor. Although rebreathing is an extremely important variable, it is impossible to describe accurately variations which occur in the degree of rebreathing by the use of such terms as semi-closed, semi-closed with absorption, partial rebreathing, etc. It appears to be agreed by most workers that semi-closed refers to partial rebreathing techniques. Thus, for example, a system which has nearly complete rebreathing of the expired gases might have the same label as a system which has almost no rebreathing. Clearly this system of nomenclature may allow erroneous interpretations concerning the actual inspired concentration or tension of any inhalation anaesthetic. In order to clarify matters so that readers of an account of a procedure reported in any paper or book can obtain an exact picture of what was actually done, regardless of variations of teaching, practice and geographical location, it is only necessary for an author to give two simple pieces of information. First, the actual equipment used needs to be described (T-piece, etc.), and second, the fresh gas flow rate should be stated. These two basic items of information need only be supplemented under certain, special circumstances. For example in certain communications it might be necessary to give details such as the exact apparatus deadspace volume, types of valves, type and location of vaporizer (in or out of the breathing circuit), etc. For the majority of communications simply stating the apparatus used and the flow rates of gases would be quite adequate. It is to be hoped that authors will adopt this simple expedient so easy exchange of accurate information so vital to patient's welfare, teaching and research, will become a possibility in veterinary anaesthesia.

FACE MASKS AND ENDOTRACHEAL TUBES

Anaesthetics given by any method must be delivered to the animal through a well fitting face mask or endotracheal tube or the anaesthetic agent will be diluted and inhaled with an unknown quantity of air.

ANAESTHETIC FACE MASKS

In domestic animals there are wide variations in the configuration and size of the face in any one species, so that it is difficult to obtain an accurate airtight fit between the face and a mask. However, this difficulty can be overcome by the use of malleable constructions of latex rubber (Figs. 9.17 & 9.18) which can be moulded around the face. Another type of mask for small animals makes use of rigid transparent cones fitted with a perforated thin rubber diaphragm to provide an air-tight seal around the face. This latter type are difficult to apply for IPPV of the lungs and should be avoided if the mask is to be left in place for any length of time for the tightly fitting rubber diaphragm cuts off the venous return from the muzzle and can cause cutaneous oedema. In small animals the lower jaw must be pushed forward into the mask for if it is displaced backwards the airway may become obstructed by the base of the tongue coming into contact with the posterior wall of the

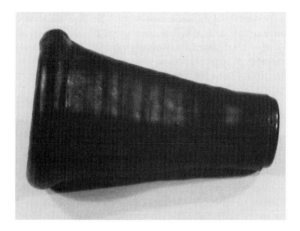

FIG. 9.17 Commercially available malleable face mask.

pharynx. Variations in face shape are not so troublesome in large animals and face masks for horses and cattle can be made from rigid material with a soft cushion to provide an air-tight seal with the muzzle, but again a variety of sizes is needed.

Whenever a face mask is used care must be taken not to cause damage to the eyes and, in species of animal that breathe through the nose rather than the mouth, it is most important to

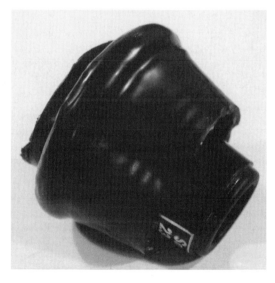

FIG. 9.18 Modification of commercially available face masks for cats and small brachycephalic dogs to reduce excessive deadspace. The masks are cut in two and the smaller diameter cemented inside the other. This telescoping produces a more rigid mask with a much smaller deadspace.

ensure that the nostrils are not obstructed by coming into contact with the mask. Some patterns of face mask are made of transparent material to allow the anaesthetist to observe the position of the mouth and nostrils.

ENDOTRACHEAL INTUBATION

The history of endotracheal intubation in animals is older than that of anaesthesia. In 1542 Vesalius passed a tube into the trachea of an animal and inflated the lungs by means of a bellows to keep the animal alive while the anatomy of its thoracic cavity was demonstrated. Similar demonstrations were given before the Fellows of the Royal Society in London by Robert Hook in 1667.

There are two methods by which inhalation anaesthetics can be administered through an endotracheal tube. The first to be used was that of 'insufflation' in which the anaesthetics are blown into the lungs near to the carina through a narrow bore tube. Respiration and the return flow of gases and vapours takes place around the tube. The insufflation technique is said to render respiratory movements unnecessary but has the great disadvantage of causing a considerable loss of heat and water vapour from the body. It has fallen into disuse but has given rise to the technique of intermittent entrainment of air to produce ventilation of the lungs of apnoeic small animal patients during rigid-tube bronchoscopy (Fig. 9.19).

A fine-bore tube (usually an 18 s.w.g. needle) mounted at the eyepiece end of a rigid bronchoscope has oxygen or a mixture of oxygen, nitrous oxide and/or a volatile agent blown through it intermittently. The jet of gas entrains air and generates enough pressure to inflate the animal's lungs which deflate as soon as the gas flow through the fine-bore tube is stopped. To-and-fro respiration takes place through one large-bore tube.

The standard endotracheal tubes used in man in the UK were designed by Magill and hence are known as 'Magill tubes'. Both 'oral' and 'nasal' are available. The oral tubes have comparatively thick walls and are intended for intubation through the mouth, while the 'nasal' tubes, designed for passage through the nostril into the trachea, have comparatively thin walls. The tubes are obtainable

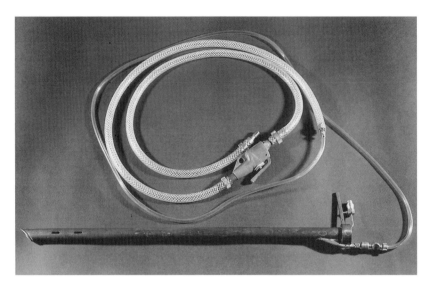

FIG. 9.19 Entrainer on rigid bronchoscope to allow ventilation of the lungs of the apnoeic patient during bronchoscopy.

in red rubber (seldom encountered today), plastic, or silicone rubber. The oral tubes may be either plain, or fitted with a cuff which can be inflated with air after the tube has been passed into the trachea. The inflated cuff provides an airtight seal between the wall of the trachea and the tube so that all respired gases must pass through the lumen of the tube. A good seal between the trachea and cuff reduces the danger of inhalation of foreign material, but over inflation must be avoided because this may result in either pressure damage to the mucous membrane of the trachea or to respiratory obstruction by pressing the wall of the tube into its lumen (Fig. 9.20).

Some of these problems may be overcome by the use of tubes which have a high volume, low pressure cuff but these tubes may be difficult to pass through the larynx. On all cuffed tubes a pilot balloon gives some guidance to the degree of inflation but does not show when an air-tight seal has been obtained. The cuff should be inflated with air until gentle compression of the reservoir gag of the anaesthetic circuit to which the patient is connected no longer causes an audible leak of gas around the tube.

Intracuff and 'leak-past' pressures of various types of tube have been measured and it has been shown that air diffuses out of the cuff irrespective of the material being red rubber, later or PVC. The

material of the cuff stretches under stress, increasing cuff volume. The 'leak-past' pressure decreases with red rubber and silicone rubber tubes but increases with PVC tubes as time passes. Pressure changes within the cuff may be caused by the dif-

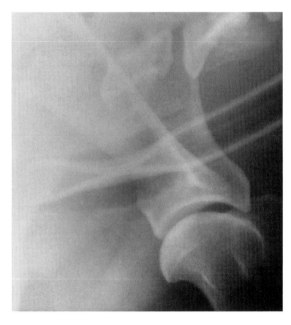

FIG. 9.20 Radiograph showing occlusion of an endotracheal tube due to over-distension of the inflatable cuff.

fusion of gases – the most important gas is oxygen and when the respired gases contain 30% oxygen the pressure in the cuff can increase by up to 90 mmHg (0.9 KPa). Ideally, the pressure inside the cuff should be monitored to prevent damage to the tracheal mucosa but in practice this is seldom done.

Length of endotracheal tubes

An endotracheal tube which is too long may be inadvertently introduced into one or the other of the main bronchi; this results in one lung providing a large 'shunt'. Most commonly the tube will enter the right main bronchus. Endobronchial intubation may give rise to persistent cyanosis and hypercapnia. It should be suspected if an animal shows cyanosis when breathing an oxygen-rich mixture through an endotracheal tube. Often very high inspired concentrations of volatile anaesthetic agent are required to keep the animal asleep.

All new Magill tubes must be cut to the correct length both to ensure that endobronchial intubation is impossible and to minimize the respiratory deadspace. They should be cut so that when their bevelled tip lies between the larynx and carina their cut end is immediately beyond the nostrils. Also, the connecting piece between the tube and anaesthetic delivery apparatus should be as short as possible. Unfortunately with many modern tubes, the tube through which the cuff is inflated is enclosed within the wall of the endotracheal tube, making it impossible to shorten.

Reinforced endotracheal tubes

Frequent use with associated cleaning and sterilization processes makes red rubber endotracheal tubes soft and plastic tubes may soften when warmed to body temperature. Soft tubes flatten out and are easily compressed by pressure. Obliteration of the lumen from either of these causes may give rise to serious obstruction of the airway. Patency of the airway, when the animal has to be placed in any position which may cause flattening or kinking of the tube, can be assured by the use of an armoured, or reinforced, endotracheal tube. These special tubes incorporate a wire or nylon spiral in their walls. They are more expens-

ive than the standard tubes, and because there are not many occasions when their use is essential, many veterinary anaesthetists consider their purchase to be unjustified. They have thicker walls than non-reinforced tubes and are difficult to cut to shorter lengths (they come with a non-reinforced end to ease their connection to the endotracheal connector). They are usually very flexible and to facilitate their introduction it is often necessary to stiffen them with a malleable stilette introduced into their lumen in such a way as not to protrude from the bevelled tip.

LARYNGOSCOPES

Although not strictly essential, a laryngoscope greatly facilitates the process of intubation in many animals and is a piece of equipment which is most desirable. A suitable laryngoscope usually holds a dry electric battery in the handle and has detachable blades of different sizes. The blades should be designed so as to enable the passage of a large bore endotracheal tube to be made as easily as possible. For veterinary purposes one standard human adult and one child size 'Magill pattern' blades and one special blade are the minimum requirements. The special blade should be of the Macintosh pattern, 3/4 inch (1.9 cm) wide, and 23 to 30 cm long. The blades should be separate from the lamp and its electrical connections so they can be sterilized by boiling without risk of damage to the electrical system. Various types are available and one suitable instrument is shown in Fig.9.21.

For small animal use, a modified penlight torch can provide an inexpensive light source which, although less satisfactory than a laryngoscope, may prove adequate in an emergency. For large animals, special laryngoscope blades are required and the Rowson blade (Rowson, 1965) has greatly simplified the intubation of small cattle, sheep and large pigs. The most attractive feature of the Rowson blade is that it makes lifting of the lower jaw to expose the laryngeal opening unnecessary. The 14 inch Wisconsin blade is excellent for llamas, large rams and goats and in these animals it may be necessary to use an introducer in the form of a stilette passed through the tube to stiffen it.

Difficult intubation may be overcome by use of a fibrescope to identify the glottis. Before passing the

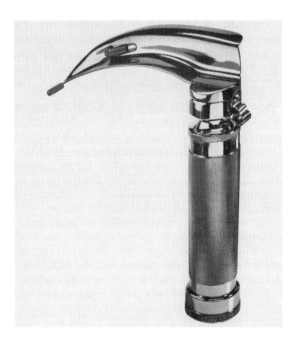

FIG. 9.21 Laryngoscope with detachable Macintosh blade – a wide variety of patterns of blade are available.

fibrescope it is introduced through an appropriate sized endotracheal tube so that this tube may be 'railroaded' into the trachea once the tip of the fibrescope is seen to be correctly placed. Because the fibrescope occupies most of the lumen of the tube it must be quickly withdrawn leaving the tube in place. Intubating flexible endoscopes (KeyMed, KeyMed House, Stock Road, Southend-on-Sea, Essex SS2 5QH) are manufactured with tougher rubber than is used in other flexible endoscopes to ensure that 'railroading' an endotracheal tube will not cause deterioration of the endoscope.

Wide-bore tubes may be introduced into the trachea in various ways and the method to be adopted in any particular case is decided by the skill and experience of the anaesthetist and the kind of animal. In the chapters dealing with anaesthesia for the various species of animal will be found descriptions of techniques which undergraduate students and anaesthetists in training have found relatively easy to master. Experienced, skilled anaesthetists should of course be able to pass an endotracheal tube in all species of animal under any circumstances and most develop their own techniques.

CLEANING AND STERILIZATION OF ANAESTHETIC EQUIPMENT

Anaesthetic equipment is obviously a potential source of cross infection from one patient to the next; ideally, all parts of the breathing systems should be capable of being sterilized between each use. Unfortunately, this is not very practical as parts of the apparatus do not tolerate many of the possible methods of sterilization and, where they do, most of the methods shorten their life. The nearer the part of the system to the patient, the greater the risk of cross infection from organisms associated with previous usage. The compromise usually adopted with anaesthetic equipment is, therefore, to sterilize the components such as endotracheal tubes or face masks after use, whilst the rest of the equipment is only regularly cleaned by washing. All equipment should, however, be sterilized periodically, or immediately following its use on a patient thought or known to be suffering from an infectious disease.

Whatever method of sterilization is to be employed, the apparatus must first be thoroughly cleaned by washing in hot water with a detergent or soap. Many parts of the breathing circuit may be damaged if subjected to autoclaving. Heat sterilization by boiling may be used for endotracheal tubes although regular treatment of this nature does shorten their life. The various means of chemical sterilization rarely damage equipment but when they are used the apparatus must be thoroughly washed afterwards because traces of chemical, particularly if remaining on face masks or endotracheal tubes, may prove to be very irritant indeed to the next patient The use of ethylene oxide gas is now a practical method of sterilization in veterinary practice and although it causes no damage to anaesthetic equipment a sufficient time (up to 7 days) must be allowed to elapse before the equipment is used again in order to allow all traces of this most irritant gas to disappear. Also, it must be remembered that some plastics which have been previously sterilized by γ irradiation (e.g. most plastic endotracheal tubes supplied in sterile packets) produce an extreme toxic substance, ethylene chlorohydrin, when subjected to ethylene oxide gas so they should never be resterilized by exposure to the agent (Dorsch & Dorsch, 1975).

REFERENCES

Clutton, R.E. (1995) The right anaesthetic breathing system for you? *In Practice* **5**: 229–237.

Dorsch, J.A. and Dorsch, S.E. (1975) *Understanding Anaesthetic Equipment*. Baltimore: Williams and Wilkins.

Humphrey, D. (1983) A new anaesthetic breathing system combining Mapleson A.D and E principles. A simple apparatus for low flow universal use without carbon dioxide absorption. *Anaesthesia* **38**: 361–372.

Hunt, K.H. (1955) Resistance in respiratory valves and canisters. *Anesthesiology* **16**: 190–205.

Kain, M.K. and Nunn, J.F. (1968) Fresh gas economics of the Magill circuit. *Anesthesiology* **29**: 964–974.

Laredo, F.G., Sanchez-Valverde, M.A., Cantalapiedra, A.G., Pereira, J.L. and Agut, A. (1998) Efficacy of the Komesaroff anaesthetic machine for delivering isoflurane to dogs. *Veterinary Record* **143**: 437–440.

Lilja, A.S., Alibhai, H.I.K. and Clarke, K.W. (1999) Evaluation of the Humphrey ADE circuit during spontaneous ventilation in dogs. *Journal of Veterinary Anaesthesia* (in press).

Mapleson, W.W. (1954) The elimination of rebreathing in various semi-closed anaesthetic systems. *British Journal of Anaesthesia* **26**: 323–332.

Miller (1995) An enclosed efferent afferent reservoir system: the Maxima. *Anaesthesia and Intensive Care*. **23**: 292–295.

Moens, Y. (1985) Introduction to the quantitative practice and the use of closed circuit in veterinary anaesthesia. *Proceedings of the 2nd International Congress of Veterinary Anesthesia, Sacramento*, p.57.

Muir, W.W. and Gadawski, J. (1998) Cardiorespiratory effects of low-flow and closed circuit inhalation anesthesia using sevoflurane delivered with an in-circle vaporizer, and concentrations of compound A. *American Journal of Veterinary Research* **59**: 603.

Rowson, L.E.A. (1965) Endotracheal intubation in the pig. *Veterinary Record* **77**: 1465.

Sykes, M.K. (1968) Rebreathing circuits. *British Journal of Anaesthesia* **40**: 666–670.

Waterman, A.E. (1985) Clinical experiences with the Komesaroff machine. *Journal of the Association of Veterinary Anaesthetists* **13**: 42–49.

Waterman, A.E. (1986) Clinical evaluation of the Lack coaxial breathing circuit in small animal anaesthesia. *Journal of small Animal Practice* **27**: 591–598.

General principles of local analgesia

10

INTRODUCTION

Many surgical procedures can be satisfactorily performed under local analgesia. Whether or not sedation is employed as an adjunct will depend on the species, temperament and health of the animal, as well as the magnitude of the procedure. In adult cattle and horses, many operations can be performed on standing animals and since sedation may induce the animal to lie down, it is often better avoided. In other animals sedation should be adopted since efficient surgery is greatly facilitated by the reduction of fear and liability to sudden movement. Local analgesics may exert a sedative action when they are absorbed from sites of injection and for surgery on the standing animal the dose of any calming sedative drug must be reduced to allow for this.

There are several features of local analgesia which render it particularly useful in veterinary practice. It enables protracted operations to be performed on standing animals and in large animals this avoids the dangers associated with prolonged recumbency. Local analgesia can also be a useful technique to reduce the depth of anaesthesia needed for major surgery during general anaesthesia. A feature which appeals to those in general veterinary practice is that the surgeon can induce local analgesia and operate without the assistance of an anaesthetist. The techniques of local analgesia are not difficult to learn and do not involve the use of expensive or complicated equipment.

ANATOMY AND FUNCTION OF THE NERVE FIBRE

The unit of nervous tissue consists of the nerve cell and its processes, the dendrites and the axon. The processes are dependent upon the intact connection with the nerve cell for survival and nutrition. Conventional theories of nerve function have long been based on the assumption that the surface membrane of nerve fibres and cells exists as a differentially permeable interface between tissue fluid and the liquid phase of the neuronal cytoplasm. However, modern cytological studies render it very unlikely that external surfaces of nerve cells and fibres are bathed directly by tissue fluid, for it now appears that most neurones are entirely, or almost entirely, covered by supporting cells applied directly to their external surfaces. Thus, the diffusion barrier surrounding neurones must be considered to involve these supporting cells and their membranes. The larger nerve cells are surrounded by a coat of fatty material – the myelin sheath. The thickness of this sheath increases with the diameter of the axon it encloses, and it is composed of a number of lipoprotein lamellae which, in the case of peripheral nerve fibres, are laid down from the Schwann cells that enclose the axons. The myelin lamellae are not continuous along the entire length of the fibre, being interrupted at more or less regular intervals (the nodes of Ranvier) to leave short segments of the axon covered by the

TABLE 10.1 **Relationship between nerve fibre size and function. The divisions are not absolute and there is a varying degree of overlap from one diameter group to the other**

Group	Fibre diameter range (μm)	Functions
I	15–25 (myelinated)	Somatic motor efferents Proprioceptive afferents
II	5–15 (myelinated)	Cutaneous afferents (except pain)
	2–5 (myelinated)	Pain efferents γmotor efferents
III <5 {	< 2 (unmyelinated)	Pain afferents Postganglionic sympathetic efferent

Schwann cells. Thus throughout the length of the unmyelinated fibres and at the nodes of Ranvier in myelinated fibres, the axon is always separated from the surrounding tissue fluid by the thickness of the Schwann cell in which it is embedded; in the internodal segments of myelinated fibres the axon is separated by the myelin lamellae also.

Peripheral nerves are composed of fibres of many different diameters, the finest of which usually have no myelin within their Schwann cells, while the larger fibres are surrounded by increasing numbers of myelin lamellae. There is some correlation between fibre size and function, and the fibres in the spinal peripheral nerves may be classified into three broad groups in terms of diameter ranges, each of these groups mediating particular functions. Such an arbitrary division does, of course, give rise to some overlap (Table 10.1).

The action of local analgesics is one of stabilization of the active membrane which surrounds the nerve fibre, and in the case of myelinated fibres occurs only at the node of Ranvier. All, including motor nerves, may be blocked and transmission at the neuromuscular junction and at the autonomic ganglia may be affected by a similar mechanism.

When a peripheral nerve is exposed to a local analgesic, conduction in its constituent fibres is blocked at a rate that is inversely proportional to their diameters. If a pool of local analgesic surrounds a peripheral nerve, function fails first in the unmyelinated fibres then in the smaller, followed by the larger, myelinated fibres. This sequence is due to the fact that the Schwann cells containing myelin are relatively impervious to local analgesic solutions compared to those which contain little or no myelin. Therefore, once a drug has penetrated through the connective tissues of the nerve into the endoneural fluid, it can act upon the entire length of any unmyelinated fibres but only on the short segments of myelinated fibres at the nodes of Ranvier. As the number of nodes per unit length of an axon is greater in fine fibres than in thick ones, there will be more of such segments within the pool of solution in the finer fibres than in the thicker ones. For this reason also, local blockade of nerve fibres becomes more rapid and effective the greater the length of the fibres exposed to the action of the drug. An alternative to employing an increased concentration of drug to accelerate local analgesia is, therefore, to infiltrate along a greater length of the nerve with a more dilute solution.

MECHANISM OF NERVE BLOCK

Most of the clinically useful local analgesics are weakly basic tertiary amines which exist in a charged (ionic) or uncharged (free base) form. The greater the alkalinity of the solution the more uncharged or free base form is present. The pKa (the pH at which the solution contains equal proportions of charged and uncharged molecules) of currently used compounds lies between 7.7 and 8.5 and commercially available solutions are always acid so they contain more charged molecules. It seems that both the unionized base (B) and the ionized cationic form (BH+) are important for actual local blocking activity. The more lipid soluble the analgesic compound, the more potent it is and protein binding is believed to determine the duration of the block produced.

It can be shown by voltage clamp experiments that local analgesics block conduction in excitable tissues by diminished entry of sodium ions during the generation of the action potential. As the local concentration of the drug is increased there is a progressive fall in the rate of rise of the spike potential causing a corresponding slowing of conduction velocity. This is because the less intense the depolarization at any point, the shorter the range of the local circuits produced. Finally there is inability to reach the threshold potential, resulting in conduction block. Although higher concentrations of the drug can decrease the exit of potassium ions this is irrelevant to the local blocking action which can occur without any change in resting potential.

CLINICALLY USEFUL LOCAL ANALGESIC DRUGS

BASIC STRUCTURE

Clinically useful local analgesics have a common chemical pattern of aromatic group–intermediate chain–amine group (Table 10.2). The aromatic group confers lipophilic properties while the amine group is hydrophilic. The intermediate chain is usually either an ester or an amide. The ester linkage can be hydrolyzed by esterases, while the amide group can only be broken down by liver enzymes. Some compounds lack the hydrophilic tail (e.g. benzocaine) and are nearly insoluble in water so that they are unsuitable for injection but they can be applied to mucosal surfaces.

Modification of the chemical structure alters activity and the physical properties of the molecule. Lengthening of the intermediate chain or addition of carbon atoms to the aromatic or amine groups results in an increase in potency up to a certain maximum, beyond which any further increase in molecular weight is followed by a decrease in activity. The addition of a butyl group to the aromatic end of the procaine molecule increases lipid solubility and gives a 10-fold increase in protein binding with an increased duration of action and systemic toxicity. Similarly, the substitution of a butyl group for the methyl group of the amine of mepivacaine gives greater potency and a more prolonged duration of activity. Once again there is an increase in lipid solubility and a greater degree of protein binding.

Cocaine

Cocaine is an alkaloid obtained from the leaves of *Erythroxylum coca*, a South American plant. It was first introduced into surgery by Koller in 1884, some 38 years after the introduction of general anaesthesia. Its toxicity and addictive properties in man led to a search for synthetic substitutes and reference to it now has become largely historical

for it has been almost entirely replaced by compounds which do not suffer from these disadvantages to the same extent. Its one remaining use is for surgery in the nasal chambers, where its property of producing intense vasoconstriction shrinks the mucous membrane, allowing more room for the surgeon and aiding haemostasis.

Procaine

Procaine was introduced in 1905 under the trade name of Novocain, and largely replaced cocaine as a local analgesic. Compared to cocaine its power of penetration of mucous membranes is poor and following injection nerve block is slow in onset.

Amethocaine

Amethocaine is a member of the procaine series of compounds which is particularly useful for desensitizing mucous membranes. A 1% solution is used for instillation into the conjunctival sac instead of proxymetacaine and a 2% solution is used for the pharyngeal, laryngeal and nasal mucous membranes.

Cinchocaine

This was first introduced as Percaine in 1929. It is known as 'Nupercaine', a name which prevents confusion with procaine, and in the United States as 'Dibucaine'. The drug is quite different from either cocaine or procaine, being a quinoline derivative – butyloxycinchoninic acid diethyl ethylene diamide. It is readily soluble in water and solutions may be boiled repeatedly for sterilization. It is decomposed by alkali, and for this reason traces of acid are added to solutions which are to be stored. For the same reason Nupercaine must always be kept in alkali-free glass containers. The drug is much more toxic than procaine, but this is counterbalanced by the smaller quantities used, for the minimal effective concentration is about one-fortieth that of procaine. In addition, the analgesia it produces lasts for very much longer. Nupercaine has been used for every type of local analgesia but has been found most useful for surface and spinal analgesia.

TABLE 10.2 Chemical structures and properties of some commonly used local analgesics

| | Chemical structure | | | | |
Aromatic end	Intermediate chain	Amino end	Lipid solubility	Anaesthetic duration	Onset time
Amino esters					
Procaine H_2N—◯—$COOCH_2CH_2$		$-N\begin{smallmatrix}C_2H_5\\C_2H_5\end{smallmatrix}$	1	Short	Slow
2-Chloroprocaine H_2N—◯(CL)—$COOCH_2CH_2$		$-N\begin{smallmatrix}C_2H_5\\C_2H_5\end{smallmatrix}$	1	Short	Fast
Tetracaine $\begin{smallmatrix}H_9C_4\\H\end{smallmatrix}N$—◯—$COOCH_2CH_2$		$-N\begin{smallmatrix}CH_3\\CH_3\end{smallmatrix}$	80	Long	Slow
Amino amides					
Lignocaine (ring with CH_3, CH_3)	$NHCOCH_2$	$-N\begin{smallmatrix}C_2H_5\\C_2H_5\end{smallmatrix}$	4	Moderate	Fast
Prilocaine (ring with CH_3)	$NHCOCH$	$-N\begin{smallmatrix}C_3H_7\\H\end{smallmatrix}$	1.5	Moderate	Fast
	CH_3				
Etidocaine (ring with CH_3, CH_3)	$NHCOCH$	$N\begin{smallmatrix}C_2H_5\\C_3H_7\end{smallmatrix}$	140	Long	Fast
	C_2H_5				
Mepivacaine (ring with CH_3, CH_3)	$NHCO$	(piperidine ring) N—CH_3	1	Moderate	Fast
Bupivacaine (ring with CH_3, CH_3)	$NHCO$	(piperidine ring) N—C_4H_9	30	Long	Moderate

Lignocaine (lidocaine)

Since its introduction into veterinary clinical practice in 1944 lignocaine (lidocaine in North America) has replaced procaine and most other compounds in every field where local analgesia is used (except for postoperative analgesia). Chemically, lignocaine is N-diethylaminoacetyl-2,6-xylidine hydrochloride and as it is not an ester it is unaffected by pseudocholinesterase (procaine esterase). It is extremely stable in solution and solutions can be stored and resterilized almost indefinitely, without fear of toxic changes or loss of potency. Compared with procaine, lignocaine has a far shorter period of onset, a more intense and a longer duration of action. Spread through the tissues is much greater with lignocaine than with procaine, and injections made in the neighbourhood of a nerve trunk penetrate more effectively. This facility for tissue penetration has some important practical applications. It is unnecessary to add hyaluronidase to solutions of lignocaine for infiltration or nerve blocking purposes (as is often recommended with other agents) since the spreading power of this agent is already adequate. Probably as another result of its tissue penetrating properties, lignocaine also has marked local analgesic activity when applied to the surface of mucous membranes or the cornea. Its activity on mucous membranes is similar to that of cocaine, while on the cornea a 4% solution of lignocaine is approximately equivalent to a 2% solution of cocaine.

The drug is rapidly absorbed from tissues and mucous surfaces. In dogs, after subcutaneous or intramuscular injection, the blood concentration of lignocaine reaches a maximum in about 30 minutes. The addition of adrenaline (epinephrine) to the injected solution approximately doubles the time required for complete absorption. Ten percent or less of an injected dose of lignocaine is excreted unchanged in the urine and the metabolism of lignocaine has, therefore, been the subject of much investigation. Liver is the only tissue which has been shown to metabolize lignocaine in significant quantities. The approximate maximum dose by infiltration before toxic signs become apparent is not known with any certainty but is thought to be 6–10 mg/kg.

Prilocaine

This substance is closely related to lignocaine and possesses the same pKa and onset time of the block in isolated nerves. However, *in vivo*, prilocaine nerve blocks do not develop as rapidly as lignocaine blocks. It is popular in equine surgery because it is claimed to produce less tissue reaction than lignocaine. It is the most rapidly metabolized amide and its metabolism releases o-toluidine, which causes methaemoglobinaemia.

Mepivacaine

This compound (Carbocaine) closely resembles lignocaine hydrochloride but is slightly less toxic. It has been found to be especially useful for the nerve blocks used in the diagnosis of equine lameness because there is less post-injection oedema than with lignocaine.

Bupivacaine

Bupivacaine (Marcain) is dl-l-butyl-2'.6'-pipecoloxylidide hydrochloride, a remarkably stable compound which is resistant to boiling with strong acid or alkali and shows no change on repeated autoclaving. It possesses, to greater or lesser degrees, the most desirable general properties of a local analgesic drug.

The local analgesic effect of bupivacaine is slower in rate of onset and similar in depth to that of lignocaine and mepivacaine, but is of much longer duration. The addition of adrenaline in low concentrations has been shown to increase both the speed of onset and the duration of analgesia so that all solutions of bupivacaine for clinical use should contain adrenaline.

Bupivacaine is approximately four times as potent as lignocaine; hence a 0.5% solution is equivalent in nerve-blocking activity to a 2% solution of lignocaine. It is generally agreed that bupivacaine provides a period of analgesia at least twice as long as that of lignocaine, and that it is exceptionally well tolerated by all tissues. Due to these properties it is increasingly used today as a component of regimens providing postoperative analgesia.

Ropivacaine

Ropivacaine, a relatively new long acting amide-type local analgesic, is the (S) enantiomer of a chain-shortened homologue of bupivacaine. It appears to provide a greater margin of safety than bupivacaine when used in equal dosage (Reiz *et al.*, 1989). It is an effective long acting drug when given epidurally and it appears to be a vasoconstrictor over a wide range of concentrations. Subcutaneous infiltration of plain ropivacaine produces cutaneous vasoconstriction equivalent to adrenaline, in contrast to bupivacaine, which produces vasodilatation.

PHARMACOKINETICS OF LOCAL ANALGESIC DRUGS

The concentration of local analgesics in the blood is determined by the rate of absorption from the site of injection or application, the rate of tissue distribution and the rate of metabolism and excretion of the particular compound. The physiological disposition and resultant blood concentration will also depend on the age of the animal, its cardiovascular status and hepatic function.

ABSORPTION

Factors which influence systemic absorption and potential toxicity of local analgesics are:

1. The site of injection
2. The dosage
3. The addition of a vasoconstrictor
4. The pharmacological profile of the agent itself.

Multiple injections (e.g. intercostal nerve blocks) may expose the agent to a great vascular area, resulting in a faster rate of absorption. The same dose of agent injected in one site results in a much lower maximum blood level. Topical application of local analgesics at various sites also results in differences in absorption and toxicity. In general, absorption occurs most rapidly after intratracheal spray for the agent is dispersed over a wide surface area, promoting vascular absorption. The rate of absorption is less after intranasal instillation and administration into the urethra and urinary bladder. Peak blood levels occur 10 minutes after intrapleural instillation. The use of ointments or gels to apply local analgesic drugs to mucous membranes tends to delay absorption.

The absorption and subsequent blood levels of local analgesics is related to the *total* dose of drug administered regardless of the site or route of administration. For most agents there is a linear relationship between the amount of drug given and the resultant peak blood level. Local analgesic solutions frequently contain a vasoconstrictor, usually adrenaline (epinephrine), in concentrations varying from $5 \mu g/ml$ to $20 \mu g/ml$, to delay the absorption and prolong the action of the agent. Although other vasoconstrictors such as noradrenaline (norepinephrine) and phenylephrine have been employed with local analgesic drugs neither seems as effective as adrenaline in a concentration of 1:200 000.

The pharmacological characteristics of the specific local analgesic also influence the rate and degree of vascular absorption. For example, lignocaine and mepivacaine are absorbed more rapidly than prilocaine from the epidural space, while bupivacaine is absorbed more rapidly than etidocaine. These differences are probably a reflection of differences in both vasodilator activity and lipid solubility.

Local analgesic drugs distribute themselves throughout the total body water. Their rate of disappearance from the blood (tissue redistribution), the volume of distribution and relative uptake by the various tissues are related to their physiochemical properties. The distribution can be described by a two or three compartment model. The rapid disappearance (α) phase is believed to be related to uptake by rapidly equilibrating tissues (i.e. those with high vascular perfusion). The slower β phase of disappearance from blood is mainly a function of distribution to slowly equilibrating tissues and the metabolism and excretion of the compound. This secondary phase may also be subdivided into distribution into slowly perfused tissues (true β phase) and a phase of metabolism and excretion (γ phase). A comparison of the three amide drugs (lignocaine, mepivacaine and prilocaine) reveals that prilocaine is redistributed at a significantly faster rate from blood to tissues than is lignocaine or mepivacaine (which have similar rates of tissue redistribution). In addition, the β disappearance phase from blood also occurs more rapidly with prilocaine, suggesting a more rapid rate of metabolism.

Local analgesics become distributed throughout all body tissues, but the relative concentration in different tissues varies. In general the more highly perfused organs show a greater concentration of local analgesic drugs than less well perfused organs. The highest fraction of an injected dose is found in the skeletal muscles since their mass makes them the largest reservoir but they have no specific affinity for these drugs.

The pattern of metabolism of the local analgesics varies according to their chemical composition. Plasma pseudocholinesterase hydrolyses the ester class agents. Chloroprocaine is hydrolysed more rapidly than procaine or tetracaine and the toxicity of these agents is directly related to their rate of degradation. Less than 2% of unchanged procaine is found in the urine but 90% of para-aminobenzoic acid, its primary metabolite, is excreted in urine. The amide class of local analgesics undergoes enzymatic degradation primarily in the liver. The rate of hepatic degradation may vary between compounds which, in turn, may influence the toxicity of the specific agent. Prilocaine undergoes the fastest rate of enzymatic metabolism and is the least toxic of the amide-type agents. Lignocaine is metabolized more rapidly than is mepivacaine. Some degradation of these amide compounds may take place in tissues other than liver cells and their metabolism is more complex than that of the ester compounds. The metabolites of local analgesics are of clinical importance since they may exert both pharmacological and toxicological effects similar to those of their parent compounds.

The excretion of amide-type compounds occurs through the kidneys. Less than about 5% of the drug is excreted unchanged. The major fraction appears in the form of various metabolites, some as yet unidentified. The renal clearance of the amide-type drugs appears to be inversely related to their protein binding abilities. Renal clearance is also inversely proportional to urinary pH, suggesting that urinary excretion occurs by non-ionic diffusion.

In animals with a pathologically low hepatic blood flow, or advanced hepatic disease, significantly higher blood concentrations of the amide agents may be expected. This is important for the disappearance of lignocaine from the blood may be markedly prolonged in animals with congestive heart failure.

SYSTEMIC AND TOXIC EFFECTS OF LOCAL ANALGESIC DRUGS

Local analgesics affect not only the nerve fibres but all types of excitable tissue including skeletal, smooth and cardiac muscle. Side effects occur when they enter the systemic circulation and the most severe follow inadvertent intravascular injection, but absorption from tissue depots can also be responsible if the rate of absorption exceeds the rate of metabolism or elimination from the body as it may be if the dose rate is too high. Cardiovascular, respiratory and central nervous disturbances are common side effects but allergic reactions occasionally occur with ester-type agents.

CENTRAL NERVOUS SYSTEM

Local analgesics have a complex effect on the central nervous system. Usually, sedation is the first obvious sign but a further increase in the brain concentration produces *grand mal* tonic-clonic seizures. One explanation given for this is that local analgesics stabilize cell membranes even at low concentrations but as the concentration increases more and more of the cells having inhibitory functions are affected and as the inhibitory pathways become blocked facilitatory neurones are released to act unopposed, thus giving rise to excitation and convulsions. As the concentration of the drug in the brain rises still higher, however, depression of both inhibitory and facilitatory systems occurs with overall loss of central nervous activity. For this explanation to be valid it would seem that there must be certain predilection sites of activity in the brain but evidence for their precise location is conflicting.

Lignocaine and other agents have anticonvulsant activity as well as the ability to produce seizures. In general, the dose giving rise to anti-convulsant activity is less than that associated with convulsions and a marked antiepileptic effect is observed. It seems probable that this antiepileptic activity is due to depression of specific hyper-excitable cortical neurones.

Seizures induced by local analgesics may be managed in several different ways but it should be remembered that many are self-limiting due to the rapid redistrubution of the drug from the brain to other tissues. *Grand mal* seizures increase the cere-bral oxygen consumption yet interfere with nor-mal pulmonary function, while hypercapnia potentiates the effect of local analgesics on the brain. Thus, whatever else is done, measures to protect the airway and ensure adequate alveolar ventilation must be taken immediately. If the seizures continue for more than 1–2 minutes diazepam (up to 0.2 mg/kg) or 5 mg/kg of thiopental should be given by i.v. injection. It has been suggested that diazepam has a specific antag-onist effect against the excitatory effects of local analgesics on the limbic brain and that it gives rise to fewer side effects than thiopental, but the barbi-turate has a shorter duration of action and in many situations this short duration of action may be desirable.

The stimulant action of local analgesics on the brain has led to their abuse by human subjects seeking to achieve the preseizive aura without using sufficient of the drug to produce a general-ized seizure, and also in the horse racing industry where they have been given to enhance perform-ance.

CARDIOVASCULAR SYSTEM

Local analgesics have both direct and indirect effects on the cardiovascular system. In experi-ments on isolated cardiac muscle preparations with concentrations of lignocaine known to con-trol arrythmias but which are not toxic, it has been shown that automaticity is strongly suppressed. The duration of the action potential and effective refractory period is shortened in both Purkinje fibres and ventricular muscle and it has been sug-gested that these effects are responsible for the sta-bilizing action which lignocaine has on cardiac irregularities. Toxic concentrations of lignocaine are associated with a decrease in the maximum rate of depolarization on Purkinje fibres and ven-tricular muscle, a reduction in amplitude of the action potential, and a marked decrease in conduc-tion velocity. On the ECG there is an increase in the P–R interval and in duration of the QRS complex. Sinus bradycardia may proceed to cardiac arrest at high lignocaine concentrations. At concentrations of lignocaine sufficient to control arrythmias there is no reduction in cardiac output or myocardial contractility. Lignocaine is particularly useful for controlling ventricular arrhythmias perhaps because it enhances the efflux of K^+ from ventricu-lar muscle and Purkinje fibres but not from atrial tissue.

The usual clinical doses of lignocaine and other analgesics used for local and regional analgesia do not give rise to blood levels which are associated with cardiodepressant effects. Accidental intravas-cular injection of excessive doses may, however, give rise to concentrations which result in signific-ant decreases in myocardial contractility or even cardiac arrest.

Cocaine is the only agent which produces vaso-constriction and it is believed that this results from uptake of catecholamines into tissue binding sites. Most other agents have a dose-related effect; low concentrations stimulate smooth muscle produc-ing vasoconstriction, while high concentrations cause vasodilatation.

Secondary effects independent of the direct actions of whatever agent is used can occur due to the regional nature of the block produced. Systemic hypotension may accompany epidural injection due to sympathetic blockade. For the heart rate to be able to compensate for falls in arter-ial pressure the cardioaccelerator fibres in the first two thoracic nerves must be unaffected and if the block reaches this level vasodilatation will occur in the forelimbs and peripheral resistance will decrease so that hypotension will be very severe. If the block affects the caudal nerves only the hypo-tension is less profound because of compensatory vasoconstriction in the rostral regions of the body.

Renal and hepatic blood flow may also decrease secondary to the effects of the drugs on the central nervous system and this will result in a decrease in both renal excretion and liver metabolism of the amide-type drugs.

RESPIRATORY SYSTEM

At subtoxic doses bronchial smooth muscle is relaxed and some respiratory depression may occur from central nervous activity.

Local toxic effects

Large doses of local analgesics cause damage to tissues such as nerves and skeletal muscles and the use of excessive amounts together with vasoconstrictors in wound areas may delay healing. Cytotoxicity is correlated with potency – the more potent the drug the greater its cytotoxic activity.

Methaemoglobinaemia has been reported in dogs following topical application of large amounts of benzocaine for relief of pruritis.

Local analgesics must always be treated with respect and it is important that in practice only minimal, accurately placed quantities are used if toxic effects are to be avoided.

INTERACTION WITH OTHER DRUGS

The duration of nerve block can be increased and the potential risk of systemic toxicity can be reduced by combining vasoconstrictor drugs with local analgesics so as to delay absorption from the injection site. As already mentioned, it is probable that adrenaline in concentrations between 1:100 000 and 1:200 000 is the most generally useful drug for this purpose. Dilute solutions of adrenaline tend to be unstable and for this reason most commercially available solutions of local analgesics contain rather more – usually about 1:80 000 – to allow for deterioration in strength during shelf-life.

Local analgesics can enhance the duration of action of both depolarizing and non-depolarizing neuromuscular blocking agents. Drugs such as the phenothiazine derivatives and pethidine may lower the threshold at which the convulsant actions of local analgesics are encountered.

FORMS OF LOCAL ANALGESIA

SURFACE ANALGESIA

Agents which cause freezing of the superficial layers of the skin are sometimes used for analgesia.

Ice is the simplest but, generally, volatile substances which cause freezing by rapid volatilization from the surface of the skin are used (e.g. ethyl chloride spray and carbonic acid snow). Their action is very superficial and transient and their use is limited to the simplest forms of surgical interference, such as the incision of small superficial abscesses. Used too freely, they may cause skin necrosis. In man, the thawing out after their use is known to be painful. Decicaine and lignocaine are sometimes incorporated in ointments and applied with friction to the skin. Some slight absorption occurs producing a local numbing which has been found to be useful for the control of pruritis but they have little use in anaesthesia. Similarly, aqueous solutions of 2% lignocaine or 4% procaine may be applied topically for the relief of pain from superficial abraded or eczematous areas.

EMLA cream (2.5% lignocaine base with 2.5% prilocaine base) and 4% amethocaine gel can be applied to the skin over the site of venepuncture to render subsequent penetration by needles and catheters painless. They are applied under an occlusive dressing and anaesthetizing the superficial skin layers takes about 60 minutes with EMLA cream but less than 30 minutes with amethocaine gel.

For analgesia of the mucous membranes of the glans penis and the vulva the application of lignocaine in carboxymethylcellulose gel is the preparation of choice. (This gel possesses very good lubricating properties and is an excellent lubricant for urethral catheters.)

For procedures in the nasal chambers of the horse, or for the transnasal passage of a stomach tube in dogs, spraying with 4% lignocaine provides satisfactory analgesia. In ophthalmic surgery 4% lignocaine is quite safe but the agent of choice for topical analgesia of the cornea is proxymetacaine hydrochloride (2-diethylaminoethyl-3-amino-4 propoxybenzoate hydrochloride), known by the trade name of 'Ophthaine'. Using a single drop, the onset of corneal analgesia occurs in about 15 seconds and persists for about 15 minutes. This compound does not produce pupillary dilatation and is non-irritant, but its solution is rather unstable, having a shelf-life of only 12 months.

INTRASYNOVIAL ANALGESIA

Surface analgesia is also employed for the relief of pain arising from pathological processes or operations involving joints and tendon sheaths. A solution of local analgesic is injected into the synovial cavity and then dispersed throughout the cavity by manipulation of the limb. If the synovial cavity is distended with fluid, it is first drained to ensure the injected solution is not excessively diluted. It is relatively simple to introduce a needle into synovial sheaths when they are distended with fluid, but entry to a normal sheath is not easy. When searching for a synovial sheath the exploring needle should be connected to a syringe containing the analgesic solution and a slight pressure maintained on the syringe plunger. As soon as the needle enters the sheath resistance to injection disappears and some of the solution enters the sheath, lifting its wall away from the underlying tendon. Analgesia develops within 5 to 10 minutes after successful injection and persists for about one hour depending on the drug employed. The injection renders the synovial membrane insensitive but it is not known whether the nerve endings in the underlying structures are affected.

Intra-articular injection of local analgesics in connection with the diagnosis of lameness was first introduced by Forssell at the Royal Veterinary College, Stockholm in 1921, and his techniques, with only slight modifications, are still in use today. Clearly, almost every joint and tendon sheath in the body can be treated in this way and the technique is now being increasingly employed for the relief of postoperative pain after arthrotomy.

INFILTRATION ANALGESIA

By this method the nerve endings are affected at the actual site of operation. Most minor surgical procedures not involving the digits, penis or teats can be performed under infiltration analgesia and the technique is also useful, in conjunction with light narcosis, for major operations in animals which are bad operative risks. Infiltration should, however, never be carried out through, or into, infected or inflamed tissues.

Suitable concentrations of lignocaine for canine and feline anaesthesia are 0.2 to 0.5%, and stronger solutions than 0.5% should never be necessary. In large animals 2% solutions of lignocaine are commonly used. Bupivacaine is used in concentrations of 0.125 to 0.250%. Care must be taken to minimize the total doses of analgesic in dogs and cats to avoid toxic reactions; maximum effective dilution of the agent is necessary. It is usual to add adrenaline (1:400000 to 1:200000) to the solution, but this vasoconstrictor should be omitted when there are circumstances present which may interfere with healing, e.g. damaged tissue, possible contamination.

A hypodermic syringe and needle is all the apparatus necessary for the administration of local infiltration analgesia. The limits of the area to be infiltrated are conveniently defined and marked for subsequent recognition by the use of intradermal weals. To produce an intradermal weal a short needle is held almost parallel to the skin surface with the bevel of its point uppermost. The needle is thrust into the skin until the bevel is no longer visible and by exerting considerable pressure on the plunger of the syringe 0.5 to 1.0 ml of local analgesic solution is injected. The resulting weal is insensitive as soon as it is formed and if punctures are repeatedly made at the periphery of such weals, a continuous weal can be produced along the proposed line of incision without an animal feeling more than the initial needle prick. Such intradermal infiltration is only easily performed in thick-skinned animals; in horses and cattle it is usual to simply mark the proposed line of infiltration by raising a weal at either end of the line.

Subcutaneous tissues are infiltrated by introducing a needle through the skin at the site of an intradermal weal. For infiltration of a straight line incision a needle about 10 cm long is introduced almost parallel to the skin surface and pushed through the subcutaneous tissue along the proposed line. Before injecting any local analgesic solution, aspiration is attempted to ascertain that the needle point has not entered a blood vessel. If blood is aspirated back into the syringe, the needle is partially withdrawn and reinserted in a slightly different direction. About 1 ml of solution is injected for every centimetre length of incision as the needle is withdrawn. If the proposed incision is longer than the needle it may be infiltrated from its middle, the needle being introduced first in one direction and then in the opposite direction. Very long incisions will necessitate more than one puncture, but the needle may be reinserted through the extremity of the area that has already been infiltrated so that the animal suffers only the sensation of one needle insertion. Care should be taken to infiltrate an adequate area at the outset, so there is no necessity for further infiltration as operation proceeds. It is always better to overdo local infiltration than to apply it inadequately and to use more of a dilute rather than less of a concentrated, solution of local analgesic. Local infiltration may also be used at the concluding stages of an operation carried out under general anaesthesia to ensure a measure of postoperative pain relief.

To infiltrate several layers of tissue, the procedure is to inject, from one puncture site, first the subcutaneous tissue and then, in succession by further advancing the needle, the deeper tissues.

REGIONAL NERVE BLOCKS

One form of regional nerve block consists of making walls of analgesia enclosing the operation field. It is accomplished by making fanwise injections in certain planes of the tissues so as to soak all the nerves which cross these on their way to the operation site. Usually the entire thickness of the soft tissue in which the nerves run is involved. In cattle and sheep, for flank coeliotomy, two linear infiltrations are made of the whole thickness of the abdominal wall, one cranial to and one dorsal to, the line of incision (Fig. 10.1).

Ring block of an extremity is another special type of regional analgesia in which a transverse plane through the whole extremity is infiltrated and particular attention is paid to the sites of large nerve trunks. In limbs the technique is more effective when the injection is made distal to a tourniquet. When used for operations on cow's teats it is important that vasoconstrictors should not be added to the analgesic solutions, for prolonged vasoconstriction may result in ischaemic necrosis of the end of the teat.

More commonly, regional analgesia is brought about by blocking conduction in the sensory nerve or nerves innervating the operation site. The

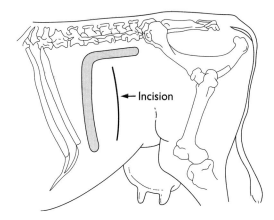

FIG. 10.1 The L-block often used for flank coeliotomy in cattle and sheep. This technique is effective but cumbersome and, if properly carried out, time consuming.

operative field itself is not touched while its sensitivity is abolished and good analgesia results from the use of small quantities of solution. The solution must, however, be brought into the closest possible contact with the nerve which is to be blocked, and special care must be taken to ensure that there is no sheet of fascia between the nerve and the site of deposition of the analgesic solution since solutions do not diffuse through fascial sheets. Success in regional nerve blocks comes only from constant practice, as does success in other techniques, but clearly it requires a thorough knowledge of the topographical anatomy of the nerves and sites of injection. Moreover, no description, however long and detailed, or however well illustrated, can ever be more than a poor substitute for demonstration and tuition by an experienced practitioner.

It is quite beyond the scope of this book to give a complete account of all the nerve blocks that can be carried out, but in the following chapters various techniques will be described, arranged more or less on a regional basis. Selection presents difficulty in a book of limited scope and must be rather arbitrary, but two considerations have been borne in mind. First, the methods described are, with one or two exceptions, comparatively easy to carry out and may be attempted without apprehension. Secondly, they are all useful techniques which are suitable for inclusion in a general textbook of anaesthesia.

INTRAVENOUS REGIONAL ANALGESIA (IVRA)

In 1908 Bier reported a technique of 'venous anaesthesia' and recorded 134 cases, but this technique seems to have been largely forgotten until recent years. After suitable modification it has been employed in canine and bovine surgery with gratifying results.

A small needle or catheter is inserted into a vein at the distal extremity of a limb and temporarily blocked with an obturator or tap. The limb is exsanguinated, usually with an Esmarch bandage, a tourniquet is inflated or tied to occlude the arterial supply at the top of the limb and the local analgesic solution is injected via the needle or catheter. Analgesia of the limb up to the lower limit of the tourniquet comes on rapidly, and when the tourniquet is released it wears off with almost equal rapidity.

The mode of action of this technique is unclear but it seems to be both safe and simple for operations on the digits, especially in ruminant animals and in dogs unfit for general anaesthesia because of a full stomach or intercurrent disease. The good analgesia and bloodless field are appreciated by the surgeon. Analgesia develops distally and progresses proximally so it is important that the injection is made as distally as possible. If the tourniquet is left in place for more than about 1.5 hours ischaemic damage may follow and pain is severe. Bupivacaine should not be used for this technique because, due to the toxicity of this local analgesic drug, cardiovascular collapse and death may occur when the tourniquet is released. Major advantages of this technique is that it requires no precise knowledge of anatomy and only one injection needs to be made.

LOCAL ANALGESIA FOR FRACTURES

A technique which does not fit readily into any classification but must be mentioned, is that of local analgesia for the relief of pain arising from fractured bones. The injection is made directly into the haematoma at the site of fracture and deposition of the solution in the correct place is essential for success. The needle should be inserted as far into the haematoma and as near the bone ends as possible. Its position should be verified by aspiration, when blood or blood clot should be drawn into the syringe. Lignocaine hydrochloride (1% solution without adrenaline) is the best agent to use. In small animal patients 2 to 5 ml, and in large animals 10 to 15 ml, of solution are required. Analgesia follows 5–10 minutes after injection. Scrupulous asepsis must be observed when injecting into a fracture site as the consequences of infection are serious. This technique is particularly suitable as a first aid measure and in the relief of pain arising from fractured ribs.

SPINAL NERVE BLOCKS

Spinal analgesia is a special type of regional block comprising the injection into some part of the spinal canal of a local analgesic solution. By coming into contact with the spinal nerves the drug temporarily paralyses them and gives rise to loss of sensation in those parts of the body from which the sensory portion of the nerves carries impulses and, when more concentrated solutions are used, paralysis of those parts supplied by the motor fibres. It is divided into two distinct types:

1. Subarachnoid injection in which the needle penetrates the dura mater and the arachnoid mater so that the analgesic solution is introduced directly into the cerebrospinal fluid.

2. Epi- (extra-) dural injection, in which the needle enters the spinal canal but does not penetrate the meninges, and the injected solution permeates along the spinal canal outside the dura mater.

In 1885 Corning found that the injection of cocaine solutions into the spinal canal of the dog was followed by paralysis of the hind limbs and loss of sensation in them. This observation received very little attention until 1899 when Bier published his observations in the injection of cocaine solutions into the subarachnoid space in man. In veterinary practice subarachnoid injections were first performed in France by Cuille and Sendrail in 1901. They demonstrated the method in the horse, ox and dog, but consequent upon its perceived difficulties and dangers it was not widely adopted. Epidural injection was introduced into the UK by Brook in 1930 and this same worker contributed an extensive review of the subject (Brooke, 1935).

Anatomy of the epidural space

Examination of the epidural space has been performed using a great number of methods. Postmortem measurements, pressure measurements involving needle and catheter introduction into the space, radiographic examination with or without contrast injection, isotopic studies of local blood circulation, computerized tomography, endoscopic examination, magnetic resonance and cryomicrotome section have all contributed to present day knowledge of this space but some studies were, regrettably, unsound. Studies claiming to show the existence of a space by the introduction of air, contrast media or endoscopes, all displaced the dura and created the space which was then studied. Acceptable studies show that the epidural space is not a cavity in the undisturbed state *in vivo*; it contains vessels, nerves and fat in dorsal and lateral compartments, i.e. it is only a *potential* space.

The spinal cord lies within the spinal canal and is covered by three membranes, the dense dura mater, the arachnoid mater and the delicate pia mater. The wall of the spinal canal is formed by the vertebral arches and bodies, the intervertebral discs and the intervertebral ligaments. The tube-like canal is somewhat flat in the lumbar region. The spinal cord and dura mater end at the lumbar enlargement and the canal itself tapers off caudal to this enlargement to end in the 4th or 5th coccygeal vertebra. In each vertebral segment the canal has lateral openings between the vertebral arches, the 'intervertebral foraminae', through which pass blood vessels and the spinal nerves.

In the cranial cavity the dura mater is arranged in two layers, the 'periosteal' and 'investing' layers, which are firmly adherent except where they split to enclose venous sinuses. The outer layer forms the periosteum of the inner surface of the cranial bones and in the spine acts as the periosteum lining the vertebral canal. The investing layer is continued from the cranium into the spinal canal but at the foramen magnum is firmly adherent to the margins of the foramen where it blends with the outer or periosteal layer. Between the two

layers in the spinal canal is the 'extra-' or 'epidural' (perhaps more strictly the 'interdural') potential space. The dorsal and ventral nerve roots issuing from the spinal canal penetrate the investing layer of dura and carry tubular prolongations (dural cuffs) which blend with the perineurium of the mixed spinal nerve.

The spinal arachnoid mater is a continuation of the cerebral arachnoid. An incomplete and inconsistent septum divides the spinal subarachnoid space along the midline of the dorsal surface of the cord. In the spinal canal the pia mater is closely applied to the cord and extends into the ventral median fissure. The blood vessels going to the cord lie in the subarachnoid space before piercing the pia mater. They carry with them into the spinal cord a double sleeve of meninges.

Although the venous plexuses of the spinal canal lie in the epidural space to form a network they can be subdivided into:

1. A pair of ventral venous plexuses lying on either side of the dorsal longitudinal ligament of the vertebra, into which the basivertebral veins drain.

2. A single dorsal venous plexus which connects with the dorsal external veins. All interconnect with one another and form a series of venous rings at the level of each vertebra. The accidental injection of local analgesic solution into these veins may occur during the performance of an epidural block and be responsible for toxic manifestations.

In addition to the venous plexuses, branches from vertebral, ascending cervical, deep cervical, intercostal, lumbar and iliolumbar arteries enter the intervertebral foramina and anastomose with one another, chiefly in the lateral parts of the epidural space. The spaces between the nerves, arteries and veins in the epidural space are filled with fatty tissue, the amount of which corresponds with the adiposity of the subject.

Each spinal nerve results from the union of two roots – a dorsal, ganglionic or sensory root and a ventral motor root. In the horse, these roots penetrate the dura mater separately and converge towards the intervertebral foramina where they join, immediately external to the point where the dorsal root has the ganglion placed on it. In the cervical, dorsal and cranial lumbar regions the bundles of both roots pass through separate openings in the dura mater in linear series before uniting into a root proper, but further caudally the bundles of each root unite within the dura mater. In the dog, union is effected within the intervertebral foramina, except in the lumbar and coccygeal regions, where it takes place within the vertebral canal. The point of fusion of the two roots is of practical significance – at any rate, in the small animals in which epidural anaesthesia is induced. It is the dorsal root which it is desired to influence and thus when injecting volumes likely to permeate in front of the cranial lumbar region it is an advantage to place the animal on its back after injection to reduce the extent of the complicating factors resulting from paralysis of vasomotor fibres emerging with the ventral root.

Spread of epidural analgesia

For a long time the clinical management of epidural blockade was based on three assumptions that seemed self-evident. First, the number of segments blocked would depend on the volume of solution injected. The space was considered to be a simple cylindrical reservoir, whose volume was determined by the length and diameter of the cylinder less the volume of the structures it contained. Thus a larger volume would be needed for animals with long backs than for those with short ones. Secondly, certain escape channels, most importantly the intervertebral foramina, drained this reservoir and the extent of spread from the injection site would depend on the leakage of solution through these escape channels. Thirdly, the quality or intensity of sensory and motor blockade would be governed by the concentration of the local analgesic solution used.

There were a number of reasons for doubting the first two of these assumptions, although the third gained more credibility from clinical observations. Brook (1935) quoted the assertion of several practitioners that, in cattle, the concentration of the solution employed affected the extent of the block. For example, 2–3 ml of 5% lignocaine injected into the caudal region of a cow blocks as many segments as 10–12 ml of 2% lignocaine. That spread could not be simply governed by volume of solution injected was indicated from a well recognized and commonly used technique for examining the bull's penis. In this technique, if the initial injection was ineffective succeeding injections of smaller volumes of solution seemed to pass cranially, tracking along in the wake of the initial ineffective injection, to extend the neural block and result in the desired extrusion of the penis from the prepuce. If volume alone was the major determinant of spread, why should this be? The inter-relationships of concentration, volume and effect were indeed difficult to explain on the basis of the prevailing assumptions and it is only in recent years that explanations have been recognized.

Other assumptions were also accepted for too many years. It was held that the dura mater was impermeable to the passage of local analgesic (or any other) drugs so that there seemed to be no logical limit to the volume of solution that could be injected into the epidural space, and excessive amounts would leak harmlessly out through the intervertebral foramina. Moreover, since the dura fused with the periosteum at the base of the skull, it was assumed that the impermeable dura would form a safety barrier preventing the entry of local analgesics from the epidural space into the intracranial parts of the central nervous system. Unfortunately, neither of these is true. It is now recognized that the dura itself appears to be permeable to drugs and it is the pia-arachnoid with its complex mixture of water (extracellular fluid and cerebrospinal fluid) and lipid (in cell membranes) which constitutes the permeability barrier (Bernards & Hill, 1990).

When a drug is administered into the epidural space it must diffuse into neuronal tissue to produce an effect. The drug may leak out through intervertebral foramina, it may get taken up into epidural fat, it may diffuse into nerve roots beyond the meningeal sleeves, and it may be removed by epidural blood flow. It may diffuse into the dorsal roots through the dural cuffs or directly through the meninges to the cerebrospinal fluid and the spinal cord itself. The site of action of local analgesics given epidurally is still controversial but the main sites are thought to be the nerve roots within the dura and nerve tracts in the superficial layers of the spinal cord. The quantity of drug actually reaching the neuronal tissues is largely, but not entirely, dependent on the lipid solubility of the drug. Hydrophilic drugs easily cross the hydrophilic component of the meningeal tissue but enter the hydrophobic lipid phase with difficulty, in contrast to hydrophobic drugs.

The precise effect of epidurally administered local analgesic drugs is not only related to lipid solubility, however. Other physiochemical properties such as the pH of the solution, the pKa of the drug and tissue and protein binding capacity are also involved. The effectiveness of block is a function of drug concentration and its duration appears to be related to its protein binding. Although it is the base form of the drug which is responsible for penetration of the lipid membrane, it is the ionic form which is responsible for blocking sodium channels and so interfering with nerve conduction.

It is well recognized that epidural block has a tendency to spread widely during pregnancy, at least at term and when labour has begun. Several factors are probably involved. One of the most important is the space occupying and massaging effects of the distended venous plexuses in the epidural space causing rhythmic pressure waves which tend to disperse solutions lying around them. Increased vascularity of the meninges and changes in the cerebrospinal fluid have also been suggested as contributing to the spread.

In the final analysis it appears that the spread of solutions in the epidural space is a function of the total mass (concentration × volume) of the particular drug used, and the site of injection. The duration of block depends on the protein binding of the drug and whether or not a vasoconstrictor such as adrenaline is mixed with the injected drug. Lignocaine and mepivacaine are less tightly protein bound than bupivacaine and ropivacaine and, consequently have a shorter duration of effect. The addition of adrenaline prolongs block due to lignocaine and mepivcaine but not that of bupivacaine or ropivacaine (Feldman & Covino, 1988).

Effects of spinal nerve blocks

Many of the spinal nerves which may be involved in spinal nerve blocks contain fibres of the autonomic nervous system. The function of these nerve fibres varies according to the site at which they leave the spinal cord.

The cranial and sacral outflow (parasympathetic) is, in general, concerned with vegetative functions such digestion and excretion, whereas the lumbar and thoracic (sympathetic) outflow is more closely concerned with protective reflex activity. Distinct from the sympathetic nervous system but running with it are afferent fibres from the viscera. These visceral afferent fibres travel with the postganglionic fibres, but run in the opposite direction, passing through the ganglia, up the white rami and into the dorsal root of the spinal nerve. Their cell bodies are located in the dorsal root ganglia and an axon passes to a synapse in the lateral horn of the spinal cord. These fibres must not be confused with the postganglionic autonomic fibres (vasoconstrictor and vasodilator fibres) which also follow the dorsal root but whose cell bodies have not yet been precisely located.

The postganglionic fibres to a limb mainly pass with the spinal nerves to reach the cutaneous blood vessels, and the sweat and sebaceous glands in its distal four-fifths. The proximal one-fifth of the limb in the groin and axilla is supplied by fibres passing directly from ganglia without joining the spinal nerves. Since the spinal nerve always carries sympathetic fibres, a peripheral nerve block always produces vasodilatation in the distal part of the limb. Physiologically, neurogenic sympathetic influences are important for the control of blood pressure by the rapid adjustment of flow resistance and cardiac output on one hand, and by stabilizing the filling of the heart via their effects on blood distribution on the other.

The largest vasomotor nerves in the body are the splanchnic, which pass to the abdominal viscera. The area supplied by them is so great that their paralysis should produce a marked fall in blood pressure. This fall should be most marked in herbivores, in which the abdominal viscera are large and their blood supply correspondingly great. It would thus seem that when the lumbar and thoracic nerves which give rise to the splanchnic nerves are blocked a marked fall in blood pressure should occur. However, since the development of indirect means of measuring arterial pressure it has become apparent that in healthy subjects this does not happen.

Cardiovascular effects of spinal nerve blocks

Most studies to date have shown that changes in arterial pressure, heart rate and cardiac output vary within ± 20% of pre-block levels, regardless of whether the upper analgesic level is above or below the T4 spinal segment. This is also true with segmental epidural blockade, which definitely eliminates sympathetic drive to the heart, so that bradycardia during major spinal blocks must be of vagal origin. Blood flow is always increased in the denervated extremities (upper and lower limbs) provided the cranial analgesic level exceeds T4. In contrast, blood flow is decreased in all other organs, despite the fact that they are deprived of neurogenic sympathetic tone. Why the blood flow of the internal organs decreases rather than increases is as yet unknown. Alternatives are that compared with the limbs, the internal organs have a low resting sympathetic tone, are also under the control of vagal vasoconstrictor tone, respond preferentially to vasoactive hormones, or their blood flow decreases when arterial pressure falls.

Physiologically, neurogenic sympathetic tone is important for the control of arterial blood pressure by the rapid adjustment of flow resistance, the cardiac output and stabilization of the filling of the heart via their effects on blood distribution. It is now apparent, however, that animals can well maintain their circulation even when the sympathetic tone is removed by autonomic blockade. Spinal nerve blockade jeopardizes primarily the filling of the heart because of blood pooling in denervated body regions, which is normally counteracted by vasoconstriction in the remaining innervated body regions and particularly by vasoconstriction in the splanchnic region. Blood loss, low blood volumes from other causes and positive airway pressure also reduce the filling of the heart which must be maintained to avoid circulatory collapse. The empty heart cannot maintain an efficient circulation and renders cardiopulmonary resuscitation ineffective (Keats, 1988).

The capacitance vessels – postarteriolar extrathoracic vessels, the venules and veins of the systemic circulation and the sinusoids of the liver and spleen – contain a large proportion of the blood which can be mobilized in favour of cardiac filling (Arndt, 1986). Although the pulmonary circulation contains a large proportion of the total blood volume it cannot be used actively to increase filling of the left ventricle because of lack of muscle fibres in the blood vessels of greater than about 0.2 mm in diameter. Consequently left ventricular filling must passively follow changes in the extrathoracic capacitance vessels.

Maintenance of cardiac filling during spinal nerve blockade of sympathetic fibres is dependent on hormonal support systems, particularly vasopressin. (Share 1988). Although angiotensin, the most effective constrictor of resistance vessels plays a dominant role in normal blood pressure regulation there is evidence that the renin-angiotensin mechanism does not respond as a blood pressure support during spinal nerve blocks (Peters et al., 1990). Renin, which controls the formation of angiotensin II, originates from the juxtaglomerular apparatus of the kidneys and is released in response to a fall in arterial blood pressure, particularly renal perfusion pressure, but also and apparently more importantly, in response to increased sympathetic drive via β_1 adrenoceptors (Ehmke et al., 1987). This drive is eliminated by spinal nerve blocks which affect the relevant nerve roots. It is, therefore, vasopressin that stabilizes the arterial pressure during spinal nerve blocks. Vasopressin plasma concentrations increase considerably during epidural blocks, especially when combined with severe hypoxaemia. In dogs, when vasopressin is prevented from acting by pretreatment with a vasopressin 1 receptor antagonist, epidural block causes a profound fall in blood pressure (Peters et al., 1990a).

Site of injection

It is now customary to classify extradural spinal blocks as epidural and caudal, according to the site of injection.

Caudal block

Caudal injection is made between the coccygeal intervertebral spaces with the object of providing analgesia over the tail and croup as far as the mid-sacral region, the anus, vulva, perineum and the caudal aspect of the thigh. If paralysis of motor fibres is produced the anal sphincter relaxes and the posterior part of the rectum balloons. Defaecation will be suspended and stretching of the vulva provokes no response. The vagina dilates and in animals at parturition 'straining' or 'bearing down' ceases while uterine contractions are uninfluenced.

Epidural block

Epidural block implies that the injection is made further cranially, usually at the lumbosacral junction or in the lumbar region, although injection is sometimes made in the thoracic region. There is usually some degree of interference with the control of the hind limbs, depending on the drugs used and their concentration. It is important to note that the motor nerve fibres need not be blocked for this to occur, for block of afferent fibres alone will suffice to destroy temporarily the integrity of the reflex arcs involved in the maintenance of muscle tone. Recently there has been considerable interest, especially in human obstetrics, in using spinal analgesia to provide sensory blocks without interfering with motor control. The mechanisms behind this differential blockade are not well understood but it can be achieved by injecting dilute solutions of the local analgesic into the epidural space. It has been suggested that differential uptake by nerve fibres firing at different frequencies may be responsible since the drugs are taken up more readily by fast firing fibres. An alternative explanation is that it is related to the action at the nerve roots – small unmyelinated C-fibres need to be bathed in solution for only a short distance to prevent impulse conduction, whereas in myelinated fibres a longer distance incorporating several nodes of Ranvier have to be involved. Bupivacaine at concentrations of less than 0.125% and ropivacaine at 0.1% appear to have the least effect on motor fibres while producing good sensory block.

The concept of differential nerve block is attractive in veterinary medicine where it is desired to avoid recumbency following epidural analgesia but it seems that the proprioceptive and sensory deficits produced may limit its application. It will be further discussed in subsequent chapters.

Drugs used in epidural injections

The efficacy of local analgesic drugs in producing epidural block may be enhanced by mixing them with other drugs such as opioids, α_2 adrenoceptor agonists, NMDA antagonists and non-steroidal anti-inflammatory drugs. Since these drugs have actions which are mostly distinct from each other it seems logical that combinations of different classes of drugs will enhance analgesia.

Opioids

In the epidural space there is a synergism between local analgesics and opioids (Wang *et al.*, 1993) and combinations are being used clinically at doses which minimize the side effects of each individual drug. The opioids are believed to act at presynaptic sites in the dorsal horn to prevent the release of substance P and on postsynaptic receptors to hyperpolarize nerve cells. Thus, they diminish nociception without having any noticeable effect on motor function. In rats the potency of different opioids given intrathecally has been shown to be a linear function of lipid solubility (Dickenson *et al.*, 1990), with decreasing potency as lipophilicity increases. Morphine has been the most useful opioid given by epidural injection because it has a high potency and a long duration of action. It has been used in dogs (Bonath & Saleh, 1985), cats (Tung & Yaksh, 1982), horses (Valverde *et al.*, 1990), and goats (Pablo, 1993). The common side effects noted in animals with epidural morphine are pruritis and urinary retention (Drenger & Magora, 1989). It is believed that only about 0.3% of epidural morphine crosses the meninges in dogs (Durant & Yaksh, 1986).

Pethidine (meperidine)

In cats pethidine given epidurally has a rapid onset of action with a duration of up to 4 hours, depending on the dose (Tung & Yaksh, 1982). It must be noted in this connexion that pethidine has local analgesic properties in addition to its opioid activity (Jaffe & Rowe, 1996) and this may have a bearing on the rapidity of onset.

Methadone

Intrathecal methadone increases urinary bladder tone and decreases bladder compliance in dogs (Drenger *et al.*, 1986). It has also been given to cats (Tung & Yaksh, (1982) by epidural injection in doses of 0.7 to 1.0 mg/kg.

Oxymorphone

Epidural oxymorphone has been given to dogs and 0.1 mg/kg was shown to more effective and to last longer (10 hours compared with 2 hours) than 0.2 mg/kg given i.m. (Popilskis *et al.*, 1991). A more recent clinical study indicated that 0.05 mg/kg epidurally gave about 7 hours of good analgesia without significant side effects (Vesal *et al.*, 1996).

Fentanyl, sufentanil

There is considerable doubt about the effectiveness of these two opioids when given epidurally.

Butorphanol

A number of studies have failed to produce good evidence that there is any advantage in administering butorphanol epidurally rather than i.v. but the epidural route may have advantages in dogs (Troncy *et al.*, 1996).

Buprenorphine

The analgesia effects of epidural buprenorphine appear similar to those of epidural morphine. The occurrence of urinary retention is less likely with buprenorphine since its intrathecal injection has minimal effects on urodynamics in dogs (Drenger & Magora, 1989).

α_2 adrenoceptor agonists

When epidural doses of α_2 adrenoceptor agonists produce analgesia it is usual to see signs of sedation as a result of systemic uptake. Of the available compounds clonidine, xylazine, detomidine and medetomidine have been administered by the epidural route.

Clonidine

Clonidine has been used quite extensively in humans and is known to produce a dose dependent duration of analgesia accompanied by some sedation and systemic hypotension. In sheep the drug gave profound analgesia and some sedation with no hypotension (Eisenach *et al.*, 1987).

Xylazine

Epidural xylazine can provide profound analgesia in some animals without interfering with motor activity (Caulkett *et al.*, 1993). In cattle and llamas the onset of analgesia occurs within 15 to 20 minutes and persists for 2 to 3 hours; in horses the onset is slower but the analgesia lasts longer. Both horses and cattle show signs of sedation and decreased intestinal activity as well as slight ataxia. In cattle the systemic signs can be antagonized without loss of analgesia by systemic tolazoline (Skarda & Muir, 1990).

Detomidine

Mainly used in horses, epidural detomidine produces profound analgesia with ataxia and loss of proprioception. Skarda and Muir (1994) reported that 60 µg/kg administered at the first intercoccygeal space induced analgesia as far cranially as the 4th thoracic segment. Onset of analgesia was within 20 minutes and was accompanied by marked sedation, a reduction in heart and respiratory rates and an increase in $PaCO_2$. Ko *et al.* (1992) failed to produce analgesia in pigs after epidural injection of massive doses of detomidine.

Medetomidine

Epidural medetomidine in cats produces sedation and, often, vomiting, which suggests that its effects are mainly systemic following absorption from the epidural space. Further evidence in favour of this is that it produces an initial increase in arterial blood pressure followed some 20 minutes later by a decrease, while heart rate and respiratory rates are both decreased.

NMDA antagonists

Ketamine is known to have activity as a local analgesic, an NMDA antagonist, an opioid agonist/antagonist and, possibly, as an antimuscarinic. These complex actions have made the evaluation of epidural ketamine difficult. In isoflurane anaesthetized dogs epidural ketamine (2 mg/kg) is associated with minimal haemodynamic effects (Martin *et al.*, 1997). Further investigation is needed before epidural ketamine can be recommended.

Miscellaneous drugs

NSAIDs, corticosteroids anticholinesterases, inhibitors of nitric oxide synthase, vasopressin and somatostatin have all been shown to have some degree of analgesic effect when administered epidurally. Currently, none is used clinically by epidural injection.

Continuous epidural block

Continuous spinal blocks can be used to provide long term analgesia and, with the correct choice of drugs and drug concentrations, animals can be kept both ambulatory and pain free after operations on the caudal limbs, perineum and tail. The technique can also be used to prevent straining in cases of rectal and vaginal prolapse. In most instances the catheter is introduced into the epidural rather than subarachnoid space and the drugs are injected from a syringe in repeated small, fractional doses, or by slow continuous infusion using a syringe pump. The introduction of commercially available sterile packs of catheters and suitable needles has made the use of continuous blocks attractive in many species of animal.

The indications, advantages, contraindications and complications associated with continuous epidural block are similar to those of single injection techniques. The additional advantages of continuous block are the ability to maintain analgesia for long periods and to maintain a route for the injection of opioids and other drugs during surgery and postoperatively.

To date, continuous epidural block has not become a routine technique in veterinary anaesthesia because of technical difficulties in catheter placement, the potential for producing damage of the spinal cord, meninges and nerves, the risk of introducing infection and catheter related problems. However, practice should render the technique safer and its accomplishment less formidable in all species of animal.

Problems and hazards of epidural block

Very few drugs are specifically marketed for epidural or spinal use and those available for intramuscular or intravenous injection contain preservatives. Common preservatives are sodium bisulphite, benzethonium chloride, chlorbutanol and disodium EDTA. Their neurotoxicity is currently largely unknown. One preservative, methylparaben, does not appear to be toxic but has been associated with allergic responses in man (Adams *et al.*, 1977). Morphine is now marketed specifically for epidural use ('Duramorph') and this preparation is free from preservatives.

Testing for entry to the epidural space by loss of resistance to injection of a small quantity of air as is often used in children (Michel & Anaes, 1991) and sheep (Hall & Clarke, 1991) may be associated with incomplete or patchy absorption of epidural drugs, postoperative neurological deficits and even air embolism. (Dalens *et al.*, 1987; Stevens *et al.*, 1989; Sethna & Berde, 1993).

Arterial hypotension is more frequently the consequence of toxic blood levels after absorption or from undetected intravenous injection than the result of sympathetic block. It seems probable from experience in a variety of animals that the safety limits are to inject no more than 10 mg/kg of lignocaine and no more than 4 mg/kg of bupivacaine, but the maximal doses produced depend on the speed of injection and the time to reach maximum plasma concentration.

Catheters can be sheared off when pulled backward through the insertion needle. When advancement is impossible the needle and catheter should be withdrawn together and the procedure repeated. The management of cases where a catheter has sheared or broken is rather controversial, but a retained fragment is rarely a problem (Hurley & Lambert, 1990).

Puncture of the dura is not dangerous if recognized and does not contraindicate a second attempt (preferably at another interspace) with a slow speed of injection. Total spinal block occurs when dural puncture is not recognized and full doses intended for epidural injection are given. The first signs are changes in respiratory rate but haemodynamic changes are minimal. The pupils first become unequal, then dilated and apnoea follows. If the animal is intubated and ventilated with pure oxygen it is usually found that total spinal block takes about one hour to wear off. If the situation is under control it is probably not necessary to postpone surgery.

The major complication of a 'bloody tap', when blood issues from the hub of a spinal needle, is the danger of intravascular injection that can result in cardiac toxicity.

REFERENCES

Adams, H., Mastri, A. and Charron, D. (1977) Morphological effects of subarachnoid methylparaben on rabbit spinal cord. *Pharmacological Research Communications* **9**: 547–551.

Arndt, J.O. (1986) The low pressure system: the integrated function of veins. *European Journal of Anaesthesiology* **3**: 343–370.

Bernards, C.M., and Hill, H.F. (1990) Morphine and alfentanil permeability through the spinal dura, arachnoid and pia mater of dogs and monkeys. *Anesthesiology* **73**: 1214–1219.

Bouarth, K.H. and Saleh, A.S. (1985) Long-term pain treatment in the dog by peridural morphine. *Proceedings of the 2nd International Congress of Anesthesia*, Sacramento, p. 161.

Brook, G.B. (1930) Spinal (epidural) anaesthesia in cattle. *Veterinary Record* **10**: 30–36.

Brook, G.B. (1935) Spinal (epidural) anaesthesia in the domestic animal. A review of our knowledge at the present time. *Veterinary Record* **15**: 549–553; 576–581; 597–606; 631–635; 659–667.

Caulkett, N., Cribb, P.H., Duke, T. (1993) Xylazine epidural analgesia for cesarian section in cattle. *Canadian Veterinary Journal* **34**: 674–676.

Dalens, B., Bazin, J.E. and Haberer, J. P. (1987) Epidural air bubbles a cause of incomplete analgesia during epidural anesthesia. *Anesthesia and Analgesia* **66**: 697–683.

Dickenson, A., Sullivan, A. and McQuay, H. (1990) Intrathecal etorphine, fentanyl and buprenorphine on spinal nociceptive neurones in the rat. *Pain* **42**: 227–234.

Drenger, B., Magora, F., Evron, S. *et al.* (1986) The action of intrathecal morphine and methadone on the lower urinary tract of the dog. *Journal of Urology* **135**: 852–855.

Drenger, B. and Magora, F. (1989) Urodynamic studies after intrathecal fentanyl and buprenorphine in the dog. *Anesthesia and Analgesia* **69**: 348–353.

Durant, P.A.C. and Yaksh, T.L. (1986) Distribution in cerebrospinal fluid, blood and lymph of epidurally injected morphine and inulin in dogs. *Anesthesia and Analgesia* **65**: 583–592.

Eisenach, J.C., Dewan, D.M., Rose, J.C. and Angelo, J.M. (1987) Epidural clonidine produces antinociception, but not hypotension in sheep. *Anesthesiology* **66**: 496–501.

Emhke, H., Persson, P.B. and Kirchheim, H.R. (1987) A physiological role for pressure-dependent renin release in long term pressure control. *Pfluegers Archive European Journal of Physiology* **410**: 450–456.

Feldman, H. and Covino, B. (1988) Comparative motor blocking effects of bupivacaine and ropivacaine, a new amino amide local anesthetic in the rat and dog. *Anesthesia and Analgesia* **67**: 1047–1052.

Hall, L. W. and Clarke, K.W. (1991) *Veterinary Anaesthesia*, 9th ed. London: Baillière Tindal, p. 263.

Hurley, R.J. and Lambert, D.H. (1990) Continuous spinal anesthesia with a microcatheter technique; preliminary experience. *Anesthesia and Analgesia* **70**: 97–102.

Jaffe, R.A. and Rowe, M.A. (1996) A comparison of the local anesthetic effects of meperidine, fentanyl and sufentanil on dorsal root axons. *Anesthesia and Analgesia* **83**: 776–781.

Keates, A.S. (1988) Anesthesia mortality – a new mechanism. *Anesthesiology* **68**: 2–4.

Ko, J.C.H., Thurmon, J.C., Benson, J.G. *et al.* (1992) Comparison of epidural analgesia induced by detomidine or xylazine in swine. *Veterinary Surgery* **21**: 82.

Martin, D.D., Tranquilli, W.J., Olson, W.A., Thurmon, J.C. and Besson, G.J. (1997) Hemodynamic effects of epidural ketamine in isoflurane anesthetized dogs. *Veterinary Surgery* **26**: 505–509.

Pablo, L.S. (1993) Epidural morphine in goats after hindlimb orthopedic surgery. *Veterinary Surgery* **22**: 307–310.

Peters, J., Kutkuhn, B., Medert, H.A., Schlaghecke, R., Schuttler, J. and Arndt, J.O. (1990) Sympathetic blockade by epidural anesthesia attenuates the cardiovascular response to severe hypoxemia. *Anesthesiology* **72**: 134–144.

Peters, J., Schlaghecke, R., Thouet, H. and Arndt, J.O. (1990a) Endogenous vasopressin supports blood pressure and prevents severe hypotension during epidural anesthesia in conscious dogs. *Anesthesiology* **73**: 694–702.

Popilskis S. Kohn, D., Sanchez J.A. and Gorman, P. (1991) Epidural vs. intramuscular oxymorphone analgesia after thoracotomy in dogs. *Veterinary Surgery* **20**: 462–467.

Reiz, S., Häggmark, S. Johansson, G. and Nath, S. (1989) Cardiotoxicity of ropivacaine – a new amide local anaesthetic agent. *Acta Anaesthesiologica Scandinavica* **33**: 93–98.

Sethna, N.F. and Berde, C.B. (1993) Venous air embolism during identification of the epidural space in children. *Anesthesia and Analgesia* **76**: 925–927.

Share, L. (1988) Role of vasopressin in cardiovascular regulation. *Physiological Reviews* **68**: 1248–1284.

Skarda, R.T. and Muir, W.W. III (1990) Influence of tolazoline on caudal epidural administration of xylazine in cattle. *American Journal of Veterinary Research* **51**: 556–560.

Stevens, R., Mikat-Stevens, M., Van Clief, M. *et al.* (1989) Deliberate epidural air injection in dogs: a radiographic study. *Regional Anesthesia* **14**: 180–182.

Troncy, E., Cuvelliez, S. and Blaise, D. (1996) Evaluation of analgesia and cardiorespiratory effects of epidurally administered butorphanol in isoflurane-anesthetized dogs. *American Journal of Veterinary Research* **57**: 1478–1482.

Tung, A.S. and Yaksh, T.L. (1982) The antinociceptive effects of epidural opiates in the cat: Studies on the pharmacology and the effects of lipophilicity in spinal analgesia. *Pain* **12**: 343–356.

Valverde, A., Little, C.B. Dyson, D.H. and Motter, C.H. (1990) Use of epidural morphine to relieve pain in a horse. *Canadian Veterinary Journal* **31**: 211–212.

Vesal, N., Cribb, P. and Frketic, M. (1996) Postoperative analgesic and cardiopulmonary effects of oxymorphone administered epidurally and intramuscularly, and medetomidine administered epidurally: a comparative clinical study. *Veterinary Surgery* **25**: 361–369.

Wang, C., Chakrabarti, M.K. and Whitwam, J.G. (1993) Specific enhancement by fentanyl of the effects of intrathecal bupivacaine on nociceptive afferent but not sympathetic efferent pathways in dogs. *Anesthesiology* **79**: 766–733.

Anaesthesia of the Species

Anaesthesia of the horse

INTRODUCTION

Probably no other species of animal presents as many special problems to the veterinary anaesthetist as the horse. Perioperative mortality rate in relation to general anaesthesia in apparently healthy horses is around 1% (Johnston *et al.*, 1995) and has remained constant over at least 30 years (Hall, 1983; Tevik, 1983; Clarke & Gerring, 1990; Young & Taylor, 1993) despite increasing sophistication of anaesthetic techniques and monitoring. However, lack of improvement in survival rates results mainly from the longer duration of many surgical procedures which, without the advances which have occurred, would have been impossible to perform. Increased duration of anaesthesia significantly increases the risk (Johnston *et al.*, 1995). The veterinary anaesthetist is faced with numerous disturbances of cardiopulmonary and skeletal muscle function associated with general anaesthesia, many of which are only very incompletely understood. Their certain prevention is currently impossible, and measures designed to overcome one problem often only result in exacerbation of another. Developments in the provision of reliable sedation has enabled a wider range of procedures to be carried out under local analgesia than was once considered practicable, but even this technique is not without risk (to horse and operator) and general anaesthesia still remains the only option in many cases.

SEDATION OF THE STANDING HORSE

It frequently is necessary to sedate horses to enable procedures to be carried out easily and safely. Horses are not good subjects for sedation for if they experience a feeling of muscle weakness or ataxia they may panic in a violent manner. Historically, the most effective sedative was, for many years, chloral hydrate, but its use required administration of large volumes of solution and panic responses to ataxia produced by it were occasionally encountered. Other drugs used included cannabis indica, bulbocapnine, bromides, and pentobarbitone (Amadon & Craige, 1936; Wright, 1942). The introduction of the mood-altering 'neuroleptic' agents, in particular the phenothiazines, followed in 1969 by xylazine (Clarke & Hall, 1969), and more recently other α_2 adrenoceptor agonists, has revolutionized equine sedation and, with the additional use of local analgesic techniques, enable many procedures to be performed in the standing animal. However, even with modern agents, sedated horses must be handled with caution for they may be aroused by stimulation and when disturbed can respond with a very well aimed kick.

PHENOTHIAZINES

Acepromazine

Acepromazine is the phenothiazine derivative most widely used in horses for both its mood-altering and sedative actions. Intravenous (i.v.) doses of 0.03 mg/kg or intramuscular (i.m.) of 0.05 mg/kg exert a calming effect within 20–30 minutes of injection and, although at these dose rates obvious sedation may only be apparent in 60% of horses, they become much easier to handle. Doses may be doubled, but the dose–response curve of acepromazine is such that the level of sedation does not always increase, although the duration will. Acepromazine (in paste or tablet forms) also may be given orally at maximally recommended doses of 0.1 mg/kg. Oral availability in horses is high and can be equal to that of the i.m. route (Hashem & Keller, 1993). Acepromazine is very long acting, and elimination may be further delayed in old or sick animals, particularly in those with even mild liver disease.

Acepromazine at the doses recommended has little effect on ventilation, but causes hypotension through vasodilation, and hypovolaemic horses may faint. Tachycardia results from the fall in arterial blood pressure (ABP), but sometimes first degree atrioventicular block is seen. A very small proportion of horses (the authors have seen two such cases) show aberrant reactions, and may become recumbent without there being any apparent cardiovascular cause; these reactions were more common with other phenothiazine agents. In male animals effective sedation with phenothiazine derivatives is associated with protrusion of the flaccid penis or, on very rare occasions, priapism. In either case, physical damage to the penis must be avoided. In the vast majority of animals the penis retracts as sedation wears off; in a very small proportion prolonged prolapse occurs. Treatment of this complication is by manual massage, compression bandage and replacement in the prepuce followed by suture of the preputial orifice. It is the opinion of the authors that the low incidence of this complication coupled with the possibility of immediate treatment means that where a phenothiazine agent is the drug of choice its use is not contraindicated in stallions or geldings.

Acepromazine has proved a very safe agent in the horse. The calming and low level sedative effects it produces make it the agent of choice for interventions such as shoeing, and when used in young animals it appears to assist in training the horse to tolerate many future procedures without

sedation. When acepromazine is combined with opioid agents deep sedation is achieved, and such combinations may be used in cases where α_2 adrenoceptor agonists alone would be inappropriate. Acepromazine is an excellent premedicant before general anaesthesia; it calms the horse prior to the insertion of catheters, lengthens the action of the anaesthetic agents, statistically reduces the anaesthetic risk in the horse (Johnston *et al.*, 1995) and its prolonged duration of action means that it contributes to a quiet recovery.

α_2 ADRENOCEPTOR AGONISTS

Xylazine

Following the introduction of xylazine for sedating horses, it rapidly gained in popularity because of the reliable sedation produced. Doses of 0.5–1.1 mg/kg i.v. are followed within 2 minutes by obvious signs of effect. The horse's head is lowered and the eyelids and lower lip droop (Clarke & Hall 1969; Kerr *et al.*, 1972). Although the horse may sway on its feet, cross its hindlegs or knuckle on a foreleg, it will remain on its feet and show no panic. Sedation is maximal after about 5 minutes and lasts 30 to 60 minutes depending on the dose. Doses of 2 to 3 mg/kg i.m. give similar effects, maximal sedation being achieved 20 minutes after injection. Xylazine has analgesic properties, particularly in colic (Pippi & Lumb, 1979; Lowe & Hilfiger, 1986; Jochle *et al.*, 1989; England & Clarke, 1996) and in colic cases analgesia is associated with the marked reduction in gut movement caused by drugs of this class. Horses sedated with xylazine remain very sensitive to touch and the apparently well sedated horse may, if disturbed, respond with a very sudden and accurate kick.

The cardiopulmonary effects of xylazine in horses have been well investigated (Muir *et al.*, 1979a; Short, 1992; England & Clarke, 1996). A transient rise in ABP peaks 1–2 minutes after i.v. injection; the pressure then slowly falls to below resting values and remains depressed for at least one hour. Concurrent with the hypertensive phase there is profound bradycardia coupled with both atrioventicular and sinoatrial heart block. Heart block is at its most intense in the first few minutes and in many cases disappears as the heart rate increases. Changes in ABP are dose dependent in intensity and duration, and following i.m. injection changes are similar but less marked. Cardiac output (CO) is significantly reduced, i.v. doses of 1.1 mg/kg causing falls of 20–40% of normal resting values. At doses of up to 1.1 mg/kg xylazine does not cause severe respiratory depression although there may be a small rise in $PaCO_2$ and a slight decrease in PaO_2. However, some upper airway obstruction may occur. Heavy coated horses may sweat as sedation is waning – this is most commonly seen if atmospheric temperatures are high. Other side effects are those typical of α_2 adrenoceptor agonists and include hyperglycaemia (Thurmon *et al.*, 1982) and diuresis. Changes in insulin production and hyperglycaemia do not appear to be a feature of xylazine action in neonatal foals (Robertson *et al.*, 1990).

When used as a premedicant, xylazine greatly reduces the amount of both injectable and volatile anaesthetic agents subsequently required. In the 30 years since its launch xylazine has become the 'gold standard' for equine sedation and premedication, particularly in North America. In Europe until the advent of generic forms and alternative agents forced prices to reduce to a realistic level, its use was limited by much higher pricing.

Detomidine

Detomidine, a very potent α_2 adrenoceptor agonist was first used as a sedative and analgesic agent by Alitalo and Vainio in 1982, and since its introduction has gained great popularity for sedation and premedication of all types of horse (Vainio, 1985; Alitalo, 1986; Clarke & Taylor, 1986; Short, 1992). Initially very high doses (up to 160 µg/kg) of detomidine were recommended but it soon became obvious that maximal sedative effects were obtained with i.v. doses of 20 µg/kg and that higher doses increased the duration rather than depth of sedation. Slightly higher doses appear necessary to provide good analgesia (Hamm & Jochle, 1984). The concentrated but non-irritant form of 10 mg/ml in which detomidine (as Domosedan or Dormasedan) is provided makes it very suitable for i.m. injection, doses approximately twice those given i.v. being required to produce the same effect.

Detomidine has some effect when injected subcutaneously (SC) and is also absorbed through mucous membranes. The latter property has been utilized by administering the drug on sugar lumps, peppermint sweets or, more effectively, squirting it under the tongue (Malone & Clarke, 1993). When given in food, the effect is less reliable as the drug is extensively metabolized by first pass through the liver. The property of easy absorption across mucous membranes must, for reasons of personal safety, be taken into account when handling the drug.

The type of sedation produced by detomidine is identical to that produced by xylazine; blind trials failed to identify which horses had been given 1 mg/kg xylazine i.v. and which 20 µg/kg detomidine i.v. (England *et al.*, 1992), except by duration of action. As with xylazine, horses under detomidine sedation are sensitive to touch and may kick. Lower doses of detomidine do not always result in maximal sedation, but may prove useful where a short period of action is required. Detomidine premedication reduces the dose of anaesthetic agents subsequently required.

The pharmacological properties of detomidine are typical of those of an α_2 adrenoceptor agonist. Following doses of 10–20 µg/kg i.v. cardiovascular changes are very similar to those following xylazine (Short, 1992), there being a marked bradycardia with heart block, coupled with arterial hypertension followed by hypotension. However, with higher doses the hypertensive phase is considerably more prolonged (Vainio, 1985; Short *et al.*, 1986). Whether this hypertension is then followed by prolonged hypotension has not been investigated – most studies terminating when sedation ceases. At clinically used doses respiration is slowed and PaO_2 is slightly decreased. Some horses snore – presumably from congestion of the nasal mucous membranes. The authors have noted occasional horses (usually those suffering from toxaemic conditions) becoming tachypnoepic for some 10–15 minutes after the administration of detomidine. Similar reactions have been observed after other α_2 adrenoceptor agonists xylazine, romifidine and medetomidine (Clarke & Gerring 1990; Bettschart *et al.*, 1999a). Other effects include reduction in gut motility, hyperglycaemia, sweating and an increase in urination. Doses above 60 µg/kg may cause swelling of the head; this problem appears to be associated with the prolonged head droop and can be prevented by propping the head in a more normal position. Occasionally urticarial reactions have been noted; these are self-limiting and regress without treatment. Moderate doses of detomidine are claimed to be safe in pregnancy and many mares have received multiple doses throughout gestation without any maternal or foetal harm resulting. Abortion has been reported in a pony mare which had received detomidine (Katila & Oijala, 1988), but the authors considered the abortion was due to other causes.

The actions of detomidine (and of other α_2 adrenoceptor agonists) can be reversed by the specific antagonist, *atipamezole*. Dose rates from 60–200 µg/kg have been used, that required depending on the degree of residual sedation (Nilsfors & Kvart 1986; Ramseyer *et al.*, 1998; Bettschart *et al.*, 1999a). At the doses of detomidine recommended it is rare that antagonism is required, but the authors have been grateful of its availability in cases of overdosage of α_2/opioid combinations where a horse has become severely ataxic or even recumbent.

Romifidine

Romifidine is a recent α_2 adrenoceptor agonist marketed for use in horses. The type of sedation produced by romifidine differs from that produced by the other α_2 adrenoceptor agonists; the horse's head does not hang so low, and there is considerably less ataxia (Voetgli, 1988; England *et al.*, 1992). Nevertheless, doses of from 40–120 µg/kg i.v. result in sedation which enables a range of clinical procedures to be performed. In clinical practice romifidine has proved very popular where ataxia is particularly unwelcome, e.g. for shoeing. When used to sedate animals for surgical procedures, romifidine is generally combined with opioid agents as indeed are most α_2 adrenoceptor agonists. The pharmacological actions of romifidine other than sedation are similar to all α_2 adrenoceptor agonists. Following i.v. administration there is bradycardia, a fall in CO, and hypertension followed by lowered blood pressure (Clarke *et al.*, 1991; Freeman, 1998). Romifidine

reduces gut motility, the duration of this effect being dose dependant (Freeman, 1998). Self-limiting urticarial reactions may occur occasionally. The degree of analgesia produced by romifidine has been questioned; Voegtli (1988) found that analgesia did occur but was not dose related or consistent, whilst other work has suggested that it is devoid of analgesic activity (Hamm *et al.*, 1995). Nevertheless, romifidine is widely used for premedication and as part of anaesthetic combinations it reduces the dose of anaesthetic agents subsequently used.

Medetomidine

Medetomidine's use has been investigated in horses (Bryant *et al.*, 1991; Bettschart *et al.*, 1999). Doses of 5–7 µg/kg i.v. are sufficient to cause very deep sedation with severe ataxia, and higher doses may result in recumbency. The marked hypnotic properties make the agent unsuitable for routine use as a sedative in horses. However, it appears to be very short acting in the horse, and its excellent analgesic and muscle relaxant properties mean that it can be a useful agent as part of an anaesthetic process.

PRACTICAL USE OF α_2 ADRENOCEPTOR AGONISTS IN THE HORSE.

The different manifestation of sedation and lack of ataxia with romifidine excepted, the remaining properties, including all side effects, appear similar with all three α_2 adrenoceptor agonists commonly used in horses (Fig. 11.1). Thus choice will depend on the duration of action required, the route of administration, and on personal preferences. For example, all three agents provide excellent analgesia in cases of colic, although the bradycardia and lack of gut motility induced must be considered in the subsequent assessment. Before a definitive diagnosis has been made in a colic case it is preferable to use xylazine or a low dose (up to 20 µg/kg) of detomidine for sedation and analgesia, as high doses may mask signs indicating the requirement for surgery. Following a decision that surgery is required, the longer acting romifidine with its lack of ataxia, may be the most suitable analgesic for transportation. Although

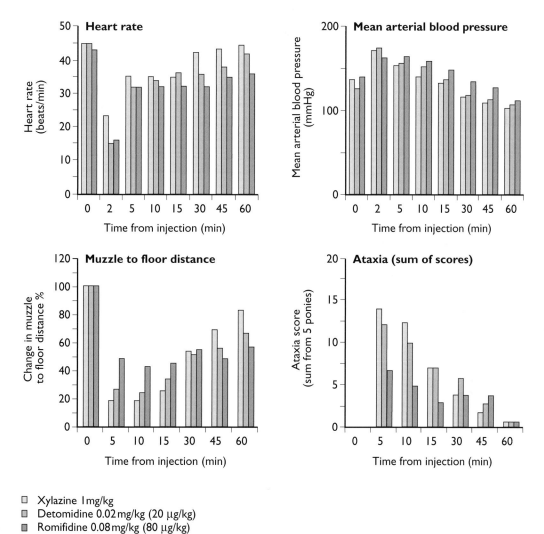

FIG. 11.1 Comparison of some of the sedative and cardiovascular effects of i.v. doses of xylazine (1 mg/kg), detomidine (20 μg/kg) and romifidine (80 μg/kg). Data from 5 ponies. SE bars are omitted for the sake of clarity (from Clarke (1988), Clarke *et al.*, 1991; England *et al.*, 1992).

there are no scientific studies of combining different α₂ adrenoceptor agonists, in practical clinical use there are many reports of changing from one to another at subsequent dosing; the effects appear to be additive as expected.

α₂ Adrenoceptor agonists have marked cardiopulmonary side effects, and it is not surprising that occasional cases of collapse, or even of death have been reported following their use. Some reported cases may have resulted from intracarotid injection, but where there is a delay between injection of the drug and the unexpected

event, then such a reaction is probably drug induced. In dogs, xylazine sensitizes the heart to adrenaline induced arrhythmias but in horse such sensitization has not been proved (W.W. Muir, personal communication). However, there are anecdotal reports of collapse in horses which are given an α₂ adrenoceptor agonist when in a high state of excitement. Unfortunately immediate sedation is necessary in many such situations, and in these cases sufficient time must be left after drug administration before further stimulation is applied. In such situations, the authors prefer combinations with acepromazine, which may reduce the risk. Clinical reports have suggested that combinations of α_2 adrenoceptor agonists and potentiated sulfonamides should be avoided, although the scientific basis of these observations is unproven.

Some authorities premedicate horses with an anticholinergic agent (atropine or glycopyrrolate) prior to the administration of an α_2 adrenoceptor agonist, but use of such combinations is controversial. Anticholinergic drugs will prevent or reverse the bradycardia caused by α_2 adrenoceptor agonists and will improve CO. However, the bradycardia protects against the hypertension caused by α_2 adrenoceptor agonist induced vasoconstriction and once pulse rate rises, so does ABP (Alibhai & Clarke, 1996). Anticholinergic drugs, if used, must be given an adequate time prior to sedation; giving the two drugs together is pointless.

Infusions of α_2 adrenoceptor agonists

Where α_2 adrenoceptor agonists are being used to provide sedation for surgery, sometimes it is necessary to increase their duration of action. Intermittent dosing, each increment being 25–50% of the original dose administered, is effective, but infusion results in a more level and controllable plane of sedation. There are few scientific studies as to the doses required; usually, the agent used is diluted in a saline drip, then, following the initial loading dose, is infused to effect. The authors have found that in conscious horses an infusion of 0.55 mg/kg/hour of xylazine provides good sedation with minimal ataxia. Detomidine infusions at 0.18 μg/kg/min have been demonstrated to provide steady sedation and to be appropriate for intraoperative infusion (Wagner et al., 1992; Daunt et al., 1993). Infusions of 3.5 μg/kg/hour of medetomidine following a loading dose of 5 μg/kg give deep sedation and have also proved effective in providing intraoperative analgesia without resulting in any delay of recovery (Bettschart et al., 1999).

Administration of α_2 adrenoceptor agonists by other routes

α_2 Adrenoceptor agonists are strong analgesics when administered by epidural or subarachnoid injection. The caudal epidural administration of 0.17 mg/kg of xylazine in 10 ml of normal saline produces safe, effective perineal analgesia of 2.5 hours duration in horses without apparent side effects (LeBlanc et al., 1988). More recently extensive investigations have been carried out into the analgesic and systemic effects of xylazine and detomidine given by this route (Skarda & Muir 1994; 1996a, b; 1998). To date there are no reports of the epidural adminstration of romifidine. Caudal epidural xylazine (0.25 mg/kg) gives perineal analgesia and variable bilateral analgesia as far forward as S3 with minimal systemic effects. In order to obtain adequate perineal analgesia with epidural detomidine, doses of 60 μg/kg were required, which resulted in variable spread of analgesia sometimes extending to the thoracic region. Systemic effects (e.g. bradycardia and sedation) suggested that a significant quantity of detomidine had been absorbed, and horses were sometimes very ataxic. However, when given by the midsacral subarachnoid route, 30 μg/kg detomidine gave good analgesia from the coccyx to the lumbar region with minimal systemic effects. Systemic effects could be antagonized with agents such as atipamezole given systemically or by the epidural route. With either α_2 adrenoceptor agonist, onset of perineal analgesia occurred within 15 minutes. Skarda and Muir (1996a, b) suggested that xylazine was exerting a local anaesthetic effect, hence the low doses required in comparison to those used when the drug is given systemically.

α_2 Adrenoceptor agonists have also been given by the epidural route in combination with opioids and/or local anaesthetic agents.

BENZODIAZEPINES

Diazepam, midazolam, climazolam and zolazepam

The anxiolytic properties of diazepam are not obvious in horses and the drug should not be used on its own as it gives rise to ataxia, sometimes associated with panic, possibly through its muscle relaxing properties (Muir et al., 1982). Another benzodiazepine, climazolam, has been found to have similar properties and the antagonist sarmazenil has been used to reverse its effects.

Although not useful as a sedatives in adult horses the benzodiazepine agents can be used in foals which will usually become recumbent following i.v. 0.1–0.25 mg/kg of diazepam or midazolam (a water soluble benzodiazepine). The muscle relaxation induced by benzodiazepine agents is useful during anaesthesia, and benzodiazepines such as diazepam, climazolam, midazolam and zolazepam have all been incorporated into anaesthetic regimes used in adult horses.

OTHER CATEGORIES

Chloral hydrate

Chloral hydrate was a popular sedative for horses but it has largely fallen into disuse because its administration poses problems and sedation is accompanied by ataxia. Details of suitable doses can be found in earlier editions of this book and it is still a useful component in some mixtures used in equine anaesthesia.

Reserpine

Reserpine has been employed for its prolonged calming action, but has many side effects and does not give the type of sedation allowing veterinary procedures to be carried out easily (Tobin, 1978).

DRUG COMBINATIONS

In the search for a completely reliable, safe method of producing sedation in standing horses a number of mixtures of drugs have been used. Appropriate doses of many of these have proved to have a more certain and profound effect than can be regularly obtained from the use of any single drug. However, the possibility of untoward reactions and appearance of as yet unrecognized drug interactions must always be considered when these mixtures are employed.

Acepromazine/α_2 adrenoceptor agonist combinations

Acepromazine (0.02–0.05 mg/kg) and α_2 adrenoceptor agonists such as xylazine (0.5–1.0 mg/kg), detomidine (10–20 µg/kg) or romifidine (50–

100 µg/kg) have often been used together for sedating horses. The prolonged calming action of acepromazine is useful in a variety of circumstances, particularly if the horse was very excited prior to sedation, both for premedication and in combination with opioids. Some North American sources have considered that acepromazine and the α_2 adrenoceptor agonists should not be used together. The pharmacological reasoning behind the suggestion that the two drugs should not be given together rests on the fact that acepromazine causes hypotension and the α_2 adrenoceptor agonist causes bradycardia. However, the maximal bradycardia occurs within 1–2 minutes of injection, and at this time is accompanied by hypertension. If detomidine is given to horses already sedated with acepromazine, there is still a hypertensive response, albeit starting from a lower base (Muir et al., 1979a). The authors have administered xylazine, detomidine or romifidine to over 4000 horses already sedated with acepromazine with no ill effects (other than an increase in ataxia) and providing both drugs are given at suitable doses there is no reason why the combination cannot be used.

Sedative/opioid combinations

The pharmacological basis for combination of sedatives with opioids has already been discussed (Chapter 4). Their use in the horse is not new (Martin & Beck, 1956; Klein, 1975) and a very large number of such combinations have been investigated and advocated for use in this species of animal (Martin & Beck, 1956; Muir et al., 1979b; Robertson & Muir 1983; Nolan & Hall, 1984; Clarke & Paton, 1988). The addition of opioids, even at subanalgesic doses, appears to enhance sedation dramatically and, in particular, diminishes the response to touch, thus reducing the likelihood of provoking well directed kicks from the sedated horse. The disadvantage is that ataxia is also increased (particularly with combinations involving methadone or butorphanol), and occasionally a horse may become recumbent. Opioid excitement reactions such as aimless walking may occur when sedation becomes inadequate and it is irrational to combine a short acting sedative such as xylazine with opioids with long actions such as buprenorphine or high doses of morphine.

TABLE 11.1 Some of the sedative/opioid combinations that have been satisfactorily used; there are many other combinations which are likely to be as satisfactory

Sedative 1	Sedative 2	Opioid
Acepromazine, 0.05–0.10 mg/kg		Methadone, 0.05–0.10 mg/kg or Butorphanol, 0.02–0.04 mg/kg
Acepromazine, 0.02–0.05 mg/kg	Xylazine, 0.5 mg/kg or Detomidine, 0.01 mg/kg or Romifidine, 0.04–0.08 mg/kg	
Acepromazine, 0.04–0.06 mg/kg	Detomidine, 0.01 mg/kg	Butorphanol, 0.01–0.02 mg/kg or Methadone, 0.05 mg/kg
Xylazine, 0.5–0.6 mg/kg or Detomidine, 0.010–0.015 mg/kg or Romifidine, 0.04–0.08 mg/kg		Butorphanol, 0.02–0.05 mg/kg or Methadone, 0.05–0.10 mg/kg.

Acepromazine has a very long action so problems are less when this is part of the combination. The incidence of opioid-induced excitement occurring can be reduced by administering sedatives first followed by opioids once sedation is apparent, although if the opioid concerned is one which has a delayed onset of action (e.g. buprenorphine), this is neither necessary nor desirable.

Table 11.1 lists some of the sedative/opioid combinations that have been satisfactorily used, but there are many other potential combinations which are likely to be as satisfactory. The dose of opioid required is considerably less than that producing analgesia (and with these combinations, local analgesia should still be employed for surgery). In recent years the most popular opioid for use in such combinations has been butorphanol, which has the advantage of not being subject to such strict control regulations as the pure agonists. In the UK the combination of i.v. detomidine (10–15 μg/kg) or romifidine (40–120 μg/kg) and butorphanol (0.02 mg/kg) has proved very suc-

cessful, particularly for clipping fractious horses. Prolonged sedation can be achieved by initial dosage of both agents followed by an infusion of the α_2 adrenoceptor; often further dosing of the opioid is not needed, although this depends on the duration of action of the agent chosen. Caution is needed to prevent cross contamination of the drugs in their multi-dose bottles; the authors have seen several cases of gross overdosage (the horse becoming very ataxic, or recumbent) where this has occurred.

ANALGESIA

As with all species, the perioperative analgesic requirements in the horse are generally met by non-steroidal analgesics, opioid analgesics and local analgesics. In certain circumstances α_2 adrenoceptor agonists and agents used as anaesthetic agents, such as ketamine, also play a part in the provision of analgesia.

NON-STEROIDAL ANTI-INFLAMMATORY ANALGESICS (NSAIDs)

Non-steroidal anti-inflammatory agents are widely used in horses for the provision of analgesia for acute pain, for their anti-inflammatory action in injury and disease, for anti-endotoxaemic actions and for the provision of analgesia in chronic pain. Although they have not been shown to provide any intraoperative analgesia (Alibhai & Clarke, 1996), they are often administered at premedication or intraoperatively so that their analgesic and anti-inflammatory actions will be effective at the time of recovery.

For many years, phenylbutazone was the NSAID of choice for equine use, and it still remains an inexpensive and very effective agent that may be given by injection in the immediate perioperative period, then orally for continuing postoperative care. Although it can cause toxic reactions, these are well known, and can be avoided with correct dosing schedules. However, currently in Europe it may not be used in food animals, and in many countries this includes horses. Other older agents used in the horse include dipyrone and meclofenic acid. In the last 10 years the most popular NSAID for use in the horse has been flunixin meglumate, which gives excellent analgesia in a wide variety of circumstances. Several of the new, very effective and potentially less toxic NSAIDs including carprofen, cedaprofen and ketoprofen are marketed in oral and/or injectable formulations for horses, and others may soon become available.

The major problem with NSAIDs is their high toxicity and fairly low therapeutic index and, although in theory the newer COX 2 sparing agents such as carprofen and vedaprofen should cause fewer problems, it will be only after some years of use that lack of toxic effects will be confirmed. The major sites of toxicity of the NSAIDs are the gastrointestinal tract, kidneys, liver and the blood cells. In horses, the gastrointestinal tract appears the organ most affected, overdose of the agent causing stomach ulceration, and also damage to other areas, including the large bowel, leading to diarrhoea. In the horse renal damage, even in the presence of hypotension, is not common, and NSAIDs are administered before or during anaesthesia without apparent problems. Liver damage due to NSAIDs has been reported in old horses maintained on NSAIDs, and blood dyscrasias have occurred in horses given high doses of phenylbutazone. Many of the injectable preparations are contraindicated for i.m. use in the horse as they cause local irritation. At least one i.v. preparation of phenylbutazone can cause severe cardiac arrhythmias if injected too fast (probably because of the solvent, rather than the drug), so in the absence of evidence to the contrary, it is best to administer all i.v. NSAIDs slowly, especially in anaesthetized horses.

The pharmacokinetics of NSAIDs vary greatly between species. In normal horses, the half-lives of some of the commonly used agents are as follows:

- Phenylbutazone: 4.5–9.0 hours
- Flunixin: 1.6–2.1 hours
- Meloxycam: 3 hours
- Carprofen: 18 hours
- Vedaprofen: 6–8 hours
- Ketoprofen: 0.7–1.0 hour.
  (Cunningham & Lees 1995; product information sheets).

Breakdown products of some agents are themselves active. Knowledge of the half-life is necessary to assess dosing schedules but efficacy may outlast effective blood levels as in some cases the NSAID is concentrated in the inflammatory fluid at the site of injury. Toxic effects, most commonly manifest by diarrhoea, are usually due to cumulation, and are most likely to occur some days into the postoperative period. It is therefore very important not to exceed the data sheet recommendations for doses and frequency of dosing, and to realise that if more than one NSAID is employed, their toxic effects will be cumulative. Even if the manufacturers guidelines are kept, toxicity may be greater than expected in a sick horse, for example in shocked animals, or in hypoproteinaemia (NSAIDs are highly protein bound).

NSAIDs are widely used as analgesics for colic but the response may be variable – sometimes there is complete relief from pain, even in cases where there is non-viable intestine, whilst another case with an identical lesion may show no remission of symptoms. NSAIDs prevent the onset of symptoms of endotoxaemia, such as the increase in pulse rate and in PCV. Prevention of these changes coupled with analgesia may prevent recognition of the onset of 'shock' and diagnosis of surgical conditions. Thus, it is better if NSAIDs are not given to horses with colic until there is a definitive diagnosis, and a decision for surgery (or not) is made. When using NSAIDs in the postoperative period in colic cases consideration must be given to the effect of altered blood protein levels, and of circulation (which may increase half-life) on their pharmacokinetics. It is difficult to distinguish whether diarrhoea following surgery for colic is due to endotoxaemia or is, itself, due to the toxicity of the NSAIDs used.

OPIOID ANALGESICS

Opioid analgesics are now widely used in the horse to provide analgesia during and after surgery, as well as in combination with sedative agents for restraint. As in all other species of animal, they cause a dose-related respiratory depression. The cardiovascular effects of high doses include tachycardia and arterial hypertension, although at clinical dose rates such responses are minimal (Muir *et al.*, 1978a). Excitement can occur following their use, depending on dosage and

TABLE 11.2 **Doses of opioids for producing analgesi; i.m. injection minimizes the risk of excitement reactions**

Opioid	Dose and route
Morphine	0.05–0.1 mg/kg i.v. or i.m. Up to 0.25 mg/kg i.m.
Methadone	0.1 mg/kg i.v. or i.m.
Oxymorphone	0.05–0.3 mg/kg i.v. or i.m.
Pethidine	1–2 mg/kg i.m. only
Buprenorphine	0.006 mg/kg i.v. or i.m.
Butorphanol	0.05–0.10 mg/kg i.v.

whether or not the horse is in pain at the time of their administration. Excitement is manifest in various ways from muzzle twitching, muscular spasms, ataxia, snatching at food, uncontrollable walking through to violent excitement. Tobin and co-workers (Tobin & Combie, 1982) developed a 'step-counting' method of measuring the walking or locomotor response and obtained dose–response curves very similar to those obtained for analgesia. It is probable that many of these responses are due to stimulation of μ(OP3) receptors.

The assessment of analgesic activity is very difficult. Drugs may affect different types of pain in different ways and despite a variety of experimental methods of assessment it is not easy to be certain of the most effective dose in any clinical circumstance. Table 11.2 lists suggested doses for some opioids but it must be remembered that the response obtained (both of analgesia and side effects) will depend on many factors such as the presence or absence of pre-existing pain and the presence of sedative or anaesthetic drugs.

Pure agonists

Morphine

Of the agonist drugs, morphine is still to be regarded as an excellent postoperative analgesic, but there is controversy as to the most effective dose. Classically, a suitable dose is said to be 0.1 mg/kg, but even this dose may cause dysphoria (Muir *et al.*, 1978a). However, Combie *et al.*, (1979; 1981) found that doses of up to 0.3 mg/kg produced minimal behavioural effects, although they did comment that any locomotor response was delayed.

Methadone

Methadone (0.1 mg/kg i.v. or i.m.) is popular for use in the horse, both as an analgesic and in sedative/opioid combinations.

Pethidine (meperidine)

Pethidine (meperidine) has been one of the most widely used opioids in horses (Archer, 1947; Combie *et al.*, 1979) especially for spasmodic colic as it has an antispasmodic action. Doses of up to 2 mg/kg have been recommended and these appear to produce good analgesia with moderate sedation. Pethidine does have several drawbacks. It is comparatively short acting (Alexander & Collett, 1974) and analgesia rarely lasts more than two hours. Following i.v. use excitement reactions are common. A small but significant number of horses suffer anaphylactoid reactions (Clutton, 1987) manifest by severe sweating, shaking and even collapse. Anaphylactoid reactions are less common and less severe when pethidine is given by i.m. injection; excitement is also less common and so this route should be considered the one of choice.

Partial agonists

The advantage of the partial agonist opioid drugs is that they are often less addictive in man and therefore subject to less control regulations than are pure agonist agents. Controversy concerning their most suitable doses for horses may be because dose–response effects occur in which higher doses antagonize analgesia already produced, so if, in clinical use, analgesia is not obtained it is inadvisable to increase the dose, and another analgesic should be used.

Pentazocine

Pentazocine has been used in horses in North America. Dose recommendations are very variable, ranging from 0.9 to 2.2 mg/kg.

Butorphanol

Butorphanol is used to provide analgesia in premedication, during surgery, for postoperative analgesia and in sedative/opioid combinations.

Again, dose recommendations vary widely. The minimal analgesic dose is 0.1 mg/kg i.v. but analgesia is transient, higher doses being required for longer effective pain relief (Robertson *et al.*, 1981; Kalpravidh *et al.*, 1984). Doses of 0.2 mg/kg i.v. have been claimed to produce effective analgesia in equine colic for up to two hours. Cardiovascular effects appear to be minimal but all studies of its use in pain-free animals found it to produce behavioural effects – nose-twitches, ataxia, shivering box walking and restlessness at doses as low as 0.1 mg/kg i.v. Differences may be due to whether or not the horse is in pain but, in the authors' experience of the use of this drug alone as an analgesic, doses of 0.1 mg/kg i.v. given to horses with mild colic pain cause the horse to walk constantly around the box for one hour (a locomotor response), and such a response could be disastrous in postoperative orthopaedic cases.

Buprenorphine

Buprenorphine, another partial agonist, gives analgesia for about eight hours although it must be remembered that even after i.v. injection onset of analgesia requires at least 15 minutes. The authors have found in clinical practice that doses of 0.006 mg/kg i.m. or i.v. to the horse in pain apparently give good analgesia for several hours.

Additional routes of administration of opioid agents

Morphine has been administered into joints following arthroscopy. This is effective in man presumably through its action on specific opioid receptors in the synovium (Lawrence *et al.*, 1992) but claims of its efficacy in the horse have yet to be substantiated. When morphine (15 mg in 5 ml of saline) is injected into the joints of ponies, the morphine plasma levels do not reach those likely to result in systemic effects, whilst morphine is still detectable in joint fluid for at least 24 hours (Raekallio *et al.*, 1997). Morphine (in a preparation which does not contain preservatives) may be given by caudal epidural injection at doses of 0.1 mg/kg. Robinson *et al.*, (1994) found that caudal epidural injection of 50 mg of morphine in 10 mls of saline resulted in analgesia of at least five

dermatomes and in some animals analgesia spread considerably further cranially. Analgesia lasted for 17 hours, but onset of analgesia was delayed for up to eight hours. When a higher dose of morphine (100 mg) was used, onset of analgesia was faster (six hours), lasted longer (19 hours) and spread further (sometimes as far as T9) but the signs of sedation, presumably through systemic absorption of the drug, were greater. There are many anecdotal reports from clinical practice as to the efficacy of epidural morphine in providing postoperative analgesia of the hind limbs and even of the abdomen of individual animals, but few mention the very prolonged onset of analgesic effects. In practice, frequently morphine is used in combination with other agents. Sysel *et al.*, (1996; 1997) demonstrated that morphine (0.2 mg/kg) and detomidine (30 µg/kg) given through an epidural catheter situated at approximately the lumbosacral junction reduced experimentally induced lameness within an a hour; that there was minimal ataxia (the horses could trot); that this analgesia lasted for at least six hours after drug administration and that incremental dosing could be used to maintain analgesia for up to 14 days.

LOCAL ANALGESIA

The many techniques of nerve block used in horses for purely diagnostic purposes and the methods for producing intrasynovial desensitization will not be considered here. Details of these techniques can be obtained from surgical textbooks or from *Die Narkose der Tiere*, volume 1, *Lokalanasthesie*, by Westhues and Fritsch (Westhues and Fristch, 1960). Those to be described here are only the ones which the authors have found useful in operative surgery or for giving pain relief (Fig. 11.2).

SPECIFIC NERVE BLOCKS

Infraorbital nerve block

The infraorbital nerve is the continuation of the maxillary division of the Vth cranial nerve and is entirely sensory. During its course along the infra-orbital canal it supplies branches to the upper molar, canine and incisor teeth on that side, and their alveoli and contiguous gum. The nerves supplying the first and second molars (PM1 and 2), the canine and incisors, arise within the canal about 2.5 cm from the infraorbital foramen and pass forwards in the maxilla and premaxilla to the teeth. The nerves to cheek teeth three to six (PM3, M1, 2 and 3) pass directly from the parent nerve trunk in the upper parts of the canal. After emerging from the foramen the nerve supplies sensory fibres to the upper lip and cheek, the nostrils and lower parts of the face.

The infraorbital nerve may be approached at two sites:

1. At its point of emergence from the infraorbital foramen: the area desensitized will comprise the skin of the lip, nostril and face on that side up to the level of the foramen

2. Within the canal, via the infraorbital foramen, when in addition the first and second premolars, the canine and incisor teeth with their alveoli and gum, and the skin as high as the level of the inner canthus of the eye, will be influenced (Fig. 11.3).

The lip of the infraorbital foramen can be detected readily as a bony ridge lying beneath the edge of the flat levator nasolabialis muscle. When it is desired to block the nerve within the canal it is necessary to pass the needle up the canal about 2.5 cm. To do this the needle must be inserted through the skin about 2 cm in front of the foramen after reflecting the edge of the levator muscle upwards. An insensitive skin weal is an advantage. For the perineural injection a needle 19 gauge (1.1 mm), 5 cm long, is suitable. The quantity of local analgesic solution required will vary from 4 to 5 ml. For blocking the nerve at its point of emergence from the canal, the needle is introduced until its point can be felt beneath the bony lip of the foramen. From 4 to 5 ml of 1% mepivacaine is injected, withdrawing the needle slightly as injection proceeds. Loss of sensation should follow in 15–20 minutes and last a further 30–40 minutes if the solution injected contains a vasoconstrictor.

Injections at site 1 may be employed for interferences about the lips and nostrils, such as suturing of wounds, removal of polypi, etc. Extraction of canine or incisor teeth is seldom required in horses, and for extraction of molar teeth general anaesthesia is usually preferred. For trephining

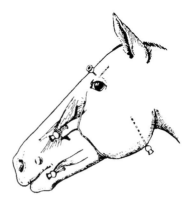

FIG. 11.2 Sites for insertion of the needle to block the supraorbital, infraorbital, mental and mandibular nerves.

the facial sinuses, local infiltration analgesia offers a good alternative.

Mandibular nerve block

The alveolar branch of the mandibular division of the Vth cranial nerve enters the mandibular foramen on the medial aspect of the vertical ramus of the mandible under cover of the medial pterygoid muscle. It traverses the mandibular canal, giving off dental and alveolar branches on that side, and emerges through the mental foramen. From this point it is styled the mental nerve. The nerves supplying the canine and incisor teeth arise from the parent trunk within the canal 3–5 cm behind the mental foramen, and pass to the teeth within the bone.

If the mandibular alveolar nerve is injected at its point of entry into the mandibular canal at the mandibular foramen, practically the whole of the lower jaw and all the teeth and alveoli on that side will become desensitized. The technique is difficult and uncertain, for the nerve enters the canal high up on the medial aspect of the vertical ramus. The foramen lies practically opposite the point of intersection of a line passing vertically downwards from the lateral canthus of the eye, and one extending backwards from the tables of the mandibular molar teeth.

A point is selected on the caudal border of the mandible about 3 cm below the temporomandibular articulation. After penetrating the skin the needle is allowed to lie in the depression between the

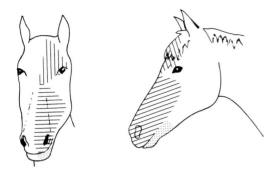

FIG. 11.3 Area of skin desensitized after blocking: the infraorbital nerve within the canal (transverse lines), the supaorbital nerve (vertical lines) and the mental nerve (spotted).

wing of the atlas and the base of the ear. The needle is advanced as its point is depressed until it passes deep to the medial border of the ramus. It is then advanced further in the direction of the point of intersection of the previously mentioned lines, keeping as close as possible to the medial surface of the mandible but, as the nerve lies medial to the accompanying artery and vein, the needle does not need to follow the bone closely. Following this method the needle should lie parallel with the nerve for a distance of 3–4 cm. About 5 ml of analgesic solution is injected along this length. German writers describe a modification: the foramen is approached from the ventral border of the ramus, just in front of the angle. The point of the needle must penetrate a distance of 1.0–1.5 cm to reach the foramen.

The chief indications are molar dental interferences in the lower jaw, but most surgeons today prefer to carry out all dental surgery under general anaesthesia and this nerve block will only be used when, for some reason, general anaesthesia is impracticable.

Mental nerve block

Suturing of wounds of the lower lip may be conveiently carried out under mental nerve block. The nerve can be injected as it emerges from the mental foramen and analgesia of the lower lip on that side will ensue (Fig. 11.3). Attempts may be made to pass the needle along a canal a distance of 3–5 cm (in which case the canine and

incisor teeth will also be desensitized) but this is not easily performed.

The mental foramen is situated on the lateral aspect of the ramus in the middle of the interdental space. It can be palpated after deflecting the pencil-like tendon of the depressor labii inferioris muscle upwards. The nerve may be detected as an emerging thick straw-like structure. From this point the technique is the same as that outlined for the infraorbital nerve.

Supraorbital nerve block

Suturing of wounds involving only the upper eyelid is easily possible after block of the supraorbital nerve (Fig. 11.3). The supraorbital (or frontal) nerve is one of the terminal branches of the ophthalmic division of the Vth cranial nerve. It emerges from the orbit accompanied by the artery through the supraorbital foramen in the supraorbital process. It supplies sensory fibres to the upper eyelid and, in part, to the skin of the forehead. The nerve is injected within the supraorbital foramen.

The upper and lower borders of the supraorbital process, close to its junction with the main mass of the frontal bone, is palpable. The foramen is recognized as a pit-like depression midway between the two borders. The skin is prepared and an insensitive weal produced. A needle, 19 gauge (1.1 mm), 2.2 cm long, is passed into the foramen to a depth of 0.5–1.0 cm and 5 ml of analgesic solution injected.

Auriculopalpebral nerve block

The auriculopalpebral nerve is a terminal branch of the facial division of the trigeminal (Vth) cranial nerve innervating the orbicularis oculi muscles. Blocking it prevents voluntary closure of the eyelids but does not in any way desensitize them. In conjunction with topical analgesia of the conjunctiva it is most useful for examination of the eye, as well as for the removal of foreign bodies from the cornea and other minor eye surgery. It may be blocked by placing 5 ml of 2% mepivacaine solution subfascially at the most dorsal point of the zygomatic arch. A 2.5 cm, 22 gauge (0.7 mm) needle is a convenient size for this injection.

Palmar/plantar nerve block

The nerves confer sensibility to the digit. The medial palmar nerve of the forelimb is one of the terminal branches of the median nerve. At the level of the proximal sesamoid bones the trunk of the nerve divides into three digital branches, and all three branches are in close relationship with the digital vessels. The dorsal branch in front of the vein distributes cutaneous branches to the front of the digit, and terminates in the coronary cushion. The middle branch, which is small and irregular, descends between the artery and vein. It is generally formed by the union of several smaller branches which cross forwards over the artery before uniting, and it terminates in the sensitive laminae and the coronary cushion. The palmar branch lies close behind the artery, except at the metacarpophalangeal joint, where the nerve is almost superposed to the artery. It accompanies the digital artery in the hoof, and passes with the palmar branch of that vessel to be distributed to the distal phalanx and sensitive laminae.

The lateral palmar nerve is formed by fusion of the termination of the ulnar nerve with one of the terminal branches of the median. In the metacarpal region it occupies, on the outside of the limb, a position on the flexor tendons analogous to that of the medial palmar nerve on the inside. Unlike the latter nerve, however, it is accompanied by only a single vessel – the lateral palmar vein – which lies in front of it. (A small artery – the lateral palmar metacarpal artery – accompanies the nerve and vein from the carpus to the metacarpophalangeal joint on the lateral aspect of the limb). At the level of the sesamoid bones it divides into three digital branches exactly as does the medial palmar nerve already described.

In the hindlimb, plantar nerves result from bifurcation of the tibial nerve when it gains the back of the tarsus. They accompany the deep digital flexor tendon in the tarsal sheath and, diverging from one another, they descend in the metatarsal region, one at each side of the deep digital flexor tendon. Each is accompanied in the metatarsus by the metatarsal vein of that side, and by a slender artery from the vascular arch at the back of the tarsus. A little below the middle of the metatarsus the medial nerve detaches a considerable branch that winds obliquely downwards and outwards behind the flexor tendons to join the lateral plantar nerve about the level of the button of the fourth metatarsal bone. At the metatarsophalangeal joint, each nerve, coming into relation with the digital vessels, resolves itself into three branches for the supply of the digit.

In the hindlimb the main artery – the dorsal metatarsal artery – passes to the back of the metatarsus by dipping under the free end of the 4th metatarsal bone, and finally bifurcates above the fetlock, between the two divisions of the suspensory ligament, to form the digital arteries. In the pastern region the disposition of the nerves and vessels is the same as in the forelimb. Plantar nerve block does not give the same results as palmar block in the forelimb. The skin and deeper tissues on the dorsal aspect of the hind fetlock and pastern are innervated by terminal branches of the fibular nerve. This may be important from a surgical standpoint although less important from a diagnostic point of view (S. Dyson, personal communication, 1991).

Technique for palmar/plantar (abaxial sesamoid) injection

Injection in both fore- and hindlimbs is where the nerves course just proximal to the metacarpophalangeal/metatarsophalangeal joint. Although the nerves divide up into three branches at about this point the injection of 2–3 ml of local analgesic solution medially and laterally still produces complete desensitization of the entire foot (Fig. 11.4) An advantage of this site is that when the limb is held up and the joint flexed, the nerves and their associated vessels can be palpated so their accurate location is easy.

A strict aseptic technique must be practised and the lateral and medial sites should be clipped and prepared as for an operation. In thin-skinned horses a 25 gauge (0.5 mm), 2.5 cm long needle is used; disposable needles can usually be introduced through the skin without the horse showing resentment.

After the injections have been completed the animal is allowed to stand quietly for 10–15 minutes. At the end of this time the limb is tested for sensation by tapping on the skin with a blunt-

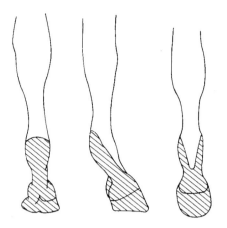

FIG. 11.4 Area of skin desensitized after bilateral plantar or palmar nerve block.

ended spike on the end of a short pole. This is a better way of detecting loss of deep sensation than pricking with a needle. Any response to tapping around the coronet and heel indicates failure to block the nerve on that side. One indication of sensation is sufficient to prove this, and successive trials only serve to agitate the animal. It may be necessary to cover the animal's eye to prevent it seeing the approach of the test instrument.

Technique of palmar/plantar metacarpal/metatarsal injection

An alternative site for blocking the palmar/plantar digital nerves is from 5 to 7 cm proximal to the metacarpophalangeal/metatarsophalangeal joint at the level of the distal enlargements of the 2nd and 4th metacarpal or metatarsal bones. This ensures that the analgesic solution is in contact with the nerve proximal to its point of division. The local analgesic is injected into the groove between the deep digital flexor tendon and the suspensory ligament. The nerve lies deep to the subcutaneous fascia immediately in front of the deep flexor tendon. A 25 gauge (0.5 mm) needle 1.2 cm long is used. The skin over the site is clipped and cleansed. In the great majority of cases the needle can be inserted without movement on the part of the animal. With the animal standing on the limb, the skin and subcutaneous fascia are tense, and it is easy to penetrate the latter and thus ensure that the subsequent injection is in direct contact with the nerve. If the limb is held raised

during insertion of the needle, the flaccidity of the skin may cause the point to enter the subcutaneous connective tissue and the method will fail. If blood escapes from the needle, it should be partially withdrawn, redirected and reinserted. It may be decided, first, to provoke an insensitive skin weal, and then pass the needle through this at the appropriate angle until its point lies beneath the fascia.

When it is intended to block both sides of the limb supplied by these nerves, the opposite side of the leg is similarly dealt with. When dealing with the medial nerve it is necessary to work around the opposite leg. With the horse standing squarely, the operator passes one hand around the front of the adjacent leg for inserting the needle, while the other is passed behind the limb for holding the syringe to the needle.

The most likely cause of failure is that the solution was injected into the subcutaneous connective tissue, and not beneath the fascia. Fortunately the skin at the site is now desensitized and a second and deeper injection can be made without restraint.

About 2.5–5.0 ml of 1% mepivacaine or 0.5% bupivacaine solution is commonly injected around each nerve. The average hunter is given 3 ml over each nerve. In the hindlimb the technique is similar, except that the procedure exposes the operator to a greater risk of injury, especially when dealing with a nervous animal. Thus, not only must the animal be twitched, but the forelimb raised in addition if the operation is to be carried out with the animal standing on the affected limb. Should the operator feel indisposed to make the injection with the hindleg free, it may be raised by an assistant, but the needle must be inserted sufficiently deeply to penetrate the fascia.

Technique of blocking palmar terminal digital nerves

The terminal divisions of the palmar and plantar nerves may be subjected to medial and lateral perineural injection in the pastern region. The site for injection is midway between the fetlock joint and coronet. The palmar or volar border of the first phalanx is located, and the dorsal edge of the (at this point flattened) deep digital flexor tendon is palpated. The nerve lies immediately dorsal to the tendon. About 2 ml of 1% mepivacaine or 0.5%

bupivacaine solution is injected SC just proximal to the collateral cartilages. The area desensitized is limited to the palmar or volar part of the foot and heel on that side.

Indications for palmar/plantar block

Palmar/plantar block is commonly used to aid diagnosis of the site of lameness, but it is also very useful to relieve the pain of acutely painful lesions about the foot, and to allow the animal to rest. The practice may be repeated daily for a few days in severe cases. Longest pain relief is obtained by using bupivacaine with a vasoconstrictor such as adrenaline at a concentration of 1:200 000.

The nerve blocks allow the painless performance of palmar and plantar neurectomy and of operations about the foot, coronet and heel, such as exposure of a corn or gathered nail track, partial operations for quittor and sandcrack. Even when operations about the foot are performed under general anaesthesia, palmar and plantar blocks can provide analgesia intraoperatively and in the recovery period. The desensitization of the foot which they produce does not seem to be an obstacle to the animal regaining its feet after general anaesthesia or to contribute to ataxia immediately afterwards.

The complete desensitization of the forelimb below the carpus

Simultaneous block of the median, ulnar and musculocutaneous (cutaneous branch) nerves desensitize the entire manus.

Median nerve

The best site at which to inject the median nerve is the one used for the operation of median neurectomy, i.e. the point on the medial aspect of the limb about 5 cm distal to the elbow joint, where the nerve lies immediately caudal to the radius and cranial to the muscular belly of the internal flexor of the metacarpus, deep to the caudal superficial pectoral muscle and the deep fascia.

With the animal standing squarely, the administrator stoops adjacent to and slightly behind the opposite forelimb. The caudal border of the radius

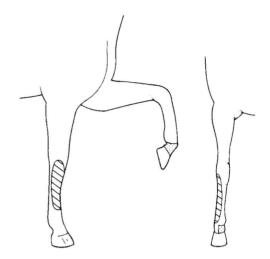

FIG. 11.5 Areas of skin desensitization after block of the ulnar (shaded) and median nerves (spotted) (S. Dyson, personal communication, 1991).

where it meets the distal edge of the caudal superficial pectoral muscle is located with a finger. The point of insertion of the needle is immediately proximal to the finger. A needle, 19 gauge (1.1 mm), 2.5–3.0 cm long, is suitable. It is directed proximally and axially at an angle of 20° to the vertical, to ensure penetration of the pectoral muscle and the deep fascia; 7.5–10.0 ml of local analgesic solution is injected. To facilitate insertion of the needle to the proper depth it is best first to induce an insensitive skin weal.

The indications for blocking the median nerve alone are limited, for the surface area desensitized is little more than that obtained with medial palmar block (see Figs 11.4 and 11.5).

Ulnar nerve

This nerve may be blocked by injection of 10 ml of local analgesic solution in the centre of the caudal aspect of the limb, about 10 cm proximal to the accessory carpal bone, in the groove between the tendons of the ulnaris lateralis and flexor carpi ulnaris, and beneath the deep fascia.

Musculocutaneous nerve

This nerve is blocked on the medial aspect of the limb where it lies on the surface of the radius halfway between the elbow and carpus, immediately adjacent to the cephalic vein. At this site, it can easily be palpated just cranial to the cephalic vein and blocked by the injection of 10 ml of local analgesic solution.

The complete desensitization of the distal hindlimb

The technique of nerve block of the hindlimb sometimes works extremely well but is unreliable, especially for removal of cutaneous sensation (Westhues & Fristch, 1960). Westhues and Fristch described techniques for blocking the tibial and peroneal (fibular) nerves.

Tibial nerve

Injection is made about 1.5 cm above the point of the tarsus, in the groove between the gastro-cnemius and the deep digital flexor tendons. Palpation of the nerve at this site is facilitated by holding up the foot and slightly flexing the leg, although the injection is best made with the limb bearing weight. Care must be taken to inject deep to the subcutaneous fascia or only the superficial branch of the nerve will be affected. Some 20 ml of local analgesic solution should be injected at this site through a 2.5 cm, 20 gauge (0.9 mm) needle that has been placed beneath the fascia.

Peroneal (fibular) nerve

The superficial and deep branches of this nerve are best blocked simultaneously in the groove between the tendons of the long and lateral digital extensors about 10 cm proximal to the lateral malleolus of the tibia. First a 3.75 cm, 22 gauge (0.7 mm) needle is introduced subcutaneously and 10 ml of the local analgesic solution injected through it to block the superficial nerve. The needle must then be inserted another 2–3 cm to penetrate the deep fascia and about 1.0–1.5 ml of local analgesic solution injected (Fig. 11.6) around the deep branch.

Saphenous nerve

The deposition of 5 ml of local analgesic solution on the dorsal aspect of the median saphenous vein

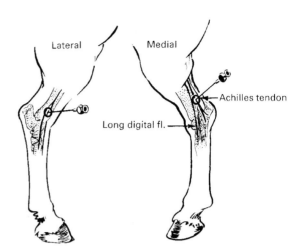

FIG. 11.6 Sites for injection about the peroneal nerve on the lateral aspect and the tibial nerve on the medial aspect of the horse's hindlimb.

proximal to the tibiotarsal joint will effectively block the saphenous nerve.

Block of the tibial nerve above the hock, and of the deep peroneal (fibular) nerve, desensitizes the plantar metatarsus, the medial and lateral aspects of the fetlock and whole digit. To produce a complete block distal to the hock, these two nerves must be injected together with the saphenous nerve, the superficial peroneal (fibular) nerve and the caudal cutaneous nerve (a branch of the tibial nerve).

Accidents and complications

Sudden movement by the animal, while inserting the needle or during injection, may cause the shaft of the needle to break from the hub. The accident is especially liable to occur if an attempt is made to carry out the operation without sedating or twitch-ing a nervous or fractious animal. A sufficient length of needle may remain exposed for it to be gripped with forceps and withdrawn. Removal will be facilitated by raising the limb, and thus eas-ing the tension of the skin. Should the needle be completely buried, it is necessary to insert another needle into the subcutaneous connective tissue, provoke an insensitive weal, and make an incision 1 cm or so long, directly over the broken needle to expose it.

Although horses can perform fast work after surgical neurectomy, care should be taken that a horse under the influence of palmar/plantar block is not exercised vigorously, for incoordinate movement after acute loss of sensation may result in bone fracture. (Cases involving the proximal and distal phalanges were reported by J. G. Wright in the 1st edition of this book.)

Local analgesia for castration

There are three methods in common use for desensitizing the scrotum, testicle and spermatic cord by injection of local analgesics but for all of them it is essential that the animal is properly restrained or sedated if the operator is not to be injured when carrying them out on the standing animal. The animal is placed with its right side against a wall or partition and if not sedated a twitch is applied to its upper lip. After preparation of the skin of the scrotum, prepuce and medial aspect of the thighs, the operator stands with his left shoulder pressed lightly against the caudal part of the animal's left chest wall. The neck of the scrotum on the right side is gripped with the left hand and the testicle drawn well down until the skin of the scrotum is tense (Fig. 11.7).

Method 1

A 19 gauge (1.1 mm) needle is quickly thrust into the substance of the testicle to a depth of 3–4 cm and 30–35 ml of 2% lignocaine injected. When an adequate amount of lignocaine has been injected the testicle feels firm. The procedure is repeated for the left testicle, and local analgesic solution is injected along the median raphe of the scrotum. After about 10 minutes has elapsed castration can be carried out painlessly.

Method 2

The spermatic cord is grasped with the fingers just above the testicle and a 5 cm 19 gauge (1.1 mm) needle thrust into the subcutaneous tissues of that region. The needle is kept stationary to avoid penetration of blood vessels and about 20 ml of 2% lignocaine injected around each spermatic cord. The scrotal skin is injected along the line of the proposed incisions. This method does not seem as effective as the one described above.

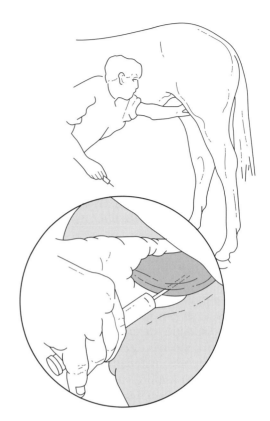

FIG. 11.7 Injection into the substance of the testicles after linear infiltration of the scrotal tissues.

Method 3

A long (12–15 cm) 19 gauge (1.1 mm) needle is thrust through the testicle and directed into the spermatic cord while 20–25 ml 2% lignocaine are being injected. After treatment of both spermatic cords the scrotal skin is infiltrated.

To infiltrate the scrotal skin it is important that the direction of the needle shall be almost parallel to the skin to ensure that its point lies in the subcutaneous connective tissue, for if it enters the dartos or the substance of the testicle itself, difficulty may be experienced in injecting the solution and, what is more important, the skin does not become analgesic. The animal usually moves as the needle is inserted and the operator must be prepared for this.

Some right-handed operators prefer to stand on the right side of the horse, with the left hand holding the scrotum or spermatic cord, so that the left arm is against the stifle and affords some measure of protection against a kick. The person holding the twitch should stand on the same side as the operator. It is interesting to note that many equine practitioners assert that a twitch applied around the upper lip appears to produce some measure of analgesia and is not simply a distraction or counter-irritant. It may be relevant that the midpoint in the midline between the upper lip and the nose is, in fact, a well-recognized acupuncture point.

PARAVERTEBRAL ANALGESIA

A thoracolumbar paravertebral block of T18, L1 and L2 segmental nerves provides useful anaesthesia of skin, muscles and peritoneum of the paralumbar fossa, and it is an excellent method of analgesia for procedures such as flank laparotomy or for laparoscopy in the standing horse (Fig. 11.8) (Moon & Suter, 1993). L3 should not be blocked, as in horses it provides some innervation to the hind limbs, and its block may cause ataxia.

The basic anatomy of the spinal nerves resembles that of cattle, each nerve bifurcating shortly after leaving the spinal canal, the dorsal branch supplying the skin and superficial tissues, whilst the ventral branch passes beneath the inter-transverse ligament, and innervates the muscle layers and peritoneum. Thus, as with cattle, it is necessary to block both dorsal and ventral branches of each spinal nerve if adequate analgesia is to be obtained. In cattle the landmarks for injection are found by palpation of the transverse process of the lumbar vertebrae, but these are almost impossible to locate in horses. However, Moon and Suter (1993) point out that a line from the most caudal portion of the last rib (easily located in almost all horses) and perpendicular to the long axis of the spine passes across the transverse process of L3. Thus, to block the spinal nerve L2, the site chosen is over the transverse process of L3, and approximately 5–6 cm lateral to the midline. A small bleb of local anaesthetic is placed in the skin, then 5 ml of 2% lignocaine (or other suitable local analgesic agent) infiltrated in the muscle. A long spinal needle (eg. 18 G × 7–15 cm) is then introduced vertically until it impinges on the transverse process; it is withdrawn a little, then redirected slightly cranially, until the inter-transverse ligament between L2 and L3 is penetrated (felt as an increase, then sudden decrease, in resistance). Following aspira-

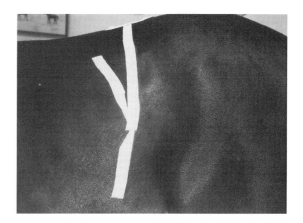

FIG. 11.8 Location of the site for paravertebral block of L2. A line extended vertically upward from the most caudal point of the last rib passes over the transverse process of L3. A needle inserted 3–6 cm (depending on size of the horse) from the midline over L3 should strike the transverse process; L2 nerve can be located by redirecting the needle to pass anterior to the process.

tion to ensure that the needle is not in a blood vessel, 20 mls of 2% lignocaine is slowly infiltrated, half 2.5 cm below the inter-transverse ligament, and the remainder 2.5 cm above to block the dorsal branch of the nerve. Skarda (1996) points out that it is easy to enter the peritoneum and that this is detected by a loss of resistance (as it penetrates the transverse ligament) and sometimes by hearing air being aspirated through the needle. Should this happen, the needle should be withdrawn to a retroperitoneal position, before the local anaesthetic is deposited. The procedure is repeated to block nerves L1 and T13. The sites for injection are located by measuring 5–6 cm anterior from the previous site (less in ponies), and confirmed by the needle impinging on a transverse process of the vertebrae.

With practice, the technique is simple and reliable, although on occasions analgesia of the ventral area of the paralumbar fossa is inadequate for surgery, and local infiltration become necessary.

EPIDURAL ANALGESIA

Caudal and more anterior blocks

In horses the caudal epidural block is performed by entering between the first and second coccygeal vertebrae (Fig. 11.9), the spinal cord and its meninges ending in the midsacral region. The depression between the first and second coccygeal dorsal spinous processes can usually be felt with the finger when the tail is raised, even in the heavy breeds, about 2.5 cm cranial to the commencement of the tail hairs, although in fat animals it may be impossible to detect any of the sacral or coccygeal dorsal spinous processes. Upward flexion at the sacrococcygeal articulation is seldom discernible; in fact, in many animals this joint is fused A line drawn over the back joining the two coxofemoral joints crosses the midline at the level of the sacrococcygeal joint. Immediately behind this may be palpated the dorsal spinous process of the first coccygeal bone, and the site for insertion of the needle is the space immediately caudal to this. The interarcual space is smaller than in the ox and may be more difficult to locate with the needle, particularly in welldeveloped or fat animals in which the root of the tail is well covered by muscle or fat. Sometimes it is possible to detect a 'popping' sensation as the interarcual ligament is penetrated. The surest evidence, however, that the canal has been entered is the almost complete absence of resistance to injection of the local analgesic solution.

Most anaesthetists introduce the needle at right angles to the general contour of the croup until the floor of the neural canal is struck, but in the method of Browne the point of the needle is inserted at the caudal part of the intercoccygeal depression and directed cranioventrally at an angle of 30° from the horizontal so that its point will glide along the floor of the neural canal and the needle can be inserted to its full length (the steep cranioventral direction of the canal at this point allows this). It is probable, however, that the first method, whereby the needle is inserted at a 60° angle from the horizontal, is easier to perform. Where it is likely that a caudal block will need extending in duration, a catheter can be placed through the needle and into the epidural space. An 18 G Tuohy needle may be placed as described above, and a 20 G epidural catheter advanced through this. Whichever type of needle is used, the skin and subcutaneous tissues should be made insensitive by the injection of a small weal of local analgesic solution.

Ten millilitres of 2% lignocaine or 5 ml of 2% mepivacaine, with or without a vasoconstrictor, is usually sufficient to produce caudal block in the

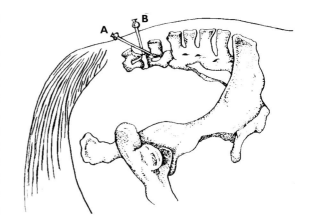

FIG. I 1.9 Caudal epidural block in the horse. The needle may be inserted at right angles to the skin surface between the first and second caudal vertebrae (**B**), or it may be introduced further caudally over the cranial boder of the second coccygeal vertebra and inclined at an angle of about 30° to the horizontal to advance up the neural canal (**A**).

largest of horses. Analgesia takes much longer to develop than in cattle and unless allowance is made for this it may be erroneously concluded that injection was not made correctly. Analgesia will usually be present after about 20 minutes and persists for 35–50 minutes depending on whether or not the solution used contained a vasoconstrictor.

Caudal block is indicated to overcome straining during manipulative correction of the simpler forms of malpresentation of the fetus, for amputation of the tail (an operation which in the UK may only be performed for surgical reasons), and for operations about the anus, perineum and vulva, suture of wounds, operation for prolapsed rectum and Caslick's operation for vaginal wind sucking.

Anterior block

Local anaesthetic agents injected epidurally at the caudal region in doses sufficient to cause anterior epidural block have no place in equine anaesthesia because of the hindlimb paralysis produced. However, with modern epidural catheters, anterior block is technically possible to perform; small quantities of local anaesthetic agents being deposited in the region of the dermatomes to be anaesthetized. Catheters inserted in the coccygeal region may be advanced at least as far forward as the lumbosacral junction (Sysel *et al.*, 1996). The technique has been used to provide long term analgesia with agents other than local anaesthetic drugs, which reduces the danger of unwanted hindlimb weakness.

Subarachnoid anaesthesia

Subarachnoid catheterization in the horse is practicable (Skarda, 1996), and enables segmental analgesia to be provided if the catheter, inserted at the lumbosacral junction, is advanced until it reaches the required dermatome. However, the technique is complicated, and paravertebral thoracolumbar analgesia is usually preferable for surgical analgesia of the sublumbar region.

Use of other agents

The use of morphine (p.257) and α_2 adrenoceptor agonists (p.252) by epidural injection has been discussed above. Where such agents are required to give surgical analgesia it is usual to combine them with small doses of local analgesics. The aim of such combinations is to combine the rapid onset of local analgesics with the prolonged pain relieving properties of opioids and α_2 adrenoceptor agonists, to reduce the dose of any single agent to below that which may cause systemic effects and, hopefully, to reduce the dose of local analgesics to that which will not cause ataxia or hindlimb paralysis.

The combination most commonly used is that of xylazine and lignocaine (Grubb *et al.*, 1992) but many similar combinations have been employed. Opioids have also been combined with local analgesics. Butorphanol (0.04 mg/kg) and lignocaine (0.25 mg/kg) given into the epidural space has been reported to give prolonged analgesia without the horses showing ataxia (Farney *et al.*, 1991). However, it must be remembered that only preservative-free solutions should be administered into the epidural space – morphine and xylazine are easily obtainable in this form, hence their popularity for use by this route.

GENERAL ANAESTHESIA

General anaesthesia in horses appears beset with more problems than are encountered in any other domestic animal. In particular, cardiopulmonary dysfunction, nerve and ischaemic muscle damage appear more pronounced and can be difficult to avoid. The problems are often inter-related and seem to follow directly from the actions of the anaesthetic agents themselves, or from interference with mechanisms existing in conscious horses to compensate for respiratory or cardiovascular changes induced by recumbency. Other problems relate to the horse's size, its temperament and its tendency to panic. It is necessary to anticipate the problems from the beginning of the anaesthetic protocol in order to take action necessary to avoid or reduce them; hence they will be considered in general at this stage.

PROBLEMS RELATING TO SIZE AND TEMPERAMENT

When handling horses the safety not only of the horse, but also of the handlers must be considered, and methods of control used must reflect the temperament of the horse and availability of well trained personnel. Sedative premedication aids placement of catheters and the smoothness of induction of anaesthesia. The sheer weight and bulk of a large horse makes it difficult to handle, transport or position for surgery without adequate manpower or mechanical aids. Many unconscious horses are transported for short distances (e.g. from the operating table to recovery box) suspended in a net or by their hobbled legs from an overhead hoist. Other methods of moving unconscious horses include trolleys which may constitute the floor of the anaesthetic induction box and may then become the operating table top.

In clinical practice anaesthesia in the adult horse is amost always induced by i.v. agents, although in young foals it may be induced with inhalation agents. Breed is often allied to temperament and must not be ignored in the selection of an anaesthetic technique. A method suitable for a phlegmatic warmblood, trotter or quarter horse may be totally unsuitable for a very excitable young Thoroughbred or Arab.

Ideally the horse should regain its feet as rapidly as possible at the first attempt, with minimal ataxia. Unfortunately this is not easily achieved following prolonged anaesthesia. Although prolonged recumbency is not desirable, it is now appreciated that in some cases ultra-fast recoveries may be of poor quality because the horse tries to arise whilst still disorientated. The best quality recoveries are seen where the drugs given during anaesthesia are eliminated in such a manner that the horse does not try to rise until it is ready, and it may be necessary to use sedation to increase the duration of recumbency. Animals which are unused to people may try to rise too soon, but the young, well handled but excitable Thoroughbred colt (which requires very careful handling for induction of anaesthesia) often remains recumbent for a considerable time, and then recovers remarkably well. Ponies exhibit poor quality recovery as often as do large horses, but it is the heavier animal which is most likely to suffer from serious injury as a result. Other causes of poor quality of recovery from anaesthesia include nerve and muscle damage induced during anaesthesia, and untreated postoperative pain.

DISTURBANCES IN CARDIOPULMONARY FUNCTION

Disturbances of cardiopulmonary function have long been recognized in anaesthetized horses but, in spite of much research, their cause remains uncertain. Because general anaesthesia necessarily involves recumbency there has been some debate as to the relative importance of the roles of recumbency and of anaesthetic agents in their genesis, but in conscious experimental animals the cardiopulmonary disturbances produced by lateral recumbency have been found to be minimal (Hall 1984; Ruch et al., 1984). The effects of posture cannot be ignored for disturbances are more severe following supine rather than lateral recumbency in anaesthetized horses; however it is probable that while various postures may magnify effects they do not initiate them.

From the evidence available today it seems likely that any disturbances resulting from recumbency are minimized in conscious animals by the operation of compensatory mechanisms that fail or become depressed when an anaesthetic is administered. Their failure or depression is manifested in several ways but probably the most important results which affect equine anaesthetic

morbidity and mortality are cardiovascular depression, the development of a large alveolar–arterial oxygen tension gradient ($(A–a) PO_2$) and, probably resulting from the first two factors, postanaesthetic myopathy.

Cardiovascular effects

Horses in which anaesthesia is maintained using volatile anaesthetic agents often suffer from hypotension, which may be the result of vasodilation and/or a fall in CO. A number of studies have investigated the effects of volatile anaesthetics alone, i.e. including volatile anaesthetic induction (Steffey & Howland, 1978a; Dunlop et al., 1987; Steffey et al., 1987a, b, c; 1990; 1993). These investigations have demonstrated that halothane depresses the equine heart in a dose-dependent fashion. Accommodation occurs and, at a given end-tidal concentration, CO and heart rate rise as anaesthesia progresses, possibly due to the release of catecholamines, although the cause of this release remains uncertain. The time course of this accommodation is more prolonged (over five or more hours) than would be encountered during normal clinical practice. Accommodation is more pronounced in spontaneously breathing animals, probably as a result of hypercapnia. Anaesthesia with isoflurane or sevoflurane (Steffey & Howland, 1980; Aida et al., 1996) also results in hypotension, mainly arising from vasodilation as, at eqi-MAC values, CO is better maintained than with halothane. However, even with these newer agents increasing the concentration still results in a dose related fall in CO.

Such experiments as detailed above provide useful pharmacological information about the volatile anaesthetic agents in horses, but are not typical of normal clinical anaesthetic practice, in which anaesthesia is induced by i.v. agents. With the i.v. techniques most commonly employed, the introduction of the volatile anaesthetic agent results in marked hypotension, in experimental situations mean arterial blood pressure (MAP) frequently falling to below 40 mmHg (Gleed & Dobson, 1990; Lee et al., 1998a). With halothane, these minimal levels are reached 30–40 minutes after anaesthetic induction, and are considerably lower than the minimal MAP of 70–80 mm Hg which occurred with 1 MAC in most of the experimental studies in which halothane was used as a sole agent. ABP slowly rises through vasoconstriction over the next hour, but CO remains unchanged or may even fall. Similar changes in MAP also occur with other volatile anaesthetics, although with these newer agents CO is better maintained. The relative effects of the different i.v. anaesthetic techniques on the subsequent cardiovascular actions of the volatile anaesthetic agents have not been fully investigated, but the fact that an induction technique itself does not cause cardiovascular depression does not mean that its combination with a volatile agent will not do so. With many total i.v. techniques, blood pressure is well maintained, but this does not mean that there is no cardiovascular depression.

In clinical practice, although hypotension may occur it is rarely as severe as that seen experimentally, as surgical stimulation causes APB to rise. However, this rise is due to vasoconstriction, and CO may fall, probably because of the increased afterload (Wagner et al., 1992). To maintain blood flow an adequate perfusion pressure must be coupled with good CO, and unfortunately CO currently is not easy to measure. Pink mucous membranes and a rapid capillary refill time indicate good peripheral blood flow. Venous blood oxygen values also give a guide as to the adequacy of perfusion. Although, ideally, mixed venous samples are necessary, in the horse the oxygen tension of jugular venous blood approximates (Wetmore et al., 1987) and values above 5 kPa (37.5 mmHg) indicate the adequacy of oygenation and therefore of perfusion of the peripheral tissue.

Pulmonary changes

A major problem encountered in equine anaesthesia is that the arterial oxygen tension (PaO_2) is always much lower than might be expected from the inspired oxygen tensions (PiO_2), i.e. there is a large (A–a)PaO_2. A normal (A–a) of about 18 mmHg (2.4 kPa) in standing horses breathing air is doubled in anaesthetized, laterally recumbent animals. Most investigations concerned with (A–a)PO_2 gradients have been carried out under halothane/oxygen anaesthesia but similar differences have been found during general anaesthesia

with other agents. The increased (A–a)PO_2 may be the result of a combination of several factors and these have been the subject of many investigations in recent years.

The PaO_2 depends on the size of the animal and its position during anaesthesia (Hall, 1983), but it is relatively unaffected by the degree of respiratory depression produced by the anaesthetic agent. Many studies have reported relative or absolute decreases in PaO_2 with or without increased $PaCO_2$ levels. Moreover, there has been shown to be no statistically significant difference in (A–a)PO_2 in a series of animals anaesthetized once with spontaneous breathing and on another occasion with IPPV to normocapnia (Hall et al., 1968a, b). One notable feature is that the (A–a)PO_2 gradient does not increase significantly with time (Gillespie et al., 1969).

When a horse is disconnected from a breathing circuit containing an O_2-rich mixture of gases and allowed to breathe air, PaO_2 of around 50 mmHg (6.5 kPa) is common. This may represent a blood O_2 saturation of around 90% (Clerbaux et al., 1986) but the steep part of the dissociation curve starts about here and any accident such as temporary obstruction of the airway can have very serious consequences. It is not uncommon for frank cyanosis to be observed in the recovery period if oxygen is not administered but it must be remembered that the PaO_2 may fall to 40 mmHg (5.3 kPa) without cyanosis becoming apparent if the blood flow to the mucous membranes is adequate. To improve the situation O_2 must be insufflated at a minimum rate of 15 l/min. The PaO_2 apparently recovers to normal levels as soon as the animal regains its feet.

Factors other than hypoventilation which may contribute to the large (A-a)PO_2 include diffusion defects in the lungs, right-to-left intrapulmonary vascular shunts, mismatching of ventilation and perfusion in the lungs, atelectasis and a fall in CO without a corresponding fall in tissue oxygen consumption.

Diffusion impairment

There is no evidence that diffusion impairment occurs so this must be regarded as an unlikely cause of hypoxaemia.

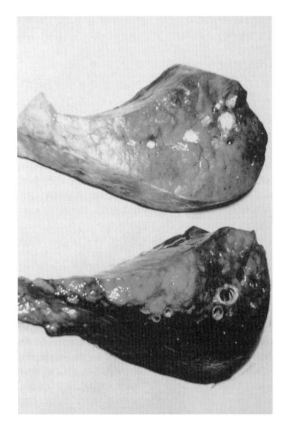

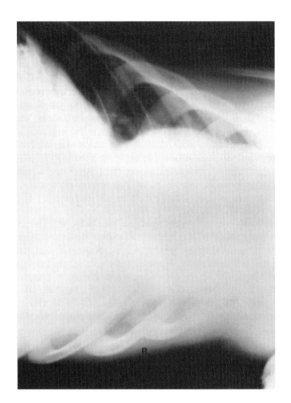

FIG. 11.11 Opacity of the lower lung seen in a radiograph taken at full expiration after 20 minutes of halothane anaesthesia in right decubitus (from McDonell, W.N., Hall, L.W & Jeffcott, L.B. (1979), with permission).

FIG. 11.10 Slices of the lungs of a large horse that died following anaesthesia. The horse had undergone 3 hours of surgery in dorsal decubitus, then been placed in lateral decubitus for recovery. The lung dependent during lateral decubitus (lower picture) shows a large region of total collapse, while the lung which was uppermost in recovery still shows considerable areas of collapse around the hilar region from the period of time in which the horse was in dorsal decubitus.

Atelectasis

Progressive atelectasis is unlikely because in horses the (A-a)PO_2 develops very soon after the induction of anaesthesia and thereafter remains relatively constant. There is no doubt, however, that atelectasis does occur for total collapse of regions of the dependent lung is commonly seen at autopsy of horses dying while anaesthetized (Fig. 11.10). This collapse is presumably due to compression of the lung by overlying abdominal and thoracic viscera. A totally collapsed lung acts as a venous–arterial shunt and can cause marked arterial hypoxaemia. A shunt of 15% of the total pulmonary blood flow has been found in laterally recumbent horses under halothane anaesthesia, compared with about 5% in the standing animal (Gillespie *et al.*, 1969). Decrease in lung volume short of collapse may not have all that an adverse effect on alveolar ventilation for the alveolar compliance curve predicts that a small alveolus will expand proportionally more for any given change in intra-alveolar pressure.

Radiographic studies (McDonell *et al.*, 1979) and blood samples drawn from pulmonary veins through implanted catheters in conscious and anaesthetized animals in lateral decubitus (Hall *et al.*, 1968b; Hall, 1979) have afforded further confirmation of the impairment of function in the lower lung. Radiographic appearances (Fig. 11.11) are suggestive of a greatly reduced volume of the lower lung in laterally recumbent animals (McDonell *et al.*, 1979; Nyman *et al.*, 1990). When a horse lies on its side a diffuse radiographic opacity of the lower lung develops within 20 minutes and may be due to alveolar collapse, regional pulmonary congestion and/or interstitial oedema. Spontaneous deep breaths or forced expansion of the lung by compression of an anaesthetic reservoir bag, both of which might be expected to reexpand collapsed alveoli, fail to alter the radiological appearance. Stolk (1979) demonstrated no significant increase in the water content of the lower lung and considered that the radiographic opacity must be due to an increased blood content. The opacity persists for some time after the horse is turned over and this raises the possibility that venous congestion may kink pulmonary veins and hinder the prompt drainage of blood from the affected lung.

Venous admixture

It would seem unlikely that total collapse of lung regions resulting in right-to-left vascular shunting accounts for all the venous admixture which occurs in anaesthetized horses. A substantial amount must be due to the occurrence of gross mismatching of ventilation and perfusion in the lungs. Some indication of this may be obtained from the physiological deadspace:tidal volume ratio. In most mammals this ratio is about 0.3 but in anaesthetized horses it is over 0.5 (Hall *et al.*, 1968a).

The large physiological deadspace: tidal volume ratio probably explains why IPPV is relatively ineffective in decreasing the $(A–a)PO_2$ in horses. The augmented tidal volume resulting from IPPV merely increases ventilation to those regions of the lung which are already overventilated in relation to their perfusion, i.e. those contributing to the physiological deadspace. While even in horses the increased ventilation will remove carbon dioxide from the lungs and keep the $PaCO_2$ within normal limits, it will not greatly increase the PaO_2.

Effect of cardiac output

CO is usually reduced under anaesthesia but tissue O_2 consumption may remain substantially unchanged. The resulting arterio-mixed venous PaO_2 tension difference, $(A–V)PO_2$, thus increases and venous blood passing through the anatomical shunt or regions of lung collapse has a greater effect on the $(A–V)PO_2$. It is important to note here that the magnitude of the reduction in CO cannot be inferred from the ABP and that IPPV may reduce CO. Indeed, the oxygen tension in mixed venous blood from the pulmonary artery (PvO_2) is lower when IPPV is used despite a slight increase in PaO_2, presumably because of an increased extraction of oxygen from the blood by the tissue – necessitated by the reduced CO – and hence rate of tissue perfusion. Because right-to-left intrapulmonary shunt increases from the normal 5% in the standing, awake horse to about 15% under halothane anaesthesia (Gillespie *et al.*, 1969), the effect of the shunted blood of lower than normal PO_2 will be to produce noticeable reduction in the mixed PaO_2 of the blood in the left atrium (PaO_2).

Lung volume

The larger the lung the greater the stretch across the airways and the less tendency for closure to occur on expiration. The lung volume at which airway closure starts to occur ('the closing volume') is important, for, if airways close, gas trapped distal to the point of closure soon becomes depleted of oxygen and the blood perfusing the region gets through unoxygenated to join the blood from other regions and reduces the mixed PaO_2. Studies strongly suggest that during general anaesthesia the horse's lung volume is reduced to a level at which airway closure may occur and that the reduction in lung volume in the laterally recumbent horse was not equally distributed between the lower and upper lungs (McDonell, 1974). In both right and left lateral decubitus there was a greater reduction in the volume of the lower lung, and pulling the legs together in hobbles reduced lung volume still further.

The effect of airway closure on PaO_2 might be mitigated by collateral ventilation from neighbouring alveoli but although anatomical studies (Tyler *et al.*, 1971) indicate that this is possible, it is unlikely to occur in horses. McDonell (1974) concluded that recumbency rather than anaesthesia was responsible for the reduction of lung volume found in anaesthetized ponies but more recent work has suggested that the anaesthetic agent may also play a part (Watney *et al.*, 1987).

Confirmation of serious impairment of expansion of the lowermost lung has been obtained from histological examination of very rapidly frozen lung regions. Also, from the histological appearances it would seem that a reduction of the tethering effect of lung parenchyma on extra-alveolar vessels might well be responsible for the increased resistance to blood flow in this lung (Hall, 1979).

It might be thought that increasing the airway pressure to above atmospheric pressure (positive end-expiratory pressure or PEEP) will, by increasing the lung volume to an amount equal to the product of the total compliance and the pressure, decrease the tendency for airways to close and thus raise the PaO_2. However, the imposition of a 10 and 20 cmH$_2$O (1 and 2 kPa) expiratory resistance by the insertion of a water trap in the expiratory limb of a circle absorber fails to improve the PaO_2 in horses breathing spontaneously under halothane/oxygen anaesthesia (Hall & Trim, 1975), and indeed usually produced immediate respiratory arrest. Broadly similar results were obtained in horses under barbiturate / guaiphenesin anaesthesia (Beadle et al., 1975), but in this second study arterial oxygen saturation was always over 95%. It is possible that some beneficial effect of expiratory resistance might be found where arterial oxygen saturation is reduced by pulmonary disease, but it seems likely that, because of its dome-like shape, only the upper part of the horse's diaphragm is susceptible to displacement by end-expiratory pressure, and thus lung volume will only increase in regions which are already well ventilated. The indiscriminate use of end-expiratory pressure certainly has no place in routine equine anaesthesia and, by reducing CO, it may even be harmful in some circumstances.

Pharmacological treatments

Hypoventilation is not the major cause of anaesthetic-induced hypoxia in the horse, and indeed in this species hypoxia, rather than hypercapnia appears to be the respiratory drive under anaesthesia (Schatzmann, 1982; Steffey et al., 1992). Thus it is not surprising that respiratory stimulants such as doxapram are ineffective at improving oxygenation in anaesthetized horses (Taylor, 1990). Gleed and Dobson (1990) reported that the β_2 agonist clenbuterol (0.8 mg/kg) was very effective in increasing PaO_2 in dorsally recumbent halothane anaesthetized horses and their work was confirmed in clinical cases (Keegan et al., 1991). Other studies failed to reproduce these

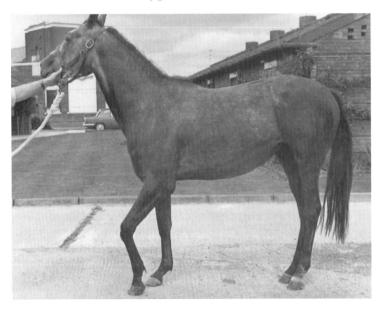

FIG. 11.12 Postanaesthetic myopathy shown in the forelimb. Characteristic posture of pain with head thrown back and up when made to walk. In this case there was hard swelling of the shoulder muscles and triceps. The posture due to pain varies with the muscles involved.

results (Doddam *et al.*, 1993; Lee *et al.*, 1998b) and it is probable that both positioning and the anaesthetic technique employed influence the efficacy of clenbuterol in raising PaO_2. In some cases the injection of clenbuterol is followed by a transient fall in PaO_2, presumably because of the increased O_2 demand associated with the side effects of sweating and tachycardia. Thus the routine use of clenbuterol to increase PaO_2 in anaesthetized horses cannot be recommended for use in clinical practice.

Muscle and nerve damage

There is an incidence of up to 6.4% of lameness following anaesthesia in the horse (Klein,1978; Richey *et al*, 1990), much of which is due to damage to nerves and muscles during recumbency. In the clinical situation it is not always easy to distingish between the two syndromes (hence the term 'radial paralysis' was once used to describe the condition now known to be caused by a triceps myopathy (Fig 11.12) and it is probable that it some cases both occur together.

Postanaesthetic myopathy (rhabdomyolysis)

It is now generally accepted that the common form of postanaesthetic myopathy is due to muscle ischaemia caused by inadequate muscle perfusion (Trim & Mason, 1973; Lindsay *et al.*, 1980; 1985; 1989). Clinical surveys (Klein, 1978; Richey *et al.*, 1990) have demonstrated that the incidence of the condition is increased by duration of anaesthesia and by periods of hypotension. In experimental circumstances it can be can be induced by prolonged (three plus hours) of hypotensive anaesthesia (Grandy *et al.*, 1987; Lindsay *et al.*, 1989). The failure of perfusion to the muscles is a typical 'compartmental syndrome'. i.e. increased pressure within the space limited by the fascial sheath of the muscle compromises the circulation. When intra-compartmental muscular pressure increases to the point at which the local circulation fails, the muscle will become ischaemic. Damage will occur at reperfusion and this results in swelling and a further increase in compartmental pressure, thus worsening the situation. The potential for continuing damage at reperfusion (Serteyn *et al.*, 1990)

explains why horses may appear unaffected when they first rise, the condition becoming apparent over the ensuing hours.

In order to limit the occurrence of myopathy, three factors are necessary:

(a) The time of anaesthesia should be kept as short as possible and anaesthetic time should never be wasted.

(b) Intracompartmental pressure should be reduced to the minimum. The intracompartmental pressure in the triceps muscles of the dependent limb in a horse positioned on a hard surface may reach as high as 50 mm Hg; positioning on a soft surface reduces this (Lindsay *et al.*, 1980; 1985). However, the weight of a horse or of one of its limbs can compress veins while patent arteries allow blood to flow into muscle capillaries, thus resulting in a rapid increase in intracompartmental pressure to that of arterial pressure (Taylor & Young, 1990) and the total failure of all muscle perfusion; this is probably the reason for myopathy in the non-dependant (or upper) limbs of laterally recumbent horses.

(c) Blood supply to the muscles should be increased. It has been routine to assume that this means increasing ABP, and certainly it is necessary to raise this above the 'closing pressure' within the muscle compartment. However, once ABP is above this 'closing pressure', then further improvement in muscle blood flow depends on increasing CO (Lee *et al.*, 1998a,b,c). Positive inotropes such as dobutamine improve CO, ABP and muscle blood flow whilst vasoconstrictor agents increase ABP but have no action on peripheral perfusion (Fig 11.13).

The condition described above fails to explain all cases of myopathy, and it is probable that the condition is multifactorial. Klein (1978) considered that there were two distinct types of anaesthetic induced myopathy, the compartmental syndrome and a more generalized form which she considered was more likely to occur in very fit animals; the authors have seen two cases of acute generalized rhabdomyolysis occurring in horses one–two days after anaesthesia, in which post-mortem findings resembled capture myopathy. The condition has much in common with equine azoturia. It has been postulated that the

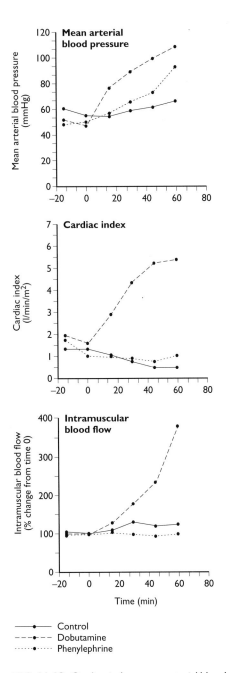

FIG. 11.13 Cardiac index, mean arterial blood pressure (MAP) and intramuscular blood flow in the dependent triceps muscle in 6 halothane-anaesthetized ponies. On different occasions the ponies were given increasing doses of infusions of one of the following: saline (control), phenylephrine or dobutamine. Dobutamine increased MAP, cardiac index and intramuscular blood flow, but whilst phenylephrine was equally effective in increasing MAP, it failed to improve either cardiac index or intramuscular blood flow (adapted from Y.H. Lee, et al., (1998)).

nutritional status and resulting intracellular pH at the time of anaesthesia is another factor involved, but no survey has found a significant link between the animals' nutritional status and anaesthetic-related myopathy. It would appear the generalized condition is sporadic and unpredictable in occurrence.

The treatment for myopathy is mainly symptomatic: analgesia (the condition is very painful), sedation if necessary, prevention of further damage, fluids (to prevent renal damage) and a great deal of tender loving care. As much of the damage occurs at reperfusion there could be a role for the administration of free radical scavengers, but as yet there is no evidence as to their efficacy. It is probable that by the time the condition is diagnosed, the damage is already present.

Neuropathy

Nerves may be damaged during the anaesthetic process by the effects of pressure, of stretching, and by ischaemia. Peripheral neuropathies (such as facial nerve damage through pressure from the headcollar (Fig 11.14) are easy to diagnose, but other cases (e.g. femoral nerve damage) may be

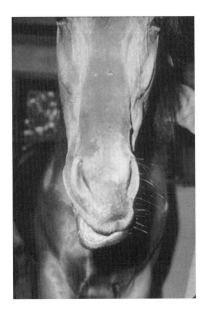

FIG. 11.14 Facial nerve paresis resulting from pressure. In this case the damage resulted from inadequate padding on the operating table, but more typically it results from pressure exerted by a head collar.

difficult to differentiate from myopathy, and indeed it is probable that the two conditions frequently occur concurrently. Neuropathy is not painful, but if it involves the motor supply to more than one limb, the horse will be unable to rise. Contused nerves may regain their function once the surrounding swelling has subsided, so symptomatic treatment should be combined with good nursing.

A very occasional but disastrous occurrence following anaesthesia is spinal malacia. The problem has only been reported to occur in young horses positioned on their back for a short procedure. Most, but not all cases have occurred in heavy horses (Brearley *et al.*, 1986; Lam *et al.*, 1995; Trim, 1997). Sometimes the horse fails to regain its feet following anaesthesia, other times it will stand, but an ascending paralysis commences. The condition appears totally painless; many cases have been maintained by good nursing for several days but the condition always progresses and euthanasia is inevitable. The cause of this condition is unknown.

PREPARATION FOR GENERAL ANAESTHESIA

The preanaesthetic examination and the general principles of preparation prior to anaesthesia described in Chapter 1 are, of course, applicable to horses, but there are some aspects of preanaesthetic preparation of these animals which warrant further consideration.

General considerations

To preserve the largest oxygen store in the body and to minimize gas trapping in the lungs, the FRC needs to be maintained at the highest possible level. Except in emergencies, it is always possible to ensure that the animal is fasted before anaesthesia. Fasting for more than 18 hours may result in acidosis, and is probably inadvisable, but it increases the FRC by up to 30%, presumably due to a reduction in the bulk of the abdominal contents through loss of ingesta and reduced gas content (McDonell, 1974). Water should always be available except for the last two hours prior to anaesthesia.

Extremely fit horses on high levels of nutrition, fed on grain-rich diets, and horses entirely grass fed seem particularly difficult to manage. They often develop abdominal distension during anaesthesia even after careful fasting and there is a clinical impression, unsupported by investigational data, that they are more prone to develop circulatory and other problems. Although there appears to be little scientific justification for it, many experienced anaesthetists and equine surgeons are firm believers in the old practice of 'letting down' an animal before subjecting it to anaesthesia and operation, i.e. reducing the protein and energy content of its diet for some 7–10 days before anaesthesia. In the authors' opinion, to postpone all but the most urgent of operations until a horse which is in full training has lost the peak of its fitness from being fed a less rich diet certainly does no harm and may have much to commend it. Unfortunately, economic considerations often demand that horses be returned to full work with the minimum of delay and this period of therapeutic inactivity is not well received by many owners.

Shoes should be removed before anaesthesia, or at least covered with adhesive plaster, to prevent damage to flooring or the animal itself in the recovery period. Surgeons may request that the horse receives prophylactic treatment for tetanus and is given antibiotics prior to the induction anaesthesia. Many of the antibiotic agents may influence the effects of anaesthetic drugs. Gentamycin and other antibiotics of this group will increase the length of action of neuromuscular blocking agents. The i.v. injection of penicillin causes marked hypotension (through vasodilation) for approximately 40 minutes (Hubbell *et al.*, 1987) and is best avoided just prior to anaesthesia. As the cardiovascular effects of most antibiotics are unknown, their i.v. use immediately prior to anaesthesia should be avoided unless absolutely essential to the overall success of the case.

In emergencies the aim of preparation for anaesthesia is to improve the physical status of the horse as much as possible, and to make any preparations which may reduce the risk of the perioperative process. To detail all such preparations is beyond the scope of this chapter. Briefly, orthopaedic cases may need support to the limb to prevent damage at anaesthetic induction, and analgesia and sedation should be chosen to avoid excessive ataxia. Most acute thoracic crises are the result of trauma and horses suffering from chest injuries may be agitated, restless and dyspnoeic, and may require an analgesic both for its sake and to reduce the risk of injury to attendants. Provided excessive doses are not used, the potential ability of analgesics to produce respiratory depression can be ignored. Air and/or fluid should be removed from the pleural cavity by the insertion of a chest drain before general anaesthesia is induced. In most emergency cases, hypovolaemia needs to be corrected before induction of anaesthesia. However, where blood loss is acute and the potential for further loss is still present (e.g. haemorrhage from the guttural pouch) such replacement should be limited prior to anaesthetic induction as an increase in blood pressure may result in the commencement of severe and uncontrollable haemorrhage. In such cases the agents used for sedation and analgesia should have minimal effects (in either direction) on blood pressure. Once the horse has been anaesthetized blood pressure will almost certainly be reduced, and it may then be necessary to administer rapidly high volumes of fluids.

Colic

The most common equine emergency case presented to the anaesthetist is that of colic. Most cases of colic presented for surgical treatment have already been treated medically and it is important to consider the drugs used, their route of administration, doses and time of dosing, for they can influence the response to subsequent anaesthesia. Pain is usually indicative of gastric and/or intestinal distension and of acute ischaemia. Its severity may make the horse unmanageable until it becomes utterly exhausted and pain must be controlled, although this is not always easy. NSAIDs, in particular flunixin, are widely used and can be so effective in reducing both the pain of colic and the signs of toxaemia as to mask the need for surgery (Moore, 1994). Opioids which are often used include butorphanol, pethidine (often in very large doses), methadone and morphine. Xylazine and detomidine are usually the most effective agents to provide analgesia in colic, but doses

should be kept low both to limit their duration of action, and their cardiopulmonary effects in an already stressed horse. The effect of these agents on gut motility is probably unimportant as it is comparatively short acting. Acepromazine, being an α-adrenergic blocker, will contribute to hypotension in dehydrated or shocked animals and is generally not advised if surgery will be necessary, although doses of up to 0.05 mg/kg are unlikely to do any harm.

The main problem in the preanaesthetic preparation of most colic cases is the replacement of fluids in the dehydrated and possibly shocked animal. Fluid replacement is extremely urgent in surgical cases if any consistent measure of success is to be obtained. Unfortunately, diagnosis is very imprecise, and there is an understandable reluctance on the part of both owners and veterinarians to spend a considerable sum of money and time on cases which may at laparotomy prove to be inoperable. To overcome this reluctance some acceptable routine which does not involve replacement of the major part of the fluid deficit prior to anaesthesia is clearly desirable. Our experience of cases in which tympany or violent intractable pain allowed only minimal preparation indicates that if really vigorous replacement is carried out once the surgeon has confirmed that surgical treatment is possible, a successful outcome is quite as likely as in cases treated before the induction of anaesthesia. Moreover, in cases of intestinal obstruction many are of the opinion that massive preoperative infusions are better avoided since much of the fluid infused accumulates in the obstructed intestine, making operation more difficult and time consuming because of the greater need for decompression of the bowel. Thus, it is possible that 'minimal' preparation can be justified on both surgical and economic grounds but it must be emphasized that for success it must be carried out in a rational manner.

Whenever possible anaesthesia should not be induced in a colic case until hypovolaemia has been improved and the packed cell volume (PCV) decreased. Tachycardia may persist, due to pain or toxaemia, even after the blood volume has been restored to normal. Hypertonic saline (4 ml/kg i.v. of 7.5%) followed by large quantities of Ringer's lactate provides an inexpensive method of treating the hypovolaemia rapidly. Other methods include the transfusion of plasma or plasma substitutes, such as starch. Acid–base disturbances are seldom a problem in the preoperative period and there is no need to administer bicarbonate at this stage. The administration of bicarbonate intraoperatively results in a very high $PaCO_2$, and the rapid exhaustion of the carbon dioxide absorbent of the anaesthetic circuit. Even in cases complicated by septic shock, the routine administration of glucocorticoids before operation is of doubtful value. Non-steroidal anti-inflammatory drugs (NSAIDs), if not already given, are usually administered both for their analgesic and antitoxaemic effects. Methods of treatment of endotoxic shock, such as the use of antibodies are very expensive and as yet there is no published data as to their efficacy in improving overall success.

Regardless of whether preoperative fluids are to be given to a colic case, at least one reliable i.v. line must be introduced into the jugular vein. A stomach tube should be passed through one nostril before the horse is anaesthetized and the stomach decompressed. It should be withdrawn into the oesophagus before the induction of anaesthesia because if left in the stomach it seems to encourage regurgitation, but it should not be completely removed for once the horse is recumbent under anaesthesia it is almost impossible to pass a tube down the oesophagus to the stomach. Gastric decompression will minimize the likelihood of the stomach rupturing during induction. Whenever possible the surgical site should be clipped and prepared while the animal is conscious and standing, for the duration of the anaesthetic period needs to be kept to a minimum in these very ill animals.

Mares nursing foals should not be separated from their offspring in the preanaesthetic period. If it is necessary to operate on the mare, the need for sedation is greatly reduced if anaesthesia is induced in the presence of the foal. Similarly, the presence of a foal's sedated mother contributes to the smooth induction of anaesthesia in the foal.

It is always safer if the weight of the animal is known and it should be determined by actual weighing, for visual appraisal, even with experience, is too inaccurate. Under field conditions it is improbable that weighing facilities will be available, and the average figures given in Table 11.3

constitute a useful guide. The weight of a horse may also be estimated with acceptable accuracy from the formula:

$$\text{Weight (kg)} = \frac{\text{Girth (inches)}^2 \times \text{Length (inches)}}{660}$$

The girth is measured just behind the elbow and the length is from the point of the shoulder to the line of the ischial tuberosity. M. Down and L. Gray (personal communication) weighed 400 horses of all ages, including geldings, stallions and mares admitted to the Cambridge Veterinary School over a 3-year period and found that the formula given above always estimated the weight to within 25 kg of the true weight. Commercially available 'weighbands' base their calculation on the girth measurement only, but still provide a useful estimate of weight.

Intravenous techniques

In horses i.v. injections are usually made into the jugular vein about half way down the neck. The horse should be handled quietly, as once forcible restraint (such as the twitch) is used many will tense their neck muscles and obscure the jugular furrow, making i.v. injection difficult and the danger of accidental intracarotid injection more likely. The usual aseptic precautions should be taken prior to insertion of a needle or catheter, the size of which depends on personal preference and on what is to be injected. A small fine needle (e.g. 23 G) does not necessarily cause the horse less pain

TABLE 11.3 **Ranges in weight for various types of animal**	
Type of animal	**Weight (kg)**
Children's ponies	150–300
Donkeys	150–200
Thoroughbred yearlings	300–350
Thoroughbred 2 y.o.	300–400
Thoroughbred 3 y.o.	400–450
Thoroughbred adults	450–550
Hunter	450–675
Warmbloods	500–750
Cart yearlings	350–450
Cart 2 y.o.	450–525
Draught cross	550–625
Heavy draught	650–850

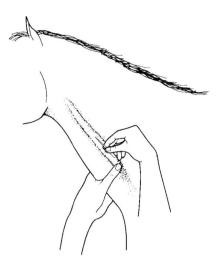

FIG. 11.15 Injection into the jugular vein of the horse. The vein is easily raised with digital pressure. 'Neck ropes' should not be employed for this purpose as they invariably displace the skin resulting in withdrawal of the needle or catheter from the vein when their compression is released.

than one of 19 G, but will reduce the damage to the vein which may be important if many such injections are anticipated. The vein is distended by pressing the thumb into the jugular furrow just below the site of venipuncture (Fig. 11.15). This tenses the skin and the distended vein is easily palpable. Two methods of placement of a needle may be used. In the first, the point of the needle is directed at an angle of 45° to the vein, slid through the skin, into the vein then advanced up the vein towards the head. In the second method the needle is held at an angle of 90° to the vein, thrust into it, then turned 90° so that it can be advanced up the vessel. It is important that a good length of needle (or catheter) is introduced into the vein otherwise there is a risk that as the vein subsides, on the release of pressure, it will retract away from the needle or that the slightest movement will cause the needle to leave the vessel. A free flow of blood indicates that the needle is well placed in the lumen of the vein. If only a few drops of blood fall either (1) the needle is in a perivascular haematoma or (2) the needle is in the vein but its lumen is partially blocked. If red blood spurts, or blood is very free flowing then the needle may be in the carotid artery and should be withdrawn, the fist being placed hard into the jugular furrow over

the point of injection and maintained there for at least 5 minutes in order to prevent the formation of a haematoma. Unfortunately intracarotid injection may not be recognized if a small bore needle is employed. Once the needle is *in situ*, its hub and the syringe should be held and pressed gently and continuously against the animal's neck during any injection so that should the animal move its neck the hand (and needle) will move with the horse and thus overcome any tendency for the needle to be pulled out of the vein.

Catheterization of the jugular vein

If larger needles or catheters are to be used in foals (which are hypersensitive to injections), or if the animal is very sensitive, it is necessary to desensitize the skin either by injecting a bleb of lignocaine subcutaneously via a very fine needle, or by using an intradermal pressure injector. EMLA cream also may be used for this purpose but it is difficult to keep the cream-covered swab in place for long enough to be effective.

Catheters are now almost routine for the administration of i.v. anaesthetic agents in the horse. Simple, short (less than 6 inches) over the needle catheters are perfectly adequate and are placed as described in Chapter 9. Once it is certain that a catheter is in the vein to its maximum length it should be secured in position with a partial skin thickness stitch and a stopcock or injection cap attached (Fig. 11.16). The catheter may be kept patent for many hours if its lumen is periodically flushed with heparin saline solution (10 IU/ml). Ideally the skin suture should be laid before venipuncture is attempted so that it may be tied securely around the catheter without risk of displacing this from the vein, but otherwise, the catheter may be fixed in place with a drop of acrylate glue which will hold it whilst the suture is completed.

There is no advantage to be gained from introducing a needle or catheter into the vein in a downwards direction away from the head except, possibly, for the infusion of large volumes of solutions such as guaiphenesin. Technical errors are much more likely to arise if attempts are made to perform venipuncture in this manner. The operation is more awkward: it is more difficult to assess

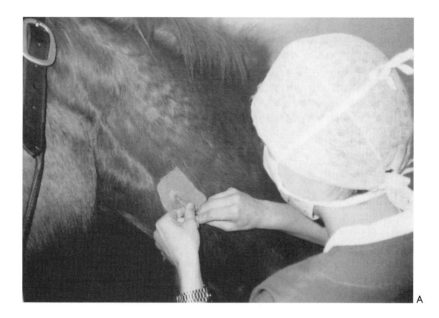

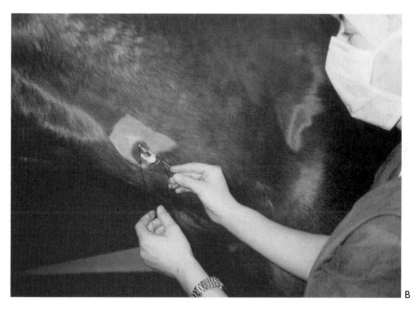

FIG. 11.16 Introduction of a catheter into the jugular vein. In (**A**) a catheter of the 'over-the-needle' variety is being introduced through an insensitive skin weal produced by the intradermal injection of 1 ml of 2% lignocaine. It is usually necessary to make a small skin incision in the centre of the weal to prevent 'belling-out' of the catheter tip, or the catheter being pushed back along its introducing needle as the skin is penetrated. After penetration of the skin the vein is distended by digital pressure and the catheter advanced well into the vein. In (**B**) the catheter and its occluding tap are being fixed in position with partial skin thickness sutures. (It is helpful if these sutures are in position before the catheter is introduced but this was avoided here for sake of clarity.)

the depth to which the needle is being inserted, it is more difficult to detect intracarotid injection and if the animal moves its neck the direction of move-

ment will be against the point of the needle thus tending to transfix the vein. Care must be taken to avoid air embolism when a needle or catheter is directed downwards since its tip will be at a lower pressure than its hub, predisposing to the aspiration of air if the hub is not closed off whenever an injection is not being made. Very little air needs to be aspirated to cause the horse to collapse – the authors have seen one case where aspiration was heard to occur for less than one second through a 23 G catheter.

Where a catheter is to remain in place for some time postoperatively, usually to enable the infusion of fluids, then long catheters are used. These catheters are usually placed over guide wires by the Seldinger technique and are always directed towards the heart. Long catheters are not ideal for i.v. induction of anaesthesia (other than by infusion techniques) nor for the very rapid administration of fluids as their length increases resistance and therefore slows the speed of injection. When catheters are left in place, there is a danger of infection and subsequent thrombophlebitis so full sterile precautions are required for their placement, and in subsequent handling of the injection ports.

PREMEDICATION

The choice and dose of any premedicant drug will depend on the physical condition and temperament of the horse, the likely duration of the proposed examination or operation and the nature of the anaesthetic technique to be employed. In many respects, the relative importance given to the premedicant drugs or the anaesthetic agents is a matter of personal preference. Some anaesthetists favour heavy sedative premedication which decreases the quantities of sedatives and anaesthetics administered later, while others habitually use light premedication and more of the anaesthetic. In the hands of their exponents both regimens appear to produce similar results.

Anticholinergics

In current practice anticholinergic drugs are not used in the routine premedication of horses, although they may be administered if required once the horse is anaesthetized, for example if the surgery is likely to provoke vagal reflexes or should bradycardia develop. Doses of 0.01–0.02

mg/kg i.v. atropine appear to be safe to use where required but nevertheless in horses, glycopyrrolate (0.005–0.010 mg/kg) is probably preferable (Singh *et al.*, 1997), for it is shorter acting and does not readily cross the blood-brain barrier, thus being less likely to cause central excitatory effects.

Sedatives

Premedication with sedative agents whilst the horse is still in its accustomed accommodation greatly improves the process of anaesthetic induction as it keeps the horse calm, reduces apprehension and fear, and makes procedures such as the placement of catheters more pleasant for both horse and anaesthetist.

Acepromazine

In many cases acepromazine (0.03–0.05 mg/kg i.m. or 0.03 mg/kg i.v.) given 30–60 minutes prior to anaesthesia is ideal for premedication; it calms the horse without making it ataxic and its long-lasting effects usually last throughout the whole perioperative period, so contributing to a calm recovery. Acepromazine reduces the dose of the parental anaesthetics used and reduces MAC of volatile anaesthetic agents (Heard *et al.*, 1986). The influence of acepromazine premedication on the amount of volatile anaesthetic agent required becomes obvious when the effects of concurrently administered short acting $\alpha_2$adrenoceptor agonists wane (usually 60–90 minutes); without acepromazine the depth of anaesthesia lightens very suddenly, necessitating a rapid increase in the inspired levels of volatile anaesthetic agents. The use of acepromazine for premedication significantly reduces the overall anaesthetic risk (Johnston *et al.*, 1995).

$\alpha_2$adrenoceptor agonists

Xylazine, detomidine and romifidine are widely used as part of the anaesthetic induction process and they reduce markedly the dose of both i.v. and inhalation anaesthetic agents. However, they may also be used as classic 'premedicants' in which case their residual action must be taken into account when deciding on doses to be used at anaesthetic induction. Doses used i.v. for premedication are approximately half those used for sedation (i.e. xylazine at 0.5 mg/kg, detomidine at 10 μg/kg and romifidine at 50 μg/kg) so that the horse is able to walk to the anaesthetic induction area. The i.m. use of α_2 adrenoceptor agonists has been much neglected, but i.m. doses of 1 mg/kg xylazine or 20 μg/kg detomidine give excellent sedation after approximately 20 minutes. If the horse is exceptionally difficult to handle, 40–50 μg/kg detomidine (chosen because of the low volume invoved) may be given i.m., the horse left quietly for at least 20 minutes, after which time, in the authors' experience, i.v. injection has always become possible, although occasionally only with the aid of a twitch. In such horses i.m. injection may be given at any convenient site (the horse often does not anticipate an injection in the pectoral muscles) as swelling rarely occurs after the use of i.m. detomidine.

Analgesics

Opioid analgesics may be used both to provide preoperative pain relief if necessary, when full analgesic doses are required, and to improve the level of sedation, when doses are usually reduced to half. Full doses may be required for difficult horses, and in these circumstances can usually mixed in the same syringe as the α_2 adrenoceptor agonist. In general mixing such combinations is not recommended by the manufacturers as the necessary tests to ensure chemical stability have not been performed, but with difficult horses there may only be one opportunity to carry out the injection. If not already given, NSAIDs may be administered so that they will be effective by the postoperative period.

INDUCTION OF ANAESTHESIA

The past 40 years have seen great improvements in equine anaesthesia but a routine method suitable for every situation has yet to be discovered. The anaesthetist must choose a suitable method with regard to the size, health and temperament of the individual horse, the cost of the procedure and the facilities and staff available.

Facilities for induction

With the exception of occasional emergency situations, anaesthesia should never be induced in horse without there being available the necessary apparatus to resuscitate the horse should it become necessary. Such apparatus includes endotracheal tubes, methods to administer O_2 and apply IPPV, and the drugs likely to be needed should cardiac arrest occur. In the hospital setting the apparatus needed to administer volatile anaesthetic agents (anaesthetic machine and absorber circuit) will fulfil this role. For field anaesthesia, a portable source of O_2 will be required. IPPV of the lungs can be satisfactorily provided by the use of a stream of oxygen directed into the trachea for the Venturi effect by a Hudson valve, or using an easily portable to-and-fro circuit.

The cardiopulmonary system of the anaesthetized horse must be monitored continuously throughout anaesthesia but the degree of sophistication with which this will be done will depend on the facilities available, and in the field may be limited to those of continuous observation, palpation of the pulse, and possibly the use of a battery operated pulse oximeter. The pulse oximeter is of variable use in the horse as many such instruments cannot function with pulse rates below 40 beats/minute. The favoured site for the probe is across the nasal septum, as it is without hair, usually without pigment, and sufficiently thin. In equine hospitals monitoring is more sophisticated and may include the electrocardiogram, ABP, peripheral pulse monitor, end-tidal gases and arterial and venous blood gases.

Methods of control at anaesthetic induction

Free fall

In this simplest method of control, one person holds the horse's head as it becomes recumbent. If the horse leans back as anaesthesia takes hold, the handler holds the head down, which steadies the fall and prevents the horse going over backwards (Fig 11.17). With the type of induction which occurs following use of the dissociative agents this is less necessary, and the handler simply has to steady the head. If induction is in a padded box,

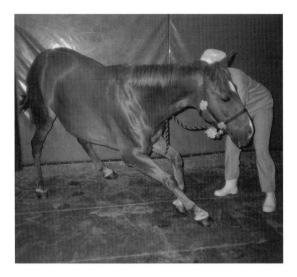

FIG. 11.17 Control of a horse during induction of anaesthesia using the 'free-fall' method.

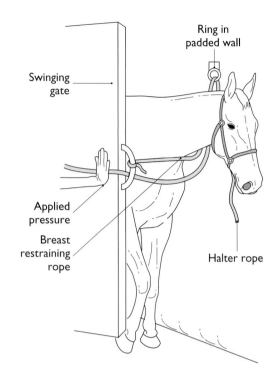

FIG. 11.18 Control of a horse during induction of anaesthesia using the 'gate' or 'swinging-door' method. Induction to recumbency is aided by two or three people applying pressure to the gate as the horse sinks towards the floor. An assistant restrains the horse's head and prevents the horse from falling forwards or backwards. The breast control rope which prevents the horse from walking forwards is slackened off as the horse becomes recumbent.

the horse may be placed with its rump to a wall so that the wall takes the weight; this makes induction very smooth, but occasionally results in a hind leg becoming trapped beneath the horse.

The free fall method requires the minimum of staff and is the only practicable method in the field.

Gate method

In this method the horse is positioned against a wall of the induction box, and restrained there by a gate. A rope, which can easily be released, holds the gate in place and prevents the horse moving forward (Fig. 11.18). Usually when available several people also press against the gate to support it. As anaesthesia is induced, the rope is released and the gate opened so that the horse may sink to the ground.

A variation of this method manages without the gate, the horse being held against the wall by a number of people. The horse is restrained and its weight supported as it becomes recumbent by head and tail ropes attached to rings in the wall of the induction box.

Tilting table

In this method the operating table top is tilted to the vertical position; the adequately premedicated or quiet animal is restrained against the table top by straps (Fig 11.19). As the horse loses consciousness during the induction process it is brought smoothly into lateral recumbency by restoring the table top to its normal horizontal position. The method usually works very well but it is only possible where an adequate number of trained personnel are available, and trouble occurs if the horse panics or a fault develops in the table mechanism at a critical stage of induction. Once the horse is unconscious, padding must be placed underneath it, so the method does not remove the necessity to lift the horse. The horse may be allowed to recover on the horizontal table top and placed on its feet as soon as it is judged able to stand by rotating the top to vertical; or the horse may be transferred to a padded recovery box.

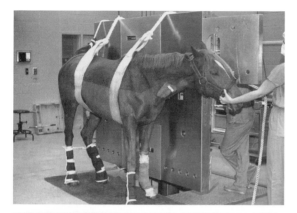

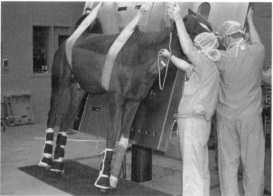

FIG. 11.19 Induction of anaesthesia using a tilting table top. The sedated horse is restrained against the table which is rotated to the horizontal position as the animal becomes unconscious and relaxed. Usually induction of anaesthesia is with guiaphenesin/thiopental or guiaphenesin/ketamine and 4 to 6 trained personnel are involved in manipulation of the table and animal.

Intravenous regimes for anaesthetic induction

In normal clinical practice anaesthesia in adult horses is induced with i.v. agents. The dose of anaesthetic required in the healthy horse will depend on the amount of sedative and opioid analgesic it has received both as premedication and just prior to anaesthetic administration. The number of possible combinations of sedative and anaesthetic agents which are suitable for anaesthetic induction are enormous, and the choice will depend on facilities, the state of the horse, and on personal preference. However, the majority of induction techniques are based on a combination of sedative drugs either with hypnotic/anaesthetic agents such as thiopental, or with dissociative

agents such as ketamine. Either method may be assisted by the use of centrally acting muscle relaxants such as guiaphenesin or the benzodiazepine agents. The following section and Table 11.4 discuss some combinations which the authors have found satisfactory. If the horse is not healthy modifications may have to be made to these protocols. For example, there may be times when the side effects of the α_2 adrenoceptor agonists are contraindicated, and conditions such as toxaemia or hypoproteinaemia reduce the quantity of anaesthetic agent required.

Hypnotic/anaesthetic agents

The manner in which a horse becomes recumbent is similar following the injection of any of the hypnotic/anaesthetic agents, and is typified by that with thiopental. Following injection of thiopental the horse tries to lean backwards and to lift its head, which must be restrained to prevent the horse losing its balance and possibly 'going over backwards' (Fig. 11.17). With restraint, the horse sinks gently to the ground. Premedication with the α_2 adrenoceptor agonists slows the circulation in a dose-dependent manner and the onset of unconsciousness is delayed for 40–120 seconds after completion of the thiopental injection. The horse may make paddling or galloping movements when it first becomes recumbent; these movements disappear within 10–20 seconds as unconsciousness deepens.

Thiopental

Thiopental is a hypnotic/anaesthetic agent commonly employed. The dose required to induce anaesthesia in the horse depends on the amount of sedation present (Table 11.4). As recovery from an induction dose of thiopental depends on redistribution rather than elimination, reduction in the dose leads to a faster and better quality recovery. Thiopental at 15 mg/kg i.v. can be given rapidly to unsedated colts for castration; induction is adequate but recovery, although rapid, may be very violent and this method cannot be recommended. Following premedication with acepromazine (0.03–0.05 mg/kg) given at least 30 minutes prior to anaesthesia, thiopental, at a dose of 10 mg/kg

TABLE 11.4 Some regimes suitable for the induction of anaesthesia prior to maintenance with volatile agents, or by TIVA. Anaesthesia results from a combination of the effects of the sedative premedicant drugs and of the induction agents. Many combinations other than those listed here can be used safely

Premedication	Anaesthetic	Maintenance by further i.v. agents (TIVA) for short duration (20–30 mins) only
Acepromazine, 0.03–0.05 mg/kg i.m. or i.v.	Thiopental, 11 mg/kg i.v. or Methohexital, 5 mg/kg i.v.	
Xylazine, 0.5 mg/kg i.v. or Detomidine, 0.01 mg/kg i.v.	Thiopental, 7–8 mg/kg i.v.	Thiopental, 1 mg/kg i.v. (recovery may be prolonged and of poor quality if total thiopentone dose exceeds 12 mg/kg)
Xylazine, 1 mg/kg i.v. or Detomidine, 0.01 mg/kg i.v.	Thiopental, 5.5 mg/kg i.v. or Methohexital, 3 mg/kg i.v.	Thiopental, 1 mg/kg i.v. (maximal dose as above)
Xylazine, 1 mg/kg i.v.	Ketamine, 2.0–2.2 mg/kg i.v. (Diazepam, 0.01–0.03 mg/kg i.v. given immediately following the ketamine will improve relaxation, but may cause apnoea)	Thiopental, 1 mg/kg i.v. (maximal dose as above) or increments of 0.5 mg/kg xylazine and 1 mg/kg ketamine i.v. as required
Detomidine, 0.015–0.02 mg/kg i.v.	Ketamine, 2.0–2.2 mg/kg i.v. (optional: diazepam, 0.01–0.03 kg/i.v. as above)	Thiopental, 1 mg/kg i.v. (maximal dose as above) or increments of 1 mg/kg ketamine i.v. as required
Romifidine 0.08–0.12 mg/kg i.v.	Ketamine, 2.0–2.2 mg/kg i.v. (optional: diazepam, 0.01–0.03 mg/kg i.v. as above)	Thiopental, 1 mg/kg i.v. (maximal dose as above) or increments of 0.02–0.04mg/kg romifidine and 1 mg/kg ketamine i.v. as required
Xylazine, 0.5–1.0 mg/kg i.v. Detomidine, 0.01–0.02 mg/kg i.v.	Tiletamine, 0.05–1.0 mg/kg i.v. and Zolazepam, 0.5–1 mg/kg i.v. (Tiletamine and zolazepam are supplied as a fixed 50:50 ratio combination)	
Acepromazine, 0.03–0.05 mg/kg i.m. or i.v.	Guaiphenesin infused i.v. (approximately 25–50 mg/kg) until ataxia, then thiopental, 5 mg/kg i.v.	Thiopental, 1 mg/kg i.v. (maximal dose as above). Extra guiaphenesin may be infused, but maximal doses should not exceed 50 mg/kg, or recovery may be delayed
Xylazine, 0.5–1.0 mg/kg i.v. or Detomidine, 0.01 mg/kg i.v. or Romifidine, 0.08 mg/kg i.v.	Guaiphenesin infused i.v. (approximately 25–50 mg/kg) until ataxia, then thiopental 5 mg/kg i.v. (Alternatively thiopentone can be mixed with the guaiphenesin, and the mixture infused until the horse becomes recumbent)	Thiopental, 1 mg/kg i.v. (maximal dose as above). Extra guiaphenesin may be infused, but maximal doses should not exceed 50 mg/kg, or recovery may be delayed
Xylazine, 1 mg/kg i.v. or Detomidine, 0.01–0.02 mg/kg i.v. Romifidine, 0.08 mg/kg i.v.	Guaiphenesin infused i.v. (approximately 15–30 mg/kg) until ataxia, then ketamine, 1.5–2.0 mg/kg mg/kg i.v.	Thiopental, 1 mg/kg i.v. or ketamine, 1 mg/kg i.v.

Additional premedication with acepromazine (<0.05mg/kg) will not reduce the dose of induction agent required, but will lengthen the duration of action. Additional premedication with an opioid (e.g., butorphanol 0.02 mg/kg) will not reduce the dose of induction agent required, but may cause additional respiratory depression. Its use may also increase the duration of effect of the anaesthetic agents.

i.v., is a satisfactory induction technique. The horse becomes unconscious and recumbent 25–30 seconds after the thiopental injection and anaesthesia lasts for an adequate time either to enable a short procedure such as castration, or to provide a smooth transition to an inhalation agent when anaesthesia is to be maintained for long periods. If no maintenance agents are given the horse regains its feet in approximately 30–40 minutes, and although there may be some ataxia, recovery is usually calm. The dose of thiopental is critical, under dosage through underestimation of weight may lead to excitement during induction, and for this reason it used to be common practice to follow the injection of thiopental with a small dose (0.1 mg/kg) of succinyl choline, but this agent is now used rarely.

The use of i.v. α_2 adrenoceptor agonists (xylazine, detomidine or romifidine) just prior to anaesthetic induction reduces the dose of thiopental required in a dose dependent manner, and also increases the therapeutic index of the drug, meaning that it is rare for underdosage to cause excitement. Xylazine 1 mg/kg or detomidine 20 µg/kg given i.v. 5 minutes prior to induction reduces the necessary dose of thiopental to about 5.5 mg/kg. Following doses of xylazine of 0.5 mg/kg or detomidine at 10 µ g/kg i.v. the dose of thiopental required is about 8 mg/kg. Anaesthesia lasts for 15–20 minutes (sufficient to enable castration) and if no further drugs are administered, the horse will regain its feet after 30–40 minutes. As yet there is little published information available as to the combination doses of romifidine and thiopental. Premedication with acepromazine prior to giving xylazine or detomidine does not appear to reduce the dose of thiopental subsequently required for anaesthetic induction. Recovery to standing (in the absence of maintenance agents) occurs in 30–40 minutes, and with less ataxia than when higher does of thiopental are employed.

Thiopental/guaiphenesin

After premedication with acepromazine, and/or α_2 adrenoceptor agonists, guaiphenesin (at concentrations of 5–15% depending on the personal preferences of the anaesthetist and the preparations available) is infused into the jugular vein until the horse shows marked ataxia (after approximately 35–50 mg/kg). A bolus i.v. dose of about 5 mg/kg of thiopental then produces recumbency and apparent unconsciousness. Panic due to muscle weakness may be seen if guaiphenesin is infused without prior administration of sufficient sedative. It is also possible to combine guaiphenesin and thiopental solutions for infusion into the jugular vein to produce recumbency but there is much less control over anaesthesia when this is done and profound respiratory depression can be produced. Recovery from these agents alone occurs in 30–40 minutes, but there may be some residual muscle weakness if high doses of guiaphenesin are used. Where anaesthesia subsequently is maintained with other agents the effects of guiaphenesin have time to wane.

Methohexital

The dose of methohexital required to induce anaesthesia appears to be half that for thiopental. For example 5 minutes after i.v. xylazine (1 mg/kg) or detomidine (15 µg/kg) anaesthesia can be induced with 2.8 mg/kg of methohexital given i.v. as a bolus dose. Lateral recumbency occurs in a similar fashion and time scale to that following thiopental. However, following the use of methohexital, the breathing rhythm is often abnormal, three deep breaths being succeeded by 30–40 seconds without any sign of respiratory activity. Similar breathing patterns occur in horses with other anaesthetic agents but the clinical impression is that they are more common during anaesthesia involving methohexital. Anaesthesia lasts for about 5 minutes and the horse usually stands up about 25 minutes later. Recovery is usually quiet and uneventful.

Propofol

A rapid injection of propofol (2 mg/kg i.v.) appears adequate for induction of anaesthesia when given 5 minutes after i.v. α_2 adrenoceptor agonists such as xylazine 0.5 mg/kg, detomidine 15–20 µg/kg, or medetomidine 7 µg/kg (Nolan & Hall, 1985; Aguiar et al., 1993; Bettschart-Wolfensberger et al., 1999a). At these doses of propofol anaesthesia appears to last for approximately 10 minutes, with recovery to standing within 30 minutes. In all studies the animals became hypoxaemic and appeared very lightly anaesthetized, but where surgery was being performed (Aguiar et al., 1993), there was no response to surgical stimulation. Without premedication a dose of 4 mg/kg propofol is necessary to induce anaesthesia and even then horses show some excitement and paddling (Mama *et al.*, 1995). With the current preparations of propofol available, it is difficult to inject even 2 mg/kg propofol sufficiently rapidly, and in large horses slow injection results in a poor quality of anaesthetic induction (Bettschart-Wolfensberger, 1999a). However, it is possible that new more concentrated preparations of propofol will become available and these may make induction of anaesthesia with this agent more practicable and perhaps, less expensive.

Etomidate and metomidate

Etomidate has apparently not been used in horses, and it is probable that current preparations would result in the volume required being too large to be practicable. However, the similar but no longer available compound, metomidate (2.25 mg/kg i.v.) following premedication with detomidine (10 μg/kg) produced excellent induction prior to maintenance of anaesthesia with halothane since significant apnoea did not occur.

Dissociative agents

When the dissociative agents, ketamine or tiletamine are given on their own to horses, they cause stimulation rather than depression of the central nervous system, with a form of excitement in which there is poor muscle relaxation, tremors and even convulsions. Many drugs have been used in attempts to suppress these most undesirable effects but only the α_2 adrenoceptor agonists and the benzodiazepines have proved to be of any real value.

The dissociative anaesthetic agents are not effective in a single brain circulation time, and therefore where sedation with an α_2 adrenoceptor agonist has preceded the i.v. injection of ketamine a large horse may take as long as 3 minutes to become recumbent. The method of achieving recumbency differs from that seen following thiopental; it is a much more gradual process, the animal often taking a step or two sideways or backwards before sitting back on its haunches and sinking to sternal recumbency. It then rolls gently over on to its side and may make one or two quite vigorous limb movements before becoming still. Once laterally recumbent, the animal settles much

more quickly and the onset of unconsciousness is more rapid when no attempt is made forcibly to restrain the head – if this is done the horse may even try to rise and can be very difficult to restrain.

Ketamine

Ketamine, following premdication with an α_2 adrenoceptor agonist produces excellent induction of anaesthesia followed by a spectacularly rapid, but usually very quiet, recovery. Xylazine 1.0–1.1 mg/kg, detomidine 20 μg/kg or romifidine 80–100 μg/kg is given i.v. and then, once maximum sedation has developed (approximately 5 minutes), a bolus of ketamine (2.2 mg/kg) is injected i.v. Lateral recumbency is assumed in 1–3 minutes after the ketamine injection, the longer time occurring with the larger animals. Anaesthesia continues to deepen for 1–2 minutes after the horse becomes recumbent, and even when eye movements cease, relaxation of the jaw muscles is not always good and it may be necessary to prise the mouth open for the passage of an endotracheal tube. Relaxation can be improved by the administration of a benzodiazepine agent i.v. (usually diazepam 0.01–0.05 mg/kg) immediately after the ketamine injection, although this tends to cause further repiratory depression and should be used with caution in situations where facilities for IPPV are not readily available. If for any clinical reason it is desirable to give a lower dose of α_2 adrenoceptor agonist, then the dose rate of the benzodiazepine can be increased to compensate. The classic signs and stages of anaesthesia are not recognizable; nystagmus and tear formation may be observed and the surest guide to the depth of anaesthesia is the presence or absence of response to surgical stimulation. When no other anaesthetic is given, depending on the degree of surgical stimulation, horses first raise their heads 10–30 minutes after the ketamine injection, roll into sternal recumbency some minutes later and stand 5 or 6 minutes after this. Termination of surgical anaesthesia is very abrupt but recovery is remarkably free from excitement and horses usually stand at the first attempt. Once standing there is very little evidence of ataxia.

The method is not without disadvantages. The very abrupt end of surgical anaesthesia when no other agents are given can lead to difficulties, and indeed this rapid 'awakening' may become evident even when anaesthesia is continued with volatile anaesthetic agents. Horses require very different handling from that used when anaesthesia is induced with the barbiturates, and this is a matter of familiarity with the regime. However, the method appears to be a very safe way of producing short periods of anaesthesia. Cardiovascular parameters are well maintained (Muir et al., 1977; Hall & Taylor, 1981; Clarke et al., 1986), respiration is adequate and continuation of anaesthesia with an inhalation agent or by total i.v. methods presents no problems.

Ketamine may also be used with other premedicant agents or in other combinations. Acepromazine premedication is inadequate prior to ketamine induction. Many dose schedules utilizing guaiphenesin together with α_2 adrenceptor agonists and ketamine have been recommended. For example, xylazine (2.2 mg/kg) is given by i.m. injection 20 minutes before 55 mg/kg of guaiphenesin is infused as a 5% solution in 5% dextrose into the jugular vein. This is followed by the i.v. injection of 1.7 mg/kg of ketamine (Muir et al., 1978b).

Ketamine can be given with benzodiazepine agents alone (i.e. with no α_2 adrenoceptor agonists). In foals diazepam or midazolam (0.10–0.25 mg/kg i.v.) followed by ketamine (2.2 mg/kg i.v.) gives a very satisfactory anaesthetic; usually foals lie down following the benzodiazepine drug. However, in adult horses the combination is more difficult to employ. Neither agent should be given alone. As both have a variable onset of action, when administered together the quality of induction is very variable depending on which agent takes effect first (Clarke et al., 1997). One study utilizing midazolam/ketamine found that even after three hours of subsequent halothane anaesthesia, recovery was complicated by muscle weakness, and in some cases it was necessary to antagonize the residual midazolam. The poor quality of induction and recovery with these benzodizepine/ketamine combinations is unfortunate as during subsequent maintenance with volatile agents, heart rate, MAP and CO are maintained at a considerably higher value than when α_2 adrenoceptor agonists are used in the induction protocol (Luna et al., 1997).

Tiletamine/zolazepam

The idea behind the combination of tiletamine with zolazepam is that there is already a benzodiazepine present to ensure muscle relaxation during subsequent anaesthesia. In the horse, however, this combination has always been used following the administration of an α_2 adrenoceptor agonist. This combination is used after xylazine (Hubbell et al., 1989) or detomidine premedication (Muir et al., 1999). Although it produces reasonably safe 'short-term anaesthesia' of a little longer duration than that seen after xylazine/ketamine/diazepam, it offers very little other advantage.

Other i.v. techniques

Etorphine

Etorphine is used in horses as 'Large Animal Immobilon', a yellow solution containing 2.45 mg etorphine hydrochloride with 10 mg acepromazine maleate per millilitre. The minimum dose for horses is 0.5 ml of the solution i.v. per 50 kg body weight. The i.m. route should only be used in dire emergencies since it results in a period of marked excitement before sedation and anaesthesia ensue. Animals made recumbent with Immobilon are very stiff, with muscle tremors, severe respiratory depression, cyanosis, tachycardia and hypertension. In male animals priapism is not uncommon. Transfer to inhalation anaesthesia is usually not required because the effects of Immobilon last about 45 minutes. Because of the marked effects in the body, Immobilon is not recommended for use in horses with cardiac problems or liver damage. Animals should not be slaughtered for consumption by humans or other animals until 28 days have elapsed.

The actions of Immobilon may be antagonized by the injection of Revivon, a blue solution containing 3 mg/ml of diprenorphine hydrochloride. A quantity of Revivon equal to the total volume of Immobilon injected should be given i.v. as soon as possible after the required period of restraint is complete. Most (but not all) horses regain their feet within a few minutes of this injection. Injection of Revivon antagonizes only the actions of etorphine, hence analgesia is lost but sedation due to the acepromazine is unaffected. Undesirable hyperexcitability may be associated with the injection of the antagonist and enterohepatic cycling may occur, causing excitement and compulsive walking 6–8 hours after remobilization. An extra half dose of Revivon given subcutaneously at the time of initial reversal may reduce the incidence of this delayed excitement, but should it still occur, a further half dose of Revivon must be given. The product information states that horses must be kept stabled for at least 24 hours after the administration of Immobilon. Donkeys appear particularly susceptible to delayed excitement with Immobilon, and the current product information no longer gives any recommendations for this species. Combinations of etorphine with other agents such as xylazine and azaperone have proved no more satisfactory in practice than Immobilon, and the attempts of some clinicians to obtain greater muscle relaxation by combining α_2 adrenoceptor agonists with Immobilon are unwise in view of the respiratory and circulatory disturbances which result.

The use of Immobilon is associated both with a degree of risk to the life of the anaesthetist and to that of even healthy horses. Large Animal Immobilon is an extremely potent neuroleptanalgesic which is highly toxic to man. In man it causes dizziness, nausea, pinpoint pupils, respiratory depression, cyanosis, hypotension, loss of consciousness and death. In the event of accidental injection, spillage on the skin or splashing into the eyes or mouth immediate treatment is essential. Any veterinarian contemplating the use of Immobilon should be thoroughly familiar with the latest treatment measures set out in the product information sheet and ensure that adequate supplies of (in date) naloxone are to hand. If it is considered for any reason that the use of Immobilon is *absolutely essential*, it is clearly most unwise to use it unless another qualified person is present.

Anaesthetic induction with inhalation agents

Although induction of anaesthesia in adult horses with volatile agents of anaesthesia is possible in experimental circumstances, it is not practicable for clinical use with the very limited exception of chloroform by Cox's mask. However, in foals anaesthesia can be induced with any suitable volatile anaesthetic agent.

Chloroform

Chloroform has little place in routine equine anaesthesia. It causes dose related liver toxicity while sensitizing the heart to adrenaline induced arrhythmias, and its safe use requires a great deal of skill. Anaesthetic chloroform is no longer available in the UK, but analytical quality chloroform is at least, if not more, pure. Despite potential problems, its use may be justified on the grounds of economy for procedures such as castration in small unbroken colts whose monetary or sentimental value is minimal. Administration of chloroform by Cox's mask to induce anaesthesia has been described in a great deal of detail in earlier editions of this book

Volatile agents in foals

An inhalation induction technique in young foals avoids the necessity of giving drugs that their immature hepatic detoxicating mechanisms may not be able to cope with. The size and lack of fat in the foal mean that induction with volatile agents is easily achieved, with minimal excitement. The mare should be sedated, but if possible allowed to remain until the foal is unconscious as to separate the two at this time will lead to great distress and high levels of circulating adrenaline in the foal, with an increased anaesthetic risk. To achieve induction of anaesthesia the standing foal is gently restrained and the inhalation anaesthetic (halothane or isoflurane) volatilized in a stream of O_2 or N_2O/O_2 administered through a face-mask applied lightly over both nostrils. The volatile agent should be introduced gradually, its concentration being increased every three or four breaths up to a maximum of $4 \times MAC$ until consciousness is lost. As the foal loses consciousness the attendants must lower it gently to the ground, the mask removed, and an endotracheal tube passed through the mouth in the usual manner. Currently there is no evidence as to the safety of using the new volatile agents, sevoflurane or desflurane, to induce anaesthesia in foal. It is anticipated that they will result in very fast effective anaesthetic induction, but their rapid speed of uptake will mean that great care is needed to prevent overdosage. The maximum concentrations required in relation to MAC will be very much lower than those recommended above for halothane and isoflurane.

An alternative to using a face-mask is to pass an endotracheal tube into the trachea via one nostril and administer the anaesthetic through this. The best endotracheal tubes for this purpose are of silicone rubber and about 55 cm long. Neonatal Thoroughbred foals can accommodate tubes of 7–9 mm internal diameter and in 6 week old foals 11 mm tubes can be passed with ease. Passage of the tube is greatly facilitated by prior preparation of the ventral nasal mucosa with lignocaine ointment or gel and lubrication of the tube with the same preparation. The possible complications of this technique have been reviewed (Webb, 1984) but with care they are rare. Anaesthetic systems designed for use in adult human subjects are adequate for foals up to 2–3 months of age.

The recent survey of anaesthetic deaths in horses (Johnston *et al.*, 1995) found that in foals induction of anaesthesia with a volatile agent resulted in a higher mortality rate than when i.v. induction methods were employed. Whether this finding represents a genuine increased risk, or whether it results from the fact that in the sickest foals anaesthesia was induced with volatile agents has yet to be elucidated.

MAINTENANCE OF ANAESTHESIA

Endotracheal intubation

In horses the passage of a Magill-type endotracheal tube (for which in the UK there is a British Standards specification) presents no great problem. With the anaesthetized horse in lateral recumbency the head is moderately extended on the neck, the mouth opened, a suitable gag or bite block put in place and the tongue pulled forward. The tube, lubricated on its outside with a suitable lubricant (e.g. K-Y Jelly, Johnson and Johnson), is introduced into the mouth with the concave side of its curve directed towards the hard palate and advanced, keeping to the midline, until its tip is in the pharynx. It is then rotated so that the concavity

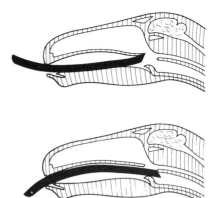

FIG. 11.20 Passage of an oral endotracheal tube in a horse.

of its curve is towards the tongue (Fig. 11.20) and at the next inspiration it is pushed rapidly on into the trachea. The rotation of the tube when its tip is in the pharynx ensures that it does not become impacted on the epiglottis.

The commonest causes for failure of the tube to enter the trachea are that the alignment of the head and neck is incorrect, that the tube is not in the midline of the orotracheal axis, or that the tip of the tube is sited ventral to the epiglottis: should any of these occur the tube should be withdrawn to clear the epiglottis, and redirected for a further attempt.

The technique for introduction of straight tubes or those with only a shallow curvature differs slightly: the head needs to be more extended on the neck and often it is easier to introduce the tube with its concavity towards the tongue, then to rotate the tube 360° once in the pharynx in order to disconnect the soft palate from the epiglottis. Once in the correct position the tube should advance down the trachea with minimal resistance; force should not be used. Resistance to passing the tube suggests either the endotracheal tube is too large, or that oesophageal intubation has occurred.

Intubation through the mouth permits the use of the largest tube which will comfortably fit the trachea. A 16.0 mm diameter tube is suitable for ponies up to about 150 kg body weight, while a 25–30 mm tube is adequate for most thoroughbreds. Heavy hunters and warmbloods often take surprisingly large tubes.

Endotracheal tubes can be passed through the inferior nasal meatus but this limits the size of the tube to that which can be accommodated by the nostril, and therefore increases resistance to breathing. The introduction and removal of nasal tubes entails the risk of damaging the turbinate bones, although with the modern soft silicone tubes this risk is reduced. Despite the limitations, nasal intubation can be very useful in cases where the surgeons require unobstructed access to the mouth. In young foals the nasal passages are relatively much larger than in adults and tubes of adequate size can be introduced through the nostril.

The cuffs of endotracheal tubes are often damaged by contact with the horse's teeth even when a reliable mouth-gag is used to keep the mouth open during intubation and extubation. Cuffed tubes made of red rubber for use in horses are very expensive, but punctured cuffs should not be repaired with patches not vulcanized on, as otherwise these patches may become detached during anaesthesia and lodge in one of the smaller air passages with disastrous results. Plastic tubes have met with only partial success; either the plastic is so hard that atraumatic intubation is difficult or, when they reach body temperature they soften so much that they become obstructed when the head is flexed on the neck. Siliconized latex rubber cuffed tubes are more successful, can be recuffed, and, although the smaller versions for foals, sheep etc. may require an 'introducer' before they can be inserted, those designed for adult horses are sufficiently stiff to enable endotracheal intubation to be performed easily. Static charges on the silicone attracts dust, and it is important that after use and cleaning it is not placed where it will attract such dirt during the induction process.

As the horse has poor laryngeal tone, the cuff of the endotracheal tube must be adequately inflated if the IPPV is to be carried out, and a good seal is exceptionally important in cases of colic to prevent inhalation of regurgitated material. Cuffs should therefore be checked for leaks by leaving them inflated for a period of time prior to use

The Cole-pattern tube (Fig. 11.21), which has no inflatable cuff, has been used in horses but these tubes have to be of the exact size needed for any given animal and accurately placed in the larynx if they are to provide an atraumatic seal which is sufficiently gas-tight for IPPV to be carried out without gross leakage of anaesthetic gases. They must

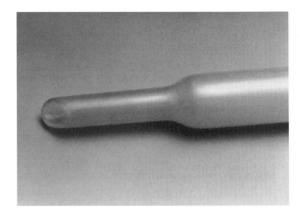

FIG. 11.21 Cole-pattern endotracheal tube for the horse.

be used with care in young animals having soft laryngeal cartilages for in them forcible dilatation with these tubes can seriously damage the larynx. They have been reported in association with acute laryngeal oedema in two adult horses although whether they were in fact the cause was not established (Trim, 1984).

Positioning

Practically the aim in positioning is:

1. to reduce to the minimum possible the pressure at all points in order to enable adequate blood perfusion to muscles and to decrease the chance of a compartmental syndrome occurring

2. to ensure that major veins are not obstructed. If this happens then pressure in the area drained by these veins will increase until it reaches arterial values, after which time there will be no further perfusion to the area

3. to avoid putting anything under tension. Nerves are particularly easily damaged by stretching as well as by direct pressure

4. to allow surgical access.

The first three aims are often at odds with the fourth, necessitating compromise and sacrifice of surgical convenience for the benefit of the horse.

It is now generally accepted that the best method to reduce pressure on the horse's body is to position it on a soft foam mattress sufficiently deep to allow the horse to sink right in (thus reducing the unit weight at any one point) without 'bot-

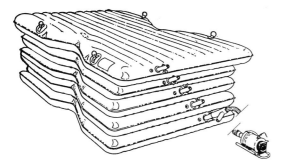

FIG. 11.22 The Snell infla-table. This is a portable, pnuematically raised table comprising of five stacked chambers. The top chamber provides the working surface and should not be fully inflated so that the horse lies on a soft, compressible surface. The lower four provide support and height adjustment. It is placed in its deflated condition alongside the anaesthetized horse which is then rolled on to it. The table is then inflated to the desired working height using an electrically powered air pump. (Manufactured by Snell-Wessex Ltd, Fosters Farm, Boyshill, Holnest, Sherborne, Dorset DT9 5PJ, UK).

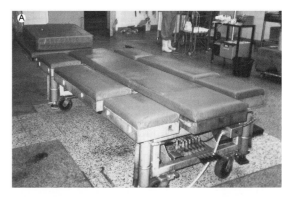

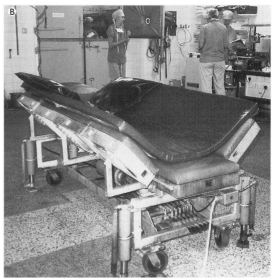

FIG. 11.23 An operating table with many sections which may slide out (**A**) thus assisting the surgeons to make a good approach to the operating site. However, the edges of hard padding around these separate sections are potential 'pressure points' and extra padding (**B**) should be provided between them and the horse.

toming' on the hard undersurface. The type of matting used in gymnastics is ideal. However, the horse has to be lifted on to such a mat. Alternatives are air or water mattresses which may be partially inflated under the horse (Fig. 11.22). It is very important that air mattresses are not fully inflated – the horse must still be able to sink in or no reduction in pressure is achieved. This is one of the times when compromise from the surgeon is necessary as operating on a horse which is lying on a soggy water or air bed is not conducive to the performance of any delicate surgery.

The edges of tables or overinflated air or water beds can cause pressure points and result in nerve or muscle damage. Operating tables may have such 'edges' in association with sections which slide out, and if so, suitable pads and matting to cover these pressure points are essential (Fig. 11.23).

When horses are positioned in lateral recumbency, the under front leg should be pulled forward, and both upper legs should be supported parallel to the body (Fig. 11.24). This support reduces pressure on the triceps muscles, brachial vessels and nerves, and also prevents obstruction of the venous drainage of the upper limbs. Supine horses may be supported by a V-shaped back support (Fig. 11.25) but where such supports are used,

care must be taken to use some soft padding or the pressure on the triceps muscle may be sufficient to induce myopathy. The legs may be supported on a hoist or tied to pillars but extending both hind legs, and in particular locking the stifle joints of dorsally recumbent horses, should be avoided unless absolutely essential to the surgery, as it may result in severe hindlimb lameness. This lameness is thought to be due to femoral nerve damage, but there may also be a component of gluteal myopathy. If bilateral, the horse will be unable to rise. The problem is unrelated to weight – the authors have seen it in miniature Shetland

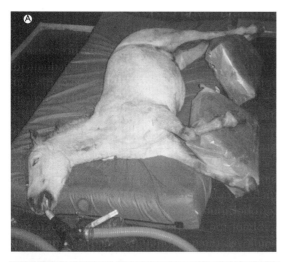

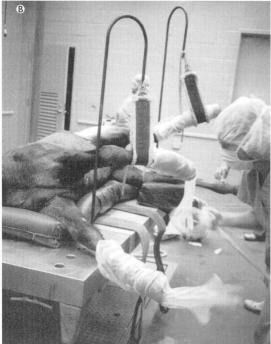

FIG. 11.24 A well positioned horse in lateral recumbency. It is placed on a deep soft foam bed, into which it sinks, thus reducing the weight at any one point. The upper limbs are supported so that venous drainage is not impaired, and the other forelimb drawn forward. When a table is not used the limbs can be positioned with cushions **A**. In **B** the limbs are supported in slings. An extra foam cushion was used to keep the head slightly elevated.

ponies, and it can occur after a comparatively short time.

The head is very liable to damage at pressure points and to avoid damage to the masseter muscle, facial nerve and eyes, care must be taken to ensure that the face is not allowed to fall over the edge of the table top or to remain in contact with sharp edges of halters or head collars. Whether in lateral decubitus or supine the head must not be over-extended (this leads to laryngeal paralysis) nor rotated on the neck. If possible the head should be slightly raised during anaesthesia to ensure good venous drainage and to avoid intense vascular congestion of the nasal passages leading to gross upper respiratory obstruction after extubation. When the anaesthetized horse has to be moved the head should be supported in a normal position in relation to the neck.

Under field conditions, the facilities may not be available to position the horse as suggested above. However, a horse in lateral decubitus may have adduction of the upper limbs prevented by supporting them on straw bales, and the undermost foreleg may be drawn as far forward as possible to minimize pressure on the brachial vessels and nerves.

AGENTS FOR THE MAINTENANCE OF ANAESTHESIA

Intravenous agents: total i.v. anaesthesia (TIVA)

Total i.v. anaesthesia for short procedures in the field (such as castration) has been used for many years, but in the past available agents had such a long duration of action that their use was very restricted. Today, drugs which are rapidly metabolized and eliminated are being introduced and TIVA can be used for more prolonged procedures as the duration of recovery after some of the more recently introduced agents and combinations is no longer than after anaesthesia with volatile agents. Also, reassessment of some of the older agents has shown that many of their disadvantages can be overcome by using them in combination with other or newer drugs.

The use of TIVA does not reduce the need for apparatus or for experienced staff. Most i.v. anaesthetic techniques cause as much, if not more respiratory depression, than do volatile anaesthetics, and

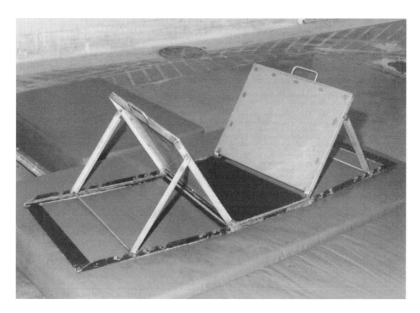

FIG. 11.25 Back support for supine horse. In use the support is covered with 3 inches (7.5 cm) thick foam padding. The weight of the horse is taken by the dorsal spine and the spines of the scapulae, thus avoiding pressure on the back muscles.

indeed overdose commonly causes respiratory arrest, so it is still essential to have a means of delivering oxygen to the horse and of providing IPPV if required. ABP is better maintained than with volatile agents, but it is now realized that this does not necessarily mean that there is no cardiovascular depression; CO still may be reduced and peripheral perfusion poor. Adequate cardiopulmonary monitoring is as necessary with i.v. as with volatile agents.

The current limitations to techniques of TIVA are those of duration and of expense. Many drugs or combinations are long acting and cumulative, so extending length of action with more drug may result in a prolonged and poor quality recovery. The ideal agents for use by infusion (propofol and some of the α_2 adrenoceptor agonists) have pharmacokinetics such that neither they nor their active metabolites are cumulative whatever the duration of administration. In a compromise between expense and the ideal agents, the techniques suitable for TIVA can be considered in three categories: those suitable for short procedures such as castration (up to 30 minutes) and which result in a very rapid recovery; those suitable for more prolonged use (up to 1.5–2.0 hours), and those which could be extended indefinitely should the surgery demand. Procedures may last far longer than anticipated, and if

necessary anaesthetists must be prepared to change technique (e.g. to introduce volatile agents, or change to different drug combinations) if required.

TIVA for short procedures (up to 30 minutes)

The techniques for i.v. induction anaesthesia described above (p. 284, Table 11.4) provide adequate anaesthesia for procedures lasting 10–15 minutes and (except for Immobilon) anaesthesia can be 'topped up' with increments of i.v. drugs for a period of time before cumulation occurs. The most commonly used combinations for short term anaesthesia are combinations of the α_2 adrenoceptors with ketamine or with thiopental. Anaesthesia is then extended with incremental doses of thiopental or ketamine.

If no additional agents are given, recovery from ketamine-based methods occurs within 20–25 minutes and is usually very smooth and well controlled. However, recovery can be abrupt, and sometimes the horse may awaken during surgery with little warning so it is essential that a rapid means to deepen anaesthesia is to hand. The duration of surgical anaesthesia can be increased by the use of local anaesthesia; this technique is particularly suitable for castration. Choice of the α_2 adrenoceptor agonist (xylazine, detomidine or romifidine) utilized prior to ketamine does not influence the quality and duration of anaesthesia, or the speed and quality of recovery (Kerr *et al.*, 1996).

With thiopental-based methods, recovery is slower (30–40 minutes), there is some hindlimb weakness, and often more that one attempt to rise is required. Nevertheless, with appropriate premedication rising is usually calm. Although the horse may still move in response to surgery (local anaesthesia is a good option to prevent this) it is easy to anticipate, and the abrupt awakenings seen with ketamine do not occur.

Agents used to extend the duration of anaesthesia

Thiopental sodium

Small doses (0.5–1.0 mg/kg i.v.) may be given to extend anaesthesia which has been induced with either thiopental or with ketamine. The major advantage of thiopental is that it acts in a circulation time and is ideal to bring an awakening animal quickly back under control. However, overdose may cause apnoea and, as the drug is cumulative, speed and quality of recovery depend on the total dose. Thus, if initial anaesthetic induction was with ketamine, more increments may be given than is possible following induction using thiopental. A total dose of 10 mg/kg still results in a calm recovery in an acceptable time; higher total doses may be safe but will lengthen recovery.

Ketamine hydrochloride

Anaesthesia induced with α_2 adrenoceptor agonists/ketamine mixtures may be prolonged with additional ketamine, but there is a danger of undesirable excitatory effects unless the α_2 adrenoceptor induced sedation is still adequate. In clinical practice, incremental doses of half the original dose of both xylazine and ketamine are given as required. There will be a delay before these agents will be effective. The xylazine/ketamine combination can be extended to give medium term anaesthesia by administration of half the initial dose of both xylazine and ketamine at approximately

20 minute intervals (Short, 1981). The combination, using infusions of the two drugs, has been used to provide approximately 90 minutes of anaesthesia (Mama *et al.*, 1998). With detomidine/ketamine combinations only a further dose of ketamine (1 mg/kg) is required initially to extend the duration, although if ketamine increments are to be given more than 30 minutes after anaesthetic induction, it is probably advisable also to administer a small dose of detomidine (approximately 5 µg/kg). With romifidine/ketamine combinations the product information sheet suggests that incremental doses of both ketamine and romifidine are given to extend anaesthesia.

To date there are no scientific reports as to the use of ketamine (1 mg/kg i.v.) to lengthen the duration of anaesthesia induced with α_2 adrenoceptor agonist/thiopental, although anecdotal reports suggest that the method is practicable.

Methohexital sodium

Methohexital (0.5 mg/kg i.v.) can be given to extend anaesthesia in the situations where increments of thiopental would otherwise be used. However, it is very respiratory-depressant and recovery is violent if the horse is not well sedated.

TIVA for medium duration procedures (30–90 minutes)

Anaesthesia which needs to be prolonged for more than 30 minutes is usually achieved by combinations of α_2 adrenoceptor agonists, ketamine, and a centrally acting muscle relaxant – guiaphenesin or a benzodiazepine. (Table 11.5). Ideally any drug used for infusion to provide long term anaesthesia should have a short half life of elimination so that there is no cumulation. Not all these agents have the ideal kinetics, hence their limitations for use beyond 90 minutes (although some extension may be possible at the expense of a more prolonged recovery).

Xylazine and detomidine have adequately rapid kinetics (the information for romifidine is currently not available), but residual guiaphenesin will cause muscle weakness in recovery, so methods which reduce the dose of this component are preferred. It benzodiazepines are used, then they

TABLE 11.5 **Some regimens of total intravenous anaesthesia (TIVA) suitable for providing anaesthesia of from 30–90 minutes duration. All agents are given i.v. unless otherwise stated. Many variations of these combinations can be used safely**

Premedication	Anaesthetic	Maintenance
Acepromazine, 0.03–0.05 mg/kg i.m. or i.v.	Chloral hydrate (10%) infused until ataxia (50–60 mg/kg), then thiopental, 5–6 mg/kg or methohexital, 2.5–3.0 mg/kg	Thiopental, 1 mg/kg (maximal total dose 12 mg/kg) or methohexital, 0.5 mg/kg. If anaesthesia needs to be extended beyond 45 minutes, more chloral hydrate may be required
Xylazine, 1 mg/kg or Detomidine, 0.02 mg/kg or Romifidine, 0.08 mg/kg	Ketamine, 2.0–2.2 mg/kg	The 'Triple Drip', a combination of guiaphenesin, α_2 adrenoceptor agonist and ketamine infused to effect. For details of how to prepare suitable mixtures, see below
Xylazine, 1 mg/kg	Ketamine, 2.0–2.2 mg/kg followed after induction by Climazolam 0.2 mg/kg	Climazolam (0.4 mg/kg/h) and ketamine (6 mg/kg/h) are infused during surgery. 20 minutes after cessation of infusion, the climazolam is reversed with sarmazenil (0.04 mg/kg)

Additional premedication with acepromazine (<0.05 mg/kg) may also be used. Additional premedication with an opioid (e.g. butorphanol 0.02 mg/kg) will not reduce the doses of agents required initially, but may lengthen their effects and may also cause additional respiratory depression. Regimens including propofol have not been included here as, at this time of writing, the costs involved mean that they are not practicable for clinical use.

must be antagonized at the end of surgery – this is expensive. Theoretically ketamine is not cumulative, but if used by infusion for periods of more than 90 minutes, prolonged and poor quality apparently hallucinatory recoveries have been seen (Bettschart-Wolfensberger et al., 1996). It is postulated that the cause of these poor quality recoveries is the cumulation of the active metabolite, norketamine. The cumulation of norketamine will depend on total dose of ketamine rather than on time, so combinations which can reduce the rate of infusion of ketamine may be used for a longer period.

α_2Adrenoceptor agonist/guiaphenesin/ ketamine – the 'Triple Drip'

The 'Triple Drip' was first used by Green et al. (1986) who used i.v. xylazine (1.1 mg/kg) followed by ketamine 2.2 mg/kg for anaesthetic induction, then maintained anaesthesia with an i.v. infusion of 2.75 ml/kg/h of a guaiphenesin/ketamine/ xylazine mixture containing 50 mg guaiphenesin, 1 mg ketamine and 0.5 mg of xylazine per ml of 5% dextrose in water. This technique, and adaptations of it using different α_2 adrenoceptor agonists are now widely used in operations of up to 90 minutes

of duration (Taylor & Luna, 1995). To make up a suitable solution for infusion 1 gram of ketamine and either 500 mg of xylazine or 10 mg detomidine are added to 500 mls of 10% guiaphenesin or 330 ml of 15% guaiphenesin. Anaesthetic induction should preferably avoid guiaphenesin in order to reduce the total dose of this long acting agent, and is then maintained by infusion to effect. The average rate of this mixture which is needed to maintain anaesthesia is 1 ml/kg/hour but, depending on the induction regime used, higher rates may be needed earlier in procedure and rates should be reduced towards the end of surgery. Recovery from prolonged infusion of the Triple Drip is not fast (often more than one hour) but is usually calm. Romifidine has been used as the α_2 adrenoceptor agonist component of the combination.

α_2Adrenoceptor agonist/benzodiazepine/ ketamine

The replacement of guaiphenesin by a benzodiazepine agent can improve the quality of recovery. The system has been most widely used in Switzerland, where both the benzodiazepine climazolam and its antagonist sarmazenil are available. Anaesthesia is induced with xylazine and ketamine, then climazolam is given at 0.2 mg/kg i.v. Anaesthesia is maintained with an infusion of climazolam 0.4 mg/kg/hour and ketamine 6 mg/kg/hour. Infusion ceases at the end of surgery, but the benzodiazepine is not antagonized with sarmazenil (0.04 mg/kg i.v.) for 20 minutes in order to give time for the ketamine effects to have waned. The system gives good cardiovascular stability and respiration is adequate but O_2 is usually given. Recovery occurs rapidly following reversal of the benzodiazepine agent (Bettschart-Wolfensberger *et al*, 1996).

Chloral hydrate/barbiturate

Chloral hydrate lost favour due to its irritant nature if injected outside the vein and to the fact that if used alone recovery is very slow. However, in combination with the barbiturates it gives good moderate term anaesthesia and administration through long i.v. catheters reduces the risk of perivascular injection. A 10% solution is infused until the horse becomes ataxic (after 40–60 mg/kg have been administered) when thiopental (5 mg/kg) or methohexital (2.5 mg/kg) is injected i.v. as a bolus. Surgical anaesthesia is maintained by injection of increments of barbiturates (thiopental 1 mg/kg or methohexital 0.5 mg/kg). If anaesthesia is to extend for more than 45 minutes, it may prove necessary to give more chloral hydrate (approximately 10 mg/kg but to effect). The need for this becomes obvious if small increments of barbiturate fail to suppress paddling movements. If no further chloral hydrate is given, the horse will stand some 50–60 minutes after anaesthetic induction and recovery is usually calm. Whilst anaesthetized, respiration is well maintained, the pulse is strong and mucous membranes are a healthy pink with a fast capillary refill time, all suggesting that there is minimal cardiovascular depression.

TIVA for long procedures (2 hours and more)

Propofol combinations

The only anaesthetic agent which is sufficiently non-cumulative in the horse to be used for very prolonged anaesthesia is propofol (Nolan *et al.*, 1996). Propofol however has several drawbacks: it is a poor analgesic, it produces severe respiratory and moderate cardiovascular depression, and its carrier results in accumulation of triglycerides in blood. In the horse there are additional disadvantages that with existing preparations, large volumes are required and at such volumes it becomes very expensive. There must also be some concern as to the dangers of triggering hyperlipaemia in susceptible individuals, although to date this complication has never occurred. Nevertheless, if TIVA is ever to become practical for anaesthesia of unlimited time in the horse, propofol is the agent most likely to be involved.

A number of studies have looked at methods to reduce the dose of propofol by providing analgesia and further sedation (Nolan & Hall, 1985; Taylor, 1989; Nolan *et al.*, 1996; Flaherty *et al.*, 1997; Carroll *et al.*, 1998; Mama *et al.*, 1998; Bettschart-Wolfensberger, 1999a; Matthews *et al.*, 1999). Most combinations utilize α_2 adrenoceptor agonists, with or without ketamine. In all studies the authors commented on the fact the horse appeared very lightly anaesthetized, yet did not respond to surgery.

Betschart-Wolfensberger (1999a) investigated the use of continuous propofol and medetomidine infusions to provide 4 hours of anaesthesia in ponies. Medetomidine was chosen for its kinetics and its marked analgesic properties. Anaesthesia was induced either with medetomidine/propofol or medetomidine/ketamine and an infusion of medetomidine at 3.5 μg/kg/hour commenced. The minimum propofol infusion required to prevent response to a noxious stimulus ranged from 0.06–0.11 mg/kg/minute and cardiovascular parameters were well maintained although oxygen supplementation was requried to prevent hypoxia. Following 4 hours anaesthesia recovery occurred in approximately 30 minutes, and was of excellent quality. Mama *et al.*, (1998) investigated the use of xylazine infusions of 35 μg/kg together with propofol at either 0.15 or 0.25 mg/kg/min for one hour; anaesthetic quality was excellent but at the higher doses there was marked hypoxia and recoveries were delayed. Flaherty *et al.*, (1997) maintained anaesthesia in ponies with an infusion of ketamine (40 μg/kg/min) and propofol

(0.124 mg/kg/min); anaesthesia was adequate for castration and recovery was smooth.

ANAESTHETIC MAINTENANCE WITH INHALATION AGENTS

Volatile agents

Halothane

Halothane's special advantages were (and still are) reasonably rapid induction and recovery, minimal excitement during induction or recovery, adequate reflex suppression and sufficient muscle relaxation to allow most surgery to be performed, lack of toxicity and ease with which anaesthesia can be controlled. Halothane causes a dose-dependent fall in ABP and CO and a rise in CVP. The fall in CO is due to a direct depressant effect of the agent on the myocardium and falls of up to 55% of the non-anaesthetized values have been recorded (Hall *et al.*, 1968). There is a marked respiratory acidosis in spontaneously breathing halothane-anaesthetized horses and while this can be overcome by IPPV this causes a further fall in CO (Steffey & Howland, 1978). Schatzmann (1982) showed that hypoxaemia causes a respiratory drive in horses anaesthetized with halothane in air, thus demonstrating that hypoxia can overcome halothane-induced respiratory depression.

In horses it is remarkably difficult to judge the depth of unconsciousness during anaesthesia with halothane (or the other volatile agents) as hypoxia from any cause results in sympathetic stimulation and signs such as nystagmus, sweating, hyperventilation and even movement. These may be taken as signs of inadequate depth of unconsciousness by the inexperienced anaesthetist, with disastrous consequences. As the MAC value for halothane is about 0.9% it is possible to monitor the depth of halothane by continuous measurement of the end-tidal concentration. The end-tidal values needed to maintain anaesthesia depend on the sedative premedication and anaesthetic induction technique employed.

Following induction of anaesthesia with thiopental, when O_2 alone is used as the carrier gas, stable maintenance of anaesthesia is usually achieved with end-tidal concentrations of 0.7–1.1% halothane; when induction is with keta-

mine, once the effect of the α_2 adrenoceptor agonist has waned end-tidal concentrations of 1.1–1.3% are frequently required. Halothane is a poor analgesic; horses which are apparently well anaesthetized may respond suddenly to surgical stimulation. Many of such responses are spinal reflexes, and are best prevented by provision of analgesia. ABP and HR during halothane anaesthesia also will depend on other agents administered. The decrease in ABP can give an indication of the depth of anaesthesia, but modern practice of treating hypotension with positive inotrope agents will counteract this fall and remove this sign.

Horses normally regain their feet within about 30 minutes following the termination of halothane administration after induction with xylazine/ketamine; after acepromazine premedication and thiopental induction, recovery takes about twice as long. Shivering is often seen during recovery; the reason is unknown – it does not seem to be related to body or environmental temperature and usually is of no importance. However, by increasing O_2 demands it may be harmful to horses suffering from respiratory and/or cardiovascular diseases which limit O_2 uptake when they are breathing air. Quality of recovery depends on the injectable drugs which have been administered, on the surgery performed and the presence or absence of pain. Recovery tends to be better following thiopental induction compared to ketamine inductions (Young & Taylor, 1993), possibly because a prolonged recovery enables more of the halothane to be eliminated before the horse tries to stand. Horses may take several attempts to rise, and show a measure of incoordination after recovery from halothane, but usually remain calm. However, horses should not be made to walk (e.g. from recovery to loose box or stall) within 10–15 minutes of standing up.

Isoflurane

Isoflurane has been used for anaesthesia in horses for approximately 15 years (Steffey *et al.*, 1977; Steffey, 1978; Steffey & Howland, 1980). In many ways it is very similar to halothane, and the signs of depth of anaesthesia in horses and the potential for a sudden response to surgery are identical with both agents. However the kinetics and the cardiopulmonary effects of isoflurane and halothane differ.

At equipotent doses isoflurane causes a smaller fall in CO than does halothane, and thus its effect on arterial hypotension mainly results from decreased peripheral resistance (Steffey & Howland, 1980). These differences between the cardiovascular effects of halothane and isoflurane are still apparent following anaesthetic induction with i.v. agents (Taylor, 1991; Lee *et al.*, 1998c). However, isoflurane is more respiratory depressant than is halothane (Steffey *et al.*, 1980) and it is advisable to perform IPPV on isoflurane-anaesthetized horses not surgically stimulated in order to avoid hypoxia and hypercapnia. The kinetics of isoflurane mean that induction and changes in depth of anaesthesia are rapid and recovery is impressively quick. However, the quality of recovery can be poor (Rose *et al.*, 1989), especially where ketamine was used for anaesthetic induction, and it is usual to administer a further dose of an α_2 adrenoceptor agonist at the end of anaesthesia to delay recovery and improve its quality.

Opinions diverge as to the relative merits of halothane and isoflurane for prolonged anaesthesia in the horse. As yet there is no evidence that isoflurane is safer than halothane; indeed in the multi-centre survey of equine deaths associated with anaesthesia (Johnston *et al.*, 1995) horses which received isoflurane were more likely to die than those receiving halothane but this may have been due to the selection of isoflurane for the more critical cases.

Enflurane

Enflurane may be used for equine anaesthesia (Steffey *et al*, 1977; 1978; Taylor & Hall, 1985), but has not gained popularity for a number of reasons. The MAC value of enflurane is about 2% and, clinically, end-tidal concentrations of about 2.3% produce satisfactory surgical anaesthesia after acepromazine premedication and thiobarbiturate induction. However, with large animals it is difficult to achieve this end-tidal concentration using the commercially available vaporizers (maximum of 5% enflurane) unless economically unacceptable high flows of fresh gas are added to the rebreathing systems. Respiratory depression with enflurane is marked, and if IPPV is used to overcome this, then hypotension can be severe or even fatal. Deep enflurane anaesthesia is associated with abnormal twitches in the muscles of the head, neck and forelimbs which become progressively more pronounced as the end-tidal concentration of enflurane increases. Recovery from enflurane anaesthesia is very rapid, but it is associated with occasional bouts of excitement and more shivering and incoordination than is recovery from halothane (Taylor & Hall, 1985).

Sevoflurane

MAC of sevoflurane in the horse is 2.3% (Aida *et al.*, 1994) and despite the fact that most commercial vaporizers currently have a maximum output of 5%, low solubility and rapid uptake means that there are no problems in achieving suitable end-tidal values. Like other volatile anaesthetic agents, sevoflurane causes dose related depression of respiration, CO and ABP (Aida *et al.*, 1996) but clinically, following anaesthetic induction with injectable agents, the cardiopulmonary depression is similar in extent to that caused by isoflurane (Grosenbaugh & Muir, 1998). The speed with which anaesthesia can be deepened means there is rarely a need to give additional injectable anaesthetic agents during anaesthesia. However, the rapidity of uptake is such that care must be taken not to overdose in the early stages of anaesthesia. Recovery from anaesthesia is very fast, but its quality is variable. Without further sedation the authors have found it to be poor, but if xylazine is administered to horses as soon as sevoflurane is terminated acceptable quality recovery occurs in about 30 minutes, and is often better than following isoflurane anaesthesia (Aida *et al.*, 1997; Matthews *et al.*, 1997).

If sevoflurane is priced at an affordable level (currently it is very expensive) it may well replace currently employed agents.

Desflurane

Trials of desflurane in the horse have been very limited. However, the few studies which have been performed suggest that desflurane has major advantages for use in this species (Jones *et al.*, 1995;

Clarke *et al.*, 1996; 1996a; Tendillo *et al.*, 1997). The kinetics of desflurane are such that the end-tidal concentration reaches inspired concentrations in a matter of minutes, even in a large horse, and recovery is equally as fast. Consequently, control of anaesthesia is very easy. The MAC of desflurane in the horse is approximately 7.5%; following i.v. induction the horse is connected to the circle circuit which has been primed with 8% desflurane in O_2. In the first 10 minutes the circle system is emptied twice to reduce the contained N_2 concentration, but after this time the circuit can be run closed – the fresh gas flow rate still containing 8% desflurane, together with enough O_2 to replace that lost by utilization and by leaks from the circuit (usually about 3 litres/minute in a large horse). The low flow rates used throughout mean that desflurane becomes comparatively inexpensive to use – in the UK it costs less than halothane. If anaesthesia is too light, the bag is emptied and refilled with a concentration 1% above the previous level, and depth of anaesthesia changes within a very short space of time. Horses anaesthetized with desflurane rarely react suddenly or violently to surgical stimulation, but occasionally if anaesthesia is too light, they exhibit muscle tremor and it is sometimes necessary to increase inspired desflurane concentration to as much as 10% to stop this. Recovery from anaesthesia is also very fast – unsedated animals attempt to rise within 6–10 minutes of withdrawal of desflurane, and although they remain calm, are still weak and may fall forward. It is now routine to administer a small dose of i.v. xylazine (0.1–0.2 mg/kg) at the end of anaesthesia, after which horses get to their feet in about 15–20 minutes in a calm and coordinated manner.

The use of desflurane is not without its problems. Cardiopulmonary depression is dose-dependent and is similar to that of equipotent doses of isoflurane (Clarke *et al.*, 1996a). At alveolar concentrations sufficient for surgery CO is well maintained, although there is marked hypotension. The rapid kinetics and very fast change in depth of anaesthesia mean that is easy to overdose, and in early work, before it was realized that the initial inspired concentration of desflurane needed to be very little higher than MAC, some horses became very hypotensive (Jones *et al.*, 1995).

Desflurane is unpopular for use in man and it is questionable as to how long it will be available. This is unfortunate, as the rapid and complete nature of recovery from desflurane means that it is an excellent anaesthetic agent in horses.

Nitrous oxide

The use of N_2O is controversial. Its analgesic properties ensures that less of the volatile agents which lack analgesic properties are required (Steffey & Howland, 1978a). The disadvantage lies in the potential for causing hypoxia. N_2O will reduce the PiO_2 and particular care needs to be taken when it is used in a rebreathing system. N_2O also passes into the gut spaces, increasing their volume and reducing FRC, thus resulting in a greater fall in PaO_2 than can be explained by the reduction in PiO_2 alone (Lee *et al.*, 1998). The use of N_2O at the phase of transfer from i.v. induction to maintenance speeds uptake of the volatile agent by the 'second gas effect'. However, increasing the alveolar concentration of volatile agent by this means will result in a greater degree of cardiopulmonary depression. N_2O can provide useful analgesia but in the horse it should be used only in situations where it is possible to monitor arterial blood gases.

General points in relation to maintenance of anaesthesia using volatile agents

Methods of administration

In equine anaesthesia volatile anaesthetic agents are administered via a circle or to-and-fro absorption system using an out-of circuit vaporizer, and for reasons of economy, they should be used with as low a flow of fresh gas as is practicable. However, the limitations to the use of minimum flows in the early phase of anaesthesia are (a) the necessity to remove N_2 from the animal and the breathing system, and (b) the need to maintain adequate inspired concentrations of volatile agent at a time when it is being taken up by the animal (Chapter 9). The simplest way to use a low-flow system is to restrict the method to the carrier gas O_2 and only one volatile anaesthetic such as halothane or isoflurane. At the outset the anaesthetic system should be primed with O_2 and up to 4% of halothane or isoflurane (less in animals with circulatory dysfunction). Following anaesthetic induction, the horse is connected to the system with fresh gas flow of 6–8 l/min (still carrying up to 4% of the anaesthetic agent). The excess of gas is vented via the (scavenged) exhaust valve, thus reducing N_2 and keeping the inspired anaesthetic agent concentration at an adequate level. The vaporizer setting is reduced in accordance with the clinical needs of the animal. At the end of 10–15 minutes, provided the reservoir bag is filling well the fresh gas flow can be reduced to about 4 l/min. At these flows rates, with a large horse given halothane the inspired concentration will be approximately half that of the vaporizer setting. The reason for this is simply that the mass of halothane delivered to the circuit at this low flow rate is insufficient in the first few hours of the anaesthetic period to make up the net losses from the breathing system to the animal's tissues. Reducing the flow rate still further (the minimum needed is that required to keep the reservoir bag filled) will increase the difference between inspired concentrations and the vaporizer setting. If the depth of anaesthesia needs to be altered, the reservoir bag should be emptied and the new concentration of agent given with a high flow of O_2 until the required depth is achieved.

The more insoluble the anaesthetic, the shorter the time required for the tissues to become saturated and therefore the closer is the inspired concentration to the vaporizer setting. Isoflurane is given in a similar manner to halothane, but since it is less soluble, the vaporizer setting and the flow rates can be reduced more rapidly; with sevoflurane these changes occur even faster, and with desflurane inspired settings are close to those of the vaporizer within minutes, even when very low flow rates are used throughout.

With all volatile anaesthetic agents difficulty can be experienced in the transition to anaesthesia after induction by an i.v. technique. When the horse is first connected to the breathing system respiratory arrest frequently occurs as a result of drug induced respiratory depression, removal of the hypoxic drive through high PiO_2 (Steffey et al., 1992) and, possibly, the sudden imposition of expiratory resistance. The problem can be overcome by IPPV,

but careful monitoring is needed to ensure that overdose does not occur. Attempts to hasten the uptake by the administration of high inspired concentrations can provoke cardiovascular collapse.

Additional analgesia

Ideally, additional analgesia should be provided to horses anaesthetized with halothane or isoflurane prior to the start of painful surgery. Local nerve blocks, where practicable, totally reduce response to surgery and may also provide postoperative analgesia. NSAIDs are often given preoperatively or intraoperatively but there no evidence that their use reduces MAC. The place of opioids is controversial; many anaesthetists consider that butorphanol (0.02–0.04 mg/kg) or morphine (0.1–0.2 mg/kg) improve the quality of anaesthesia and prevent movement in response to surgery, but in some individual animals even under anaesthesia their effect is to produce excitement and the dose of volatile anaesthetic needs to be increased to counteract this. Experimental studies have failed to demonstrate an action of opioids on MAC in the horse (Matthews & Lindsay, 1990; Pascoe et al., 1993). Once the horse has responded to surgery, a small dose of thiopental (0.05–0.10 mg/kg) will rapidly regain control, although it may cause a fall in ABP and transient apnoea. Incremental doses of ketamine (0.1–0.2 mg/kg i.v.) may be given for additional analgesia, but the total dose should not exceed 2 mg/kg, and should not be given in the last half hour of anaesthesia. Other options are α_2 adrenoceptor agonists given as bolus injections (0.1 mg/kg xylazine or 2 µg/kg detomidine) or by infusion.

TREATMENT OF CIRCULATORY DEPRESSION

In the horse, hypotension is common during anaesthesia with volatile agents, and as this parameter is easy to measure, it has usually been routine practice to equate such hypotension with cardiovascular depression. However, it is now realised that, although it is essential that ABP is adequate to perfuse vital organs, once this 'opening' pressure is reached then, as discussed above perfusion and peripheral blood flow depend on CO. Improving ABP by vasoconstriction may result in a fall in CO, presumably as the result of increased afterload (Wagner *et al.*, 1992; Lee *et al.*, 1998a). The aim of cardiovascular support is, therefore, to increase ABP to an acceptable level (usually taken as a MAP of 65–70 mmHg) by the improvement of CO and blood flow. A number of methods of providing such support have been advocated and investigated in horses anaesthetized with volatile agents. Often the findings concerning efficacy and dosage at different centres do not agree, probably because of differing responses in individual animals. In clinical practice more than one of these methods of support may be needed. Few studies have examined such treatments in horses anaesthetized with i.v. agents although it is now recognized that cardiovascular support still may be required if good peripheral perfusion is to be maintained.

Increase in circulating fluid volume

An increase in the circulating fluid volume to match the increased volume of the dilated vascular bed will restore the venous return. The simplest method entails the i.v. infusion of 5–20 litres of isotonic fluid (usually lactated Ringer), depending on the size of the animal, as rapidly as possible immediately after the induction of anaesthesia, although over-enthusiastic adminstration may cause peripheral oedema. The use of hypertonic saline (4 ml/kg) in anaesthetized horses has been reviewed by Gasthuys (1994). When given prior to anaesthesia and followed by a slower infusion of lactated Ringer it improves blood pressure during anaesthesia (Dyson & Pascoe, 1990). However, Gasthuys *et al.* (1994) found that when hypertonic saline was given to halothane anaesthetized ponies, the improvement in CO and ABP was significant only at a time point 5 minutes after the cessation of infusion. During the actual infusion of hypertonic saline ABP fell, and these workers suggest that the method is not ideal where hypotension already is severe. Gelatin-based compounds are not suitable as volume expanders in the normovolaemic horse (Taylor, 1998) as the volumes required are too great, but starch solutions have proved very effective in clinical practice for improving the circulation in endotoxic horses (Bettschart-Wolfensberger, personal communication, 1999).

Positive inotropes

Many of the sympathomimetic agents are easily oxidized to inactive compounds on exposure to air, and thus should be prepared to the required dilution just prior to use. This property may explain differing results and differing recommendations as to dosage and efficacy. Fortunately, in clinical practice some changes in potency are acceptable as the drugs are administered to effect by infusion.

The pharmacological action of dopamine, dobutamine and similar agents is to increase heart rate, yet if given too fast to anaesthetized horses bradycardia or even heart block may occur. This appears to be a vagally mediated reflex to the improving ABP, and if these drugs are given after treatment with an anticholinergic agent, tachycardia and a rise in ABP occurs with very low doses of the sympathomimetic. Bradycardia can be avoid by commencing the infusion of sympathomimetic slowly, then gradually increasing the dose as required.

Dopamine

Dopamine is a naturally occurring precursor of noradrenaline which exerts its action at α_1, β_1 and β_2, and dopaminergic adrenoceptors. In horses infusions of 2.5–5.0 mg/kg/min improve CO whilst causing vasodilation. Renal perfusion is increased (Trim *et al.*, 1985; 1989) and both CO and ABP improved in horses with endotoxic shock (Trim *et al.*, 1991). Higher doses may cause vasoconstriction via α_1 activity. Signs of overdose are tachycardia and associated arrhythmias, and trembling (Lee *et al.*, 1998a) but these effects cease as soon as the infusion rate is reduced.

Dobutamine

Dobutamine exerts its actions at both α and β adrenoceptors (β actions predominating at low doses), but is devoid of action at dopaminergic receptors. In anaesthetized horses infusions of from 0.5–5.0 mg/kg have been found to improve both CO and ABP (Swanson *et al.*, 1985; Donaldson, 1988; Gasthuys *et al.*, 1991a; Lee *et al.*, 1998a). Overdose of dobutamine causes tachycardia with associated arrhythmias (which may be dangerous in the presence of hypercapnia) but lack of dopinergic activity means that muscle tremors do not occur.

Dopexamine

Dopexamine is a new synthetic catecholamine which has marked activity at β_2 receptors with a lesser action at β_1 and dopaminergic sites. It improves CO through a positive inotropic effect, whist causing vasodilation, reducing afterload and improving renal perfusion. Muir (1992; 1992a) demonstrated in conscious and anaesthetized horses that at doses of $1\,\mu g/kg/min$ or more, CO and HR increased, whilst systemic vascular resistance decreased. In conscious horses ABP changes were minimal but in anaesthetized animals dopexamine infusion caused a dose-dependent increase. These advantageous cardiovascular effects in anaesthetized horses have been confirmed by other workers (Young et al., 1997; Lee et al., 1998), but in these later studies under halothane anaesthesia dopexamine was found to cause unacceptable side effects. The initial response to infusion of the drug was a fall in end-tidal anaesthetic agent (presumably because the vasodilation had opened under-perfused areas which then took up the halothane) and great difficulty was encountered in keeping the animals unconscious. Higher doses caused sweating, tachycardia and tremor. When infusion was stopped, ABP and heart rate continued to rise, and side effects did not abate for a considerable period of time. The quality of recovery was poor and in one study two horses developed postanaesthetic colic. The cardiovascular effects of dopexamine are ideal for circulatory support, and the side effects almost certainly result from overdosage, but considerably more experimental work is required to elucidate the correct dose before this agent can be recommended for use in clinical practice.

Phenylephrine and methoxamine

Phenylephrine and methoxamine both act as α_2 adrenoceptor agonists, and increase arterial blood pressure by vasoconstriction. An infusion dose of phenylephrine of $0.25–2.00\,\mu g/kg/min$ in anaesthetized horses raises blood pressure but CO and muscle blood flow fall or are unchanged (Lee et al., 1998). These vasoconstrictor agents should not routinely be used to treat hypotension in anaesthetized horses but may have a role where all other methods have failed.

Calcium

The use of calcium to counteract anaesthetic induced cardiovascular depression has been advocated for many years but much of the evidence as to dose and efficacy is anecdotal, and the differing availability of elemental calcium in preparations of different calcium salts sometimes makes comparisons between studies difficult (Gasthuys et al., 1991b; Grubb et al., 1994). Calcium borogluconate, being readily available in veterinary practice, is a common choice and up to 300 ml of a 40% w/v solution may be given prior to or during anaesthesia by slow i.v. infusion. Another recommendation is an infusion of $0.25–2.00\,ml/kg/min$ of 10% calcium gluconate (Daunt, 1990). In clinical practice calcium infusions tend either to be very effective or almost totally ineffective in improving ABP and peripheral blood flow. The rationale of the use of calcium is that plasma calcium levels fall during anaesthesia with volatile agents. Whether calcium has any effect in improving CO depressed by i.v. agents is not known.

Anticholinergic agents: glycopyrrolate and atropine

The advantages and disadvantages of the use of anticholinergic agents in equine anaesthesia has been discussed above. However, during anaesthesia with volatile anaesthetic agents bradycardia may contribute to the fall in CO and this is particularly likely to be the case if α_2 adrenoceptor agonists have been used in the anaesthetic protocol. Atropine ($0.01\,mg/kg$) or glycopyrrolate ($0.005\,mg/kg$) given i.v. often do not increase heart rate, but following their use, small doses of dopamine or dobutamine do, with a spectacular effect on CO.

USE OF MUSCLE RELAXANTS

Centrally acting muscle relaxants

Guaiphenesin

Where guiaphenesin has been used as part of the anaesthetic induction technique, it will improve muscle relaxation for an hour or more. Doses of guaiphenesin of 3 g and 5 g/ 50 kg may be given to the anaesthetized horse and will produce some relaxation without interfering with respiratory activity but when given in this way it causes a marked fall in ABP, probably through a negative inotropic effect (Pascoe *et al.*, 1985).

Benzodiazepines

Benzodiazepines may also be administered intra-operatively for their muscle relaxant properties. However, when given to horses already anaesthetized with volatile anaesthetic agents, benzodiazepines cause marked respiratory depression.

Neuromuscular blocking agents

For many years neuromuscular blocking agents have been used sparingly in equine anaesthesia (other than suxamethonium at induction of anaesthesia), the major fear being that residual muscle weakness when the horse tried to rise would adversely affect the quality of recovery. The advent of the short acting easily reversed competitive relaxant atracurium changed this, and neuromuscular blocking agents are now widely used not only to aid abdominal, ophthalmic and thoracic surgery, but in general and orthopaedic surgery to prevent the sudden reflex responses which sometimes occur.

The rules for the use of neuromuscular blocking agents are, as for any species: (a) that the facilities which enable immediate and sustained IPPV are available, and (b) that it is possible to be certain that the horse will be unconscious throughout the duration of their effect.

There is a wide variation among individuals in the response to a given dose of neuromuscular blocking agent and in rate of recovery from blockade. Also, some antibiotic agents such as gentamycin greatly reduce the dose of relaxant required. For this reason no attempt should be made to administer them in fixed doses; they should always be given so as to produce just the desired effect. An incremental dosage regimen enables this to be done; about one-half the anticipated full dose is given initially and further increments of half this initial dose are given at 3–5 min intervals until the desired degree of relaxation is obtained. Only small doses are needed to suppress unwanted muscle movements during general anaesthesia (e.g. in eye surgery) but large doses will be required to produce the nearly complete blockade demanded by some surgical procedures. In every case the aim should be to use only a minimum dose and to ensure a complete recovery of neuromuscular function before the termination of anaesthesia. If unwanted muscle tone is returning towards the end of a surgical procedure it is usually wiser to restore relaxation by a slight deepening of anaesthesia rather than the administration of more neuromuscular blocker.

Clinical monitoring of neuromuscular block is facilitated by the use of a peripheral nerve stimulator (Chapter 7) which may be used on the facial or superficial peroneal nerves and the strength of contraction of the relevant muscles estimated by manual sensing at the muzzle or toe. If this facility is not available, myoneural block may be monitored by careful observation of the breathing and general muscular activity of the anaesthetized horse. Signs of partial blockade include brief, weak inspiratory movements, without holding of inspiration, and feeble, unsustained withdrawal responses to painful stimulation. One extremely simple objective test is measurement of airway pressure with a water manometer when the endotracheal tube is occluded before an inspiratory effort. No significant degree of myoneural block is present if the horse can generate a pressure in the occluded airway of more than 25 cm H_2O (2.5 kPa) below atmospheric pressure. If a degree of block is present during anaesthetic recovery the horse is unable to stiffen the neck or hold up the head when attempting to sit in sternal recumbency, or it may make brief, weak attempts to stand followed by shaking of the limb muscles and collapse.

Dosage and duration of action of neuromuscular blocking drugs

Atracurium

The relatively short duration of action of activity and the lack of cumulative neuromuscular blocking effect make atracurium particularly suitable for use in horses in doses of 0.12–0.20 mg/kg (Hildebrand *et al.*, 1986; 1989). The authors recommend an initial dose of 0.1 mg/kg followed, if this does not produce the desired degree of relaxation as indicated by train-of-four stimulation, by doses of 0.01 mg/kg at 2 minute intervals until the block is judged to be adequate (reduction of initial twitch height). Edrophonium 0.5–1.0 mg/kg will antagonize any residual neuromuscular blocking effects at the end of the procedure for which it is given and prior administration of atropine or glycopyrrolate is unnecessary provided the antagonist is injected slowly over more than 1 minute. Atracurium has also been given by continuous infusion at 0.17 mg/kg/h after an initial bolus dose of 0.05 mg/kg (Hildebrand *et al.*, 1989). Cardiovascular stability is good but there may be some slowing of heart rate after an initial increase in ABP in response to edrophonium.

d-Tubocurarine chloride

In halothane-anaesthetized animals with end-tidal concentrations of halothane of about 1.0%, doses of the order of 0.22–0.25 mg/kg d-tubocurarine chloride produce good relaxation with respiratory arrest. The use of d-tubocurarine in horses suffering from asthma or alveolar emphysema may be associated with the production of bronchospasm, presumably due to histamine release. It is seldom possible to restore adequate spontaneous breathing by the use of anticholinesterases in less than 35–40 minutes after d-tubocurarine has been given in doses which produce respiratory arrest. Limb movements are not seen during this period unless the depth of anaesthesia is allowed to become inadequate.

Pancuronium bromide

During light anaesthesia doses of 0.06 mg/kg produce complete relaxation with apnoea of about 20 min duration, but it is more usual to give doses of 0.1 mg/kg to be certain of producing apnoea with complete relaxation of respiratory muscles so that IPPV can be performed with the lowest possible airway pressures (Hildebrand & Howitt, 1984). The delay in achieving maximum effect after i.v. injection is much less than that of d-tubocurarine chloride and no cases of relapse into neuromuscular block have been encountered following neostigmine. The lack of histamine release makes this drug of value in cases where the

administration of d-tubocurarine might be dangerous.

Vecuronium

Doses of 0.1 mg/kg produce neuromuscular block of some 20–30 minutes duration in horses lightly anaesthetized with halothane. Although experience with this drug is limited it appears to be well suited for use in horses in that there is no evidence of histamine release and complete antagonism of block is readily obtained about 20 minutes after attainment of full relaxation with depression of the first twitch height in train-of-four stimulation of the superficial peroneal nerve. There then is no evidence of muscle weakness in the anaesthetic recovery period.

Suxamethonium chloride

The use of suxamethonium for casting and restraint of horses is considered by the vast majority of veterinary anaesthetists to be an extremely inhumane practice, it is unnecessary and it is unsafe on pharmacological grounds. In the past, suxamethonium had a place in the provision of very short term muscle relaxation in anaesthetized horses but it has now been almost totally replaced by the short acting competitive blocking agent atracurium.

Termination of neuromuscular block

There is no effective antidote to suxamethonium, but neostigmine is an efficient antidote to the nondepolarizing relaxants. In horses its use should be preceded by the i.v. injection of 10 mg atropine sulphate or, better, 5 mg glycopyrrolate, and it is then given in incremental doses up to a total dose of 10 mg. A period of 2–3 minutes should be allowed between increments and the effect of each carefully assessed before the next is given. Edrophonium or neostigmine should be given while IPPV is continued so that there is no danger of hypoxia or hypercapnia because if given to hypoxic or hypercapnic animals neostigmine may cause serious arrhythmias. As a general rule, the dose of neostigmine needed to restore full spontaneous breathing should be noted and a further dose of half this amount given to be completely sure of full antagonism of all the effects of the relaxant drug. Care must be taken not to confuse the weakness of respiratory activity due to deep inhalation anaesthesia, hypothermia or metabolic alkalosis from excessive bicarbonate administration, with that due to residual neuromuscular block.

Intermittent positive pressure ventilation (IPPV)

Careful thought is needed before IPPV is used in horses. Since blood gas measurements have become readily available during anaesthesia, many anaesthetists have thought it advisable to institute IPPV whenever the $PaCO_2$ increases by about 15 mmHg (2 kPa). Often in these circumstances IPPV is commenced under inhalation anaesthesia without the use of muscle relaxants, the chest wall is stiff due to tone in the intercostal muscles and diaphragm so that compliance is low and high airway pressures are needed to expand the lungs. These high inspiratory pressures raise the mean intrathoracic pressure and can have a most deleterious effect on the circulation. Lower ABPs during IPPV than during spontaneous ventilation have often been erroneously attributed to lowering of the $PaCO_2$. A decline in PaO_2 is frequently observed in anaesthetized horses when muscle tone is returning after the use of neuromuscular blockers and airway pressures are increased to maintain the respiratory tidal volume. In these cases restoration of the PaO_2 requires nothing more than the administration of a further dose of the relaxant.

Normally, any increase in mean intrathoracic pressure is countered by peripheral venoconstriction which raises the peripheral venous pressure and restores the pressure gradient to the right atrium. This has the effect of increasing the venous return and hence the CO. In hypovolaemic horses (e.g. many colic cases), and where the inhalation anaesthetic agents block the effect of sympathetic discharge, the peripheral venoconstriction may be inadequate to counter the rise in mean intrathoracic pressure due to IPPV so that venous return falls and the CO declines. Diagnosis of hypovolaemia in horses is not always easy and even when correctly diagnosed there may be insuffi-

cient time for full replenishment of the blood volume by transfusion before anaesthesia has to be induced. For these reasons many anaesthetists claim that equine colic cases which may be hypovolaemic fare better if allowed to breathe spontaneously during anaesthesia even if their $PaCO_2$ rises to 60–70 mmHg (8.0–9.5 kPa). (In this connection it must be noted that there is no evidence that $PaCO_2$ increase to these levels is harmful—indeed it may be beneficial by increasing tissue perfusion.) The picture is, however, not quite as simple as this for spontaneous ventilation must produce an adequate tidal volume and many horses with bowel obstruction only ventilate satisfactorily once the abdomen has been surgically decompressed. If there is any delay in this decompression it may be essential to institute IPPV as soon as anaesthesia is induced. IPPV is, of course, essential for thoracotomy or the repair of penetrating wounds of the chest.

Ideally, monitoring of end-tidal CO_2 and/or analysis of arterial blood samples drawn after about 20 minutes after the commencement of IPPV will enable adjustments to be made to the imposed tidal volume and/or rate of ventilation so that an adequate PaO_2 is maintained with as near as possible normal $PaCO_2$. Unfortunately, in many cases facilities for blood gas estimation are not readily available and the setting of the ventilator has to be made from simple clinical observation of the horse. Excursion of the chest wall should be somewhat greater than might be expected in the spontaneously breathing horse, the respiratory frequency should be between 8 and 10 breaths/min, the tidal volume about 10 ml/kg; the airway pressure should be kept as low as is consistent with adequate expansion of the chest wall and the inspiratory time should be between 2 and 3 seconds. Experience is often the only reliable guide to proper pulmonary ventilation in any individual horse. Whenever possible, the ABP should be monitored so that any embarrassment of the circulation can be recognized before too much harm results from an unsuitable pattern of lung inflation.

Assisted ventilation, in which the horse triggers the ventilator which then delivers a prescribed tidal volume, is a very useful compromise in equine anaesthesia as long as the ventilator has a 'fail safe' mechanism, whereby if the horse does not trigger a breath within a certain time, the ventilator switches to automatic mode.

ANAESTHETIC RECOVERY PERIOD

Ideally horses should recover from anaesthesia calmly and quietly, and in as fast a time as possible, but these aims cannot always be achieved. The quality of recovery will depend on a number of factors including the sedative and anaesthetic drugs used throughout the perioperative process, the degree of postoperative pain, the comfort of the horse, its temperament, and limitation to standing caused by surgery or onset of anaesthetic induced myopathy or neuropathy.

It is important that the horse does not try to rise until it is able to do so. Following prolonged anaesthesia with volatile agents it has now common practice to administer additional sedation (e.g., xylazine at increments of 0.1 mg/kg i.v.) in the early recovery period. Such sedation is less necessary with halothane than with the newer agents or if, after suitable premedication, thiopental (which provides residual sedation) was used as the induction agent.

Horses anaesthetized under 'field conditions' may be left to recover in a grassy field or on a thick straw bed; no attempt should be made to induce an animal to stand before it tries to do so of its own accord. However, in equine hospitals animals are usually moved to a quiet, dimly-lit, well-padded room to minimize the chance of serious injury as they regain their feet. It is important that the floor of this box is not slippery, even if wet. In some hospitals horse are placed on thick soft mats – this makes it difficult for the horse to regain sternal recumbency, and this, together with the extra comfort, encourage it to remain recumbent until fully ready to stand. Assuming there are no surgical contraindications, an animal which has been supine should be placed on its left side in the recovery area. However the positioning of an animal which has been lying on its side is controversial; turning to the other side enables under-perfused muscles to be reoxygenated, but results in atelectasis of the lung lobes which are still expanded.

In major orthopaedic cases a decision may be made to assist recovery but such recoveries should only be carried out by experienced staff. Handlers prevent the horse from rising by controlling its head, and by administering small doses of xylazine as required, until the effects of the volatile agent have waned. The time required before the horse should be allowed to attempt to rise depends on the kinetics of the volatile agent employed – the authors sometimes restrain horses given halothane for up to two hours, whilst following desflurane 30 minutes is sufficient. In many hospitals ropes are used to assist the horse to rise but in most cases slings should not be used unless the horse is already accustomed to their use.

In most cases adequate analgesia for the immediate postoperative period will have been administered at the end of anaesthesia. However, if not already given, NSAIDs may be administered i.v., and i.m. doses of pethidine (1 mg/kg), do not add to recovery time (Taylor, 1986). Local nerve blocks given at the end of surgery on the digits for postoperative analgesia do not seem to cause problems for the horse attempting to stand up. Unless catheterized, the bladder of male animals given fluid i.v. during operation may become distended and cause considerable abdominal pain; catheterization of the bladder produces immediate relief. This problem does not occur in female animals because urine will seep from the bladder during anaesthesia, but catheterization will prevent urine from spilling on to the floor.

The timing of removal of the endotracheal tube is controversial. Some anaesthetists leave the tube in place until the horse has arisen, but this is only possible with an adequate mouth gag, and even then authors have seen recovering animal occlude the tube by biting on it. Respiratory obstruction caused in this way can be difficult to relieve and expensive tubes may be ruined. In addition, stimulation of the trachea by the tube has been associated with cardiac arrest, presumably through a vagal mechanism, as anaesthesia lightens. Following prolonged anaesthesia, respiratory obstruction is frequently observed after removal of the endotracheal tube, probably due to hypostatic congestion of the nasal and pharyngeal mucous membranes, and the horse makes a characteristic snoring noise. Ideally, it is prevented by keeping the horse's head slightly elevated during anaesthesia, but if this has not been done, the obstruction can be relieved by passing a small-bore endotracheal tube through one nostril. Unless properly secured such a tube may be aspirated into the tracheobronchial tree.

A rare complication in recovery is obstruction due to laryngeal paralysis; this probably results from neuronal damage from stretching the head on the neck. Should this occur the horse will obstruct as soon as the nasal tube is removed, and an emergency tracheotomy may be required. O_2 can be given through the nasal endotracheal tube, although to produce any significant improvement of PaO_2, it must be administered into the trachea at a flow rate of at least 15 1/min. It has been suggested that an O_2 demand valve may be used to administer oxygen during the recovery period (Reibold *et al.*, 1980) but others have found this rather unsuitable (Watney *et al.*, 1985).

REFERENCES

Aguiar, A., Hussni, C.A., Luna, S.P. *et al.* (1993) Propofol compared with propofol/guaifenesin after detomidine premedication. *Journal of Veterinary Anaesthesia* **20**: 26–28.

Aida, H., Mizuno, Y., Hobo, S. *et al.* (1994) Determination of the minimal alveolar concentration (MAC) and physical response to sevoflurane inhalation in horses. *Journal of Veterinary Medical Science* **56**: 1161–1165.

Aida, H., Mizuno, Y., Hobo, S. *et al.* (1996) Cardiovascular and pulmonary effects of sevoflurane anesthesia in horses. *Veterinary Surgery* **25**: 164–170.

Aida, H., Kawashima, K., Yokota, M. *et al.* (1997) Recovery characteristics of sevoflurane anesthesia in racehorses. *Proceedings of the 6th International Congress of Veterinary Anaesthesiology*, p. 125.

Alexander, F. and Collett, R.A. (1974) Pethidine in the horse. *Research in Veterinary Science* **17**: 136–137.

Alibhai, H.I. and Clarke, K.W. (1996) Influence of carprofen on minimum alveolar concentration of halothane in dogs. *Journal of Veterinary Pharmacology and Therapeutics* **19**: 320–321.

Alitalo, I. (1986) Clinical experiences with Domosedan in horses and cattle. A Review. *Acta Veterinaria Scandinavica Supplement* **82**: 193–196.

Amadon, R.S. and Craige, A.H. (1936) Observations on the use of bulbocapnine as a soporific in horses. *Journal of the American Veterinary Medical Association* **41**: 737–754.

Archer, R.K. (1947) Pethidine in Veterinary Practice. *Veterinary Record* **59**: 401–402.

Beadle, R.E., Robinson, N.E. and Sorensen, P.R. (1975) Cardiopulmonary effects of postitive end-expiratory pressure in anesthetized horses. *American Journal of Veterinary Research* **36**: 1435–1438.

Bettschart-Wolfensberger, R., Taylor, P.M., Sear, J.W. *et al.* (1996) Physiologic effects of anesthesia induced and maintained by intravenous administration of a climazolam-ketamine combination in ponies premedicated with acepromazine and xylazine. *American Journal of Veterinary Research* **57**: 1472–1477.

Bettschart, W.R., Clarke, K.W., Vainio, O. *et al.* (1999) Pharmacokinetics of medetomidine in ponies and elaboration of a medetomidine infusion regime which provides a constant level of sedation. *Research in Veterinary Science* **67**: 41–46.

Bettschart-Wolfensberger, R. (1999a) Total intravenous anaesthesia in horses using medetomidine and propofol. *PhD thesis*. London: Royal Veterinary College, University of London.

Brearley, J.C., Jones, R.S., Kelly, D.F. *et al.* (1986) Spinal cord degeneration following general anaesthesia in a Shire horse. *Equine Veterinary Journal* **18**: 222–224.

Bryant, C.E., England, G.C. and Clarke, K.W. (1991) Comparison of the sedative effects of medetomidine and xylazine in horses. *Veterinary Record* **129**: 421–423.

Carroll, G.L., Hooper, R.N., Slater, M.R. *et al.* (1998) Detomidine-butorphanol-propofol for carotid artery translocation and castration or ovariectomy in goats. *Veterinary Surgery* **27**: 75–82.

Clarke, K.W. and Hall, L.W. (1969) Xylazine–a new sedative for horses and cattle. *Veterinary Record* **85**: 512–517.

Clarke, K.W. and Taylor, P.M. (1986) Detomidine: a new sedative for horses. *Equine Veterinary Journal* **18**: 366–370.

Clarke, K.W., Taylor, P.M. and Watkins, S.B. (1986) Detomidine/ketamine anaesthesia in the horse. *Acta Veterinaria Scandinavica* (Suppl): **82**: 167–179.

Clarke, K.W. (1988) *D. Vet. Med. Thesis*. London: University of London.

Clarke, K.W. and Paton, B.S. (1988) Combined use of detomidine with opiates in the horse. *Equine Veterinary Journal* **20**: 331–334.

Clarke, K.W. and Gerring, E.E.L. (1990) Detomidine as a sedative and premedicant in the horse. *American Association of Equine Practitioners* **35**: 629–635.

Clarke, K.W., England, G.C.W. and Goossens, L. (1991) Sedative and cardiovascular effects of romifidine alone and in combination with butorphanol in the horse. *Journal of Veterinary Anaesthesia* **18**: 25–29.

Clarke, K.W., Alibhai, H.I.K. and Hammond, R.A. (1996) Desflurane anaesthesia in the horse: Minimal alveolar concentration following induction with xylazine and ketamine. *Journal of Veterinary Anaesthesia* **23**: 56–59.

Clarke, K.W., Song, D.Y., Alibhai, H.I. *et al.* (1996a) Cardiopulmonary effects of desflurane in ponies, after induction of anaesthesia with xylazine and ketamine. *Veterinary Record* **139**: 180–185.

Clarke, K.W., Freeman, S., Alibhai, H.I.K. *et al.* (1997) Cardiopulmonary actions of alpha 2 adrenoceptor agonists administered to ponies during anaesthesia. *Proceedings of the 6th International Congress of Veterinary Anaesthesiology*, p. 123.

Clerbaux, T., Sertyn, D., Willems, E. *et al.* (1986) Determination de la courbe de dissociation standard de l'oxyhemoglobine du cheval et influence, sur cette courbe, de la temperature, du pH et du diphosphoglycerate. *Canadian Journal of Veterinary Research* 50: 188–192.

Clutton, R.E. (1987) Unexpected responses following intravenous pethidine injection in two horses. *Equine Veterinary Journal* 19: 72–73.

Combie, J., Dougherty, J., Nugent, E. *et al.* (1979) The pharmacology of narcotic analgesics in the horse. *Journal of Equine Medicine and Surgery* 3: 377–385.

Combie, J., Shults, T., Nugent, E. *et al.* (1981) The pharmacology of narcotic analgesics in the horse; selective blockade of narcotic induced locomotor activity. *American Journal of Veterinary Research* 42: 716–721.

Cunningham, F.M. and Lees, P. (1995). Non-steroidal anti-inflammatory drugs. In: Higgins, A.J. and Wright, I.M. (eds) *Equine Manual*. London: W.B. Saunders, pp. 229–237.

Daunt, D.A. (1990) Supportive therapy in the anaesthetized horse. *Veterinary Clinics of North America* 6: 557–574.

Daunt, D.A., Dunlop, C.I., Chapman, P.L. *et al.* (1993) Cardiopulmonary and behavioral responses to computer-driven infusion of detomidine in standing horses. *American Journal of Veterinary Research* 54: 2075–2082.

Doddam, J.R., Moon, R.E., Olsen, N.C. *et al.* (1993) Effects of clenbuterol hydrochloride on pulmonary gas exchange and hemodynamics in anesthetized horses. *American Journal of Veterinary Research* 54: 776–782.

Donaldson, L.L. (1988) Retrospective assessment of dobutamine therapy for hypotension in anesthetized horses. *Veterinary Surgery* 17: 53–57.

Dunlop, C.I., Steffey, E.P., Miller, M.F. *et al.* (1987) Temporal effects of halothane and isoflurane in laterally recumbent ventilated male horses. *American Journal of Veterinary Research* 48: 1250–1255.

Dyson, D.H. and Pascoe, P.J. (1990) Influence of pre-induction methoxamine, lactated Ringer solution, or hypertonic saline solution infusion or post-induction dobutamine infusion on anesthetic-induced hypotension in horses. *American Journal of Veterinary Research* 51: 17–21.

England, G.C., Clarke, K.W. and Goossens, L. (1992) A comparison of the sedative effects of three alpha 2–adrenoceptor agonists (romifidine, detomidine and xylazine) in the horse. *Journal of Veterinary Pharmacology and Therapeutics* 15: 194–201.

England, G.C. and Clarke, K.W. (1996) Alpha 2 adrenoceptor agonists in the horse – a review. *British Veterinary Journal* 152: 641–657.

Farney, J., Blaise, D., Vaillancourt, D. *et al.* (1991). Caudal epidural analgesia with butorphanol in the mare. *Proceedings of the 4th International Congress of Veterinary Anaesthesia.*

Flaherty, D., Reid, J., Welsh, E. *et al.* (1997) A pharmacodynamic study of propofol or propofol and ketamine in ponies undergoing surgery. *Research in Veterinary Science* 62: 179–184.

Freeman, S.L. (1998) Studies on romifidine in the standing and anaesthetised horse. *PhD thesis.* London: Royal Veterinary College, University of London.

Gasthuys, F., DeMoor, A. and Parmentier, D. (1991a) Influence of dopamine and dobutamine on the cardiovascular depression during halothane anaesthesia in dorsally recumbent ventilated ponies. *Journal of the Veterinary Medical Association* 38: 494–500.

Gasthuys, F., Demoor, A. and Parmentier, D. (1991b) Cardiovascular effects of low dose calcium chloride infusions during halothane anaesthesia in dorsally recumbent ventilated ponies. *Journal of the Veterinary Medical Association* 38: 728–736.

Gasthuys, F. (1994) The value of 7.2% hypertonic saline in anaesthesia and intensive care: myth or fact? *Journal of Veterinary Anaesthesia* 21: 12–14.

Gasthuys, F., Messerman, C. and Moor, A.D. (1994) Cardiovascular effects of 7.2% hypertonic saline solution in halothane anaesthetised ponies. *Journal of Veterinary Anaesthesia* 21: 60–65.

Gillespie, J.R., Tyler, W.S. and Hall, L.W. (1969) Cardiopulmonary dysfunction in anesthetized, laterally recumbent horses. *American Journal of Veterinary Research* 30: 61–72.

Gleed, R.D. and Dobson, A. (1990) Effect of clenbuterol on arterial oxygen tension in the anaesthetised horse. *Research in Veterinary Science* 48: 331–337.

Grandy, J.L., Steffey, E.P., Hodgson, D.S. *et al.* (1987) Arterial hypotension and the development of postanesthetic myopathy in halothane-anesthetized horses. *American Journal of Veterinary Research* 48: 192–197.

Greene, S.A., Thurmon, J.C., Tranquilli, W.J. *et al.* (1986) Cardiopulmonary effects of continuous intravenous infusion of guaifenesin, ketamine, and xylazine in ponies. *American Journal of Veterinary Research* 47: 2364–2367.

Grosenbaugh, D.A. and Muir, W.W. (1998) Cardiorespiratory effects of sevoflurane, isoflurane, and halothane anesthesia in horses. *American Journal of Veterinary Research* 59: 101–106.

Grubb, T.L., Riebold, T.W. and Huber, M.J. (1992) Comparison of lidocaine, xylazine, and xylazine/lidocaine for caudal epidural analgesia in horses. *Journal of the American Veterinary Medical Association* 201: 1187–1190.

Grubb, T.L., Benson, G.B., Thurmon, J. *et al.* (1994) Effects of ionised calcium on cardiovascular function in horses anesthetized with halothane or isoflurane. *Proceedings of the 5th International Congress of Anaesthesiology, Guelph.*

Hall, L.W., Gillespie, J.R. and Tyler, W.S. (1968) Alveolar-arterial oxygen tension differences in anaesthetized horses. *British Journal of Anaesthesia* **40**: 560–568.

Hall, L.W., Senior, J.E.B. and Walker, R.G. (1968a) Sampling of equine pulmonary vein blood. *Research in Veterinary Science* **9**: 487–488.

Hall, L.W. and Trim, C.M. (1975) Positive end-expiratory pressure in anaesthetized spontaneously breathing horses. *British Journal of Anaesthesia* **47**: 819–824.

Hall, L.W. (1979) Oxygenation of pulmonary vein blood in conscious and anaesthetised ponies. *Equine Veterinary Journal* **11**: 71–75.

Hall, L.W. and Taylor, P.M. (1981) Clinical trial of xylazine with ketamine in equine anaesthesia. *Veterinary Record* **108**: 489–493.

Hall, L.W. (1983) Equine anaesthesia: discovery and rediscovery. *Equine Veterinary Journal* **15**: 190–195

Hall, L.W. (1984) Cardiovascular and pulmonary effects of recumbency in two conscious ponies. *Equine Veterinary Journal* **16**: 89–92.

Hamm, D. and Jochle, W. (1984) Sedation and analgesia in horses treated with various doses of Domosedan: Blind studies on the efficacy and the duration of effects. *American Association of Equine Practitioners* **30**: 235–242.

Hamm, D., Turchi, P. and Jochle, W. (1995) Sedative and analgesic effects of detomidine and romifidine in horses. *Veterinary Record* **136**: 324–327.

Hashem, A. and Keller, H. (1993) Disposition, bioavailability and clinical efficacy of orally administered acepromazine in the horse. *Journal of Veterinary Pharmacology and Therepeutics* **16**: 359–368.

Heard, D.J., Webb, A.I. and Daniels, R.T. (1986) Effect of acepromazine on the anesthetic requirement of halothane in the dog. *American Journal of Veterinary Research* **47**: 2113–2115.

Hildebrand, S.V. and Howitt, G.A. (1984) Dosage requirement of pancuronium in halothane-anesthetized ponies: a comparison of cumulative and single-dose administration. *American Journal of Veterinary Research* **45**: 2441–2444.

Hildebrand, S.V., Howitt, G.A. and Arpin, D. (1986) Neuromuscular and cardiovascular effects of atracurium in ponies anesthetized with halothane. *American Journal of Veterinary Research* **47**: 1096–1100.

Hildebrand, S.V., Holland, M., Copland, V.S. et al. (1989) Clinical use of the neuromuscular blocking agents atracurium and pancuronium for equine anesthesia. *Journal of the American Veterinary Medical Association* **195**: 212–219.

Hubbell, J.A., Muir, W.W., Robertson, J.T. et al. (1987) Cardiovascular effects of intravenous sodium penicillin, sodium cefazolin, and sodium citrate in awake and anesthetized horses. *Veterinary Surgery* **16**: 245–250.

Hubbell, J.A., Bednarski, R.M. and Muir, W.W. (1989) Xylazine and tiletamine-zolazepam anesthesia in horses. *American Journal of Veterinary Research* **50**: 737–742.

Jochle, W., Moore, J.N., Brown, J. et al. (1989) Comparison of detomidine, butorphanol, flunixin meglumine and xylazine in clinical cases of equine colic. *Equine Veterinary Journal* Suppl: 111–116.

Johnston, G.M., Taylor, P.M., Holmes, M.A. et al. (1995) Confidential enquiry of perioperative equine fatalities (CEPEF-1): preliminary results. *Equine Veterinary Journal* **27**: 193–200.

Jones, N.Y., Clarke, K.W. and Clegg, P.D. (1995) Desflurane in equine anaesthesia: a preliminary trial. *Veterinary Record* **137**: 618–620.

Kalpravidh, M., Lumb, W.V., Wright, M. et al. (1984) Analgesic effects of butorphanol in horses: dose-response studies. *American Journal of Veterinary Research* **45**: 211–216.

Katila, T. and Oijala, M. (1988) The effect of detomidine (Domosedan) on the maintenance of equine pregnancy and foetal development: ten cases. *Equine Veterinary Journal* **20**: 323–326.

Keegan, R.D., Gleed, R.D., Sanders, E.A. et al. (1991) Treatment of low arterial oxygen tension in anesthetized horses with clenbuterol. *Veterinary Surgery* **20**: 148–152.

Kerr, C.L., McDonell, W.N. and Young, S.S. (1996) A comparison of romifidine and xylazine when used with diazepam/ketamine for short duration anesthesia in the horse. *Canadian Veterinary Journal* **37**: 601–609.

Kerr, D.D., Jones, E.W., Huggins, K. et al. (1972) Sedative and other effects of xylazine given intravenously to horses. *American Journal of Veterinary Research* **33**: 525–532.

Klein, L.V. (1975) Standing sedation in the horse using xylazine and morphine. *Proceedings of the 20th World Veterinary Congress* **2**: 739.

Klein, L. (1978) A review of fifty cases of post-operative myopathy in the horse. *American Association of Equine Practiners* **24**: 89–94.

Lam, K.H.K., Smyth, J.B.A., Clarke, K. et al. (1995) Acute spinal cord degeneration following general anaesthesia in a young pony. *Veterinary Record* **136**: 329–330.

Lawrence, A.J., Joshi, G.P., Michalkiewicz, A. et al. (1992) Evidence for analgesia mediated by peripheral opioid receptors in inflamed synovial tissue. *European Journal of Clinical Pharmacology* **43**: 351–355.

LeBlanc, P.H., Caron, J.P., Patterson, J.S. et al. (1988) Epidural injection of xylazine for perineal analgesia in horses. *Journal of the American Veterinary Medical Association* **193**: 1405–1408.

Lee, Y.H., Clarke, K.W., Alibhai, H.I. et al. (1998) Effects of dopamine, dobutamine, dopexamine, phenylephrine, and saline solution on intramuscular blood flow and other cardiopulmonary variables in halothane-anesthetized ponies. *American Journal of Veterinary Research* **59**: 1463–1472.

Lee, Y.H., Clarke, K.W. and Alibhai, H.I. (1998a) The cardiopulmonary effects of clenbuterol when administered to dorsally recumbent halothane-anaesthetised ponies—failure to increase arterial oxygenation. *Research in Veterinary Science* **65**: 227–232.

Lee, Y.H., Clarke, K.W. and Alibhai, H.I. (1998b) Effects on the intramuscular blood flow and cardiopulmonary function of anaesthetised ponies of changing from halothane to isoflurane maintenance and vice versa. *Veterinary Record* **143**: 629–633.

Lindsay, W.A., McDonell, W. and Bignell, W. (1980) Equine postanesthetic forelimb lameness: intracompartmental muscle pressure changes and biochemical patterns. *American Journal of Veterinary Research* **41**: 1919–1924.

Lindsay, W.A., Pascoe, P.J., McDonell, W.N. *et al.* (1985) Effect of protective padding on forelimb intracompartmental muscle pressures in anesthetized horses. *American Journal of Veterinary Research* **46**: 688–691.

Lindsay, W.A., Robinson, G.M., Brunson, D.B. *et al.* (1989) Induction of equine postanesthetic myositis after halothane-induced hypotension. *American Journal of Veterinary Research* **50**: 404–410.

Lowe, J.E. and Hilfiger, J. (1986) Analgesic and sedative effects of detomidine compared to xylazine in a colic model using i.v. and i.m. routes of administration. *Acta Veterinaria Scandinavica* **82** (Suppl): 85–95.

Luna, S.P., Taylor, P.M. and Massone, F. (1997) Midazolam and ketamine induction before halothane anaesthesia in ponies: cardiorespiratory, endocrine and metabolic changes. *Journal of Veterinary Pharmacology And Therapeutics* **20**: 153–159.

Malone, J. and Clarke, K.W. (1993) A comparison of the efficacy of detomidine by sublingual and intramuscular administration in ponies. *Journal of Veterinary Anaesthesia* **20**: 73–77.

Mama, K.R., Pascoe, P.J., Steffey, E.P. *et al.* (1998) Comparison of two techniques for total intravenous anesthesia in horses. *American Journal of Veterinary Research* **59**: 1292–1298.

Mama, K.R., Steffey, E.P. and Pascoe, P.J. (1995) Evaluation of propofol as a general anesthetic for horses. *Veterinary Surgery* **24**: 188–194.

Martin, J.E. and Beck, J.D. (1956) Some effects of chlorpromazine hydrochloride in horses. *American Journal of Veterinary Research* **17**: 678–686.

Matthews, N.S. and Lindsay, S.L. (1990) Effect of low-dose butorphanol on halothane minimum alveolar concentration in ponies. *Equine Veterinary Journal* **22**: 325–327.

Matthews, N.S., Hartsfield, S.M., Carroll, G.L. *et al.* (1997) Maintenance and recovery from anesthesia with sevoflurane in 40 equine clinical cases. *Proceedings of the 6th International Congress of Veterinary Anaesthesiology, Thessaloniki*, p. 125.

Matthews, N.S., Hartsfield, S.M., Hague, B. *et al.* (1999) Detomidine-propofol anesthesia for abdominal surgery in horses. *Veterinary Surgery* **28**: 196–201.

McDonell, W.N. (1974) *PhD thesis*. Cambridge: University of Cambridge.

McDonell, W.N., Hall, L.W. and Jeffcott, L.B. (1979) Radiographic evidence of impaired pulmonary function in laterally recumbent anaesthetised horses. *Equine Veterinary Journal* **11**: 24–32.

Moon, P.F. and Suter, C.M. (1993) Paravertebral thoracolumbar anaesthesia in 10 horses. *Equine Veterinary Journal*, **25**: 304–308.

Moore, J.M. (1994) Endotoxaemia; recent advances in pathophysiology and treatment. *Journal of Veterinary Anaesthesia* **21**: 77–81.

Muir, W.W., Skarda, R.T. and Milne, D.W. (1977) Evaluation of xylazine and ketamine hydrochloride for anesthesia in horses. *American Journal of Veterinary Research* **38**: 195–201.

Muir, W.W., Skarda, R.T. and Sheehan, W.C. (1978) Cardiopulmonary effects of narcotic agonists and a partial agonist in horses. *American Journal of Veterinary Research* **39**: 1632–1635.

Muir, W.W., Skarda, R.T. and Sheehan, W. (1978a) Evaluation of xylazine, guaifenesin, and ketamine hydrochloride for restraint in horses. *American Journal of Veterinary Research* **39**: 1274–1278.

Muir, W.W., Skarda, R.T. and Sheehan, W.C. (1979) Hemodynamic and respiratory effects of a xylazine-acetylpromazine drug combination in horses. *American Journal of Veterinary Research* **40**: 1518–1522.

Muir, W.W., Skarda, R.T. and Sheehan, W.C. (1979a) Hemodynamic and respiratory effects of xylazine-morphine sulfate in horses. *American Journal of Veterinary Research* **40**: 1417–1420.

Muir, W.W., Sams, R.A., Huffman, R.H. *et al.* (1982) Pharmacodynamic and pharmacokinetic properties of diazepam in horses. *American Journal of Veterinary Research* **43**: 1756–1762.

Muir, W.W. (1992) Cardiovascular effects of dopexamine HCl in conscious and halothane-anaesthetised horses. *Equine Veterinary Journal* Suppl: 24–29.

Muir, W.W. (1992a) Inotropic mechanisms of dopexamine hydrochloride in horses. *American Journal of Veterinary Research* **53**: 1343–1346.

Muir, W.W. Gadawski, J.E. and Grosenbaugh, D.A. (1999) Cardiorespiratory effects of a tiletamine/zolazepam-ketamine-detomidine combination in horses. *American Journal of Veterinary Research* **60**: 770–774.

Nilsfors, L. and Kvart, C. (1986) Preliminary report on the cardiorespiratory effects of the antagonist to detomidine, MPV-1248. *Acta Veterinaria Scandinavica* **82** (Supp;): 121–131.

Nolan, A.M. and Hall, L.W. (1984) Combined use of sedatives and opiates in horses. *Veterinary Record* **114**: 63–67.

Nolan, A.M. and Hall, L.W. (1985) Total intravenous anaesthesia in the horse with propofol. *Equine Veterinary Journal* **17**: 394–398.

Nolan, A.M., Reid, J., Welsh, E. *et al.* (1996) Simultaneous infusions of propofol and ketamine in ponies premedicated with detomidine: a pharmacokinetic study. *Research in Veterinary Science* **60**: 262–266.

Nyman, G., Funkquist, B., Kvart, C. *et al.* (1990) Atelectasis causes gas exchange impairment in the anaesthetised horse. *Equine Veterinary Journal* **22**: 317–324.

Pascoe, P.J., Steffey, E.P., Black, W.D. *et al.* (1993) Evaluation of the effect of alfentanil on the minimum alveolar concentration of halothane in horses. *American Journal of Veterinary Research* **54**: 1327–1332.

Pascoe, P.J., McDonell, W.N. and Fox, A.E. (1985). *Proceedings of the 2nd International Congress of Veterinary Anesthesiology, Sacramento*, p. 61.

Pippi, N.L. and Lumb, W.V. (1979) Objective tests of analgesic drugs in ponies. *American Journal of Veterinary Research* **40**: 1082–1086.

Raekallio, M., Taylor, P.M. and Bennett, R.C. (1997) Preliminary investigations of pain and analgesia assessment in horses administered phenylbutazone or placebo after arthroscopic surgery. *Veterinary Surgery* **26**: 150–155.

Ramseyer, B., Schucker, N., Schatzman, U. *et al.* (1998) Antagonism of detomidine sedation with atipamezole in horses. *Journal of Veterinary Anaesthesia* **25**: 47–51.

Reibold, T.W., Evans, A.T. and Robinson, N.E. (1980) Evaluation of the demand valve for resuscitation of horses. *Journal of the American Veterinary Medical Association* **176**: 623–626.

Richey, M.T., Holland, M.S., McGrath, C.J. *et al.* (1990) Equine post-anesthetic lameness. A retrospective study. *Veterinary Surgery* **19**: 392–397.

Robertson, J.T., Muir, W.W. and Sams, R. (1981) Cardiopulmonary effects of butorphanol tartrate in horses. *American Journal of Veterinary Research* **42**: 41–44.

Robertson, J.T. and Muir, W.W. (1983) A new analgesic drug combination in the horse. *American Journal of Veterinary Research* **44**: 1667–1669.

Robertson, S.A., Carter, S.W., Donovan, M. *et al.* (1990) Effects of intravenous xylazine hydrochloride on blood glucose, plasma insulin and rectal temperature in neonatal foals. *Equine Veterinary Journal* **22**: 43–47.

Robinson, E.P., Moncada-Suarex, J.R. and Felice, L. (1994) Epidural morphine analgesia in horses. *Veterinary Surgery* **23**: 78.

Rose, R.J., Rose, E.M. and Peterson, P.R. (1989) Clinical experiences with isoflurane anaesthesia in foals and adult horses. *American Association of Equine Practitioners*. 34: 555–569.

Ruch, K.S., Garner, H.E., Hatfiels, D.G. *et al.* (1984) Arterial oxygen and carbon dioxide tensions in conscious laterally recumbent ponies. *Equine Veterinary Journal* **16**: 185–188.

Schatzmann, U. (1982) The respiration of the horse under different anaesthetic medications. *Proceedings of the Association of Veterinary Anaesthetists* **10** (Suppl): 112–118.

Serteyn, D., Mottart, E., Deby, C. *et al.* (1990) Equine postanaesthetic myositis: a possible role for free radical generation and membrane lipoperoxidation. *Research in Veterinary Science* **48**: 42–46.

Short, C.E. (1981) Intravenous anaesthesia; drugs and techniques. *Veterinary Clinics of North America: Equine Anaesthesia* **3**: 195–208.

Short, C.E., Matthews, N.S., Harvey, R. *et al.* (1986) Cardiovascular and pulmonary function studies of a new sedative/analgesic (detomidine/Domosedan) for use alone in horses – or as a pre-anesthetic. *Acta Veterinaria Scandinavica* **82** (Suppl): 139–155.

Short, C.E. (1992). Alpha 2– agents in animals. Sedation, analgesia and anaesthesia. Santa Barbara: Veterinary Practice Publishing Company, pp. 21–39.

Singh, S., McDonell, W., Young, S. *et al.* (1997) The effect of glycopyrrolate on heart rate and intestinal motility in conscious horses. *Journal of Veterinary Anaesthesia* **24**: 14–19.

Skarda, R.T. and Muir, W.W. (1994) Caudal analgesia induced by epidural or subarachnoid administration of detomidine hydrochloride solution in mares. *American Journal of Veterinary Research* **55**: 670–680.

Skarda, R.T. (1996). Local and regional anesthetic and analgesic techniques: horses. In: Thurmon, J.C., Tranquilli, W.J. and Benson, G.J. (eds) *Lumb and Jones' Veterinary Anaesthesia*. Baltimore: Williams and Wilkins, pp. 461–462.

Skarda, R.T. and Muir, W.W. (1996a) Analgesic, hemodynamic, and respiratory effects of caudal epidurally administered xylazine hydrochloride solution in mares. *American Journal of Veterinary Research* **57**: 193–200.

Skarda, R.T. and Muir, W.W. (1996b) Comparison of antinociceptive, cardiovascular, and respiratory effects, head ptosis, and position of pelvic limbs in mares after caudal epidural administration of xylazine and detomidine hydrochloride solution. *American Journal of Veterinary Research* **57**: 1338–1345.

Skarda, R.T. and Muir, W.W. (1998) Influence of atipamezole on effects of midsacral subarachnoidally administered detomidine in mares. *American Journal of Veterinary Research* **59**: 468–477.

Steffey, E.P., Howland, D. Jr. Giri, S. *et al.* (1977) Enflurane, halothane, and isoflurane potency in horses. *American Journal of Veterinary Research* **38**: 1037–1039.

Steffey, E.P. (1978) Enflurane and isoflurane anesthesia: a summary of laboratory and clinical investigations in horses. *Journal of the American Veterinary Medical Association* **172**: 367–373.

Steffey, E.P. and Howland, D. Jr. (1978) Cardiovascular effects of halothane in the horse. *American Journal of Veterinary Research* **39**: 611–615.

Steffey, E.P. and Howland, D. Jr. (1978a) Potency of halothane- N₂0 in the horse. *American Journal of Veterinary Research* **39**: 1141–1146.

Steffey, E.P. and Howland, D. Jr. (1980) Comparison of circulatory and respiratory effects of isoflurane and halothane anesthesia in horses. *American Journal of Veterinary Research* **41**: 821–825.

Steffey, E.P., Dunlop, C.I., Farver, T.B. *et al.* (1987) Cardiovascular and respiratory measurements in awake and isoflurane- anesthetized horses. *American Journal of Veterinary Research* **48**: 7–12.

Steffey, E.P., Farver, T.B. and Woliner, M.J. (1987a) Cardiopulmonary function during 7 h of constant-dose halothane and methoxyflurane. *Journal of Applied Physiology* **63**: 1351–1359.

Steffey, E.P., Kelly, A.B. and Woliner, M.J. (1987b) Time-related responses of spontaneously breathing, laterally recumbent horses to prolonged anesthesia with halothane. *American Journal of Veterinary Research* **48**: 952–957.

Steffey, E.P., Woliner, M.J. and Dunlop, C. (1990) Effects of five hours of constant 1.2 MAC halothane in sternally recumbent, spontaneously breathing horses. *Equine Veterinary Journal* **22**: 433–436.

Steffey, E.P., Willits, N. and Woliner, M. (1992) Hemodynamic and respiratory responses to variable arterial partial pressure of oxygen in halothane-anesthetized horses during spontaneous and controlled ventilation. *American Journal of Veterinary Research* **53**: 1850–1858.

Steffey, E.P., Dunlop, C.I., Cullen, L.K. *et al.* (1993) Circulatory and respiratory responses of spontaneously breathing, laterally recumbent horses to 12 hours of halothane anesthesia. *American Journal of Veterinary Research* **54**: 929–936.

Stolk, P.W. (1979). *PhD thesis*. Cambridge: University of Cambridge.

Swanson, C.R., Muir, W.W., Bednarski, R.M. *et al.* (1985) Hemodynamic responses in halothane-anesthetized horses given infusions of dopamine or dobutamine. *American Journal of Veterinary Research* **46**: 365–370.

Sysel, A.M., Pleasant, R.S., Jacobson, J.D. *et al.* (1996) Efficacy of an epidural combination of morphine and detomidine in alleviating experimentally induced hindlimb lameness in horses. *Veterinary Surgery* **25**: 511–518.

Sysel, A.M., Pleasant, R.S., Jacobson, J.D. *et al.* (1997) Systemic and local effects associated with long-term epidural catheterization and morphine-detomidine administration in horses. *Veterinary Surgery* **26**: 141–149.

Taylor, P.M. and Hall, L.W. (1985) Clinical anaesthesia in the horse: comparison of enflurane and halothane. *Equine Veterinary Journal* **17**: 51–57.

Taylor, P.M. (1986) Effect of postoperative pethidine on the anaesthetic recovery period in the horse. *Equine Veterinary Journal* **18**: 70–72.

Taylor, P.M. (1989) Adrenocortical response to propofol infusion in ponies: a preliminary report. *Journal of the Association of Veterinary Anaesthetists* **17**: 32–34.

Taylor, P.M. (1990) Doxapram infusion during halothane anaesthesia in ponies. *Equine Veterinary Journal* **22**: 329–332.

Taylor, P.M. and Young, S.S. (1990) The effect of limb position on venous and intracompartmental pressure in the forelimb of ponies. *Journal of the Association of Veterinary Anaesthetists* **17**: 35–37.

Taylor, P.M. (1991) Stress response in ponies during halonthone on isoflurane anaesthesia after induction with thropentone or xylazine/ketamine. *Journal of association of Veterinary anaesthesia* **18**, 8–14.

Taylor, P.M. and Luna, S.P.L. (1995) Total intravenous anaesthesia in ponies using detomidine. ketamine and guaifenesin: pharmacokinetics, cardiopulmonary and endocrine effects. *Research in Veterinary Science* **59**: 17–23.

Taylor, P.M. (1998) Endocrine and metabolic responses to plasma volume expansion during halothane anesthesia in ponies. *Journal Of Veterinary Pharmacology And Therapeutics* **21**: 485–490.

Tendillo, F.J., Mascia, A. and Santos, M. *et al.* (1997) Anesthetic potency of desflurane in the horse: determination of minimal alveolar concentration. *Veterinary Surgery* **26**: 354.

Tevik, A. (1983) The role of anesthesia in surgical mortality in horses. *Nordisk Veterinarmedicin* **35**: 175–179.

Thurmon, J.C., Neff-Davis, C., Davis, L.E. *et al.* (1982) Xylazine hydrochloride-induced hyperglycemia and hypoinsulinemia in thoroughbred horses. *Journal of Veterinary Pharmacology and Therapeutics* **5**: 241–245.

Tobin, T. (1978) A review of the pharmacology of reserpine in the horse. *Journal of Equine Medicine and Surgery* **2**: 433–438.

Tobin, T. and Combie, J.D. (1982) Performance testing in horses: a review of the role of simple behavioral models in the design of performance experiments. *Journal of Veterinary Pharmacology and Therapeutics* **5**: 105–118.

Trim, C.M. and Mason, J. (1973) Post-anaesthetic fore-limb lameness in horses. *Equine Veterinary Journal* **5**: 71– 76.

Trim, C.M. (1984) Complications associated with the use of the cuffless endotracheal tube in the horse. *Journal of the American Veterinary Medical Association* **185**: 541–542.

Trim, C.M., Moore, J.N. and White, N.A. (1985) Cardiopulmonary effects of dopamine hydrochloride in anaesthetised horses. *Equine Veterinary Journal* **17**: 41–44.

Trim, C.M., Moore, J.N. and Clark, E.S. (1989) Renal effects of dopamine infusion in conscious horses. *Equine Veterinary Journal* Supp;: 124–128.

Trim, C.M., Moore, J.N., Hardee, M.M. *et al*. (1991) Effects of an infusion of dopamine on the cardiopulmonary effects of Escherichia coli endotoxin in anaesthetised horses. Research in Veterinary Science **50**: 54–63.

Trim, C.M. (1997) Postanesthetic hemorrhagic myelopathy or myelomalacia. *Veterinary Clinics of North America. Equine Practice* **13**: 73–77.

Tyler, W.S., Gillespie, J.R. and Nowell, J. (1971) Modern functional morphology of the equine lung. Equine Veterinary Journal **3**: 84–94.

Vainio, O. (1985) Detomidine, a new sedative and analgesic drug for veterinary use. Pharmacological and clinical studies in laboratory animals, horses and cattle. *PhD thesis*. Helsinki: University of Helsinki.

Voetgli, K. (1988). Studies on the sedative and analgesic effects of an alpha 2 adrenoceptor agonist (STH 2130) in horses. *D.V et. Med. Thesis*. Berne: University of Berne.

Wagner, A.E., Dunlop, C.I., Heath, R.B. *et al*. (1992) Hemodynamic function during neurectomy in halothane-anesthetized horses with or without constant dose detomidine infusion. *Veterinary Surgery* **21**: 248–255.

Watney, G.C., Watkins, S.B. and Hall, L.W. (1985) Effects of a demand valve on pulmonary ventilation in spontaneously breathing, anaesthetised horses. *Veterinary Record* **117**: 358–362.

Watney, G.C.J., Jordan, C. and Hall, L.W. (1987) The effect of halothane, enflurane and isoflurane on bronchomotor tone in anaesthetized ponies. *British Journal of Anaesthesia* **59**: 1022–1026.

Webb, A.I. (1984) Nasal intubation in the foal. *Journal of the American Veterinary Medical Association* **185**: 48–51.

Westhues, M. and Fristch, R. (1960). *Die narkose der Tierre*, Berlin: Paul Darey.

Wetmore, L.A., Derksen, F.J., Blaze, C.A. *et al*. (1987). Mixed venous oxygen tension as an estimate of cordiac output in anesthetized horses. *American Journal of Veterinary Research* **48**: 971.

Wright, J.G. (1942) *Veterinary Anaesthesia*. London: Ballière Tindall and Cox.

Young, L.E., Blissitt, K.J., Clutton, R.E. *et al*. (1997) Temporal effects of an infusion of dopexamine hydrochloride in horses anesthetized with halothane. *American Journal of Veterinary Research* **58**: 516–523.

Young, S.S. and Taylor, P.M. (1993) Factors influencing the outcome of equine anaesthesia: a review of 1,314 cases. *Equine Veterinary Journal* **25**: 147–151.

Anaesthesia of cattle

12

INTRODUCTION

Cattle are by no means good subjects for heavy sedation or general anaesthesia. Regurgitation followed by aspiration of ruminal contents into the lungs can easily occur. Once a ruminant animal is in lateral or dorsal recumbency, the oesophageal opening is submerged in ruminal material, normal eructation cannot occur, and gas accumulates. The degree of bloat depends on the amount of fermentation of the ingesta and on the length of time that gas is allowed to accumulate. Gross distension of the rumen becomes a hazard if anaesthesia or recumbency is prolonged and regurgitation can follow from this. In addition, the weight of the abdominal viscera and their contents prevents the diaphragm from moving freely on inspiration and ventilation becomes shallow, rapid and inefficient for gas exchange within the lungs.

The danger of regurgitation and inhalation of ingesta is always present but the likelihood of it occurring can be minimized by:

1. Withholding all food for 24 to 48 hours before anaesthesia. Optimum duration for starvation is up for discussion, with some recommending that 24 hours is not only sufficient but also produces the best consistency of rumen contents to minimize regurgitation. A longer period of starvation may result in formation of a more liquid ruminal content which may be regurgitated more easily.

2. Withholding water for 8 to 12 hours before anaesthesia.

3. When the animal is in lateral recumbency during anaesthesia arranging that the occiput is above general body level and that the head slopes so that saliva and any regurgitated material runs freely from the mouth (Fig. 12.1).

4. At the end of anaesthesia, cleaning solid material from the pharynx and leaving the endotracheal tube in the trachea with the cuff inflated until the animal is in sternal recumbency, is swallowing and, most importantly, can withdraw its tongue back into its mouth.

An additional procedure to prevent regurgitation that has been tried but not often used is to pass a modified stomach tube as far down the oesophagus as possible. The tube has a balloon firmly attached to its end that can be inflated to

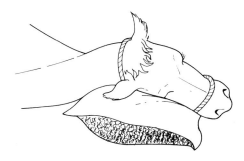

FIG. 12.1 Animal's head inclined over a support to allow saliva and any regurgitated rumenal content to drain out of the mouth.

obstruct flow of ingesta from the rumen into the pharynx.

Regurgitation occurs during both light and deep anaesthesia so that it is probable that two mechanisms are involved in the process. During light anaesthesia ingesta may pass up the oesophagus into the pharynx as a result of an active, but uncontrolled, reflex mechanism. It is then a matter of chance whether or not the protective reflexes, e.g. laryngeal closure, coughing, etc., are active and can or cannot prevent aspiration. Fortunately, laryngeal closure often occurs but, as hypoxia develops, at some point the animal will take a large breath and any ingesta accumulated in the pharynx will be aspirated. The order in which the reflexes of laryngeal closure, coughing, swallowing, and regurgitation disappear as anaesthesia is deepened differs from one anaesthetic drug combination to another but the relative safety of the various agents is not documented. During deep anaesthesia, on the other hand, regurgitation is a passive process. The striated muscle of the oesophagus loses its tone and any increase in the intraruminal pressure – whether from pressure on the abdominal wall from a rope or belly band or from gas accumulation in the rumen itself – may force ingesta up into the pharynx. The protective reflexes are not active and aspiration may occur easily.

Tracheal intubation is not always performed in all sedated or anaesthetized recumbent bovine animals and regurgitation does not always occur. However, some animals will regurgitate, and this has an unreasonably high risk for fatal outcome. Should regurgitation occur during the induction of anaesthesia before endotracheal intubation has been accomplished, the endotracheal tube may be immediately passed into the oesophagus and its cuff inflated so that the regurgitated material passes along the tube and out of the mouth. The trachea can then be intubated with a second tube, taking care to cover the end of the tube to avoid scooping material into its lumen. In actuality, the presence of one endotracheal tube in the pharynx often makes passage of a second tube nearly impossible due to the small size of the bovine pharynx. One option is to intubate the trachea with a stomach tube and attempt to feed the second endotracheal tube over the stomach tube. An alternative is to wait until the flow of ingesta stops,

remove the tube from the oesophagus and to rapidly intubate the trachea. However, if the conditions initiating the regurgitation such as ropes tight around the thorax and abdomen have not been removed, or the depth of anaesthesia is light, regurgitation may recommence during the removal of the endotracheal tube from the oesophagus.

Salivation continues as a copious flow throughout general anaesthesia but the loss of saliva is unlikely to produce a significant effect on acid–base status. Antisialagogues are not of much use for they make the secretion more viscid in nature and do not significantly reduce its production. It is important to arrange the head of the anaesthetized animal so that saliva drains from the mouth and does not accumulate in the pharynx. Intubation with a cuffed endotracheal tube will prevent inhalation of saliva.

In two reports involving restraint of unsedated cows or bulls in dorsal or lateral recumbency, a decrease in PaO_2 from an average standing value of 11.4 kPa (86 mmHg) to less than 9.3 kPa (70 mmHg) was measured, with a decrease to below 6.6 kPa (50 mmHg) in some individuals (Semrad *et al.*, 1986; Klein & Fisher 1988). Arterial PCO_2 remained at or slightly below 5 kPa (38 mmHg). In another investigation of cows from which food was withheld for 18 h, mean PaO_2 in standing animals was 14.5 kPa (109 mmHg) (Wagner *et al.*, 1990). Significant decreases in PaO_2 occurred in both lateral and dorsal positions but only in dorsal recumbency did values decrease to below 9.3 kPa (70 mmHg). These changes indicate that even in unsedated cattle, recumbency creates abnormalities of ventilation and perfusion that are not counter-balanced by normal compensatory mechanisms. It is not surprising that cattle sedated with xylazine and breathing air will develop decreased oxygenation or hypoxaemia (DeMoor & Desmet, 1971; Raptopoulos & Weaver 1984).

Withholding feed before sedation and anaesthesia may reduce pressure on the diaphragm, limit lung collapse and modify the decrease in PaO_2. In a study of fed and non-fed cows anaesthetized with halothane and breathing oxygen, cows fed before anaesthesia had a progressive decrease in PaO_2, reaching hypoxaemic levels after an hour of anaesthesia, whereas cows that were starved before anaesthesia were well oxygenated (Blaze *et al.*, 1988). Severe hypercapnia was measured in both groups with a greater increase measured in the fed cows. Thus, hypoxaemia may develop in recumbent non-starved cattle even when inhaling high O_2 concentrations but supplementation of inspired air with O_2 may prevent hypoxaemia if the cow has been starved first. Respiratory acidosis usually develops in anaesthetized cattle.

Normal values for cardiovascular parameters in unsedated healthy cattle are approximately 73 ± 14 beats/min (mean $\pm$ SD) for heart rate, 150 ± 27 mmHg for mean arterial pressure, and 64 ± 14 ml/kg/min for cardiac output (Wagner *et al.*, 1990). Withholding feed for 48 h has been determined to cause significant decreases in heart rates in cattle (Rumsey & Bond, 1976; McGuirk *et al.*, 1990).

RESTRAINT

The majority of bovine clinical surgery is carried out under local analgesia, frequently in the standing animal. Surgical procedure is made easier by use of appropriate sedation and/or restraining 'crushes' or 'chutes'. Ropes are useful additions for restraining sedated or unsedated cattle and anyone in cattle veterinary practice soon becomes expert at tying quick-release knots, tying bowline knots for rope loops, applying Reuff's method of casting a mature bovine by squeezing with a neck loop and two half-hitches around the body, and assembling figure of eight ties to secure flexed front and hind limbs.

Electroimmobilization

Electrical devices are available to immobilize cattle by causing muscle tetanus from application of an electrical current between electrodes at the lip and rectum. There are concerns that this technique is neither humane nor analgesic. Holstein cows trained to be lead with a halter and enter a set of stocks were observed for behavioural and physiological responses to either immobilization by application of an electric current for 30 s from a commercially available electroimmobilizer or to an intramuscular injection with an 18 gauge needle (Pascoe, 1986). The electrical immobilization was associated with significant aversive behaviour and evidence of distress and the results led the authors to believe that electroimmobilization was a strong noxious stimulus that was remembered for several months.

SEDATION

AGENTS USED IN BOVINE ANAESTHESIA

Xylazine

Xylazine has for a long time been the most effective sedative available for cattle. The dose rate of xylazine in cattle, 0.02–0.20 mg/kg, with the highest dose intended for i.m. use, is one-tenth of that used in horses. Intravenous injection results in deeper sedation than i.m. administration. Cattle may assume recumbency even at the lowest dose rates, although breed differences in sensitivity to xylazine have been reported. In an investigation comparing Hereford and Holstein cattle, 84% of Herefords spontaneously lay down after xylazine administration, whereas only 22% of Holsteins did so (Raptopoulos & Weaver, 1984). Furthermore, the average duration of recumbency in the Herefords was 90 min compared with 50 min in the Holsteins. The environmental conditions under which xylazine is administered may influence the response. In a study comparing the effects of xylazine in Holstein heifers under a thermoneutral condition compared with a hot environment (temperature approximately 33 °C and relative humidity 63%), the time to standing was increased from 41 min to an average of 107 min during heat stress (Fayed *et al.*, 1989). Xylazine causes contraction of the bovine uterus similar to oxytocin (LeBlanc *et al.*, 1984), and premature birth has been reported after administration to heavily pregnant cows. Today it is generally acknowledged that use of xylazine in pregnant cows in the last trimester of pregnancy is contraindicated.

Xylazine may cause mild to severe decreases in PaO_2 and moderate increases in $PaCO_2$ in mature cattle (DeMoor & Desmet, 1971; Raptopoulos & Weaver, 1984). Xylazine administration induces bradycardia, decreased MAP and CO, and increased peripheral resistance (Campbell *et al.*, 1979). Campbell *et al.* (1979) also noted second degree atrioventricular heart block in one out of five calves receiving xylazine.

Xylazine has a number of side effects that may have an adverse effect on the animal. It abolishes the swallowing reflex so that regurgitation can result in pulmonary aspiration. The inability of the cow or bull to withdraw its tongue into its mouth and swallow may persist until after the animal regains the standing position. Thus, it is advisable to withhold food and water from cattle before giving xylazine. Gastrointestinal motility is decreased and bloat may develop, while diarrhoea may be observed 12–24 hours after sedation (Hopkins, 1972). Hyperglycaemia persisting for about 10 hours develops after xylazine administration and this is associated with a decrease in serum insulin concentration (Symonds & Mallinson, 1978; Eichner *et al.*, 1979). The decrease in serum insulin is believed to be due to a decrease in production (Fayed *et al.*, 1989). Increased urine production occurs within 30 minutes of administration and continues for two hours (Thurmon *et al.*, 1978) due to suppression of antidiuretic hormone (ADH) release. Use of xylazine in animals with urethral obstruction may be responsible for rupture of the urinary bladder or urethra.

Minor surgical procedures have been performed on cattle sedated with xylazine but, whenever possible, local infiltration techniques or nerve blocks should be utilized to ensure sufficient analgesia.

Detomidine

In contrast to xylazine, the dose rates for detomidine in cattle are similar to those used in horses. Dose rates of 0.03–0.06 mg/kg i.m. have been used in clinical trials, however lower doses may provide sufficient sedation for combination with local analgesic techniques for surgery. Elimination is mainly by metabolism as there is negligible excretion of the drug in urine. No detomidine was detectable in milk 23 h after dosing and tissue concentrations measured 48 h after dosing were less than 3% of the original dose (Salonen *et al.*, 1989). Detomidine, 0.04 and 0.06 mg/kg, increases electrical activity of the bovine uterus, although administration of detomidine, 0.05 mg/kg, to a group of pregnant cows was not followed by abortions (Vainio, 1988).

A lower dose rate of detomidine, 0.02 mg/kg, decreased electrical activity of the uterus and sedation at this dose rate may be safe in the pregnant animal (Vainio 1988).

The pharmacologic effects of detomidine in cattle are very similar to those of xylazine in that it causes bradycardia, hyperglycaemia, and increased urine production. An exception is that detomidine causes arterial hypertension which is dose-dependent in duration.

Medetomidine

Deep sedation without recumbency can be obtained with intravenous doses of medetomidine, 0.005 mg/kg, while 0.01 mg/kg produces recumbency and sedation equivalent to that obtained with intravenous doses of 0.1–0.2 mg/kg xylazine (G. C. W. England and K. W. Clarke, unpublished observations). Medetomidine, 0.04 mg/kg, has been given intravenously alone or with ketamine for anaesthesia in calves (Raekallio *et al.*, 1991; Ranheim *et al.*, 1998). Medetomidine, 0.015 mg/kg, has been administered by epidural injection for analgesia in cows (Lin *et al.*, 1998).

Antagonists to the α_2 adrenoceptor agonists

As prolonged recumbency causes so many problems in cattle, the availability of α_2 adrenoceptor antagonists is of particular value. These antagonists not only cause the animal to awaken, they also antagonize the majority of the side effects of the agonists, including restoring ruminal motility to normal.

Almost all the α_2 adrenoceptor antagonists have been used in cattle sedated with xylazine. Yohimbine, 0.125 mg/kg, with aminopyridine, 0.3 mg/kg, will awaken cattle sedated with 0.2–0.3 mg/kg of xylazine, but will not restore a normal state of consciousness. Idazoxan at dose of 0.01–0.10 mg/kg is reported to be effective against xylazine in calves, with no relapse to sedation. Tolazoline at 0.2 mg/kg reverses the suppression of ruminal motility induced by xylazine but higher doses, 0.5–2.0 mg/kg, are required for full reversal of sedation. Care must be taken to administer tolazoline slowly as intravenous injection has been associated with abrupt adverse haemodynamic changes. One experimental study of xylazine administered by intramuscular and lumbosacral epidural routes concluded that the technique did not provide adequate analgesia for umbilical surgery in calves (Lewis *et al.*, 1999). In this study, reversal of sedation with tolazoline caused transient sinus bradycardia and sinus arrest, accompanied by severe systemic arterial hypotension.

Atipamezole in doses of 25 and 50 µg/kg, intravenously or intramuscularly, causes awakening in cows sedated with 0.2 mg/kg of xylazine, with restoration of ruminal motility to normal. Two hours later some relapse occurs although resedation should not be so deep as to cause recumbency. Relapse does not occur after i.m. injection of the antagonist. Atipamezole, 60 µg/kg, given either as the entire dose i.v. or as half the dose i.v. and half i.m. to antagonize medetomidine in calves results in a rapid smooth recovery to ambulation (Raekallio *et al.*, 1991). Calves sedated with medetomidine, 0.04 mg/kg, and injected with atipamezole, 200 µg/kg i.v. 60 minutes later, became resedated on average 80 min after the injection of atipamezole and this lasted an average of 240 min (Ranheim *et al.*, 1998). These authors suggested that the relapse into sedation could not be explained by differences in pharmacokinetic parameters of medetomidine and atipamezole. It may be that the elimination of medetomidine from the sites of action is slower than elimination of the drug from plasma. Atipamezole given to unsedated cattle, or as medetomidine sedation is waning, may induce a state of hyperactivity, kicking and bucking.

Acepromazine

Acepromazine may be given in doses of 0.05 mg/kg i.v. or 0.1 mg/kg i.m. to induce mild tranquillization. Acepromazine will decrease the dose rate of subsequently administered anaesthetics and may increase the risk of regurgitation.

Chloral hydrate

Although some of the more recently introduced agents, such as the α_2 adrenoceptor agonist xylazine, may have some advantages, including easier administration, chloral hydrate is still a perfectably acceptable, inexpensive sedative for adult cattle. It may be given by mouth or i.v. injection. To obtain a recumbent, very lightly unconscious adult cow, the drug is usually administered by drench, or preferably by stomach tube, in doses of 30–60 g as a 1 in 20 solution in water. Sedation attains its maximum depth in a period of 10–20 min and local analgesics may be injected for nerve blocks while sedation is developing. As cows can generally be cast and restrained without difficulty, i.v. administration will generally be in this position with the head and neck extended. The external jugular vein can be readily distended by finger pressure and the use of choke cords is unnecessarily distressful for the animal. The dose required is between 80 and 90 mg/kg of a 10% solution and it should be remembered that narcosis will continue to deepen after the i.v. injection is completed. The induction and recovery periods are excitement free.

Young bulls present no particular difficulties provided their temperament is such that they can be safely and effectively restrained for drenching or precise i.v. injection. In older bulls the precise i.v. injection of drugs in the standing position may not only be uncertain on account of difficulties in satisfactorily introducing the needle into the vein but sometimes impossible because of movement by the animal.

In many instances the temperament of the bull is such that large doses have to be given by mouth in order to obtain sufficient sedation to allow application of casting tackle. The further administration of the drug by the i.v. route after casting gives rise to danger of overdose consequent on continued absorption from the stomach. When, without any previous medication, chloral hydrate is given to a bull by i.v. injection at the usual rate, the dose required to induce deep narcosis is the same as for the big cow – about 90–100 mg/kg. When the drug is given by the mouth a dose of 140–200 g (or even more) may be required to induce a degree of sedation whereby the animal can be handled safely and even after such a quantity the animal may still be able to stand.

The bull which is running free in the yard or a loose-box may be quite dangerous even to approach. In such cases it is generally advised that drinking water be withheld for 36 hours and that the animal then be offered water containing 90 to 120 g of chloral hydrate in 12 litres. It is often taken and, if it is, the degree of sedation is such that, with care, the bull can be approached and a leading pole applied.

Pentobarbital

Nervous or excitable cattle may be restrained by the slow i.v. injection of a 20% solution of pentobarbital. To make the animal sway slightly on its hind legs while being able to walk unaided, a dose of 1–2 g is needed for the adult cow. A dose of about 3 g/500 kg usually makes an adult cow recumbent and almost unconscious.

Small doses (15–20 ml of a 6.5% solution, i.e. 1.00–1.25 g) may be given to prolong narcosis induced with chloral hydrate. It is injected i.v. as soon as the chloral hydrate effect becomes inadequate and provided the injection is made slowly, and to effect, no harmful effects occur. The period of recumbency is much less than if additional doses of chloral hydrate are administered and recovery is not associated with struggling and excitement. More than one injection of pentobarbital may be given during the course of long operations.

Butorphanol

Administration of butorphanol to healthy unsedated cows will not predictably induce sedation and may induce behaviour changes including restlessness and bellowing. Butorphanol, 0.02–0.03 mg/kg, may provide sedation in cattle that are sick and may increase the quality of sedation when administered in conjunction with xylazine. Butorphanol can be detected in the milk for up to 36 hours following administration (Court *et al.*, 1992)

LOCAL ANALGESIA

SPECIAL NERVE BLOCKS

Auriculopalpebral nerve block

This nerve supplies motor fibres to the orbicularis oculi muscle. The nerve runs from the base of the ear along the facial crest, past and ventral to the

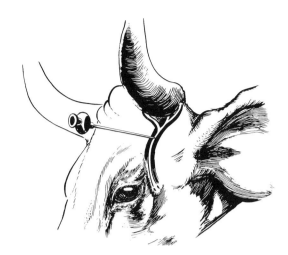

Fig. 12.2 Auriculopalpebral nerve block.

eye, giving off its branches on the way. This block is used to prevent eyelid closure during examination or surgery of the eye. It does not provide analgesia to the eye or eyelids and should be used in conjunction with topical analgesia or other nerve blocks for painful procedures.

The needle is inserted in front of the base of the ear at the end of the zygomatic arch until its point lies at the dorsal border of the arch (Fig. 12.2). About 10–15 ml of 2% lignocaine is injected beneath the fascia at this point.

Cornual nerve block

The horn corium and the skin around its base derive their sensory nerve supply from a branch of the ophthalmic division of the 5th cranial nerve. The nerve emerges from the orbit and ascends just behind the lateral ridge of the frontal bone. This latter structure can be readily palpated with the fingers. In the upper third of the ridge the nerve is relatively superficial, being covered only by skin and a thin layer of the frontalis muscle.

The site for injection is the upper third of the temporal ridge, about 2.5 cm below the base of the horn (Fig. 12.3). The needle (18 gauge, 2.5 cm long) is inserted so that its point lies 0.7–1.0 cm deep, immediately behind the ridge, and 5 ml of 2% lignocaine solution injected. The needle must not be inserted too deeply, otherwise injection will be made beneath the aponeurosis of the temporal muscle and the method will fail. In large animals

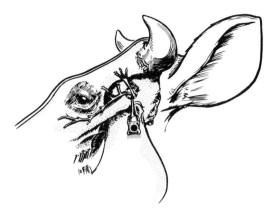

FIG. 12.3 Injection of the nerve to the horn core. In some animals the branch to the caudal part leaves the parent trunk proximal to the normal site for injection.

with well developed horns, a second injection should be made about 1 cm behind the first to block the posterior division of the nerve (Fig. 12.3). Loss of sensation develops in 10–15 minutes and lasts about 1 hour. This nerve block has been widely used for the dishorning of adult cattle but the block is not always complete. Variability in the curvature of the lateral ridge of the frontal bone makes exact determination of the site of the nerve difficult. In a struggling animal, it may be difficult to ensure that the point of the needle is at the correct depth. A third injection may be required in adult cattle with well developed horns; it is made caudal to the horn base to block the cutaneous branches of cervical nerves.

Petersen eye block

A 22 gauge, 2.5 cm needle is used to infiltrate local analgesic solution subcutaneously, about 5 ml of 2% lignocaine, within the notch formed by the supraorbital process cranially, the zygomatic arch ventrally and the coronoid process of the mandible caudally (Fig. 12.4). A 12 or 14 gauge, 2.5 cm needle placed as far rostral and ventral as possible in the desensitized skin of the notch serves as a cannula and a 18 gauge, 10 or 12 cm needle is introduced through it. The long needle is directed in a horizontal and caudal direction until it strikes the coronoid process of the mandible. It is then redirected towards the pterygopalatine fossa rostral to the orbitorotundum foramen at a depth of about 8–10 cm from the skin and 10–15 ml of 2% lignocaine solu-

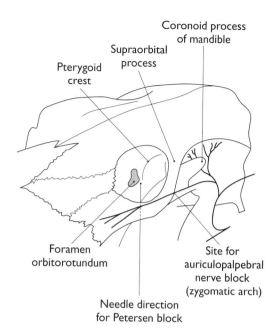

FIG. 12.4 Schematic drawing of the Petersen nerve block to block the nerves emerging from the foramen orbitorotundum, together with the auriculopalpebral nerve block on the zygomatic ridge. This is an alternative to the retrobulbar block but requires more skill to perform.

tion injected. This blocks the oculomotor, trochlear, abducens nerves and the three branches of the trigeminal nerve as they emerge from the foramen orbitorotundum. The needle is withdrawn to the subcutaneous tissue and redirected caudally and laterally to block the auriculopalpebral nerve on the zygomatic ridge by the injection of 5–10 ml of the local analgesic solution. The Petersen technique requires more skill to perform than a retrobulbar block but it may be safer.

Peribulbar and retrobulbar block

Retrobulbar injection is achieved by introduction of a curved needle through the skin about 1 cm lateral to the lateral canthus, or through the conjunctiva. The needle is first directed straight back and away from the eyeball until the point is beyond the globe and then turned inward to penetrate the muscle cone. When no blood is obtained after aspiration, lignocaine is deposited behind the eye.

Peribulbar anaesthesia is produced by inserting the needle and injecting lignocaine in 2 to 4 quadrants within the orbit but outside the ocular muscles. Injection of 20–30 ml of 2% lignocaine (or its equivalent) will produce corneal analgesia, mydriasis, and proptosis and paralysis of the eyeball. Anaesthesia is produced after spread of the anaesthetic agent; thus a larger volume of lignocaine is required for peribulbar anaesthesia, the onset of block is longer, and the larger volume of solution causes a greater increase in ocular pressure.

Recommendations vary over the use of sharp hypodermic or blunt (e.g. spinal needle) needles for ocular blocks, but penetration of the globe has been reported in human patients with both sharp and blunt needles (Hay, 1991; Wong, 1993). Blunt needles are not considered to be safer than sharp needles. Visual outcome is not a factor when penetration of the globe occurs during nerve block for enucleation. However, bacterial contamination of the orbit is possible.

Potentially adverse effects of both the Petersen block and the retrobulbar block include bradycardia, hypotension, asystole, respiratory depression, apnoea, perforation of the globe and intraorbital or retrobulbar venous haemorrhage. Symptoms of local anaesthetic spread to the central nervous system vary but respiratory arrest is a usual sign of brainstem anaesthesia. When the block is used for other purposes, care must be taken to ensure that the corneal surface does not become dry because of loss of tear formation for several hours.

Inverted L block

Infiltration of the skin, subcutaneous and deeper tissues in an inverted L shape with 60 ml of 2% lignocaine solution is a commonly used technique to provide analgesia for a flank laparotomy in a standing cow (Chapter 10). It is also used in recumbent animals to block the site for a paramedian incision, or repeated in a mirror image to form a U shape and analgesia for a midline incision. Injections must be made both subcutaneously and down to the peritoneum to produce a total block. The block can be achieved by making isolated injections at intervals of about 1 cm, which relies on lateral diffusion of the analgesic solution. Alternatively, a wall of local analgesic solution can be created by inserting a long needle to its depth, and injecting anaesthetic solution in a steady stream as the needle is withdrawn.

Paravertebral nerve block

Paravertebral block involves the perineural injection of local analgesic solution about the spinal nerves as they emerge from the vertebral canal through the intervertebral foramina. This technique is commonly used to provide analgesia for laparotomy. It offers a major advantage over use of field infiltration in that the abdominal wall including the peritoneum is more likely to be uniformly desensitized. Additionally, the abdominal wall is relaxed.

The area of the flank bounded cranially by the last rib, caudally by the angle of the ilium and dorsally by the lumbar transverse processes, is innervated by the thirteenth and first and second lumbar nerves. In addition, the third lumbar nerve, although it does not supply the flank, gives off a cutaneous branch which passes obliquely backwards in front of the ilium. Operations involving the ventral aspect of the abdominal wall will require additional desensitization of the dorsal nerves cranial to the thirteenth. The last dorsal and first lumbar intervertebral foramina in cattle are occasionally double. The last dorsal foramen lies immediately caudal to the head of the last rib and on a level with the base of the transverse process of the first lumbar vertebra. The lumbar foramina are large and are situated between the base of the transverse processes and approximately on the same level. The spinal nerves, after emerging from the foramina, immediately divide into a smaller dorsal and a larger ventral branch. The dorsal branch supplies chiefly the skin and muscles of the loins, but some of its cutaneous branches pass a considerable distance down the flank. The ventral branch passes obliquely ventrally and caudally between the muscles and comprises the main nerve supply to the skin, muscles, and peritoneum of the flank. The ventral branch is also connected with the sympathetic system by a ramus communicans. Paralysis of the nerves at their points of emergence from the intervertebral foramina will provoke desensitization of the whole depth of the flank wall and complete muscular relaxation. Block of the rami communicantes will result in splanchnic vasodilatation and potential for hypotension.

The number of nerves to be blocked will depend on the site and extent of the proposed inci-

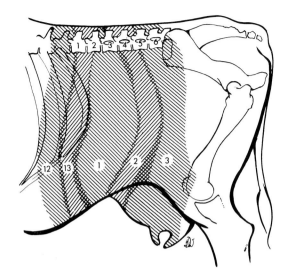

FIG. 12.5 Regions of the flank involved after paravertebral block of the respective nerves.

sion. The areas involved by blocking of respective nerves are illustrated in Fig. 12.5. Therefore, for rumenotomy, using an incision parallel with and about 7 cm caudal to the last rib, analgesia of the thirteenth thoracic and first and second lumbar nerves is required. The third lumbar nerve must be blocked for a more caudal incision and for relaxation of the internal oblique muscle.

A number of different techniques for blocking the respective nerves have been described but the most reliable relies on directing the needle towards the cranial border of the transverse process of the vertebra behind the nerve to be blocked. For example, to block the 1st lumbar nerve the needle should be directed to strike the cranial broder of the 2nd lumbar vertebra about 5–6 cm from the animal's midline. At such sites the cranial borders of the transverse processes are usually in the same cross sectional plane of the body as the most prominent parts of their lateral borders.

To block the thirteenth thoracic and first, second and third lumbar nerves skin weals should be raised in line with the most obvious parts of the transverse processes of the second, third and fourth lumbar vertebrae, 5–6 cm from, the midline of the body. Location of the transverse process of the first lumbar vertebra is usually difficult (particularly in well-muscled or obese animals) so in most cases the site for infiltration around the thir-

teenth thoracic nerve is found by simple measurement. The distance between the skin weals over the second and third lumbar transverse processes is measured and another skin weal is produced at a distance equal to this, cranial to the anterior weal, to mark the site where the needle is to be introduced to strike the cranial border of the first lumbar transverse process. A stout needle (7 cm long, 3 mm bore) is inserted through each skin weal and the underlying longissimus dorsi muscle infiltrated with 2–3 ml of 1% lignocaine (lidocaine) or other local analgesic solution as they are advanced to a depth of about 4 cm from the skin surface. This infiltration is omitted by some workers but it does serve to counteract spasm of the longissimus dorsi during the subsequent insertion of the longer needle used to deposit analgesic solution around the main nerve trunks. The needles used for injection around the nerves (10 cm long, 2 mm bore) are introduced, after an appropriate pause, through the holes made in the skin by the stout needles used for infiltration of the longissimus dorsi muscle, and advanced to strike the anterior border of the transverse process. Each needle is then redirected cranially over the edge of the transverse process and advanced until it is felt to penetrate the intertransverse ligament. Penetration of the intertransverse ligament is made more obvious if the needles used have 'short-bevel' points. Injection of 15 ml of local analgesic solution is made immediately below the ligament and a further 5 ml is injected as the needle is withdrawn to just above the ligament. During final withdrawal of the needle the skin is pressed downwards to prevent separation of the connective tissue and aspiration of air through the needle.

It is important to ensure that the needles shall be vertical when contact is first made with the cranial border of the transverse processes for, if they are not, redirection over the edge of the processes may cause their points to lie well away from the course of the nerves. Successful infiltration around the nerves is indicated first by the development of a belt of hyperaemia which causes a distinct and appreciable rise in skin temperature. Full analgesia develops in about ten minutes and when lignocaine with adrenaline 1:400 000 is used it persists for about 90 minutes. When a unilateral block is fully developed it produces a curvature of the

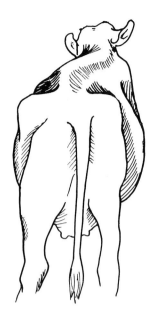

FIG. 12.6 Unilateral analgesia with either a paravertebral block or lumbar epidural producing spinal curvature towards the affected side.

spine, the convexity of which is towards the analgesic side (Fig. 12.6).

An alternative method of lumbar paravertebral block utilizing a lateral approach to the nerves is favoured by some. About 10 ml of local analgesic solution is injected beneath each transverse process towards the midline. The needle is then withdrawn a short distance and then redirected first cranially, then caudally, with more analgesic solution being injected along each line of insertion. A total of about 20 ml of solution is used for each site and the last portion of each 20 ml is injected slightly dorsal and caudal to the transverse process to block dorsolateral branches of the nerves. With this technique analgesic solution may be injected below fascial sheets and thus be prevented from bathing the nerves.

It is inevitable that failure or at least partial failure will sometimes attend attempts to inject local analgesic solution in the immediate vicinity of a series of nerves situated at a depth of 5–7 cm from the body surface, however careful the technique of injection and no matter which approach is adopted. Among the factors which reduce the precision of the method are: the nerves traverse the intertransverse spaces obliquely; in some ani-

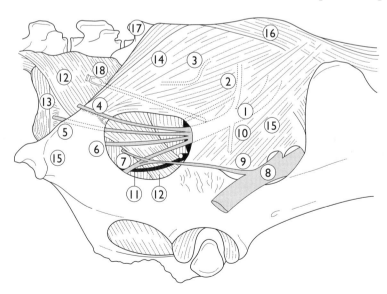

FIG. 12.7 Pudendal nerve block. Lateral view of the pelvis with the sacrosciatic ligament removed to show distribution of the sacral spinal nerves. 1: Pudic nerve; 2: middle haemorrhoidal nerve; 3: caudal haemorrhoidal nerve; 4, 5: proximal and distal cutaneous branches of pudic nerve; 6: deep perineal nerve; 7: nerve that becomes the dorsal nerve of the penis; 8: sciatic nerve; 9: branch connecting sciatic nerve with branch of pudic nerve 7; 10: pelvic nerve; 11: internal pudic artery; 12: coccygeus muscle; 13: external anal sphincter; 14: sacrosciatic ligament; 15: tuber ischii; 16: sacrum; 17: first coccygeal vertebra; 18: needle in position.

mals the nerve roots are double, emerging from double foramina; it is difficult to ensure that the site of injection is the same as that assessed from the body surface; penetration of the muscular mass of the back tends to cause spasmodic contraction of the muscles with consequent modification of the needle track. Precise location of the injection sites is also more difficult in the newer large breeds of cattle.

Pudic (internal pudendal) block

While epidural block is a reliable means of provoking exposure of the penis in the bull, it must be acknowledged that the method also has disadvantages, particularly in heavier individuals. The chief of these is that the volume of analgesic solution required to cause complete exposure may result in severe interference with the motor power of the hindlimbs, and in order to prevent injury to the limbs and pelvis it becomes necessary to keep the animal cast and restrained for several hours. But prolonged recumbency in a heavy bull, often associated with struggling, may result in injury elsewhere. A most useful alternative to produce analgesia of the penis for examination and surgical procedures is a bilateral pudic (internal pudendal) block.

The pudic (internal pudendal) nerve consists of fibres arising from the ventral branches of the third and fourth sacral nerves. It passes ventrally and caudally on the medial surface of the sacrosciatic ligament, where it is associated with the middle haemorrhoidal nerve, to cross the lesser sacrosciatic foramen where it is accompanied by the internal pudic vessels; they then pass along the floor of the pelvis to the ischial arch supplying motor fibres to the urethra and the erector and retractor muscles of the penis, the middle haemorrhoidal nerve and sensory fibres to the skin on either side of the midline from the anus to the scrotum. Between the sacrosciatic ligament and the rectum in the region of surgical approach to the nerve lies the sheet-like coccygeal muscle. The pudic nerve lies between the ligament and the muscle, while the accompanying middle haemorrhoidal nerve lies deep to the muscle, that is between it and the rectal wall. The lesser sacrosciatic foramen is closed by a sheet of fascia which is an extension of

the fascia of the coccygeal muscle. In addition to the pudic and middle haemorrhoidal nerves some fibres which enter into the dorsal nerve of the penis are obtained from a branch of the sciatic nerve which, leaving the parent nerve on the outer aspect of the sacrosciatic ligament, passes into the lesser sacrosciatic foramen and anastomoses with the ventral branch of the pudic nerve where that lies immediately above the internal pudic vessels close to the ventral border of the foramen (Fig. 12.7).

The pudic nerve is located per rectum, the hand being introduced as far as the wrist and the fingers directed laterally and ventrally to detect the lesser sacrosciatic foramen. Its outline is not clearly identifiable, but its position is recognized by the softness and depressability of the pelvic wall at this point. Moreover, the internal pudic artery which can readily be detected running along the lateroventral aspect of the pelvic cavity passes out of the pelvis at the cranial part of the foramen. Care should be taken not to advance the hand too far, for on entering the rectum the foramen lies immediately ventrolateral to the fingers. The nerve can readily be felt, the size of a straw, lying on the sacrosciatic ligament immediately rostral and dorsal to the foramen.

The site of insertion of the needle is at the point of deepest depression of the ischiorectal fossa and it is directed rostral and slightly ventral in direction. During the whole procedure a hand is kept in the rectum. When the needle has penetrated to a depth of 5–7 cm, it will be palpable through the rectal wall and its point should be directed to the position of the nerve a little rostral to the foramen. Here some 20–25 ml of 2% lignocaine hydrochloride (or its equivalent) is injected. A further 10–15 ml is injected a little caudal and dorsal to this point to block also the middle haemorrhoidal nerve which may carry some sympathetic fibres to the penis. A third injection should be made after redirecting the needle a little ventrally just inside the lesser sciatic foramen where the ventral branch of the pudic nerve can be palpated distal to its anastomosis with sciatic nerve branches. The onset of adequate exposure of the penis is delayed for a period of 30–45 min after injection of the nerves.

Another approach to pudendal nerve block is a lateral one. One injection is made over the pudendal nerve just as it passes medial to the dorsorostral quadrant of the lesser sciatic foramen and a second injection is performed between the posterior haemorrhoidal and pudendal nerves. This latter injection necessitates penetration of the sacrosciatic ligament. The site of insertion of the needle is determined by using the cranial tuberosity of the tuber ischii as a fixed point and the length of the sacrotuberous ligament as a radius. The distance is used to establish the site on a line drawn parallel to the midline anterior to the fixed point. After clipping, cleaning and disinfecting the skin the site is marked by the s.c. injection of 2 ml of 2% lignocaine or equivalent drug solution. This injection makes subsequent manipulations less painful and renders the subject more amenable to handling. Either hand is then introduced into the rectum and the lesser sciatic foramen located. A 12 cm long, 1.8 mm bore needle is introduced through the skin site and directed towards the middle finger held in the foramen until it can be felt to lie alongside the nerve. About 10 ml of the local analgesic solution is injected at this point. The needle is withdrawn 4–5 cm and redirected caudally and dorsally so that it penetrates the sacrosciatic ligament at a point about 2.5 cm above and behind the first site of injection. About 5 ml of solution is injected at this point, the needle is withdrawn and the sites massaged to spread the solution in the tissues. Similar injections are carried out on the other side of the animal.

Local analgesia for castration

For castration the site of the proposed incision in the scrotum may be desensitized by the s.c. infiltration of local analgesic solution but this does not, of course, block the nerve fibres running in the spermatic cord. These fibres can be blocked by the direct injection of 5–10 ml of local analgesic solution into each cord at the neck of the scrotum or by injecting 5–25 ml (depending on the size of the animal) into the substance of each testicle. In the latter method the drug is assumed to pass out from the testicle along the lymph vessels and to block, after diffusion, the nerve fibres present in the cord. The bulk of the drug is carried on in the lymph to enter the blood stream and for this reason excessive dosage must be avoided or intoxication will occur.

For the closed or bloodless (Burdizzo) castration the skin of the neck of the scrotum must be infiltrated by s.c. injection and the spermatic cord itself is also infiltrated at the same site. About 10–20 ml of 2% lignocaine is a suitable dose on each side.

Caudal epidural analgesia

The spinal cord ends in the region of the last lumbar vertebra but the meningeal sac is continued as far as the junction of the 3rd and 4th sacral segments. The diameter of the neural canal as it passes through the sacrum is approximately 1.8 cm in the caudal part and 2 cm in the cranial. In the lumbar regions the dimensions of the canal are much greater, its width at the last segment being 4 cm. This helps to explain why paralysis of the spinal nerves as far forward as the first sacral is effected with comparatively small quantities of local analgesic solution (20 ml), whereas paralysis of the cranial lumbar nerves necessitates the injection of much larger quantities (100 ml).

Caudal epidural block is performed by insertion of the needle between the 1st and 2nd coccygeal vertebrae, i.e. beyond the termination of the spinal cord and its meninges (Fig. 12.8). This site is larger and more easily penetrated and, in some animals, more easily located than the sacrococcygeal space. One or more of the following methods may be used:

1. The tail is gripped about 15 cm from its base and raised 'pump-handle' fashion. The first obvious articulation behind the sacrum is the first intercoccygeal space.

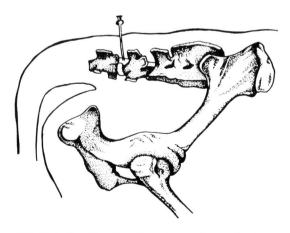

FIG. 12.8 Caudal epidural injection made into the first intercoccygeal space.

2. Standing on one side of the animal and observing the line of the croup, the prominence of the sacrum is seen. Moving the eye back towards the tail, the next prominence to be observed is the spine of the first coccygeal bone. The site is the depression immediately behind it.

3. The caudal prominence of the tuberosity of the ischium is palpated and the point selected 10–11 cm in front of it. A line drawn directly over the back from this point passes, in a medium-sized animal, through the depression between the first and second coccygeal spines.

The dimensions of the opening in the dorsal wall of the neural canal are approximately 2 cm transversely, 2.5 cm craniocaudally and about 0.5 cm in depth.

The canal is occupied by six caudal nerves, together with a vein on each side. The aperture between the two vertebral arches is closed by the interarcual ligament and the space between the spines occupied by connective tissue. Surmounting the spines is a variable amount of fat covered by skin. The floor comprises, about the centre of the space, the intervertebral cartilaginous disc and, in front and behind this, the surface of the vertebral centrum.

An insensitive skin weal is made with the object of preventing movement during insertion of the injection needle and thus ensuring that the latter is introduced in the correct position and direction. For insertion of the epidural needle the tail is allowed to hang naturally. The point of the needle is applied to the centre of the depression between the 1st and 2nd coccygeal spines, taking care that it is precisely in the midline. The needle is advanced ventrally and cranially at an angle of 15° with the vertical, until its point impinges on the floor of the canal. Often, contact with a caudal nerve causes the animal to move suddenly, and the anaesthetist should be prepared for this.

Provided the needle has been correctly introduced there is usually no doubt but that it has entered the epidural space. Sometimes, however, the point of the needle will tranverse the space and penetrate the intervertebral disc. This is detected, on attaching the syringe and attempting to inject solution, by a great resistance offered to the syringe plunger. Should this error occur, the needle should be slightly withdrawn, the syringe re-applied and injection attempted. When the point of the needle is correctly placed in the neural canal there is, for all practicable purposes, no resistance and injection can be made quite easily. Sometimes blood issues from the needle due to penetration of a vein but experience indicates that injection can still be injected without harm. If thought preferable the needle can be withdrawn, cleansed of blood clot and reintroduced.

The rate of injection should be rather slow, a volume of 15 ml being given over 10–15 seconds; 2% lignocaine hydrochloride is now almost universally used but the duration of block can, if needed be increased by using 0.5% bupivacaine.

Production of caudal block means that motor control of the hindlimbs is uninfluenced. When 2% solutions of lignocaine are used the total dose lies between 5 and 10 ml depending on the size of the animal. Provided that the concentration of the solution used is sufficient to paralyse the sensory fibres, skin analgesia will develop in the tail and croup as far as the mid-sacral region, the anus, vulva and perineum and the posterior aspect of the thighs. Paralysis of motor fibres will cause the anal sphincter to relax and the posterior part of the rectum to balloon. Defaecation will be suspended, stretching of the vulva will produce no response and the vagina will dilate. During parturition straining ceases but uterine contractions are uninfluenced.

The onset of muscular paralysis of the tail occurs from 60–90s after injection and affords reliable evidence that the injection has been made correctly. When lignocaine is used analgesia attains its maximum extent over 5–10 min, and persists for about an hour after which there is progressive recovery. The block completely disappears by the end of the second hour from the time of injection.

The introduction of caudal epidural analgesia was immediately followed by its use as a means of causing relaxation and exposure of the penis in bulls. For this, a minimum dose should be given, the epidural needle left in place and if extrusion of the penis does not occur after the elapse of an appropriate length of time additional small doses can be given until it does. The dose necessary for penile extrusion is very close to that causing some degree of motor incoordination of the hind limbs.

As yet, there is no way of determining the effective dose in relation to weight or other measurements and it is necessary to wait for at least 25 min before concluding that the dose administered was inadequate. For this particular purpose caudal block has, nowadays, been replaced to a large extent by pudic nerve block, sympathetic blockade or by the use of tranquillizers such as acepromazine, or the α_2 adrenoceptor agonists.

Many other drugs are now commonly administered into the epidural space at the caudal site. Xylazine, 0.05 mg/kg diluted to 5 ml in 0.9% saline, is used to provide analgesia of the perineum and to reduce straining during parturition. Xylazine will induce bilateral analgesia of dermatomes supplied by the caudal, caudal rectal, perineal, pudendal, and caudal cutaneous femoral nerves (StJean *et al.*, 1990). Analgesia develops by 20 min after administration and persists for 2 h. The tail will be flaccid and mild ataxia may be present. Sufficient xylazine is absorbed to induce mild sedation, decreased ruminal motility (bloat), bradycardia and decreased MAP. These side effects may have a significantly adverse effect in sick animals. A slightly higher dose of xylazine, 0.07 mg/kg in 7.5 ml of 0.9% saline, has been used by caudal epidural injection to provide analgesia for castration in mature bulls (Caulkett *et al.*, 1993). Sedation was evident in these animals and moderate ataxia, with recumbency, was observed in 14%. Surgery was performed 30 minutes after injection and surgical analgesia was judged to be good in 81% of animals but pain or discomfort during emasculation was apparent in the remaining bulls.

Medetomidine, 0.015 mg/kg diluted with 0.9% saline to a volume of 5 ml, has been evaluated for epidural analgesia in cows (Lin *et al.*, 1998). Results of this investigation showed that medetomidine induced analgesia within 10 minutes and lasted 412 ± 156 min (mean $\pm$ SD) – significantly longer than lignocaine, 0.2 mg/kg, which lasted 10 to 115 min (mean 43 ± 37 min). Systemic effects of absorbed medetomidine included mild to moderate sedation and mild ataxia.

Lumbosacral epidural analgesia

Injection of local analgesic solutions in the caudal region affords a method of inducing epidural anal-gesia, but when lumbar epidural block is required it is not always possible to produce satisfactory cranial spread from the caudal injection site. Consequently, some make the injection at the lumbosacral foramen although needles introduced here may enter the subarachnoid space and once this has been done it is no longer really safe to proceed with the induction of an epidural block until the puncture in the dural has become sealed. The patency of the hole in the dura persists for several hours and if an immediate spinal block is essential, a deliberate, controlled subarachnoid block must be performed. However, a subarachnoid block can only be managed in relatively small animals, where full use can be made of gravity to control the extent of neural blockade, so injection at the lumbosacral foramen is normally only employed in sheep, goats, small pigs and dogs.

Injection into the epidural space in the lumbar region can be employed to produce analgesia of a number of body segments in cattle. By careful control of the dose of local analgesic injected it is possible to produce a belt of analgesia around the animal's trunk without interfering with control of the hind limbs. Although not easy to perform, in expert hands it can be most effective.

With the animal standing, the site for insertion of the needle is just to the right of the lumbar spinous process on a line 1.5 cm behind the cranial edge of the 2nd lumbar transverse process. An initial skin weal is produced using a fine needle and a longitudinal skin incision some 2–3 cm is made to facilitate penetration by the spinal needle. The spinal needle (14 gauge, 12 cm long) is directed ventrally and medially at an angle of 10–13 ° with the vertical for a distance of 7.5 cm – at which point the needle enters the neural canal. Even when small quantities of local analgesic are injected along the track of the needle, penetration of the interarcual ligament is apparently painful and thus the animal needs adequate restraint. The intervertebral space through which the needle must pass to enter the epidural space is actually an interosseous canal formed by the bases of the spinous processes cranially and caudally and by the intervertebral articular processes laterally. Immediately the needle is felt to penetrate the interarcual ligament the stilette is withdrawn and if air is heard to enter the needle it is certain that the epidural space has been entered. Alternatively, in the absence of air aspiration and if no fluid flows from the needle, a trial injection is made. If the needle is correctly placed in the epidural space scarcely any pressure on the syringe plunger is needed. If on removing the stilette, cerebrospinal fluid flows from the needle, the latter must be quickly but gently withdrawn until the flow ceases and then injection made (Fig. 12.9).

The cardiovascular response to segmental block (T13–L1) is associated with a reduction in MAP, and an increase in CO due to an increase in HR in response to decreased vascular resistance. These changes appear to be of no clinical significance and

it seems generally agreed that the sympathetic blockade caused by segmental epidural injection is well tolerated by non-sedated healthy cows.

Digital nerve blocks

The nerve supply of the digits of cattle is more complex than in the horse and regional analgesia is more difficult to produce. The skin below the carpus and tarsus is tense and the subcutaneous tissue fibrous, so that precise location of the nerves is not easy.

Analgesia may be produced in the forelimb by injection at the sites indicated in Fig. 12.10. The

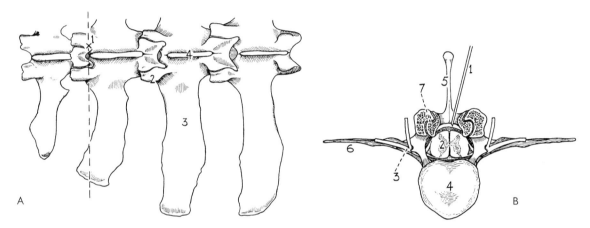

FIG. 12.9 Segmental epidural block. **A** First four lumbar vertebrae viewed from above. 1: Point of insertion of spinal needle through skin; 2: articular process; 3: transverse process; 4: spinous processes. **B** Transverse section through the joints between the articular processes of the 1st and 2nd lumbar vertebrae. The body of the 1st lumbar segment is viewed from its caudal aspect. 1: Needle in position; 2: spinal cord surrounded by meninges; 3: left 1st lumbar nerve; 4: body of 1st lumbar vertebra; 5: spinous process; 6: transverse process; 7: sectioned interlocking articular processes.

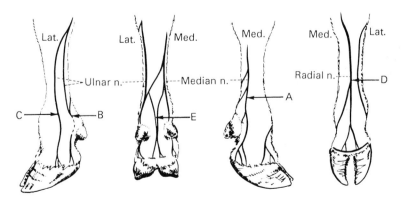

FIG. 12.10 Nerve block of the forelimb. To block the whole digit, injections must be made at A, B, C, D and E. To block the medial digit, inject at A, D and E. To block the lateral digit, inject at points B, C, D and E.

dorsal metacarpal nerve is located by palpation at about the middle of the metacarpus, medial to the extensor tendon. The dorsal branch of the ulnar nerve is blocked about 5 cm above the fetlock on the lateral aspect of the limb, in the groove between the suspensory ligament and the metacarpal bone. At this point, the palmar branch of the ulnar nerve may also be blocked, the two nerves being respectively situated in front of, and behind the suspensory ligament. The axial palmar aspect of the digits may be rendered analgesic by an injection in the midline just above the fetlock. The injection will reach the lateral branch of the median nerve before it divides, or if it has already divided its two branches will still be close to each other. The two branches may also be simultaneously blocked on the midline just below the level of the dew claws, i.e. after they have passed from below the fibrous plate of the dew claws. The medial branch of the median nerve is blocked on the medial side of the limb in the groove between the suspensory ligament and the flexor tendons about 5 cm above the fetlock. Blocking the median nerve higher up the limb before it divides is not practical as at this point the nerve lies beneath the artery and vein.

An alternative technique that is less precise is to perform a ring block of the limb with local anaesthetic solution in an attempt to block all nerve branches at the same level.

The hindlimb can be blocked to provide loss of sensation below the hock. The peroneal nerve is blocked immediately behind the caudal edge of the lateral condyle of the tibia, over the fibula. The nerve is blocked before it dips down between the extensor pedis and flexor metatarsi muscles to divide into the deep and superficial peroneal nerves. The bony prominence can easily be palpated in most animals, and in some, the nerve itself can be rolled against the bone as it passes superficially, obliquely downwards and cranially, at this point. An 18 or 20 gauge, 2.5 cm, needle is inserted through the skin, the subcutaneous tissue and the aponeurotic sheet of the biceps femoris until its point just touches the bony landmark. Lignocaine, approximately 20 ml of 2% for an adult, is injected at this point. Onset of analgesia is in 20 minutes.

The tibial nerve is blocked about 10–12 cm above the summit of the calcaneous on the medial

aspect of the limb, just in front of the gastrocnemius tendon. The gastrocnemius tendon is grasped between the thumb and index finger of one hand while a needle, about 2.5 cm long, is inserted immediately below the thumb until its point can be felt just under the skin by the index finger. About 15 ml of local analgesia solution is injected at this site. A further 5 ml of solution should be injected on the medial side of the leg to block a small cutaneous nerve. The block takes 15 minutes to develop.

An alternative method for desensitization of the hindlimb below the fetlock involves blocking the superficial and deep peroneal nerves separately. The superficial peroneal nerve is blocked in the upper third of the metatarsus where it lies subcutaneously over the midline of the dorsal aspect of the metatarsal bone (Fig. 12.11). The deep peroneal nerve accompanies the dorsal metatarsal vessels in a groove on the cranial aspect of the metatarsal bone under cover of the extensor tendons. Injection is made halfway between the hock and the fetlock. The needle is inserted from the lateral aspect of the bone and the point directed beneath the edge of the tendon.

The plantar metatarsal nerves are blocked on the medial and lateral sides of the limb in the depression between the suspensory ligament and

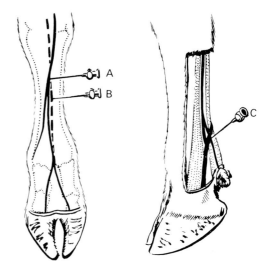

FIG. 12.11 Nerve block of the distal part of the hindlimb. **A:** injection of the superficial peroneal nerve. **B:** injection of the deep peroneal nerve. **C:** injection of the plantar metatarsal nerves.

the flexor tendons, about 5 cm proximal to the fetlock joint and deep to the superficial fascia (Fig. 12.11). Five ml of local analgesia solution is injected over each nerve.

INTRAVENOUS REGIONAL ANALGESIA

Intravenous regional analgesia (IVRA) is a simple and commonly used technique to provide analgesia of the limb or digits. It is achieved by injecting local analgesic solution into a superficial vein in a limb isolated from the general circulation by a tourniquet. The limb distal to the site of application of the tourniquet becomes analgesic and remains so until the tourniquet is released.

The animal is restrained in lateral recumbency, with or without sedation. The hair over a prominent vein on the relevant limb is clipped and the skin prepared for injection (Fig. 12.12). A tourniquet of stout rubber tubing or a wide flat rubber band is applied above the carpus or hock, or above the fetlock, to occlude arterial blood flow. The flat

tourniquet is preferable as it appears to cause the animals less discomfort than rubber tubing; consequently, they are less likely to be restless. When the tourniquet is to be placed on the hind limb above the hock in an adult animal, rolls of bandage should be placed either side of the limb beneath the tourniquet in the depression between the tibia and the gastrocnemius tendon to ensure occlusion of all blood vessels (Fig. 12.12). A 19 gauge needle or butterfly needle is inserted into a vein with its point towards the foot. If the limb is to be exsanguinated by application of an Esmarch bandage, the vein may be difficult to locate after application of the bandage; the needle should be placed first and kept patent with heparin-saline solution. In adult cattle, 30 ml of 2% lignocaine (without adrenaline) is injected into the vein after first aspirating blood to confirm location of the needle within the lumen of the vessel. Some veterinarians may follow that injection with saline to encourage spread of the local anaesthetic through the limb. Analgesia distal to the tourniquet will develop in 15–20 minutes and persist until the tourniquet is removed. Provided that 10 minutes or more have elapsed since the injection, no adverse effect from the local analgesic solution should be observed when the tourniquet is removed. Analgesia dissipates very rapidly in almost all animals.

Occasionally, the foot is analgesic everywhere except for the skin between the digits. This can be blocked by injection of 5 ml of 2% lignocaine midline on the dorsal aspect of the fetlock and a further 5 ml of solution on the caudal aspect of the fetlock between the dew claws.

The duration of analgesia is limited only by the time it is considered safe to leave a tourniquet in place. Intravenous regional analgesia is safe for up to at least 1.5 hours and this is long enough for most procedures done on the bovine foot.

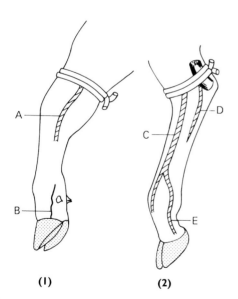

(1)   **(2)**

FIG. 12.12 Easily recognized veins of the distal parts of limbs that can be used in placing needles or cannulae for intravenous regional analgesia. (**1**) Medial view of the right foreleg. A: radial vein; B: medial palmar digital vein. (**2**) Lateral view of the right hindleg. C: lateral branch of lateral saphenous vein; D: lateral plantar vein; E: lateral plantar digital vein.

GENERAL ANAESTHESIA

Clearly, choice of technique depends in large part on the circumstances surrounding the need for sedation or anaesthesia. For example, management of a dairy cow for caesarian section is different from management of a beef or feedlot heifer that has not been handled. Sedating a bull for a foot trim or radiographs may be more difficult when done on the farm than when performed in the clinic.

Regurgitation during anaesthesia is a real hazard with potential consequence of pulmonary aspiration of ruminal fluid and material, asphyxia, pulmonary abscesses, or pneumonia. Food is customarily withheld from cattle older than 3 months of age before elective anaesthesia for 36 (24–48) hours, water for 8–12 hours, to decrease the volume of the rumen contents. This reduction in gastrointestinal volume has an added benefit of improving oxygenation during recumbency. Animals less than 2 months of age are likely to develop hypoglycaemia if food and milk are withheld for several hours. One recommendation is to prevent the calves from eating solid food for several hours and to withhold milk or milk replacer for 30 to 60 minutes before anaesthesia.

Choice of drugs may be influenced by current legislature concerning use of anaesthetic agents in food-producing animals. In this chapter information on the pharmacological effects of various agents and their combinations is given in order that informed decisions can be made about their use in all situations. Some of the anaesthetic agents mentioned may be unsuitable in some countries for use in animals for subsequent slaughter because of presumed persistence of drug residues.

ANAESTHETIC TECHNIQUES

Anaesthesia can be induced in the standing animal with only one assistant holding the head during injection, or the cow or bull can be first cast with ropes or strapped to a tilting table and anaesthetized in standing or lateral position. There is a clinically obvious difference in response to anaesthetic drugs between *Bos taurus* breeds and breeds crossed with *Bos indicus*. Dairy breeds in particular are relatively tolerant of the effects of anaesthesia. Breeds such as the Beefmaster, Santa Gertrudis, and Brahman often require a much lower dose of anaesthetic agents.

Premedication is not essential prior to injection of thiopental or thiopental-guaiphenesin. Administration of acepromazine or xylazine will decrease the dose rate of induction drug, alter the cardiovascular parameters, and slow recovery from anaesthesia. Premedication with xylazine or

TABLE 12.1 Drug combinations used in cattle anaesthesia

Drugs	Dose	Comments
Thiopental	11 mg/kg i.v.	Premedication decreases dose rate
Guaiphenesin 5% + Thiopental	50–100 mg/kg i.v. + 3–4 mg/kg	Dose rate decreases > 600 kg bodyweight; premedication decreases dose rate
Xylazine + Ketamine	0.1–0.2 mg/kg/ i.m. or i.v. + 2 mg/kg i.v.	15–20 min duration; prolong with 1 g ketamine in 1 litre 5% guaiphenesin at 1.5–2.0 ml/kg/h
Xylazine 100 mg/litre + Guaiphenesin 50 g/litre + Ketamine 1 g/litre	Infuse 1–2 ml/kg of the mixture i.v.	

medetomidine is usual prior to anaesthesia with ketamine, except in young calves in which anaesthesia can be induced with diazepam-ketamine.

Intravenous injection

Use of an indwelling catheter is preferable to avoid perivascular injection of irritant drugs, such as thiopental or guaiphenesin, and to facilitate supplemental injections. A 14 gauge, 13 cm long catheter is suitable for insertion in the jugular vein, although a 10 gauge catheter is better for administration of guaiphenesin solutions in bulls. The skin of bulls may be 0.5–1.0 cm thick over the jugular vein and insertion of the catheter is easier through a small incision made with a scalpel blade through an intradermal bleb of local analgesic (usually lignocaine).

Endotracheal intubation

There are a variety of techniques that can be used to facilitate endotracheal intubation in adult cattle. In cattle up to about 300 kg, intubation can be accomplished under direct vision of the larynx

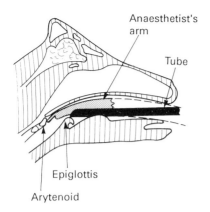

Anaesthetist's arm

Tube

Epiglottis

Arytenoid

FIG. 12.13 Intubation by palpation.

using a laryngoscope with a blade suitable for intubating a large dog. The animal is supported in sternal position, the head and neck extended, and the laryngoscope positioned at the corner of the animal's mouth with the tip of the blade on the dorsum of the tongue. The trachea is intubated with an endotracheal tube of 11–18 or 20 mm internal diameter (ID), with a technique similar to that used in dogs. Care must be taken in smaller calves not to use the blade of the laryngoscope as a lever with the incisor teeth acting as a fulcrum.

In large bovine animals, a longer laryngoscope blade will be needed to view the laryngeal opening. A stiff stomach tube or a 2 m metal rod with a blunted end is passed through the mouth and into the trachea. The laryngoscope is withdrawn and the endotracheal tube is fed over the tube or rod and into the trachea, whereupon the tube or rod is removed. One problem is that the tube may catch on the epiglottis unless it is rotated at the appropriate moment.

Intubation by palpation is a technique commonly employed for cows and bulls. The mouth of the anaesthetized animal must be held open securely using a wedge-shaped gag inserted between the molar teeth or any other gag suitable for ruminants. A 25 mm or 30 mm ID endotracheal tube is used for adult cattle. The anaesthetist grasps the end of the endotracheal tube and inserts the arm and tube into the cow's mouth, taking care to remain midline so that the endotracheal tube cuff does not brush against the sharp edges of the molar teeth and tear (Fig. 12.13). The forefinger is used to depress the epiglottis and the

free hand is used to advance the endotracheal tube onto the epiglottis. The arm inside the mouth is then advanced a further 5 cm and the forefinger and middle finger are used to spread the arytenoids and open the larynx. The free hand is used to advance the endotracheal tube into the larynx and trachea. If the endotracheal tube catches at the entrance of the larynx, the forefinger should be swept around the tube to free it for insertion. The anaesthetist's arm is removed and the endotracheal tube inserted its full length. The endotracheal tube cuff should be inflated immediately and the tube secured with gauze to the speculum, the halter, or by lengths of gauze around the head or horns. When there is insufficient room for both the anaesthetist's arm and the endotracheal tube, a stomach tube or metal rod can be inserted in a manner just described and then the endotracheal tube fed over the tube or rod and into the trachea after removal of the anaesthetist's arm.

Endotracheal tubes may be passed 'blind' by the anaesthetist gripping the larynx with one hand and feeding the endotracheal tube into the larynx with the other hand. This is not an easy technique but the success rate of this technique increases with practice.

The lubricant applied to any endotracheal tube used in ruminant animals should never contain a local analgesic drug for if it does the mucous membrane of the trachea and larynx may remain desensitized for some time after the tube is withdrawn. The protective cough reflex will then be absent and foreign material may be inhaled into the bronchial tree.

INJECTABLE ANAESTHETIC AGENTS

Thiopental

Thiopental may be used in adult cattle either alone to provide full anaesthesia for operations of short duration or to induce anaesthesia that is then maintained by inhalation agents. In the unpremedicated animal thiopental, 5% or 10% solution, is injected rapidly into the jugular vein in a dose of 11 mg/kg estimated body weight; if xylazine premedication has been used a dose of 5–6 mg/kg is usually adequate. The animal sinks quietly to the ground within 20–30 seconds of injection and there is a brief period of apnoea. Apnoea seldom lasts for more than 15–20 seconds and artificial respiration is not required. Surgical anaesthesia of about 10 minutes is followed by recovery which is complete within 45 minutes. Recovery is usually quiet and free from excitement. The animal can be propped up, and will maintain a position of sternal recumbency, about 12–15 min after injection of the drug. The period of surgical anaesthesia is brief but adequate for operations of very short duration or for endotracheal intubation prior to maintenance of anaesthesia with an inhalation agent.

Apart from the usual risks of anaesthesia in ruminant animals the method is safe in healthy cattle. Overdosage may occur when there is a gross error in estimation of body weight. Underdosage is more frequent and the animal may remain standing, but excitement does not occur. Failure to induce anaesthesia may be the result of the injection being made too slowly or because of perivascular injection. Additional thiopental may be injected i.v. immediately to achieve anaesthesia provided that i.v. access can be guaranteed. Perivascular injection should be treated by infiltration of the area with 1–2 mg/kg of 2% lignocaine and several hundred ml of 0.9% saline in an attempt to avoid tissue necrosis and abscesses.

Thiopental should not be administered by this rapid injection technique to sick animals or animals with compromized cardiovascular function. Young calves up to 2.5 months of age are not good subjects for thiopental anaesthesia and the use of even small doses for induction of anaesthesia cannot be recommended.

Thiopental-guaiphenesin

Approximately 80–100 mg/kg of 5% guaiphenesin on it own is needed to produce recumbency in cattle. If pain-producing procedures are to follow, a combination of guaiphenesin and thiopental should always be used (50 g of guaiphenesin to 2 g thiopental sodium). The mixture is run rapidly into a catheterized vein (perivascular injection will cause tissue necrosis and sloughing) to produce the desired effect; the prior use of xylazine greatly diminishes the necessary quantity of the combination necessary. Administration of the mixture results in a decrease in respiratory tidal volume and

ABP, and an increase in respiratory and heart rates.

The dose rate in unpremedicated cattle up to 500 kg is approximately 2 ml/kg and this rate decreases substantially on a mg/kg basis, with even large bulls seldom requiring more than 1500 ml of the mixture for anaesthesia adequate for endotracheal intubation. Administration of xylazine premedication greatly reduces the dose rate required for anaesthesia.

The drugs may also be administered separately, in which case, guaiphenesin is first infused i.v. at 50 mg/kg followed by a bolus injection of 3–4 mg/kg of thiopental.

Methohexital

Because recovery after methohexital (methohexitone) is so much more rapid than it is after thiopental, it might appear to be the better of the two compounds for use in cattle. However, the action of methohexitone is, for unknown reasons, rather unpredictable and the rapid i.v. injection of a computed dose cannot be recommended. Given to adult cows by slow i.v. injection, assessing the effects produced as injection proceeds, the agent has proved to be quite satisfactory although muscle tremors occur as unconsciousness supervenes. These muscle tremors appear to have no clinical significance.

Methohexital appears to produce better conditions for endotracheal intubation than are produced by thiopental. The jaw is more relaxed for a given degree of unconsciousness and the laryngeal and cough mechanisms appear to be less active. Recovery from methohexital anaesthesia is smooth and extremely rapid but occasionally it is accompanied by a return of the muscle tremors seen during induction of anaesthesia.

Doses of 1 mg/kg by rapid i.v. injection are sufficient to enable endotracheal intubation to be carried out in young calves and can be used for castration of calves whose ages range from 6 weeks to 10 months.

Pentobarbital

Toosey (1959) found that 1.9–3.8 mg/kg of i.v. pentobarbital produced sedation in adult animals which remained standing, but swaying, on their feet. Thirty years later, Valverde *et al.* (1989) confirmed that 2 mg/kg i.v. produces reliable sedation in standing adult cattle. These doses produce moderate sedation for 30 min and mild sedation for a further 30 min. Respiratory rate is significantly decreased but no changes have been measured in arterial blood gases.

Full general anaesthesia may be induced in small bovine animals by the slow i.v. injection of pentobarbital, taking some 4 min over the injection. Induction is quiet and the dose for the production of light anaesthesia varies from 1.00 to 1.45 g/50 kg. Surgical anaesthesia persists for about 30 min and is followed by slow recovery taking up to 3 h before the animal can regain its feet. For the very young calf – animals up to 1 month old – pentobarbital is quite unsuitable. In these young animals unconsciousness lightens slowly over more than 2 days and there is a grave danger that during this period the animal will succumb from pulmonary oedema, or that it may subsequently develop pneumonia.

Ketamine

Ketamine alone will not cause seizures in cattle but the quality of anaesthesia obtained by it is poor. Premedication with xylazine produces quiet, smooth induction of anaesthesia with good muscle relaxation and a smooth recovery from anaesthesia. In young calves, premedication with xylazine may be substituted with diazepam or acepromazine, with or without butorphanol. The dose rate of ketamine is usually higher in calves than in mature animals.

Xylazine is given to adult cattle either i.m. at 0.1–0.2 mg/kg or i.v. at 0.05–0.10 mg/kg to produce deep sedation, often with recumbency. Ketamine is then given i.v. in doses of 2 mg/kg to induce anaesthesia. Often, endotracheal intubation can be performed soon after the xylazine injection and before ketamine is given and whenever possible this should be done, for ketamine appears to produce copious salivation or an inability to swallow the normal saliva volume. The duration of anaesthesia is about 15 min.

In smaller animals of about 200–350 kg body weight, xylazine, 0.1–0.2 mg/kg, is given intramuscularly 5–8 min before ketamine at either 6 mg/kg by intramuscular injection or 4 mg/kg by

intravenous injection. In calves, xylazine, 0.1 mg/kg, and ketamine, 10 mg/kg, can be given intramuscularly at the same time, or ketamine may be administered after a few minutes intravenously at 4–6 mg/kg. Intramuscular administration of xylazine and ketamine will provide 25–30 min of anaesthesia. Anaesthesia can be maintained after any of these combinations by intermittent injections or infusion of guaiphensin-ketamine, 1 gram of ketamine in 1 litre of 5% guaiphenesin, or by inhalation agents.

The combination of diazepam and ketamine will produce less cardiovascular depression in calves than xylazine and ketamine. Diazepam, 0.2 mg/kg, and ketamine, 5 mg/kg, can be combined and injected intravenously as a bolus or in increments to achieve the desired effect. This combination will provide about 15 min of anaesthesia. Butorphanol, 0.1–0.2 mg/kg, can be included with this combination to increase analgesia and muscle relaxation. Anaesthesia may be prolonged by intermittent injections of diazepam and ketamine, or by inhalation agents.

Medetomidine, 0.02 mg/kg, and ketamine, 0.5 mg/kg, given together intravenously is a combination that has been described to produce deep sedation lasting 30 min in calves that could be combined with local analgesia for surgery (Raekallio *et al.*, 1991). As might be expected, hypoxaemia developed in the calves in dorsal recumbency. Administration of atipamezole, 20–60 μg/kg, produced a rapid smooth recovery. It should be noted that in another study of medetomidine sedation in calves, injection of antipamezole, 200 μg/kg, to reverse sedation induced transient severe hypotension and even sinus arrest (Ranheim *et al.*, 1998). Therefore, reversal agents should be given cautiously while monitoring the patient closely. Relapse of sedation may occur 90 minutes later.

Ketamine-guaiphenesin

A similar technique to that for thiopental/guaiphenesin employs a mixture of 1 g of ketamine mixed with 50 g of guaiphenesin, infused i.v. to effect.

Anaesthesia can also be induced and maintained by i.v. infusion of xylazine, guaiphenesin and ketamine. Xylazine, 100 mg and ketamine 1000 mg are added to 1 litre of 5% guaiphenesin and the mixture infused i.v. at 1–2 ml/kg. Alternatively, after induction of anaesthesia with xylazine and ketamine anaesthesia can be maintained by intermittent or continuous infusion of a mixture of guaiphenesin-ketamine (1000 mg ketamine added to 1 litre of 5% guaiphenesin) at approximately 2 ml/kg /h – there is no need to add xylazine to the maintenance anaesthetic combination because in cattle the half life of xylazine is longer than ketamine. When anaesthesia is prolonged supplementation with O_2 is advisable.

Propofol

It would seem because of rapid and complete recovery, irrespective of the duration of anaesthesia, that propofol should be the ideal agent for general anaesthesia in cattle. However, there are very few reports of its use in these animals, probably due to cost making its use impractical in adults. In calves inhalation anaesthesia is easily managed and much less expensive so that there has been little incentive to use an expensive i.v. agent.

Personal experience (LWH) has been that one i.v. injection of propofol (5–6 mg/kg) provides, in non-premedicated calves up to 3 months of age, perfectly acceptable general anaesthesia of 4–9 min duration, with a smooth, excitement-free awakening. Further work to establish the dose–response to propofol alone, and after α_2 adrenoceptors agonists is needed.

Tiletamine-zolazepam

The combination of tiletamine-zolazepam, 4 mg/kg, and xylazine, 0.1 mg/kg, injected i.m. in sequence produced anaesthesia within minutes in calves (Thurmon *et al.*, 1989). Analgesia lasted on average 70 min and the calves were able to walk in 130 ± 18 min from the time of the last injection. When higher doses of xylazine were used in another group of calves some became apnoeic. Although not measured in this study, clinical experience has been that calves anaesthetized with tiletamine-zolazepam become hypoxic when placed in dorsal recumbency.

INHALATION ANAESTHESIA

Mask induction with halothane or isoflurane is possible with little difficulty in calves up to 2 months of age. A small animal circle system can be used to deliver O_2 and anaesthetic initially through a well-fitting mask. The calf can be unpremedicated or sedated with a combination of diazepam, 0.1 mg/kg, butorphanol, 0.05–0.10 mg/kg, and xylazine, 0.02 mg/kg. With the calf standing the mask is applied with the O_2 flowing at 3–4 l/min, the vaporizer setting starts at zero and is increased by 0.5% increments every few breaths. As its legs begin to relax the calf is allowed to subside to the ground and it is supported in sternal recumbency. The trachea is intubated under direct vision of the larynx using a laryngoscope. The mouth can be held open using lengths of gauze looped around the upper and lower jaws and the tongue pulled to the opposite side of the mouth to the laryngoscope. After intubation the cuff is inflated and the tube secured by tying gauze around the tube and then around the back of the calf's head. Subsequently the calf can be positioned or lifted onto the operating table.

Halothane

Halothane is a useful inhalation anaesthetic for cattle and is usually administered by low-flow methods with a precision vaporizer and CO_2 absorption. Endotracheal intubation is first accomplished after administration of xylazine or thiopental or ketamine, with or without guaiphenesin. Tracheal intubation is associated with increased circulating catecholamine concentrations (Semrad *et al.*, 1986) and premature ventricular contractions may develop in some animals after intubation, particularly when anaesthesia is not deep. The prevalence of arrhythmias decreases over 15 minutes. Halothane induces a significant decrease in ABP with increasing depth of anaesthesia but ABP is usually high during halothane anaesthesia in mature male cattle.

Isoflurane

Isoflurane is often chosen for anaesthesia of young calves. MAP may fall due to peripheral vasodilatation, mucous membrane colour and capillary refill time remaining good. Induction of anaesthesia is normally as smooth as it is with halothane while recovery is said to be more rapid than after halothane, although this is scientifically unsubstantiated. Isoflurane anaesthesia is satisfactory in adult cattle.

Sevoflurane and desflurane

The safe use of sevoflurane and desflurane in cattle has still to be established. Administration of anaesthesia with sevoflurane is similar to halothane and isoflurane except that higher inspired concentrations are required to overcome its lower potency. Desflurane anaesthesia is easily controlled and, although expensive, its use in a closed system may prove to be commercially acceptable.

Nitrous oxide

N_2O/O_2 mixtures are not often used in cattle because of the progressive movement of N_2O into the rumen and intestines which results in bloat. N_2O is not sufficiently potent to induce or maintain anaesthesia when given on its own and it is, therefore, administered with another agent such as halothane or isoflurane.

NEUROMUSCULAR BLOCKING DRUGS

The fact that in cattle peripheral nerve blocks are easily used to produce skeletal muscle relaxation means that neuromuscular blocking drugs are seldom necessary in clinical anaesthesia. Such further muscle relaxation as may be needed is usually provided by the i.v. injection of guaiphenesin.

In experimental studies pancuronium (0.1 mg/kg) has been found to produce relaxation of some 30–40 min duration. As in horses, but in contrast to other species of animal, the facial muscles are more resistant to neuromuscular block than are the limb muscles. Monitoring of block should, therefore, be carried out by stimulation of nerves to limb muscles.

MONITORING

Monitoring the anaesthetized animal is discussed in Chapter 2 but there are some differences from the general descriptions that should be noted. The bovine eye rotates with increasing depth of anaesthesia into a ventral rather than rostroventral position and only the sclera can be seen; it then rotates back into a central position during deep anaesthesia. The pupil usually constricts to a horizontal slit but some pupillary dilatation may occur after ketamine administration. The presence of a palpebral reflex indicates that anaesthesia is light. During ketamine anaesthesia increased muscle tone may result in a centrally placed eye and strong palpebral reflex.

Respiratory rate may be rapid (20–40 breaths/min) and the depth shallow. Mature bulls and cows develop high $PaCO_2$ during inhalation anaesthesia and IPPV is often necessary to prevent severe hypercapnia, which manifests as tachycardia. A rate of 10 breaths/min and a tidal volume of 10 ml/kg (5–6 l for an adult cow or bull) will usually maintain a $PaCO_2$ of around 5.3 kPa (40 mmHg). Spontaneously breathing calves usually seriously hypoventilate when supine and IPPV with tidal volumes of 12–15 ml/kg, at rates of 12 breaths per min and an inspiratory pressure of 30 mmHg may be necessary to keep the $PaCO_2$ at about 5.3 kPa (40 mmHg). Oxygenation when anaesthesia is being maintained with i.v. agents can be provided by endotracheal intubation and connection to an anaesthetic system or a demand valve for assisted or controlled ventilation. Insufflation of O_2 at 15 l/min through a small bore tube down an endotracheal tube may prevent hypoxaemia.

Mature bulls and cows usually maintain HRs of 60–80 beats/min during anaesthesia. Bulls and adult cows develop hypertension during anaesthesia and systolic pressures of >200 mmHg are not uncommon. Values obtained by indirect methods of measurement are often incorrect, but ABP is easily and accurately measured by direct means using a 20 or 22 gauge catheter placed in the middle or caudal auricular artery (Fig 2.15) and connected to a manometer or electrical transducer. Hypotension should be treated in the usual manner, namely, by decreasing the rate of anaesthetic administration, infusing balanced electrolyte solution and infusion of either dopamine or dobutamine. For prolonged anaesthesia or major surgery it is common practice to give 10 ml/kg/h of balanced electrolyte solution while calves less than 3 months of age should be given 2–5 ml/kg/h of 5% dextrose in water to prevent the development of hypoglycaemia.

In calves ABP is similar to that in other small ruminant animals. The MAP should be >60 mmHg and values less than this warrant treatment. Premedication with acepromazine or xylazine may contribute to low ABPs.

POSITIONING

Correct positioning and padding is important as radial nerve damage may develop in the under-most forelimb in cattle that have been lying in lateral recumbency for more than about 20 min. Padding (e.g. inflated tractor tyre inner tubes) should be inserted under the shoulder and fore-arm. Position of the limbs in cattle is the same as in anaesthetized horses, but the difference in the shoulders makes it difficult to pull the lower fore-limb forward to the same extent. The upper limbs should be elevated into a horizontal position and the head should be positioned with a pad under the poll so that the nose is lower than the crown, allowing saliva and any regurgitated material to drain from the pharynx. The horns should be pro-tected from breakage.

RECOVERY FROM ANAESTHESIA

Cattle should be moved into sternal recumbency and propped up in this position as soon as anaes-thesia is terminated to allow eructation for the expulsion of ruminal gases which impair respira-tory function. The endotracheal tube should not be removed until the animal is swallowing and vol-untarily withdraws its tongue into its mouth. This may not occur for some time after coughing and chewing movements return. O_2 administration by insufflation down the endotracheal tube, or through a facemask, should be carried out when-ever possible. In animals that have been intubated, the tube should be removed with the cuff still par-tially inflated. Cattle often remain sitting for some time after consciousness has returned and the process of standing is much more deliberate than it is in horses. After sevoflurane anaesthesia recov-ery to standing is rapid.

Cattle may be allowed to eat and drink within a few hours of recovery to consciousness, the precise time depending, to some extent, on the anaesthetic agents administered. Calves are usually prevented from suckling for an hour and hypoglycaemia should be ruled out if recovery is slow.

REFERENCES

Blaze, C.A., LeBlanc, P.H. and Robinson, N.E. (1988) Effect of withholding feed on ventilation and the incidence of regurgitation during halothane anesthesia of adult cattle. *American Journal of Veterinary Research* **49**: 2126–2129.

Campbell, K.B., Klavano, P.A., Richardson, P. and Alexander, J.E. (1979) Hemodynamic effects of xylazine in the calf. *American Journal of Veterinary Research* **40**: 1777–1780.

Caulkett, N.A., MacDonald, D.G., Janzen, E.D., Cribb, P.N. and Fretz, P.B. (1993) Xylazine hydrochloride epidural analgesia: a method of providing sedation and analgesia to facilitate castration of mature bulls. *Compendium for Continuing Education* **15**: 1155–1159.

Court, M.H., Dodman, N.H., Levine, H.D., Richey, M.T., Lee, J.W. and Hustead, D.R. (1992) Pharmacokinetics and milk residues of butorphanol in dairy cows after single intravenous administration. *Journal of Veterinary Pharmacology and Therapeutics* **15**: 28–35.

DeMoor, A. and Desmet, P. (1971) Effect of Rompun on acid-base-equilibrium and arterial O_2 pressure in cattle. *Veterinary Medical Reviews* **2**: 163–169.

Eichner, R.D., Prior, R.L. and Kvasnicka, W.G. (1979) Xylazine-induced hyperglycemia in beef cattle. *American Journal of Veterinary Research* **40**: 127–129.

Fayed, A.H., Abdalla, E.B., Anderson, R.R., Spencer, K. and Johnson, H.D. (1989) Effect of xylazine in heifers under thermoneutral or heat stress conditions. *American Journal of Veterinary Research* **50**: 151–153.

Hay, A. (1991) Needle penetration of the globe during retrobulbar and peribulbar injections. *Ophthalmology* **98**: 1017–1024.

Hopkins, T.J. (1972) The clinical pharmacology of xylazine in cattle. *Australian Veterinary Journal* **48**: 109–112.

Klein, L. and Fisher, N. (1988) Cardiopulmonary effects of restraint in dorsal recumbency on awake cattle. *American Journal of Veterinary Research* **49**: 1605–1608.

LeBlanc, M.M., Hubbell, J.A.E. and Smith, H.C. (1984) The effects of xylazine hydrochloride on intrauterine pressure in the cow. *Theriogenology* **21**: 681–690.

Lewis, C.A., Constable, P.D., Huhn, J.C. and Morin, D.E. (1999) Sedation with xylazine and lumbosacral epidural administration of lidocaine and xylazine for umbilical surgery in calves. *Journal of the AmericanVeterinary Medical Association* **214**: 89–95.

Lin, H.C., Trachte, E.A., DeGraves, F.J., Rodgerson, D.H., Steiss, J.E. and Carson, R.L. (1998) Evaluation of analgesia induced by epidural administration of medetomidine to cows. *American Journal of Veterinary Research* **59**: 162–167.

McGuirk, S.M., Bednarski, R.M. and Clayton, M.K. (1990) Bradycardia in cattle deprived of food. *Journal of the AmericanVeterinary Medical Association* **196**: 894–896.

Pascoe, P.J. (1986) Humaneness of an electroimmobilization unit for cattle. *American Journal of Veterinary Research* **47**: 2252–2256.

Raekallio, M., Kivalo, M., Jalanka, H. and Vainio, O. (1991) Medetomidine/ketamine sedation in calves and its reversal with atipamezole. *Journal of Veterinary Anaesthesia* **18**: 45–47.

Ranheim, B., Soli, N.E., Ryeng, K.A., Arnemo, J.M. and Horsberg, T.E. (1998) Pharmacokinetics of medetomidine and atipamezole in dairy calves: an agonist-antagonist interaction. *Journal of Veterinary Pharmacology and Therapeutics* **21**: 428–432.

Raptopoulos, D. and Weaver, B.M. (1984) Observations following intravenous xylazine administration in steers. *Veterinary Record* **114**: 567–569.

Rumsey, T.S. and Bond, J. (1976) Cardiorespiratory patterns, rectal temperature, serum electrolytes and packed cell volume in beef cattle deprived of feed and water. *Journal of Animal Science* **42**: 1227–1238.

Salonen, J.S., Vaha-Vahe, T., Vainio, O. and Vakkuri, O. (1989) Single-dose pharmacokinetics of detomidine in the horse and cow. *Journal of Veterinary Pharmacology and Therapeutics* **12**: 65–72.

Semrad, S.D., Trim, C.M. and Hardee, G.E. (1986) Hypertension in bulls and steers anesthetized with guaifenesin-thiobarbiturate-halothane combination. *American Journal of Veterinary Research* **47**: 1577–1582.

StJean, G., Skarda, R.T., Muir, W.W. and Hoffsis, G.F. (1990) Caudal epidural analgesia induced by xylazine administration in cows. *American Journal of Veterinary Research* **51**: 1232–1236.

Symonds, H.W. and Mallinson, C.B. (1978) The effect of xylazine and xylazine followed by insulin on blood glucose and insulin in the dairy cow. *Veterinary Record* **102**: 27–29.

Thurmon, J.C., Nelson, D.R., Hartsfield, S.M. and Rumore, C.A. (1978) Effects of xylazine hydrochloride on urine in cattle. *Australian Veterinary Journal* **54**: 178–180.

Thurmon, J.C., Lin, H.C., Benson, G.J., Tranquieli, W.J. and Olson, W.A. (1989) Combining telazal and xylazine for anesthesia in calves. *Veterinary medicine* **84**: 824–830.

Toosey, M.B. (1959) The uses of concentrated pentobarbitone sodium solution in bovine practice. *Veterinary Record* **71**: 24–27.

Vainio, O. (1988) Detomidine (letter to the editor). *Veterinary Record* **123**: 655.

Valuesde, A., Doheny, T.J., Dyson, D. and Valliant, A.E. (1989) Evaluation of pentobarbital as a drug for standing sedation in castle. *Veterinary Surgery* **18**: 235–238.

Wagner, A.E., Muir, W.W. and Grospitch, B.J. (1990) Cardiopulmonary effects of position in conscious cattle. *American Journal of Veterinary Research* **51**: 7–10.

Wong, D.H.W. (1993) Regional anaesthesia for intraocular surgery. *Canadian Journal of Anaesthesia* **40**: 635–657.

Anaesthesia of sheep, goats and other herbivores

13

INTRODUCTION

Anaesthetic management of sheep and goats is usually uncomplicated with the notable exception that regurgitation with potentially fatal pulmonary aspiration is always a risk of sedation or general anaesthesia. Furthermore, intubation can be technically difficult, particularly in large rams, because the animals' narrow jaws leave little room to view the larynx during insertion of the endotracheal tube. Two factors should be considered in selection of anaesthetic protocols for these ruminants. First, dose rates of some anaesthetic agents differ from those in other species. Secondly, animals that are not used to being handled or isolated may not exhibit signs commonly associated with sickness or pain. These animals will have a reduced requirement for anaesthesia and failure to recognize this may result in overdosage.

This chapter describes techniques and drug combinations that can be used to anaesthetize sheep, goats, and llamas in a variety of clinical settings. Local analgesia is useful in these species and details on the techniques are included. Some information on methods of anaesthesia of deer, camels and elephants has been provided at the end of the chapter.

LOCAL ANALGESIA

Local analgesia techniques are highly useful in sheep and goat practice because equipment involved is inexpensive, cardiovascular and respiratory depression are less than produced by general anaesthesia, and the risk of regurgitation and aspiration is decreased. The immediate post surgical recovery time may or may not be shorter than after general anaesthesia, depending on the agents and techniques used. Local anaesthetic agents may induce toxic symptoms when used inappropriately, especially when an excessive volume of local anaesthetic is injected. Limiting the initial administration of lignocaine to 6 mg/kg has been found to be safe; administration of lignocaine in excess of 10 mg/kg can result in sufficiently high blood levels to cause cardiovascular depression and central nervous system stimulation. This section will also discuss techniques of local nerve blocks involving use of opioids or α_2 adrenoceptor agonists.

APPLICATIONS OF LOCAL ANAESTHESIA

Cornual nerve blocks for dehorning

The cornual branches of the lachrymal and infratrochlear nerves provide sensory innervation to the horns. The cornual branch of the lachrymal nerve emerges from the orbit behind the root of the supraorbital process. The nerve, covered by a thin frontalis muscle, divides into several branches, two of which supply mainly the lateral and caudal parts of the horn. The main trunk of the infratrochlear nerve emerges from the orbit dorsomedially and divides into two branches, the dorsal

341

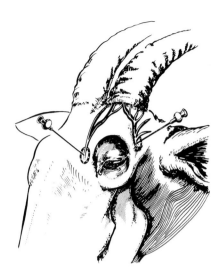

FIG. 13.1 Nerve blocks for dehorning of goats. The cornual branches of both the lachrymal and infratrochlear nerves must be blocked. Care must be taken in young kids to ensure that attempts to block both nerves do not lead to injection of toxic quantities of local analgesic solution.

or cornual branch and the medial or frontal branch. The cornual branch soon divides, one division coursing to the dorsal aspect of the base of the horn and ramifying dorsally and dorsomedially. The other division passes to the medial aspect of the base of the horn and gives off branches to the medial and caudomedial parts of it. Both divisions are covered in part by the orbicularis and in part by the frontalis muscle.

The site for producing block of the cornual branch of the lachrymal nerve is caudal to the root of the supraorbital process (Fig. 13.1). The needle should be inserted as close as possible to the caudal ridge of the root of the supraorbital process to a depth of 1.0–1.5 cm in adult goats. The syringe plunger should be withdrawn before injection to check that the tip of the needle has not penetrated the large blood vessel located at this site.

The site for blocking the cornual branch of the infratrochlear nerve is at the dorsomedial margin of the orbit (Fig. 13.1). In some animals the nerve is palpable by applying thumbnail pressure and moving the skin over this area. The needle should be inserted as close as possible to the margin of the orbit and under the muscle to a depth of about 0.5 cm. Local analgesic solution such as 2% Lignocaine should be injected at each site, up to a

maximum of 6 mg/kg or about 2–3 ml per site for adult animals.

Care must be taken with young goats not to exceed the toxic dose of Lignocaine or to inadvertently inject local anaesthetic intravenously. Alternative analgesic techniques for dehorning include administration of xylazine for sedation, or production of light general anaesthesia with diazepam and ketamine, Saffan®, propofol, or an inhalant. It must be remembered that when inhalation anaesthesia is employed, the oxygen must be switched off and the facemask removed before application of a hot iron.

Castration

In the UK the Protection of Animals (Anaesthetics) Act specifies that castration of male sheep over 3 months of age and of male goats over 2 months of age must be carried out under local or general anaesthesia. All of the methods described for cattle are applicable.

Caudal block

Injection of 2 (1–4) ml of 2% lignocaine solution into the epidural canal through the sacrococcygeal space will provide caudal epidural analgesia for obstetrical procedures involving the vagina, vulva, and perineum. A smaller volume of local anaesthetic, 0.75 to 1.0 ml of 1% lignocaine, will provide analgesia for the docking of lambs' tails. Strict attention must be paid to aseptic technique to avoid complications and several minutes must be allowed for analgesia to develop.

The wool must be clipped from over the sacrum and the base of the tail. The site for needle placement is located by moving the tail up and down and palpating the most cranial point of articulation. A 20 gauge hypodermic needle is inserted midline approximately at a 45° angle to the curvature of the rump so that the tip of the needle enters the vertebral column and may even thread for a few mm cranially. Addition of xylazine, 0.05 mg/kg, will prolong analgesia for up to 36 hours.

Continuous caudal block can be employed to provide relief of conditions of the vagina and rectum which provoke severe and continuous straining. Continuous block is facilitated by placement

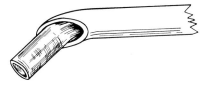

FIG. 13.2 Catheter emerging from tip of Tuohy needle.

TABLE 13.1 Epidural analgesia for flank laparotomy in goats. A lower dose rate, such as 1 ml/7 kg, is sufficient for analgesia of the hindlimbs or perineal surgery			
Treatment	**Onset (min)**	**Duration (h)**	**Standing (h)**
Lignocaine 2% with adrenaline, 1 ml/5 kg	25	2	3.5–5.0
Bupivacaine 0.5% or 0.75%, 1 ml/4 kg	45	4–6	8–12

of an epidural catheter. Threading of the catheter into the epidural space is performed using a Tuohy needle, which has a curved end that directs the catheter (Fig. 13.2). The needle is withdrawn after the catheter has been advanced 6–8 cm in the epidural space. Local analgesic solution is injected through the catheter whenever the animal shows signs of returning sensation. Extreme care must be taken to secure the catheter in position and to ensure sterile injections by protecting the free catheter end – capped and wrapped in sterile gauze, for example.

Digital nerve block

Digital nerves are easily blocked with lignocaine at the sites described for cattle. (Chapter 12)

Epidural block

Epidural block can be produced by injection of local anaesthetic solution into the epidural space at the lumbosacral junction. Complete analgesia and paralysis can be induced in the hindlimbs and abdomen to allow surgery, depending on the volume of local anaesthetic injected (Trim, 1989). The dose rates for different drugs and their times for onset of action are listed in Table 13.1. The dose rates listed are to produce analgesia for flank laparotomy. The dose should be decreased if the animal is old, obese, or pregnant. A lower dose of lignocaine, such as 1 ml/7 kg, is sufficient for perineal or hindlimb surgical procedures, and for caesarian section. The long duration of hindlimb paralysis from bupivacaine block for caesarian section interferes with nursing of the newborn, and for that reason lignocaine with adrenaline is usually preferred.

The lumbosacral junction is easy to palpate in thin animals but recognition of landmarks will be necessary to identify the point of needle insertion in muscled or fat animals. Epidural block can be performed with the goat or sheep standing or in lateral recumbency. An imaginary line between the cranial borders of the ilium crosses between the spinous processes of the last lumbar vertebrae (Fig. 13.3). The caudal borders of the ilium, where the angle bends to parallel midline, are level with the cranial edge of the sacrum. The point of needle insertion is midline halfway between the spinous process of the seventh lumbar vertebra and the sacrum. If the spinous process of the last lumbar vertebra can be palpated, the next depression caudal to it is the lumbosacral space. This area must be clipped and the skin prepared with a surgical scrub.

A spinal needle should be used because it has a stilette to prevent injection of a core of subcutaneous tissue into the epidural space. The notch on the hub of the needle indicates the direction of the bevel. Thus the anaesthetist can ensure that injection of local anaesthetic solution is towards the head of the animal.

When epidural nerve block is to be performed on the conscious animal, 1–3 ml 2% lignocaine should be injected subcutaneously with a fine needle at the site intended for insertion of the spinal needle. For lambs, kids, and pygmy goats, a 22 gauge 3.7 cm spinal needle can be used. For adult animals a sturdier needle, such as an 18 gauge 6.25 cm spinal needle, is recommended. The needle should be inserted midline perpendicular to the curvature of the hindquarters and perpendicular to the midline sagittal plane of the animal, i.e. not necessarily parallel or perpendicular to the floor or table top (Fig. 13.4).

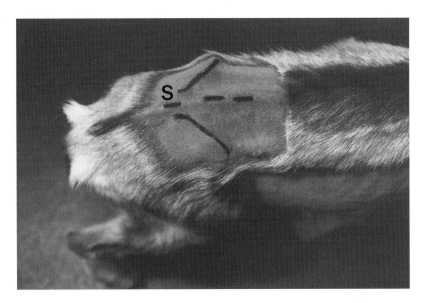

FIG. 13.3 Black pen has been used to identify the landmarks used to locate the lumbosacral space in a goat. An imaginary line between the cranial edge of the ilium crosses midline between the spinous processes of the last two lumbar vertebrae. The wings of the ilium angle obliquely towards midline and the sacrum (S).

Considerable pressure may be needed to introduce the needle through the skin and supraspinous ligament and it may be preferable to puncture the skin first with a larger, sharp hypodermic needle. Once introduced, the spinal needle should be advanced gently for two reasons. First, to be able

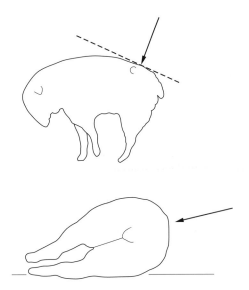

FIG. 13.4 Direction of insertion of needle for lumbar epidural injection in sheep in lateral recumbency.

to appreciate the resistance then penetration of the interarcuate ligament which lies over the epidural space, described as a 'pop', and secondly, to control introduction of the tip of the needle into the epidural space so that movement of the needle can be stopped immediately. Further introduction of the needle will penetrate the spinal cord and the animal, if conscious, will jump and may dislodge the position of the needle. If the tip of the needle strikes bone and the needle does not appear to be deep enough to be in the epidural space, the needle should be withdrawn until the tip is just under the skin and redirected in a cranial direction. If unsuccessful, the procedure should be repeated with the needle advanced in a caudal direction.

After correct placement of the needle, the stilette should be removed and placed on a sterile surface. A 3 ml syringe containing 0.5 ml air should be attached to the spinal needle and the plunger withdrawn to test for aspiration of cerebrospinal fluid (CSF) or blood. Attempts at aspiration should reveal only a vacuum and aspiration of air means that the syringe is not tightly attached to the needle. When no cerebrospinal fluid or blood is aspirated, a test injection of a small amount of air should be made. Injection should be easy when the needle is in the epidural space. After correct placement of the needle, the 3 ml syringe should be detached and the syringe containing the local anaesthetic solution attached. Injection of the drug should be made over at least 30 seconds. Faster injections result in increased intracranial pressure which, if the animal is conscious, manifest as opisthotonus, nystagmus, and collapse. After injection, the spinal needle should be withdrawn. If analgesia of one side or leg is required the animal should be placed in lateral recumbency with the side to be desensitized underneath. When bilateral analgesia is required, the animal should be positioned either prone or supine so that the vertebral canal is horizontal. The goat or sheep should not be allowed to 'dog-sit', otherwise analgesia will not develop cranially.

The spinal cord may project into the sacrum in sheep and goats and penetration of the dura will result in aspiration of CSF. Injection into the subarachnoid space of the same volume of local anaesthetic intended for epidural analgesia will result in the block extending further cranially and respiratory arrest. Usually, the volume for subarachnoid injection is half the epidural dose. There is some risk of local anaesthetic solution entering CSF through the puncture hole if the spinal needle is partly withdrawn and redirected into the epidural space a few mm distant from the original insertion. If the entry of the needle into a venous sinus is not detected by aspirating blood, intravenous injection may result in cardiovascular depression. The local anaesthetic solution should be warmed when the epidural injection is to be made in the conscious animal. Injection of a cold solution will stimulate receptors in the spinal cord and the animal will jump, possibly dislodging the needle. Indwelling catheters can be inserted into the epidural space at the lumbosacral junction using a 16 gauge Tuohy needle as described for caudal analgesia.

Placement of a venous catheter is a sensible precaution when epidural analgesia is to be used for surgery. Epidural injection of local anaesthetic solution causes paralysis of the splanchnic nerves and results in a decrease in blood pressure. Hypotension may develop, especially in hypovolaemic animals, such as for caesarian section, or animals positioned in such a way as to promote pooling of blood in the hindlimbs. In these animals, treatment should include expansion of blood volume with intravenous administration of fluid and injection of ephedrine, 0.06 mg/kg, or methoxamine, 5–10 mg. Animals with urethral obstruction being given epidural analgesia for perineal urethrostomy or cystotomy may already have a distended urinary bladder at risk of rupture. Nonetheless, administration of fluid intravenously is important to restore blood volume and cardiovascular function. One option is to decrease the size of the bladder by cystocentesis. Alternatively, fluid infusion can begin at the time of epidural administration so that surgical relief of distension can be accomplished before a substantial increase in urine production occurs.

Approximately 50% of human patients experience visceral pain during caesarian section under epidural block with bupivacaine and describe the pain as poorly localized, dull pain, or as a feeling of heaviness or squeezing (Alahuhta *et al.*, 1990). Sheep or goats may respond by movement or vocalization to manipulation of viscera during laparotomy under epidural analgesia with lignocaine or bupivacaine. The animals may be made more comfortable by i.v. butorphanol, 0.1 mg/kg, diazepam, 0.05–0.10 mg/kg, or xylazine, 0.02 mg/kg. Disadvantages of adjunct drug administration include respiratory depression, pharyngeal relaxation that may promote regurgitation and pulmonary aspiration, and depression of the lambs or kids delivered by caesarian section.

Sensory block may extend several dermatomes cranial to the level of motor block. Limb movement is possible even when the animal is sufficiently analgesic for surgery. During recovery from epidural block, the ability to move the hindlimbs may develop before analgesia is lost, although the ability to stand may not return until long after analgesia is gone.

Respiratory paralysis can occur if local anaesthetic solution travels cranially to the neck. This will occur if a too large volume is injected, i.e. inaccurate calculation of dose. In this event, general anesthesia must be quickly induced, the trachea intubated and IPPV applied until the animal is able to breathe again.

During recovery from epidural block produced by local anaesthetic solutions, the animal should be allowed to recover quietly. It will be able to maintain sternal recumbency but there is potential for injury to the hindlimbs if it makes uncoordinated attempts to rise.

Epidural morphine

Epidural injection of morphine, 0.1 mg/kg used as a 1 mg/ml preservative-free solution, or 15 mg/ml diluted in saline to 0.15–0.20 ml/kg, at the lumbosacral junction will produce analgesia without paralysis. This technique can be used to decrease the requirement for general anaesthetic agents and to provide postoperative analgesia. Its beneficial effects were documented by a study during which it was noted that goats given epidural morphine after stifle surgery vocalized less and were less likely to grind their teeth than goats that had not (Pablo, 1993). Epidural morphine also provides pain relief for 6 hours after abdominal surgery (Hendrickson *et al.*, 1996).

Epidural xylazine

Xylazine, 0.05 mg/kg, diluted with saline to 0.1 ml/kg may be used as an adjunct to general anaesthesia for surgery. Systemic effects of sedation and decreased gastrointestinal motility may accompany epidural administration of xylazine in ruminants. A higher dose of xylazine, 0.4 mg/kg, has been injected at the lumbosacral junction of rams to produce analgesia for surgery involving lateral deviation of the penis (Aminkov & Hubenov 1995). Analgesia extended to T5–T6 within 10 minutes and lasted for 120–140 minutes. Although sedation was judged to be poor,- heart rates decreased moderately, the ability to swallow was decreased, and the rams urinated frequently, and these are all signs indicative of systemic absorption. The rams were supine during the surgical procedure but changes in PaO_2 and $PaCO_2$ were clinically insignificant. Hindlimb motor block lasted an average of 224 minutes.

Paravertebral nerve block

In sheep and goats lumbar paravertebral nerve block is carried out using techniques similar to those employed in cattle. For operations carried out through the flank the thirteenth thoracic and first three lumbar nerves are blocked. For each of these nerves up to 5 ml of 1 or 2% lignocaine is used, divided and injected above and below the intertransverse ligament, up to a maximum total dose of 6 mg/kg lignocaine. Onset of analgesia may be as fast as 5 minutes. Duration of analgesia is an hour, or longer when lignocaine with adrenaline is used.

Inverted L block

Flank laparotomy can be performed using local infiltration of lignocaine in an inverted L pattern 2 to 3 cm cranial and dorsal to the intended skin incision site. Blebs of lignocaine must be injected subcutaneously and deep in the abdominal muscle at approximately 1.5 cm intervals along the injection site. The maximum dose of lignocaine to be injected at one time is 6 mg/kg and dilution of 2% solution to 1% solution may be necessary to provide sufficient volume for injection. The duration of analgesia is about 1.5 hours.

Intravenous regional analgesia

Surgery on the limbs can be performed using intravenous regional analgesia (Chapter 10). In sheep and goats the tourniquet or sphygmomanometer cuff is usually placed on the forelimb above the elbow (taking care not to pinch skin in the axilla) and on the hindlimb above the hock (leaving sufficient length of the saphenous vein for injection) (Fig. 13.5). A tourniquet must be sufficiently tight to block arterial flow without being excessively tight, and a sphygmomanometer cuff used as a tourniquet must be inflated to above the systolic blood pressure. Injection of 4 mg/kg lignocaine without adrenaline should be made slowly through a 25 gauge needle directed towards the foot. Care must be taken to keep the needle immobile within the vein during injection. Blood should be aspirated before injection to confirm needle placement within the vein. Onset of action is in 15–20 minutes. Analgesia will persist as long as the tourniquet is in place but sensation will rapidly return after the tourniquet is removed. The tourniquet should not be released within 10 minutes of

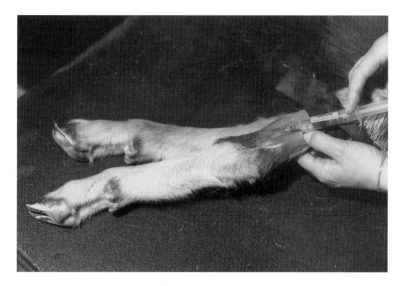

FIG. 13.5 Intravenous regional analgesia in the hindlimb of a goat. A tourniquet is tied around the limb proximal to the intravenous injection of lignocaine.

the initial injection to allow time for the lignocaine to diffuse into tissues. Thereafter, releasing the tourniquet has no clinical effect on the animal. No long lasting effect has been noted in sheep or goats when the tourniquet has been in place for 2 hours.

Peroneal and tibial nerve block

Analgesia of the hindlimb below the hock can be achieved by peroneal and tibial nerve blocks. The peroneal nerve is blocked by injection of 5 ml 2% lignocaine where the nerve runs obliquely cau-dodorsally to cranioventrally approximately 2.5 cm below the lateral condyle of the tibia. The nerve can often be palpated by using thumbnail pressure to move the skin and underlying tissues. Analgesia of the dorsum of the foot is obvious from the animal's stance (Fig. 13.6).

The tibial nerve is blocked by infiltration of 4 ml of 2% solution of lignocaine on the medial side of the leg at the hock between the flexor tendons and the gastrocnemius tendon. A further 1 ml is inject-ed at a similar site on the lateral side of the limb to block a small cutaneous nerve, a branch of the common peroneal nerve originating at the middle of the thigh. Onset of analgesia should be within 15 minutes and is accompanied by straightening of the hock (Fig. 13.6).

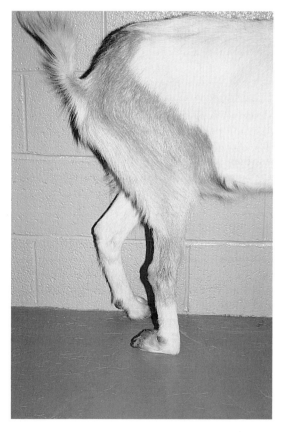

FIG. 13.6 Peroneal and tibial nerve block produces analgesia distal to the hock. The hock will straighten and the goat will stand on the dorsum of the fetlock.

SEDATION

SEDATIVE AGENTS EMPLOYED IN SHEEP AND GOATS

Acepromazine

Acepromazine, 0.05–0.1 mg/kg, can be used to provide mild tranquilisation in sheep and goats.

α_2 Adrenoceptor agonists and antagonists

Xylazine, detomidine, medetomidine, or romifidine provide light to heavy sedation according to the dose rate administered. Use of these agents alone provides satisfactory sedation for restraint or they can be used for premedication prior to induction of anaesthesia with other anaesthetic agents. Dose rates for xylazine range from 0.02 to 0.2 mg/kg, the largest dose producing profound sedation for many hours. Animals that are young or sick will only require a low dose to induce sedation. Variation in the analgesic effects of xylazine has been noted in different breeds of sheep, for example, analgesia after xylazine was less in Welsh mountain sheep than in Clun sheep (Ley et al., 1990). The average weight of the Welsh Mountain was 46 kg compared with 69 kg for the Clun and the authors hypothesized that the difference may have been the result of dosing according to body weight rather than body surface area.

This group of sedatives induces marked physiological changes. A comparison of i.v. xylazine, 0.15 mg/kg, detomidine, 0.03 mg/kg, medetomidine, 0.01 mg/kg, and romifidine, 0.05 mg/kg, indicated that all caused a significant decrease in PaO_2 (hypoxaemia) for 45 minutes with no alteration in $PaCO_2$, and that respiratory rate increased (Celly et al., 1997). These observations are in general agreement with previously published investigations. The authors suggested that, since the hypoxaemia was not due to hypoventilation or change in body position, a possible cause might be an increase in shunt fraction occurring from segmental airway obstruction, areas of pulmonary atelectasis, or opening of previously closed vascular connections. Of further clinical interest, the hypoxaemia outlasted the duration of sedation. Further investigation has confirmed that in sheep xylazine causes severe pulmonary parenchymal damage, including capillary endothelial damage, intra-alveolar haemorrhage, and interstitial oedema (Celly et al., 1999). Xylazine administration has occasionally been associated with the development of clinical signs of pulmonary oedema in sheep.

Xylazine induces a short-lived decrease in heart rate and a mild decrease in mean arterial pressure (MAP). Detomidine, medetomidine and romifidine induce significant bradycardia whereas detomidine and romifidine increase MAP (Celly et al., 1997). The impact of these cardiovascular changes will depend on the dose rate of the agent, concurrent administration of other anaesthetics, and the physical status of the patient.

The effects of xylazine can be reversed by intravenous administration of yohimbine, 0.1 mg/kg, tolazoline, 2 mg/kg, or doxapram, 0.5 mg/kg. Atipamezole 25 to 50 μg/kg i.v. can also be used to antagonize the effects of this group of sedatives.

Diazepam and midazolam

Intravenous administration of these agents alone may produce some sedation and ataxia in sheep and goats for 15–30 minutes, but the degree of sedation is unpredictable in healthy animals. Midazolam, 0.2 mg/kg i.v. significantly decreased the response of sheep to a mechanical painful stimulus for 20 minutes (Kyles et al., 1995). Increasing the dose rate to 0.3 mg/kg extended the duration of antinociception but not the intensity. Administration of flumazenil, 0.02 mg/kg, markedly attenuated the sedation and analgesia induced by midazolam but did not abolish it completely. Diazepam, 0.2 mg/kg, i.v. can be used to produce mild sedation for transdermal tracheal wash.

Opioids

A variety of opioids have been used in sheep and goats to provide intraoperative and postoperative analgesia. Pethidine (meperidine) has been used for many years as an adjunct to anaesthesia in sheep and goats. Butorphanol, 0.05–0.20 mg/kg, i.m. or i.v. is useful to increase sedation from xylazine, acepromazine, or diazepam. Butorphanol has a rapid onset of action and given 5–10 minutes before diazepam and ketamine facilitates a smooth and relaxed induction of anaesthesia.

The duration of effect appears to be 1 to 2 hours. Buprenorphine, 0.006–0.010 mg/kg, given intramuscularly 30 minutes before induction of anaesthesia, appears to decrease the concentration of inhalation agent required for anaesthesia. Buprenorphine can be repeated in 4 hours for treating postoperative pain.

Buprenorphine, 0.006 and 0.012 mg/kg i.v. in experimental sheep produced analgesia from 40 minutes to 3.5 hours against a thermal stimulus but no detectable relief from pressure-induced pain (Waterman *et al.*, 1991). This difference in effect against different types of pain, which has not been observed with pethidine or fentanyl, may be related to the fact that buprenorphine is a partial agonist at the μ opioid receptor. Buprenorphine, 0.006 mg/kg, did not cause any significant change in pHa, $PaCO_2$ or PaO_2.

Etorphine and carfentanil

These opioids are used for immobilization of non-domestic animals. A study comparing intramuscularly administered etorphine or carfentanil, 10, 20, and 40 μg/kg of body weight, in instrumented goats described similar effects for both drugs (Heard *et al.*, 1996). The goats were rapidly immobilized, more quickly with carfentanil ($\leq$ 5 minutes) than with etorphine (5–10 minutes) and etorphine always induced transient struggling. Immobilization was characterized by limb and neck hyperextension with occasional vocalization and bruxation. The goats were partially recovered by an hour after etorphine administration but were unable to stand at 2 hours after carfentanil. Both drugs significantly increased blood pressure and decreased heart rates without changing cardiac outputs. Arterial O_2 content was not decreased and the goats did not regurgitate.

GENERAL ANAESTHESIA

PREPARATION

Withholding food from small ruminants before anaesthesia is not a universal practice. However, most anaesthetists prefer to withhold food for 24 hours and water for 6 to 12 hours before anaesthesia whenever possible to decrease pressure of the rumen on the diaphragm and aid ventilation, to decrease the severity of bloat, and to decrease the prevalence and volume of regurgitation. Lambs and kids should be prevented from suckling for 30 to 60 minutes before anaesthesia.

When heavy sedation or general anaesthesia is to be administered to an unfasted ruminant, rapid-sequence induction of anaesthesia and intubation of the trachea should be performed.

It is doubtful if atropine has any value as a general premedicant in sheep and goats. The doses necessary to prevent salivation completely (0.2–0.8 mg/kg) produce undesirable tachycardia and ocular effects, while smaller doses merely make the saliva more viscid and hence more difficult to drain from the oropharynx. Bradycardia develops seldom during anaesthesia but may be treated by i.v. atropine, 0.02 mg/kg, or glycopyrrolate, 0.005 mg/kg.

Premedication is not essential before general anaesthesia in small ruminants, as excitement at induction is uncommon. Administration of an opioid, such as butorphanol, 0.05–0.20 mg/kg, or buprenorphine, 0.01 mg/kg, i.m. or i.v., will improve muscle relaxation and will provide essential analgesia for orthopaedic procedures. Xylazine is an important part of induction of anaesthesia with a xylazine and ketamine combination. Diazepam is often administered concurrently with ketamine at the time of induction.

ANAESTHETIC TECHNIQUES

Intravenous injection

The site of venepuncture in sheep and goats depends mainly on the assistance available and the personal preference of the anaesthetist. The cephalic vein in the forelimb (Fig.13.7) and the saphenous vein in the hindlimb are easily viewed after the wool or hair over them has been clipped. It should be noted that the cephalic vein is more oblique on the limb than in the dog (Fig.13.8). A catheter (18 gauge, 5 cm long) can be inserted into either vein, capped, flushed with heparinized saline, and secured to the leg with adhesive tape. A butterfly needle (21 gauge or 19 gauge) can be used in the cephalic vein.

Goats have relatively long, thin necks with obvious jugular veins so that jugular venepuncture

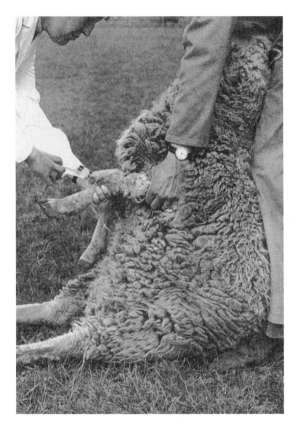

FIG. 13.7 Restraint of sheep for injection into the cephalic vein. For jugular venepuncture the sheep is similarly restrained in the sitting position but it is not easy to place the needle correctly in the vein with the sheep in this position and hence the injection of irritant substances into the jugular vein of the sitting sheep is to be avoided.

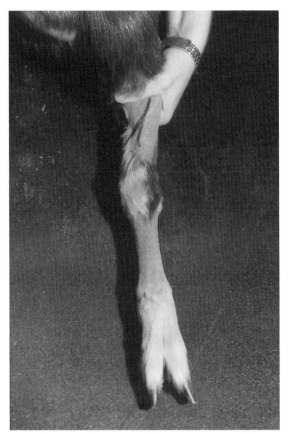

FIG. 13.8 The cephalic vein in a goat is short and oblique across the forearm (black pen has been used to identify the location of the left cephalic vein in this animal).

or catheterization may be carried out with the goat standing, as described for horses. A 14 gauge 8 cm long catheter is suitable for mature animals. Sheep have relatively short, thick necks and jugular catheterization is less easy.

The ear veins are easily observed after the hair is clipped, especially in goats, and can be used for intravenous injection.

Endotracheal intubation

After induction of anaesthesia, the sheep or goat should be held in a sternal, head up position to minimize the likelihood of regurgitation until the trachea is intubated and the endotracheal tube cuff inflated. If regurgitation occurs during the process of intubation, the animal should be turned into

lateral recumbency and the head lowered to allow drainage. Regurgitated rumen material should be quickly scooped out of the mouth before tracheal intubation is attempted. When difficulty is encountered in intubating the trachea, turning the animal into dorsal recumbency with its head off the end of the table may facilitate the process by overextending the head and neck. Note that this position will impair ventilation and may promote regurgitation.

Endotracheal intubation is best performed under direct vision with the aid of a laryngoscope. Full extension of the head and neck is essential to place the pharynx and trachea in a straight line (Fig. 13.9). Strips of gauze around the upper and lower jaws may be used to hold them open and keep the assistant's fingers out of the anaesthetist's view. The assistant holds the tongue in a gauze

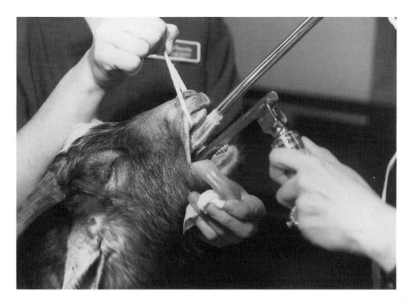

FIG. 13.9 Intubation of the trachea is facilitated by extending the head and neck to form a straight line and use of a laryngoscope to view the laryngeal opening.

sponge for better grip and draws it out of the mouth. Endotracheal tubes with 11–12 mm internal diameter are used for adult sheep and goats, and up to 16 mm for large breeds of sheep. A metal or plastic covered stilette inside the endotracheal tube may be used to stiffen it and provide more control over the tip of the tube. The tip (last 2 cm) of the stilette should be bent down at a 30 degree angle. The laryngoscope blade should be used to depress the dorsum of the tongue and the tip of the blade must be positioned at the base of the tongue in front of the epiglottis. Downward pressure on the length of the blade will expose the laryngeal entrance. Care must be taken to avoid damaging the incisor teeth. The tip of the endotracheal tube is placed on the epiglottis and used to flatten it against the tongue before the tube is advanced into the larynx and trachea. Slight resistance may be felt as the tube passes by the vocal cords. A length of gauze is tied tightly around the tube behind the incisors and then secured around the back of the head behind the ears, or around the bottom jaw. The cuff is inflated to produce an airtight seal within the trachea.

Alternative methods of intubation include inserting a half-metre blunt-ended, thin metal rod into the trachea under direct vision, removing the laryngoscope, then feeding the endotracheal tube over the rod into the larynx and trachea, whereupon the rod is withdrawn. The tube may have to be rotated 360° as it enters the pharynx in order for the tip to pass over the epiglottis and enter the larynx. Utilizing another method, some anaesthetists are able to pass the endotracheal tube into the trachea blindly. The endotracheal tube (which must have a good curvature to it) is introduced into the mouth with one hand and the tip fed into the larynx, which is gripped externally by the anaesthetist's other hand.

Tubes lubricated with an analgesic jelly may also be passed through the nostril. The ventral nasal meatus is relatively large in sheep and goats and although tubes passed via the nostril must be smaller than those introduced through the mouth reasonably adequately sized ones can be used. If the tube passed up the nostril cannot be introduced blindly through the larynx a laryngoscope is used to view the tip of the tube in the pharynx. The tip of the tube is grasped with forceps and assisted into the laryngeal opening as the tube is advanced through the nostril.

INJECTABLE ANAESTHETIC AGENTS

Major surgery and prolonged diagnostic procedures in sheep and goats are best performed under inhalation anaesthesia, using injectable anaesthetic agents only for induction and to facilitate endotracheal intubation. The greatest disadvantage to use of injectable anaesthetics for maintenance as well as induction of anaesthesia is the high likelihood of hypoxaemia developing. Further, with the exception of propofol, extending anaesthesia time beyond 30 minutes with injectable agents is often accompanied by prolongation of recovery. Use of preanaesthetic drugs whose actions can be antagonized, such as the α_2 agonist sedatives or opioids, may shorten recovery but they also contribute to greater respiratory depression and hypoxaemia.

Thiopental

Thiopental has been extensively used to induce anaesthesia in sheep and goats. Onset of anaesthesia is fast and the drug can be titrated to achieve the desired effect. The dose range to induce anaesthesia in the unpremedicated animal is wide, 7 to 20 mg/kg, and the low or high dose does not seem to correlate with any particular patient characteristic, not age nor conformation nor degree of ill health. To avoid overdosage, an initial bolus dose of 5–7 mg/kg of 2.5% thiopental should be injected. Within 30 seconds the degree of central nervous system depression can be assessed and further small boluses of drug administered every 20 seconds until the jaws are relaxed for endotracheal intubation. The duration of anaesthesia is short, at 5 to 10 minutes, depending on the dose of thiopental administered. Recovery is usually smooth. Preanaesthetic sedation decreases the dose rate proportionately to the degree of sedation.

Methohexital

In both sheep and goats the intravenous injection of 4 mg/kg of a 2.5% solution of methohexital produces anaesthesia of 5–7 minutes' duration. Recovery to standing position is complete within 10–14 minutes of the injection but the recovery is usually associated with violent jerking or convulsive movements and excitement if the animal is disturbed by noise during this period. Recovery excitement may be prevented by premedication with diazepam or xylazine. Premedication

will decrease the induction dose of methohexital to 2 mg/kg.

Pentobarbital

Many years ago Phillipson and Barnett (1939) reported the experimental use of pentobarbital in sheep. The approximate dose rate in adult sheep is 30 mg/kg when given by slow intravenous injection but there is great variation in response to the drug and anaesthesia time is short – about 15 minutes. In contrast to its effects in other species, detoxification of pentobarbital in sheep is rapid. The dose rate for pentobarbital in goats is similar to that in sheep with a variable but longer duration of anaesthesia.

It is important to note that commercially available solutions of pentobarbital may contain propylene glycol and this causes haemolysis and haematuria in goats and sheep. Clinically, injectable anaesthetic agents other than pentobarbital are now usually used for anaesthesia.

Ketamine

Ketamine can be used for anaesthesia in sheep and goats without fear of causing convulsions. Muscle relaxation is poor, but may be improved by sedatives such as diazepam or xylazine (Table 13.2). Ketamine alone or when given in low dose rates with diazepam appears to produce a state of sedation in which there is profound analgesia with only partial depression of the swallowing and cough reflexes. Large dose rates have been used but a lower dose is all that is needed to accomplish endotracheal intubation. A useful drug combination for induction of anaesthesia is diazepam, 0.25 mg/kg i.v., and ketamine, 5 mg/kg (4–6 mg/kg) i.v., administered at the same time. In many animals, half of this calculated dose is sufficient for endotracheal intubation. Better muscle relaxation is achieved when i.v. butorphanol, 0.05–0.10 mg/kg, is administered before the diazepam and ketamine. A different opioid or a small dose of xylazine, 0.02–0.05 mg/kg, can be given as an alternative to butorphanol. Acepromazine, 0.05 mg/kg, i.v. or i.m. can be substituted for the diazepam but sufficient time should be allowed for onset of action before injection of ketamine, 6 mg/kg.

TABLE 13.2 **Injectable drug combinations for general anaesthesia in goats and sheep**

Drugs	Dosage (mg/kg)	Duration	Comments
Diazepam + Ketamine	0.2 to 0.3 mg/kg i.v. + 5.0 to 7.5 mg/kg i.v.	10–15 min	Can include butorphanol 0.1 mg/kg
Xylazine + Ketamine	0.1 mg/kg i.m. + 6 mg/kg i.v. or 11 mg/kg i.m.	30 min	Additional xylazine can be added if depth of anaesthesia not adequate
Thiopental	7 to 20 mg/kg i.v.	10 min	Not < 3 months age. Dosage varies: inject 5 mg/kg i.v. initially and titrate additional drug 'to effect'
Xylazine + tiletamine-zolazepam	0.1 mg/kg i.m. + 4 mg/kg i.v.	45–60 min	Higher xylazine dose may cause apnoea
Propofol	About 4 mg/kg i.v.	Short; can be maintained by incremental injections or infusion	Quality of anaesthesia improved by premedication

The combination of xylazine and ketamine is easy to use and produces a longer duration of anaesthesia. In goats, onset of anaesthesia is approximately 5 minutes after i.m. xylazine, 0.1 mg/kg, and ketamine, 11 mg/kg. If attempts at intubation induce chewing movements, an additional injection of xylazine, 0.1 mg/kg, should induce complete relaxation. The duration of surgical anaesthesia is 30–40 minutes. Alternatively, xylazine can be administered i.m. 5 minutes before induction of anaesthesia by i.v. ketamine, 2–4 mg/kg. The duration of anaesthesia is shorter after i.v. compared with i.m. administration. A disadvantage to the use of xylazine and ketamine is that MAP and cardiac output are decreased. This is particularly apparent when xylazine and ketamine are administered prior to halothane or isoflurane, when the combined effects often result in low arterial blood pressure.

A combination of medetomidine, 0.02 mg/kg, and ketamine, 2 mg/kg, has been used to anaes-thetize sheep and the effects reversed by injection of atipamezole, 0.125 mg/kg (Laitinen, 1990; Tulamo *et al.*, 1995). In one study, anaesthesia was continued by a further injection of medetomidine, 0.01 mg/kg, and ketamine, 1 mg/kg, 25 minutes after the first injection (Tulamo *et al.*, 1995). Administration of atipamezole 45 minutes after induction of anaesthesia resulted in the sheep standing on average 15 minutes later. With this anaesthetic protocol hypoxaemia and moderate hypoventilation develop, and cardiac arrest at induction has been reported (Tulamo *et al.*, 1995). Endotracheal intubation and supplementation with oxygen is advisable during anaesthesia.

Tiletamine-zolazepam

Intravenous administration of tiletamine-zolazepam produces longer lasting anaesthesia than diazepam-ketamine. Tiletamine-zolazepam may not provide sufficient analgesia for laparotomy and an additional drug should be included for analgesia. In one report, i.v. butorphanol, 0.5 mg/kg, and tiletamine-zolazepam, 12 mg/kg i.v. resulted in 35 minutes of anaesthesia (25–50 minutes) (Howard *et al.*, 1990). Mean arterial pressures and heart rates were sustained at acceptable values, and cardiac output decreased by an average of 30%. Apnoea was present immediately after induction for up to 72 seconds followed by apneustic breathing patterns and hypoxaemia was present for the first 10 minutes of anaesthesia. Mild hypoventilation persisted for longer than the anaesthesia time.

The combination of i.v. tiletamine-zolazepam, 6.6 mg/kg, with i.v. ketamine, 6.6 mg/kg, and xylazine, 0.11 mg/kg, resulted in a longer duration of anaesthesia, 83 ± 27 min (mean and standard deviation), and a protracted recovery, mean 4 hours (Lin *et al.*, 1994). Hypotension was present 30 minutes after induction and persisted for the remainder of anaesthesia. Blood gas analyses were not performed, however, it is probable that hypoxaemia developed in these animals.

Saffan

Anaesthesia may be induced in healthy sheep and goats by the intravenous injection of 3 mg/kg

Saffan and this is sufficient for intubation and a smooth transition to inhalation anaesthesia. When Saffan is to be used as sole agent in lambs and kids for disbudding, recommended intravenous dose rates are 4–6 mg/kg.

The effects of Saffan on the heart rate, arterial blood pressure (ABP) and respiratory rate are dose-dependent. Saffan at 2.2 mg/kg i.v. produces a short-lived decrease in heart rate and ABP with some slowing of respiration. This dose may produce about 10 minutes of surgical anaesthesia with recovery to the standing position about 20 minutes after injection. A dose of 4.4 mg/kg Saffan may produce a longer duration of decreased heart rate and ABP, and about 15 minutes of anaesthesia with complete recovery after a further 30 minutes.

Propofol

Propofol has a licence for clinical use in dogs and cats. Its chief advantage lies in its rapid detoxification and elimination resulting in rapid recovery from anaesthesia, even after multiple supplements. Propofol, 5–7 mg/kg i.v. in unpremedicated sheep and goats will induce anaesthesia sufficient for endotracheal intubation (Pablo *et al.*, 1997). Apnoea is common but regurgitation should not be a problem if food and water have been withheld before anaesthesia. Premedication with acepromazine, 0.05 mg/kg, and papaveretum, 0.4 mg/kg, (Correia *et al.*, 1996), or detomidine, 0.01 mg/kg, and butorphanol, 0.1 mg/kg (Carroll *et al.*, 1998), all given i.m. decreased the dose of propofol for intubation to approximately 4 mg/kg.

Anaesthesia can be maintained with an inhalant anaesthetic or maintained by continuous infusion of propofol. The cardiopulmonary effects during anaesthesia maintained with halothane or isoflurane will reflect the influence of the inhalant. Recovery from anaesthesia is usually smooth and rapid.

The infusion rate of propofol to maintain anaesthesia for surgery is within the range 0.3 to 0.6 mg/kg/min and depends on the presence or absence of premedication and the intensity of the surgical stimulus. The animals should be less responsive to the surgical stimulus when they have been premedicated with a sedative or a sedative and opioid combination. Moderate to severe

hypoventilation occurs in sheep and goats during continuous propofol anaesthesia, resulting in hypercapnia (Lin *et al.*, 1997; Carroll *et al.*, 1998). Consequently, endotracheal intubation and supplementation with O_2 is recommended, either by insufflation of O_2 at 50–100 ml/kg/min into the endotracheal tube or by giving 100% O_2 from an anaesthesia machine. MAP may be low after induction of anaesthesia with propofol but should progressively rise with time. Recovery from anaesthesia is rapid with the animals standing 10 to 20 minutes after propofol infusion is discontinued.

Combination of propofol with ketamine is an alternative technique for total intravenous anaesthesia that has been tried in sheep (Correia *et al.*, 1996). Induction was achieved with propofol, 3 mg/kg, and ketamine, 1 mg/kg. Anaesthesia was maintained for the first 20 minutes with a combined infusion of propofol, 0.3 mg/kg/min, with ketamine, 0.2 mg/kg/min. This infusion rate was subsequently decreased to 0.2 mg/kg/min of propofol and 0.1 mg/kg/min of ketamine. Recovery from anaesthesia was rapid and free from excitement.

Guaiphenesin (guaifenesin, glyceryl guaiacolate, GGE)

Maintenance of anaesthesia with an infusion of guaiphenesin and ketamine after induction with xylazine and ketamine is a common protocol for total intravenous anaesthesia (TIVA) in cattle over 200 kg body weight (see Chapter 12). Guaiphenesin is not often used in sheep and goats because of its cost, but it can be used. One report described anaesthesia of sheep with an infusion of guaiphenesin, 50 mg/ml, ketamine, 1 mg/ml, and xylazine, 0.1 mg/ml, combined in 5% dextrose in water. Anaesthesia was induced by rapid administration of 1.2 ml/kg of the mixture and maintained by infusion at 2.6 ml/kg/h (Lin *et al.*, 1993). The sheep were intubated and breathing air. Respiratory rates were fast and the animals were severely hypoxaemic with an average PaO_2 of 4.8 kPa (36.4 mmHg) at 30 minutes of anaesthesia. Heart rates and MAPs remained within acceptable ranges of values. Recovery was smooth with time from termination of infusion to standing of 96 ± 50 minutes. The advantage of the technique is the constant level of anaesthesia that can be produced by a continuous infusion. Nonetheless, the severity of the decrease in PaO_2 introduces potential for a fatal outcome unless O_2 administration is included in the technique.

INHALATION ANAESTHESIA

Inhalation anaesthesia is a popular and reasonably safe technique for providing anaesthesia for surgery and medical diagnostic procedures. Halothane/O_2 and isoflurane/O_2 are the most commonly used inhalation anaesthetics in ruminants. They offer advantages over injectable agents of easy control of the depth of anaesthesia, O_2 that usually prevents hypoxaemia, and rapid recovery from anaesthesia. The greatest disadvantages are the production of respiratory and cardiovascular depression that may require treatment with IPPV and vasoactive drugs.

Tracheal intubation prior to halothane or isoflurane anaesthesia is usually accomplished after anaesthesia is first induced with injectable agents. Induction of anaesthesia with the inhalant delivered through a facemask is less desirable in an adult sheep or goat. The longer time for induction allows accumulation of saliva in the pharynx and increases the time before endotracheal intubation, during which regurgitation and aspiration can occur. Induction with an inhalant also requires that deep anaesthesia is induced to facilitate endotracheal intubation, and this is often accompanied by a significant decrease in ABP. Furthermore, induction using a mask is often physically resented by the adult animal. In contrast, young lambs and kids are easily induced with halothane or isoflurane via facemask.

Anaesthetic breathing systems that are used for dogs can be used for sheep and goats. The initial vaporizer setting will depend on the anaesthetic agents used for induction of anaesthesia and the type of breathing system. For example, after induction and intubation in animals anaesthetized with acepromazine and thiopental, or butorphanol, diazepam and ketamine, and connection to a circle circuit, a halothane vaporizer (vaporizer out of circle) may be set at 1.5% or the isoflurane vaporizer at 2.0 or 2.5% with an oxygen flow rate of 1 to 2 l/min. In contrast, after induction of anaes-

thesia with xylazine and ketamine, or with tiletamine-zolazepam, the central nervous system depression is greater and the vaporizer setting should be lower, for example, 0.50 to 0.75% halothane or 1% isoflurane. In either case, as the depth of anaesthesia changes with time and onset of surgery, the vaporizer setting can be adjusted up or down as needed. After about 20 minutes, when the blood anaesthetic concentrations are more stable, O_2 flow can be reduced to 1.0 or 0.5 l/min, if desired, to limit wastage of inhalant agent.

Lambs and kids may be connected to a T-piece or Bain circuit. The inspired anaesthetic concentration is the same as the vaporizer setting and thus during maintenance of anaesthesia should be about 1.0 to 1.5 % for halothane or 1.4 to 1.8% for isoflurane, depending on the degree of preanaesthetic sedation provided.

Halothane, isoflurane, and sevoflurane

All these agents cause dose-dependent decreases in ABP and cardiac output. MAC value for sevoflurane has been reported as 3.3% in sheep and 2.7% in goats (Clarke, 1999).

Nitrous oxide (N_2O)

A major disadvantage of N_2O is that it rapidly diffuses into the rumen and causes bloat and respiratory compromise. However, N_2O can be used as an adjunct to injectable anaesthesia or used to supplement and decrease the requirement for halothane or isoflurane. Low flows must not be used with N_2O and a circle rebreathing system. Gas flows for a small sheep or goat should be 1 l/min each of O_2 and N_2O, with an increase to 2 l/min of each for very large animals.

ANAESTHETIC MANAGEMENT

Positioning

During anaesthesia, the head and neck should be positioned so that the nose is lower than the pharynx for drainage of saliva and any regurgitated ruminal fluid. Salivation will continue throughout anaesthesia and saliva ceases to flow from the mouth only when it is accumulating in the pharynx or because a deep plane of anaesthesia has decreased production.

Fluid therapy

Balanced electrolyte solution, such as lactated Ringer's solution at 10 ml/kg/h, should be infused i.v. when surgery is being performed or when anaesthesia time becomes extended. Animals less than age 3 months should also receive 5% dextrose in water at 2 to 5 ml/kg/h. Occasionally an adult ruminant develops hypoglycaemia, and this should be suspected any time that recovery is more prolonged, or after recovery from the immediate effects of the anaesthetic if the animal is more lethargic than anticipated.

Monitoring

The position of the eyeball during inhalation anaesthesia in goats and sheep is similar to the pattern observed in anaesthetized dogs; the eye rolls rostroventral between light and medium depth anaesthesia, and returns to a central position during deep plane of anaesthesia. Occasionally during light anaesthesia the eye will rotate dorsally ('star gazing'). The palpebral reflex is lost in medium to deep anaesthesia. The pupil should be merely a slit during an adequate plane of inhalation anaesthesia and dilates in light or deep anaesthesia. The pupil dilates after ketamine administration although, if the dose rate is low, the pupil may close down during inhalation anaesthesia.

Respiratory rates are usually 15–30 breaths/minute; higher rates are associated with hypoventilation or hypoxaemia. Oxygen saturation and pulse rate can be monitored using a pulse oximeter with a probe on the tongue. The depth of each breath is impaired when these animals are supine and moderate to severe hypercapnia usually develops during inhalation anaesthesia. Oxygenation is usually adequate when the inspired gas is O_2 rich. Rumen bloat may develop during anaesthesia despite preoperative fasting, pressing on the diaphragm and further impairing ventilation. Bloating can often be relieved by passage of a wide bore tube through the mouth into the rumen, but the tube may become blocked. Tachycardia, and sometimes hypertension, may develop as a con-

sequence of the hypercapnia and these will return to normal values after the onset of controlled ventilation. Other potential consequences of hypoventilation are the lack of adequate anaesthesia during inhalation anaesthesia despite a high vaporizer setting, and hepatic ischaemia as a result of hypercapnia-induced splanchnic vasoconstriction. A near normal $PaCO_2$ results when IPPV is applied at 12 breaths/min and an inspiratory pressure of 20–25 cmH$_2$O or tidal volume of 15 ml/kg.

Peripheral arteries that are easily palpated or can be used for indirect methods of blood pressure measurement are on the caudomedial side of the forelimb above or below the carpus and on the hindlimb on the dorsal surface of the metatarsus (Fig. 13.10). The median and caudal auricular arteries on the outside surface of the ear can be used for needle or catheter placement for direct

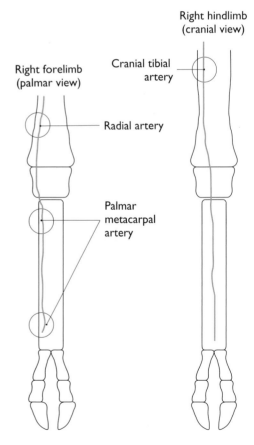

FIG. 13.10 Schematic drawing of the arteries on fore- and hindlimbs for palpation of pulses and indirect blood pressure measurement.

measurement of arterial pressure and for collection of blood for pH and blood gas analysis (see Chapter 2, Fig. 2.15). Heart rates are most frequently between 60 and 120 beats/minute. Heart rates less than 55 beats/min should be considered to constitute bradycardia and heart rates greater than 140 beats/min should be investigated for possible abnormal cause. MAP should be above 70 mmHg during anaesthesia.

It is not uncommon for the animal's temperature to decrease to 37.2 °C (99 °F) before anaesthesia after 24 hours without food. Hypothermia may develop during anaesthesia and efforts should be made to prevent heat loss. Sheep and goats require external application of heat when rectal temperature decreases to 35.5 °C (96 °F) to avoid prolonged recovery. Conversely, anaesthesia in a hot environment may result in hyperthermia.

Treatment of hypotension

Mean pressures below 65 mmHg should be treated appropriately according to the suspected cause of hypotension. Treatment might include a 10 to 20 ml/kg bolus of electrolyte solution intravenously and lightening the depth of anaesthesia. Cardiovascular stimulation may be achieved by administration of a catecholamine, such as an intravenous bolus of ephedrine, 0.03–0.06 mg/kg, or an infusion of dopamine or dobutamine at 5–7 μg/kg/min of a 100 μg/ml solution in 0.9% saline. Blood loss can be treated initially by infusion of lactated Ringer's solution at 2 to 3 times the volume of blood lost and by decreasing anaesthetic administration.

Recovery

The animal should be placed prone at the end of anaesthesia. When bloat is present ruminal gas should be heard and smelled at the mouth. Regurgitation during anaesthesia is not a problem when the endotracheal tube is present and the cuff inflated to produce an airtight seal. Solid rumen material should be removed from the pharynx before the end of anaesthesia. It must be remembered that regurgitation may occur when the animal is waking up. Consequently, the endotracheal tube must not be removed until the animal is chewing, swallowing, and can withdraw its tongue

back into its mouth; this may be a considerable time after the animal is able to lift up its head. Recovery is usually quiet and, unlike horses, ruminants may be in no hurry to stand after anaesthesia. Full control of swallowing and gastrointestinal motility may not return for several hours after xylazine administration and feeding must be delayed. Hay or grass and water may be allowed 3 hours after anaesthesia with most other agents used in these species.

Pain relief

The relief of postoperative pain demands the same care in goats and sheep as in all other animals. Signs of pain are not as obvious as in some other species. Shivering may be a sign of anxiety. Immobility, vocalization, or grinding the teeth may be indicators that the animal is experiencing pain. Systemic administration of opioids may include i.m. 2 to 4 mg/kg of pethidine, 0.2 mg/kg of butorphanol, or 0.006 to 0.010 mg/kg of buprenorphine. Epidural injection of 0.1 mg/kg of morphine will provide analgesia for procedures on the hindlimbs or abdomen.

OTHER HERBIVORES

LLAMAS (*lama glama*) AND ALPACAS (*lama pacos*)

Llamas may weigh up to 200 kg and live up to 20 years. Alpaca males weigh on average 60 kg. These animals should be handled with care as llamas can kick, swinging the limb forward and out, and males may bite. Use of side rails is not advised, as a leg can be broken. Some commercial llama chutes incorporate straps which are passed under the animal's thorax and caudal abdomen to prevent the animal assuming sternal recumbency. Most llamas and alpacas tolerate a halter with a rope lead. Suggestions for manual restraint include holding the haltered head and exerting the full force of your weight on the hindlimbs to force the animal into a sternal recumbent submissive position (cush) (Jessup & Lance, 1982). This works because the forelimbs are the main weight bearers and the hindlimbs cannot be locked up. Tapping

TABLE 13.3 Comparison of mean times for onset and duration of epidural analgesia with 2% lignocaine, 0.22 mg/kg, and diluted 10% xylazine, 0.17 mg/kg, in six llamas (Grubb et al., 1993)

Treatment	Onset (min)	Duration (min)
Lignocaine	3	71
Xylazine	21	187
Lignocaine/xylazine	4	326

behind the knee of the forelimb may help. Weanling or yearlings should not be tied as they may struggle and injure cervical vertebrae. Aggressive handling or striking an animal will result in fear, distrust and spitting.

Caudal epidural analgesia

Caudal epidural injection of lignocaine, xylazine, or a combination of these has been evaluated in llamas (Grubb et al., 1993). Injections were made into the sacrococcygeal space where the epidural space is shallow and easily entered. The procedure was performed with a 20 gauge, 2.5 cm long needle inserted at a 60° angle to the base of the tail. Onset of action was rapid after injection of lignocaine and analgesia lasted longest when a combination of lignocaine and xylazine was used (Table 13.3). Ataxia did not develop, although the llamas tended to lie down. The dose rate of xylazine used in this study was toward the high end of the dose range used in ruminants and from which some systemic effects are to be expected. Mild sedation developed in half the llamas given xylazine, beginning about 20 minutes after injection and lasting for 20–30 minutes. The synergistic effect on duration of analgesia caused by combining xylazine with lignocaine is similar to that in horses.

Local analgesia for castration

A technique for castration in the standing llama has been performed in more than 100 animals without complications (Barrington et al., 1993). Butorphanol, 0.1 mg/kg, i.m. was administered 15 minutes before applying a surgical scrub to the perineal region. Lignocaine, 2–5 ml of a 2% solu-

tion, was injected into each testicle until it became turgid and a further 1–2 ml was deposited subcutaneously at the site of the proposed incision as the needle was withdrawn. The lower dose of lignocaine is recommended for llamas weighing less than 30 kg. These authors noted that llamas given butorphanol are not sedated but also that they do not exhibit the signs of discomfort and restlessness during the procedure that have been observed in animals castrated with only local analgesia.

Preparation for anaesthesia

A number of publications are available documenting the reference ranges for haematological and biochemical values in llamas and alpacas (Fowler & Zinkl, 1989; Hajduk, 1992). In comparison with common domestic ruminants, llamas and alpacas may have higher erythrocyte counts ($11-14 \times 10^{12}$/litre) and small mean corpuscular volume, with packed cell volumes of 0.25–0.45 litres/litre. Blood glucose levels of 108 to 156 mg/dl were measured in nursing 2 to 6 month old llamas compared with 74 to 154 mg/dl in adult llamas.

Preparation for anaesthesia is the same as for sheep and goats. Bloat, regurgitation, and aspiration can occur in llamas and, therefore, the animals should be fasted for 24 hours and water withheld for 8 to 12 hours before elective anaesthesia. Young calves (cria) may take solid food as early as 2 weeks but weaning may not occur until age 4 to 7 months. Fasting is not usually done in paediatric patients because of the risk of hypoglycaemia except that suckling is prevented for 30 to 60 minutes before anaesthesia. A rapid induction and intubation sequence is necessary for emergency procedures in animals that are not fasted.

Severe bradycardia may develop during halothane anaesthesia (Riebold et al., 1989) and there is some justification for premedication with atropine, 0.02 mg/kg, in contrast to recommendations for sheep and goats.

Anaesthetic techniques

Venepuncture

Jugular venepuncture for collection of blood or placement of a catheter is not as easy as in sheep

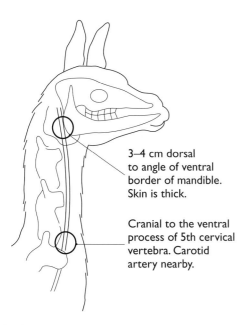

3–4 cm dorsal to angle of ventral border of mandible. Skin is thick.

Cranial to the ventral process of 5th cervical vertebra. Carotid artery nearby.

FIG. 13.11 Schematic drawing showing the landmarks for jugular vein puncture in llamas.

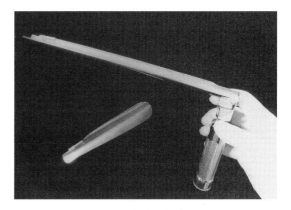

FIG. 13.12 The long 35 cm Wisconsin laryngoscope blade is useful for intubation of adult llamas; seen here in comparison with a blade used for intubation in large dogs.

Endotracheal intubation

The technique for endotracheal intubation is similar to that in sheep and goats. Viewing the laryngeal opening is difficult in adult llamas and a laryngoscope with a long blade is essential (e.g. 35 cm Wisconsin blade, Anesthesia Medical Specialties, Santa Fe Springs, California 90670) (Fig. 13.12). A 10 mm internal diameter tube can be used in a 60 kg llama and a 12 mm in a llama of 100 kg. Intubation in large animals is made easier by inserting a metal rod inside the endotracheal tube to stiffen it.

Llamas are obligate nasal breathers and airway obstruction may occur during anaesthesia in llamas that are not intubated due to dorsal displacement of the soft palate, and during recovery from anaesthesia due to nasal oedema and congestion. Nasotracheal intubation has been recommended in llamas to provide a clear airway during any phase of anaesthesia (Riebold *et al.*, 1994). A long tube will be needed, such as the 40 to 55 cm long tubes manufactured for nasotracheal intubation in foals (Bivona, Gary, Indiana 46406). The internal diameter will be about 2 mm less than the size of tube chosen for orotracheal intubation. The tube should be well lubricated, and lubricant containing phenylephrine can be used to cause vasoconstriction in the nasal mucosa and limit haemorrhage. The tip of the tube is inserted medially and ventrally into the ventral nasal meatus as in horses, with the bevel directed laterally to minimize trauma to the conchae. It is important to keep

and goats. Two sites are recommended (Fig. 13.11) (Amsel *et al.*, 1987). One site is high in the neck at the level of the mandible. An imaginary line is drawn continuous with the ventral border of the mandible and the point of needle insertion is 3 to 4 cm dorsal from its angle in an adult animal. Disadvantages to this site are that the overlying skin is very thick, and movement of the head may dislodge a needle or kink a catheter. The second site is lower on the neck where the ventral processes of the fifth cervical vertebra can be palpated. Placing a thumb in the depression just medial to the ventral process can raise the jugular vein. The overlying skin is less thick, facilitating catheter insertion. A disadvantage to this site is that the carotid artery is nearby and can be penetrated. Observation of pulsatile blood flow through the needle or catheter confirms that the catheter is in the carotid artery and should be withdrawn. A 14 gauge or 16 gauge, 13 cm long catheter is inserted in adult llamas, although prominent valves in the vein may hinder threading of the catheter. Other veins, such as an ear vein, cephalic vein, or saphenous vein can be used in depressed, sedated, or anaesthetized animals.

a finger on the tube inside the nares to ensure that the tube remains in the ventral meatus while the tube is advanced slowly and without twisting. If the tube is in the middle meatus it will impact on the ethmoid and cause significant haemorrhage. A further obstruction to intubation in llamas is the large diverticulum, 1 cm wide and 2 cm deep, at the caudodorsal angle of the nasopharynx. If the tip of the tube is level with the pharynx and it cannot be advanced then the tube should be withdrawn several cm, redirected and advanced again. The arytenoid cartilages and epiglottis protrude above the soft palate into the nasopharynx. Hyperextension of the head and neck may allow the nasotracheal tube to enter the larynx. Alternatively, a laryngoscope can be inserted into the mouth to view the tip of the tube. While the tube is slowly and gently advanced its tip is gripped with forceps or hooked rostrally with a bent stilette and directed into the larynx. Extubation after anaesthesia should be delayed, as in other ruminants, until the animal can withdraw its tongue into its mouth, and this may occur long after the first swallowing and chewing movements are observed.

Anaesthetic agents

Xylazine

Xylazine is often used as a sedative in doses of 0.4–0.6 mg/kg intravenously. This dose will provide 30 to 45 minutes of recumbency. Bradycardia will be induced with little change in blood pressure. Sedation can be reversed with yohimbine but not doxapram. Medetomidine produces dose-dependent light to heavy sedation in llamas, with 0.03 mg/kg i.m. inducing heavy sedation for 1 to 2 hours. The sedative effects of medetomidine can be reversed by i.v. atipamezole, 0.125 mg/kg.

Lower doses of xylazine are adequate for premedication to general anaesthesia. A common anaesthetic combination to provide 30 minutes of anaesthesia in healthy llamas is xylazine, 0.25 mg/kg, i.v. followed in 10 to 15 minutes by injection of ketamine, 2.5 mg/kg i.v. or 5 mg/kg i.m. Butorphanol, 0.1 mg/kg i.m., can be administered at the same time as the xylazine or, 0.05 mg/kg i.v.,

shortly before the ketamine. An alternative combination is xylazine premedication followed by induction of anaesthesia with i.v. diazepam, 0.1–0.2 mg/kg, and ketamine 2.5 mg/kg.

Guaiphenesin

Guaiphenesin, up to 0.5 ml/kg of a 5% solution, is a useful adjunct to anaesthetic induction with ketamine in large llamas. Premedication facilitates the procedure and can consist of a low dose of xylazine, or a combination of diazepam, 0.1 mg/kg, and butorphanol, 0.1 mg/kg. Guaiphenesin is most easily injected into the catheter using a 60 ml syringe and a 14 gauge needle. The llama will usually assume sternal recumbency before ketamine, 2.5 mg/kg, is injected to complete induction of anaesthesia. Dose rates of anaesthetic agents must be decreased for animals that are ill, for example, from urethral obstruction, peritonitis, or intestinal obstruction. Xylazine should be avoided in animals with urethral obstruction.

Propofol

Propofol can be used to anaesthetize llamas but the technique is expensive for large animals. Induction of anaesthesia can be accomplished by 2.0–3.5 mg/kg i.v. Anaesthesia may be maintained with an inhalation agent or by continuous infusion of propofol, 0.4 mg/kg/min. In an investigation of continuous propofol anaesthesia in llamas, MAP remained high and cardiac output was not depressed (Duke *et al.*, 1997). Hypoxaemia did not develop even though the animals were breathing air. Additional analgesia, systemic or local, will be necessary if the procedure is painful.

Inhalation agents

Halothane or isoflurane can maintain anaesthesia and is recommended for major surgery. Injectable agents are used to induce anaesthesia in adults, but induction with the inhalant using a facemask is easy in paediatric animals, particularly after premedication with diazepam and butorphanol. Anaesthetic management is as for sheep and goats described previously in this chapter. The palpebral reflex is usually retained during anaesthesia adequate for surgery. Crinkling of the lower eyelid is an indication of light anaesthesia. Llamas breathe spontaneously at 10 to 30 breaths/minute and appear to ventilate better during anaesthesia than horses or adult cattle, although IPPV should be used if monitoring identifies severe hypoventilation.

DEER

There are detailed recommendations for handling farmed deer, including recommendations for design of deer yards and raceways, deer crushes and chutes, and physical and chemical restraint (Chapman *et al.*, 1987; Fletcher, 1995). The purpose for this section in this textbook is to describe some basic principles of anaesthesia in deer and to refer to articles for further reading on the subject.

Some general guidelines for working with deer include talking to the deer to alert them as to your location and to avoid walking through the middle of a group of deer (Fletcher, 1995). There are recommendations that, except for adult stags, deer are best examined in groups, as they may become frantic when isolated. Deer may become aggressive and kick with their forelimbs, and occasionally bite or kick backward with their hindlimbs (Fletcher, 1995).

There are considerations of special significance to the anaesthetist. Not only are there differences in responses between farmed deer and wildlife, in that wild deer will require higher doses, but also there are differences between the species in their responses to both physical management and anaesthetic agents. An example given in a concise article on deer handling explains that fallow deer (*Dama dama*), unlike red deer (*Cervus elaphus*), respond favourably to darkened holding pens (Fletcher, 1995). Another author notes that while roe deer (*Capreolus capreolus*) or fallow deer may lie impassive when blindfolded and with their legs tied, the technique is not suitable for muntjac (*Muntiacus reevesi*). Muntjac are small excitable deer that will writhe, struggle and jerk violently against restraint. Extraordinary care in the method of capture of these deer has been described (Chapman *et al.*, 1987). Specifically, general anaesthesia was induced with the ultra-short acting barbiturate, methohexital.

Anaesthetic agents

Anaesthetic agents for sedation are frequently administered by darts propelled by a gun or blowpipe, or from a syringe attached to a pole. The dose rate for xylazine varies between the breeds and response to xylazine varies between individuals within a breed. Xylazine alone can be administered i.m. for sedation in penned red or fallow deer at 0.5 to 1.5 mg/kg (Fletcher, 1995), 1 mg/kg for wapiti (*Cervus canadiensis*), and 2 to 3 mg/kg for white-tailed deer (*Odocoileus virginianus*) and mule deer (*Odocoileus hemionus*) (Caulkett, 1997). A lower dosage of xylazine, 0.7 mg/kg, was satisfactory for capturing 104 free-ranging mule deer (Jessup *et al.*, 1985). Reversal of sedation is achieved by administration of yohimbine, 0.1 to 0.2 mg/kg, given half i.v. and half i.m., or tolazoline, 2 to 4 mg/kg.

Xylazine and ketamine have been used to immobilize deer. Dosages of xylazine, 4 mg/kg, and ketamine 4 mg/kg, administered intramuscularly in adult fallow deer induced recumbency in less than 5 minutes (Stewart & English, 1990). Administration of yohimbine 30 minutes later produced satisfactory reversal for release after several minutes. Another recommendation is to mix 400 mg of ketamine with 500 mg of dry xylazine powder and to dose red deer at 1 to 2 ml and fallow deer up to 3 ml (Fletcher, 1995). Xylazine and ketamine may be administered separately. The deer are sedated first with xylazine administered by dart and then ketamine, 1 to 2 mg/kg, injected i.v. when the deer is first approachable (Caulkett, 1997). This decreases the dose of ketamine and there is less chance of central nervous system excitement occurring when the xylazine sedation is reversed. Additional ketamine may be administered as needed.

Detomidine and medetomidine, 60 to 80 μg/kg i.m., administered with ketamine, 1–2 mg/kg i.m., have been used to sedate deer. The effects of detomidine or medetomidine can be reversed by injection of atipamezole at a dose rate of up to five times the medetomidine dose.

Etorphine and acepromazine (Immobilon LA), etorphine and xylazine, and etorphine, acepromazine and xylazine combinations have been used to immobilize a variety of species of deer (Jones, 1984). Excitement has been observed with the etorphine and acepromazine combination (Jones,

1984). A high number of cardiac arrests occurred in fallow deer immobilized with these combinations (Pearce & Kock, 1989).

Other opioid combinations that have been used in deer include carfentanil and xylazine and, available in New Zealand, a premixed solution of fentanyl, azaperone, and xylazine.

Anaesthesia can be deepened for major surgery by the administration of halothane or isoflurane. The vaporizer settings are low for maintenance of anaesthesia, 1% for halothane and 1.5% for isoflurane, particularly when detomidine or medetomidine have been administered.

Rectal temperature should be measured immediately and throughout the procedure. Hyperthermia will develop in animals immobilized outside in the heat of the day. Monitoring pulse rate and oxygen saturation is easily done with a pulse oximeter and a probe applied to the tongue. ABP can be measured non-invasively using the oscillometric technique and the cuff placed around the forelimb above the carpus or by using the Doppler technique and the probe over the coccygeal artery. Direct measurement of ABP can be done with a catheter in an auricular artery.

Local analgesia

Local analgesia is required for harvesting antlers. Investigation of the innervation of the antler pedicle in wapiti and fallow deer identified the infratrochlear and zygomaticotemporal nerves as the largest nerves travelling to the pedicle (Woodbury & Haigh, 1996). In some animals, the auriculopalpebral nerve supplied prominent dorsal branches to the lateral or caudal aspects of the pedicle. There should be no sensory fibres in this nerve. However, there have been reports that block of the auriculopalpebral nerve has achieved local anaesthesia in a small number of deer in which inadequate analgesia was produced by conventional nerve block. No other nerves were found to innervate the antler. Branches of the second cervical nerve were observed to terminate near the base of the ear (Woodbury & Haigh, 1996). Thus, recommendations for nerve block are the conventional block as described earlier for sheep and goats, increasing the volume of lignocaine at each site to 5 ml and depositing the solution deeper, 2 to 3 cm,

for the zygomaticotemporal nerve. Local anaesthetic solution can also be injected over the zygomatic arch, halfway between the base of the ear and the lateral canthus. A ring block can be included should additional analgesia be needed for antler removal.

CAMELS

Handling camels can be dangerous and particular caution must be observed during the breeding season when males may be intractable and vicious. Males may press a person to the ground with their neck and body, a crushing effect, or they may bite, causing severe even fatal injuries (Ogunbodede & Arotiba, 1997). Most experienced anaesthetists prefer whenever possible to work on domesticated camels made by their handlers to sit for this reduces the risk to personnel and to the animal. Tying the forelimb is a common mode of restraint (Fig. 13.13) in animals not trained to lie down on command. Also of interest to the anaesthetist, camels may be susceptible to toxicity from some drugs at doses used commonly in other ruminants. Although the pharmacokinetics of a variety of non-steroidal drugs and antibiotics have been published in recent years, very little information is available about anaesthetic agents.

Heart rates in unsedated resting camels are 40–50 beats/min, mean arterial pressures 130–140 mmHg, and respiratory rates 6–16 breaths/min. Hematologic and biochemical blood values for camels (*Camelus dromedarius*) have been published (Snow *et al.*, 1988; Nazefi & Maleki, 1998).

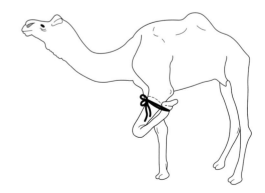

FIG. 13.13 Camels not trained to lie down on command can often be restrained by hobbling the front leg.

Measurements made after racing show that, in contrast to dogs and horses, no significant increase in haematocrit occurs after exercise due to release of red cells from the spleen. Although packed cell volume is on average 0.33 litres/litre, camel erythrocytes have a very high mean corpuscular haemoglobin concentration.

Voluntary regurgitation of rumen contents may occur in agitated camels and withholding of roughage for 48 hours and concentrate for 24 hours before anaesthesia has been recommended. Domestic camels may sit on command (couched) which avoids the need for casting or the risk of injury with ataxia or falling after administration of anaesthetic agents.

Local and regional analgesia

Nerve blocks of the hindlimb in camels have been described, including the topographical anatomy and technique to block the peroneal, tibial, and plantar nerves (Dudi *et al.*, 1984). Desensitization of the digit can also be achieved using intravenous regional analgesia by injecting 60 ml of 2% lignocaine (without adrenaline) distal to a tourniquet (Purohit *et al.*, 1985). Xylazine sedation has been combined with a line block with 2% lignocaine to provide satisfactory restraint and analgesia for caesarian section to remove dead foetuses (Elias, 1991).

Xylazine, 0.4 mg/kg i.m. , given to healthy adult camels (*Camelus dromedarius*) (Peshin *et al.*, 1980) and *Camelus bactrianus* (Custer *et al.*, 1977)) results in sternal recumbency in 11–15 minutes and a recumbency time of 1–2 hours. The cardiovascular effects of xylazine administration are qualitatively similar to those in sheep and goats in that xylazine induces bradycardia, an increase in CVP, and a small but statistically significant decrease in MAP, bottoming out at 45 minutes.

Smaller doses of xylazine, 0.25 mg/kg, have been used in combination with ketamine, 2.5 mg/kg i.m., for sedation and analgesia in the dromedary camel (White *et al.*, 1987). Loss of facial expression, drooping of the lower lip, weaving of the head, and drooling of saliva occur at the onset of sedation. Most camels lay their head and neck on the ground and would assume lateral recumbency if allowed.

In six camels (*Camelus dromedarius*) satisfactory anaesthesia for tracheal intubation was achieved with a mean thiopental dose of 7.25 mg/kg (Singh *et al.*, 1994). Subsequent maintenance of anaesthesia with halothane resulted in hypoventilation and a significant decrease in ABP. The camels recovered from anaesthesia on average 40 minutes after the halothane was discontinued. The authors noted that O_2 supplementation was necessary during recovery from anaesthesia to prevent hypoxaemia. Anaesthesia can also be induced with a mixture of thiopental and guaiphenesin prior to halothane anaesthesia. In camels injected i.m. with xylazine, 0.25 mg/kg, 30 minutes previously, 1.0–2.3 ml/kg of thiopental-guaiphenesin (2 g thiopental in 1 litre 5% guaiphenesin) given rapidly i.v. produces sufficient relaxation for intubation (White *et al.*, 1986). IPPV was employed to treat hypoventilation and MAPs were satisfactory.

Intubation of the trachea can be done manually using the same techniques that are used in cattle. Male dromedary camels have a dulaa (palatal flap or goola pouch) which extends from the soft palate (White *et al.*, 1986).

ELEPHANTS

Trained elephants are usually relatively quiet and intravenous injection can be made into an ear vein. Drug administration to free-ranging animals is by dart gun. Accurate estimates of body weight are useful when calculating drug dosages in an attempt to produce consistent anaesthetic effects. Body measurements from 75 Asian elephants (*Elephas maximus*) from 1 to 57 years of age were used to calculate correlations with body weight (Hile *et al.*, 1997). The authors concluded that in Asian elephants the heart girth is the best predictor of weight. Heart girth (cm) was measured just behind the front legs using cotton twine. Weight was predicted using the equation:

$$\text{Weight (kg)} = 18.0\,(\text{heart girth}) - 3336.$$

Measurement of pad circumference was not a useful predictor of weight.

Immobilization

Etorphine has frequently been used to immobilize elephants. Free ranging African elephants

(*Loxodonta africana*) were immobilized by i.m. injection by darts with 9.5 ± 0.5 mg etorphine (Osofsky, 1997) or 3, 6, or 9 mg of etorphine and 30, 60, or 100 mg of azaperone according to size in juvenile elephants (mean weight 672 kg) (Still *et al.*, 1996). The mean time to recumbency was 9 minutes. Additional etorphine had to be administered intravenously to maintain immobilization for transportation. All elephants recovered uneventfully after reversal by i.v. diprenorphine at approximately three times the dose of etorphine administered. In another report, etorphine, 0.002 mg/kg, was given i.m. or i.v. to provide satisfactory immobilization for laparotomy for castration (Foerner *et al.*, 1994). Supplements of 1 mg of etorphine were injected as needed to maintain immobilization.

Up to one-third of the elephants immobilized with etorphine are reported to be hypoxaemic as determined by pulse oximetry or blood gas analysis. At an average respiratory rate of 9 breaths per minute, $PaCO_2$ was only mildly to moderately increased. The average PaO_2 of the immobilized elephants in one study, 10.0 ± 1.7 kPa (75 ± 13 mmHg) (Still *et al.*, 1996), was lower than previously reported for recumbent elephants, 11.2 ± 0.4 kPa (84 ± 3 mmHg), or standing unpremedicated elephants, 12.8 ± 0.3 kPa (96 ± 2 mmHg) (Honeyman *et al.*, 1992). Hypoxaemia occurred only in elephants with a body mass <600 kg (Still *et al.*, 1996). The authors suggested that this effect in the smaller elephants may have been due in part to administration of a relatively larger dose of anaesthetic agents. A possible explanation proposed for the adequacy of ventilation in the larger animals is that the anatomical features of elephants oppose collapse of lung. These features include the lack of a pleural space and presence of a well-developed supportive system of elastic fibres in the lungs and pulmonary vessels.

ABP was measured from a 20 gauge catheter in an auricular artery in another group of six, adult male African elephants, weighing approximately 5000 kg, immobilized with etorphine, 8 mg. MAP during immobilization without stimulation was 186 ± 15 mmHg. This value was higher than the value of 145 ± 3 mmHg reported for standing elephants (Honeyman *et al.*, 1992).

Inhalation anaesthesia

General anaesthesia can be maintained in elephants with halothane or isoflurane when the equipment is available. In a series of anaesthetic episodes in juvenile (3–5-year-old) African elephants weighing 308 ± 93 kg, premedication consisted of xylazine, 0.1 mg/kg, and ketamine, 0.6 mg/kg, administered intramuscularly (Heard *et al.*, 1988). Induction of anaesthesia was accomplished 45 minutes later by i.m. etorphine, 0.0019 ± 0.00056 mg/kg, which produced recumbency in a mean time of 20 minutes. Endotracheal tubes of 18, 22, and 26 mm were used in elephants weighing 250–304 kg, 204–350 kg, and 280–636 kg, respectively. Wads of food were seen in the oropharynx in these animals despite food having been withheld for 24 hours. After removal of food from the oropharynx, the trachea was intubated blindly or by manual palpation of the larynx and guiding the endotracheal tube into the trachea. Halothane was administered via a large animal rebreathing circle system using low vaporizer settings (0.5–1.0%).

Respiratory arrest occurred in one animal after induction of anaesthesia and was treated with a half dose of diprenorphine i.v. (Heard *et al.*, 1988). ABP was lower than recorded for etorphine alone with recorded mean systolic blood pressure of 106 ± 19 mmHg and heart rate of 50 ± 12 beats per minute. Administration of dobutamine was necessary in one animal to treat hypotension. Increases in blood pressure and increases in trunk muscle tone or ear flapping were indicators that the depth of anaesthesia was becoming light. Diprenorphine i.v. was given at twice the original etorphine dose about 10 minutes after halothane was discontinued.

An anaesthetic delivery system for isoflurane was devised for an adult 3500 kg African elephant by joining two standard large animal anaesthesia machines in parallel (Dunlop *et al.*, 1994). The elephant was anaesthetized on three occasions, twice with etorphine and once with etorphine and azaperone. The trachea was intubated with a 40 mm ID tube by digital palpation in a manner similar to that used to intubate adult cattle and the aid of a stomach tube as a guide. Tachycardia and hypertension were recorded initially, but these values decreased to within normal ranges after administration of isoflurane. Anaesthesia times were from 2.4 to 3.3 hours and the elephant recovered satisfactorily after each episode. O_2 was insufflated at 60 l/min into the endotracheal tube during recovery from anaesthesia. Residual etorphine was reversed by administration of diprenorphine 25 to 40 minutes after isoflurane was discontinued.

REFERENCES

Alahuhta, S., Kangas-Saarela, T., Hollmen, A.I. and Edstrom, H.H. (1990) Visceral pain during caesarian section under spinal and epidural anaesthesia with bupivacaine. *Acta Anaesthesiologica Scandinavica* **34**: 95–98.

Aminkov, B.Y. and Hubenov, H.D. (1995) The effect of xylazine epidural anaesthesia on blood gas and acid-base parameters in rams. *British Veterinary Journal* **151**: 579–585.

Amsel, S.I., Kainer, R.A. and Johnson, L.W. (1987) Choosing the best site to perform venipuncture in a llama. *Veterinary Medicine* **82**: 535–536.

Barrington, G.M., Meyer, T.F. and Parish, S.M. (1993) Standing castration of the llama using butorphanol tartrate and local anesthesia. *Equine Practice* **15**: 35–39.

Carroll, G.L., Hooper, R.N., Slater, M.R., Hartsfield, S.M. and Matthews, N.S. (1998) Detomidine-butorphanol-propofol for carotid artery translocation and castration or ovariectomy in goats. *Veterinary Surgery* **27**: 75–82.

Caulkett, N.A. (1997) Anesthesia for North American cervids. *Canadian Veterinary Journal* **38**: 389–390.

Celly, C.S., McDonell, W.N., Young, S.S. and Black, W.D. (1997) The comparative hypoxaemic effect of four α2 adrenoceptor agonists (xylazine, romifidine, detomidine and medetomidine) in sheep. *Journal of Veterinary Pharmacology and Therapeutics* **20**: 464–471.

Celly, C.S., Atwal, O.S., McDonell, W.N. and Black, W.D. (1999) Histopathalogic alterations induced in the lungs of sheep by use of alpha2-adrenergic receptor agonists. *American Journal of Veterinary Research* **60**: 154–161.

Chapman, N.G., Claydon, K., Cl;aydon, M. and Harris, S. (1987) Techniques for the safe and humane capture of free-living muntjac deer (*Muntiacus reevesi*). *British Veterinary Journal* **143**: 35–43.

Clarke, K.W. (1999) Desflurane and sevoflurane. New volatile anesthetic agents. *Veterinary Clinics of North America Small Animal Practice* **29**: 793–810.

Correia, D., Nolan, A.M. and Reid, J. (1996) Pharmacokinetics of propofol infusions, either alone or with ketamine, in sheep premedicated with acepromazine and papaveretum. *Research in Veterinary Science* **60**: 213–217.

Custer, R., Kramer, L., Kennedy, S. and Bush, M. (1977) Hematologic effects of xylazine when used for restraint of bactrian camels. *Journal of the American Veterinary Medical Association* **171**: 899–901.

Dudi, P.R., Chouhan, D.S., Choudhary, R.J., Deora, K.S. and Gahlot, T.K. (1984) A study of topographic anatomy and nerve blocks of hindlimb in camels (*Camelus dromedarius*). *Indian Veterinary Journal* **61**: 848–853.

Duke, T., Egger, C.M., Ferguson, J.G. and Frketic, M.M. (1997) Cardiopulmonary effects of propofol infusion in llamas. *American Journal of Veterinary Research* **58**: 153–156.

Dunlop, C.I., Hodgson, D.S., Cambre, R.C., Kenny, D.E. and Martin, H.D. (1994) Cardiopulmonary effects of three prolonged periods of isoflurane anesthesia in an adult elephant. *Journal of the American Veterinary Medical Association* **205**: 1439–1444.

Elias, E. (1991) Left ventrolateral cesarean section in three dromedary camels (*Camelus dromedarius*). *Veterinary Surgery* **20**: 323–325.

Fletcher, J. (1995) Handling farmed deer. *In Practice* **17**: 30–37.

Foerner, J.J., Houck, R.I., Copeland, J.F., Byron, H.T. and Olsen, J.H. (1994) Surgical castration of the elephant (*Elephas maximus and Loxodonta africana*). *Journal of Zoo and Wildlife Medicine* **25**: 355–359.

Fowler, M.E. and Zinkl, J.G. (1989) Reference ranges for hematologic and serum biochemical values in llamas. *American Journal of Veterinary Research* **50**: 2049–2053.

Grubb, T.L., Riebold, T.W. and Huber, M.J. (1993) Evaluation of lidocaine, xylazine, and a combination of lidocaine and xylazine for epidural analgesia in llamas. *Journal of the American Veterinary Medical Association* **203**: 1441–1444.

Hajduk, P. (1992) Haematological reference values for alpacas. *Australian Veterinary Journal* **69**: 89–90.

Heard, D.J., Kollias, G.V., Webb, A.I., Jacobson, E.R. and Brock, K.A. (1988) Use of halothane to maintain anesthesia induced with etorphine in juvenile African elephants. *Journal of the American Veterinary Medical Association* **193**: 254–256.

Heard, D.J., Nichols, W.W., Buss, D. and Kollias, G.V. (1996) Comparative cardiopulmonary effects of intramuscularly administered etorphine and carfentanil in goats. *American Journal of Veterinary Research* **57**: 87–96.

Hendrickson, D.A., Kruse-Elliot, K.T. and Broadstone, R.V. (1996) A comparison of epidural saline, morphine, and bupivacaine for pain relief after abdominal surgery in goats. *Veterinary Surgery* **25**: 83–87.

Hile, M.E., Hintz, H.F. and Erb, H.N. (1997) Predicting body weight from body measurements in Asian elephants (*Elephas maximus*). *Journal of Zoo and Wildlife Medicine* **28**: 424–427.

Honeyman, V.L., Pettifer, G.R. and Dyson, D.H. (1992) Arterial blood pressure and blood gas values in normal standing and laterally recumbent African (*Loxodonta africana*) and Asian (*Elephas maximus*) elephants. *Journal of Zoo and Wildlife Medicine* **23**: 205–210.

Howard, B.W., Lagutchik, M.S., Januszkiewicz, A.J. and Martin, D.G. (1990) The cardiovascular response of sheep to tiletamine-zolazepam and butorphanol tartrate anesthesia. *Veterinary Surgery* **19**: 461–467.

Jessup, D.A. and Lance, W.R. (1982) What veterinarians should know about South American camelids. *California Veterinarian* **11**: 12–18.

Jessup, D.A., Jones, K., Mohr, R. and Kucera, T. (1985) Yohimbine antagonism to xylazine in free-ranging mule deer and desert bighorn sheep. *Journal of the American Veterinary Medical Association* **187**: 1251–1253.

Jones, D.M. (1984) Physical and chemical methods of capturing deer. *Veterinary Record* **114**: 109–112.

Kyles, A.E., Waterman, A.E. and Livingston, A. (1995) Antinociceptive activity of midazolam in sheep. *Journal of Veterinary Pharmacology and Therapeutics* **18**: 54–60.

Laitinen, O.M. (1990) Clinical observations on medetomidine/ketamine anaesthesia in sheep and its reversal by atipamezole. *Journal of the Association of Veterinary Anaesthetists* **17**: 17–19.

Ley, S., Waterman, A. and Livingston, A. (1990) Variation in the analgesic effects of xylazine in different breeds of sheep. *Veterinary Record* **126**: 508.

Lin, H.-C., Purohit, R.C. and Rowe, T.A. (1997) Anesthesia in sheep with propofol or with xylazine-ketamine followed by halothane. *Veterinary Surgery* **26**: 247–252.

Lin, H.-C., Tyler, J.W., Welles, E.G., Spano, J.S., Thurmon, J.C. and Wolfe, D.F. (1993) Effects of anesthesia induced and maintained by continuous intravenous administration of guaifenesin, ketamine, and xylazine in spontaneously breathing sheep. *American Journal of Veterinary Research* **54**: 1913–1916.

Lin, H.C., Wallace, S.S., Tyler, J.W., Robbins, R.L., Thurmon, J.C. and Wolfe, D.F. (1994) Comparison of tiletamine-zolazepam-ketamine and tiletamine-zolazepam-ketamine-xylazine anaesthesia in sheep. *Australian Veterinary Journal* **71**: 239–242.

Nazefi, S. and Maleki, K. (1998) Biochemical analysis of serum and cerebrospinal fluid in clinically normal adult camels (*Camelus dromedarius*). *Research in Veterinary Science* **65**: 83–84.

Ogunbodede, E.O. and Arotiba, J.T. (1997) Camel bite injuries of the orofacial region: report of a case. *Journal of Oral and Maxillofacial Surgery* **55**: 1174–1176.

Osofsky, S.A. (1997) A practical anesthesia monitoring protocol for free-ranging adult African elephants (*Loxodonta africana*). *Journal of Wildlife Diseases* **33**: 72–77.

Pablo, L.S. (1993) Epidural morphine in goats after hindlimb orthopedic surgery. *Veterinary Surgery* **22**: 307–310.

Pablo, L.S., Bailey, J.E. and Ko, J.C.H. (1997) Median effective dose of propofol required for induction of anesthesia in goats. *Journal of the American Veterinary Medical Association* **211**: 86–88.

Pearce, P.C. and Kock, R.A. (1989) Physiological effects of etorphine, acepromazine and xylazine on the black fallow deer (*Dama dama*). *Research in Veterinary Science* **46**: 380–386.

Peshin, P.K., Nigam, J.M., Singh, S.C. and Robinson, B.A. (1980) Evaluation of xylazine in camels. *Journal of the American Veterinary Medical Association* **177**: 875–878.

Purohit, N.R., Chouhan, D.S., Chaudhary, R.J. and Deora, K.S. (1985) Intravenous regional anaesthesia in camel. *Indian Journal of Animal Sciences* **55**: 435–436.

Riebold, T.W., Kaneps, A.J. and Schmotzer, W.B. (1989) Anesthesia in the llama. *Veterinary Surgery* **18**: 400–404.

Riebold, T.W., Engel, H.N., Grubb, T.L., Adams, J.G., Huber, M.J. and Schmotzer, W.B. (1994) Orotracheal and nasotracheal intubation in llamas. *Journal of the American Veterinary Medical Association* **204**: 779–783.

Singh, R., Peshin, P.K., Patil, D.B., Sharda, R., Singh, J., Singh, A.P. and Sharifi, D. (1994) Evaluation of halothane as an anaesthetic in camels (*Camelus dromedarius*). *Zentralblat Veterinarmed* **41**: 359–368.

Snow, D.H., Billah, A. and Ridha, A. (1988) Effects of maximal exercise on the blood composition of the racing camel. *Veterinary Record* **123**: 311–312.

Stewart, M.C. and English, A.W. (1990) The reversal of xylazine/ketamine immobilisation of fallow deer with yohimbine. *Australian Veterinary Journal* **67**: 315–317.

Still, J., Raath, J.P. and Matzner, L. (1996) Respiratory and circulatory parameters of African elephants (*Loxodonta africana*) anaesthetised with etorphine and azaperone. *Journal of the South African Veterinary Association* **67**: 123–127.

Trim, C.M. (1989) Epidural analgesia with 0.75% bupivacaine for laparotomy in goats. *Journal of the American Veterinary Medical Association* **194**: 1292–1296.

Tulamo, R.-M., Raekallio, M. and Ekblad, A. (1995) Cardiovascular effects of medetomidine-ketamine anaesthesia in sheep, with and without 100% oxygen, and its reversal with atipamezole. *Journal of Veterinary Anaesthesia* **22**: 9–14.

Waterman, A.E., Livingston, A. and Amin, A. (1991) Further studies on the antinociceptive activity and respiratory effects of buprenorphine in sheep. *Journal of Veterinary Pharmacology and Therapeutics* **14**: 230–234.

White, R.J., Bark, H. and Bali, S. (1986) Halothane anaesthesia in the dromedary camel. *Veterinary Record* **119**: 615–617.

White, R.J., Bali, S. and Bark, H. (1987) Xylazine and ketamine anaesthesia in the dromedary camel under field conditions. *Veterinary Record* **120**: 110–113.

Woodbury, M.R. and Haigh, J.C. (1996) Innervation and anesthesia of the antler pedicle in wapiti and fallow deer. *Canadian Veterinary Journal* **37**: 486–489.

Anaesthesia of the pig

14

INTRODUCTION

Surgery may be carried out on the farm using either local analgesia or general anaesthesia but, where economically possible, for all other than minor surgery it is better to have the pig transported to a place with complete surgical facilities. Where local analgesia is used, the pig is usually first heavily sedated or even lightly anaesthetized to prevent the loud squealing noises which these animals make when restrained. When general anaesthesia is employed under farm conditions, simple methods giving short-term anaesthesia suffice, as surgery is usually limited in complexity. However, the pig is now also often used as an experimental animal in research projects involving long and complicated surgery and sophisticated techniques, possibly even including cardiopulmonary bypass, may be required.

Pigs presented for anaesthesia range in size from small newborn piglets to adult boars weighing 350 kg, and the methods of restraint and administration of anaesthetics must be varied accordingly. Whilst small pigs are easily restrained, large sows and boars may prove both difficult and dangerous. Large pigs are usually restrained by a rope or wire snare around the upper jaw, behind the canine teeth (Fig. 14.1).

In most cases the pig will try to escape by pulling back against this rope or snare and thus immobilizes itself, but this method does not work if the animal moves forward to attack (as a sow

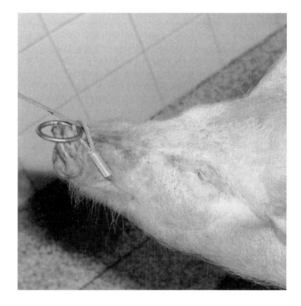

FIG.14.1 Restraint of the pig by a snare applied around the upper jaw.

attempting to defend her litter may do). Smaller pigs are usually restrained on their sides by grasping the undermost legs and leaning on the body. Pigs are easily trained and, at a research establishment, the problems of restraint are greatly reduced by very frequent, regular handling. In a large intensive farming unit, however, there is a lack of individual handling and some animals may be extremely difficult to control by physical means.

Most anaesthetists consider that when general anaesthetics are administered with due care pigs are good subjects. Although they resent restraint, as is shown by the struggling and loud squeals which they produce, this does not seem to result in adrenaline release with the attendant dangers during subsequent anaesthesia. Recovery from anaesthesia is usually calm. As they have little body hair, pigs are liable to develop hypothermia when sedated or anaesthetized, but this lack of hair does enable the anaesthetist to assess the state of peripheral circulation by monitoring the skin colour. Pigs tend to be fatter than most other farm animals and adipose tissue forms a depot for anaesthetics. The fatty nature of the tissue also makes accurate i.m. injections more difficult in these animals and necessitates the use of long needles to reach the muscle through the fatty tissue. The shape of the pig's head, together with the fat in the pharyngeal region (especially in Vietnamese Pot-bellied pigs) coupled with the small larynx and trachea, makes respiratory obstruction likely in both sedated and anaesthetized animals. Patency of the airway in the absence of endotracheal intubation is best maintained by applying pressure behind the vertical ramus of the mandible and thus pushing the jaw forward, while the tongue is drawn out between the incisor teeth (Fig. 14.2).

Salivation, even if not excessive, can contribute to airway obstruction so anticholinergic premedication is usually given before general anaesthesia unless there are contraindications such as pre-existing tachycardia or pyrexia.

PORCINE MALIGNANT HYPERTHERMIA

Although in the vast majority of pigs general anaesthesia presents few problems other than those associated with the maintenance of a clear airway, some strains and breeds suffer from a biochemical myopathy which manifests itself during general anaesthesia with some anaesthetic and ancillary agents. Hall *et al.* (1966) reported its occurrence in Landrace cross pigs following the use of suxamethonium during halothane anaesthesia, but it was later found that it could occur without the administration of suxamethonium.

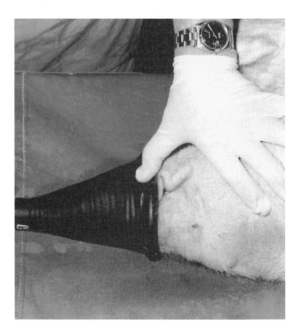

FIG.14.2 Maintaining a clear airway by pushing forward on the vertical ramus of the mandible with the tongue drawn forward on the mouth. For ease of photography, in this illustration the mask is held firmly on the face by the thumb, but the position of the hand is usually reversed, the thumb being used to push on the mandible and the fingers to hold the mask on the face.

Breeding experiments with Landrace cross pigs showed the abnormality to be inherited as an autosomal dominant with variable penetrance, occasional litters being found without susceptible animals. In some litters, however, piglets died before testing with a non-lethal test procedure which had been developed (Hall *et al.*, 1972) so this finding must be treated with some reserve. It is also possible that two genes might have been involved but, unfortunately, due to withdrawal of funding, further investigation of this was impossible.

The abnormal response of these pigs to anaesthetic and other drugs is characterized by the development of generalized muscle rigidity, a severe and sustained rise in body temperature, hyperkalaemia and metabolic acidosis. Since the first report of the porcine syndrome there have been numerous other reports of similar abnormal responses to anaesthetic agents, both in humans and animals and it is generally agreed that the syndrome has certain resemblances to the 'stress

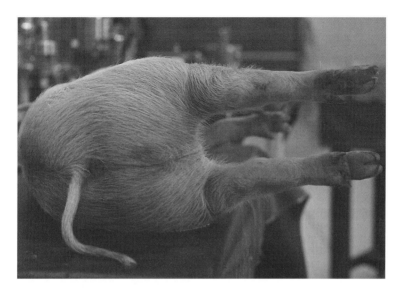

FIG. 14.3 Rigidity of limbs in a pig with developed porcine malignant hyperthermia.

reaction' seen in Pietrain and Poland-China pigs. There are, however, some striking differences between the syndrome as manifested in various pig breeds and strains. For example, in the Poland-China and Pietrain breeds dyspnoea, hyperthermia and immediate rigor mortis can be induced by environmental stress associated with exercise, transportation and high environmental temperatures, whereas Landrace and Landrace cross pigs develop the syndrome only when anaesthetized.

It has been suggested that malignant hyperthermia in man could be a syndrome resulting from more than one defect, and the same may be true for the porcine syndrome. It seems likely that it is resistance or susceptibility to triggering factors which differs, and that the final metabolic derangement which leads to death is common to all. While the pig has proved to be a valuable experimental animal for the study of this condition, great caution is needed in attempting to transpose results obtained in one breed or strain of pigs to another breed or strain, to another species of animal, or to man.

Early clinical findings suggested that the primary abnormality lies in the voluntary muscle of affected animals and attempts have been made to find a biochemical 'marker' which could support this suggestion and which might serve to identify experimental animals (and more particularly human beings) at risk. Raised serum creatine phosphokinase (CPK) occurs in a number of myopathies both in humans and in experimental animals and serum levels of this enzyme were studied in Landrace cross pigs by Woolf et al. (1970) who found that raised CPK levels in unanaesthetized animals had a fair predictive value for the development of abnormal muscle contracture following induction of anaesthesia with halothane and challenge with suxamethonium (Hall et al., 1972). Of 34 closely related pigs studied, 25 had serum CPK levels > 250 units/ml and 20 of these were subsequently found to react positively to challenge. Clearly finding of a CPK level of < 250 units/ml does not rule out the possibility of an abnormal reaction, but the chances of this happening are much lower.

It must be emphasized that the clinical veterinary anaesthetist is very unlikely to encounter cases of porcine malignant hyperthermia except in the Poland-China and Pietrain breeds, but it may occur in Large White and Landrace pigs (particularly in view of the modern practice of breeding from boars known to carry the trait because of the belief that their offspring may have faster growth rates). However, anaesthetists should be aware of the existence of this condition, be able to recognize its development during anaesthesia and, where possible, treat it. In a typical case, where a susceptible pig is given a triggering agent, its muscles develop contracture making the animal very stiff or even rigid (Fig. 14.3). Often the first sign the

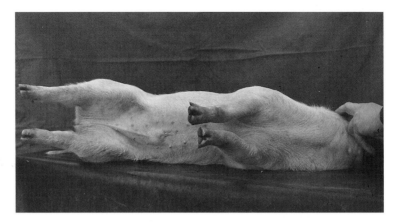

FIG.14.4 Spreading apart of the digits in a pig developing porcine malignant hyperthermia.

anaesthetist notices is a spreading apart of the digits (Fig. 14.4). Next, the body temperature starts to rise and the skin often shows blotchy reddening. If no attempt is made to treat the condition, the body temperature continues to rise (rectal temperatures of over 108° F have been recorded); eventually respiration ceases and death ensues. Presumably death is due to cellular hypoxia, for at temperatures above 42°C oxygen utilization exceeds oxygen supply.

Dantrolene sodium, a skeletal muscle relaxant, given orally in doses of 2 to 5 mg/kg 6 to 8 hours before the induction of anaesthesia, may prevent the onset of the syndrome in susceptible pigs and i.v. in doses of 2 to 10 mg/kg, has proved of some use in treating the established condition. Unfortunately dantrolene sodium is expensive. It has a very limited shelf-life and, in general, keeping it in readiness for the treatment of this uncommon porcine condition cannot be justified on economic grounds although it certainly is for man.

Induction of anaesthesia with Saffan affords some protection against the development of the syndrome in some strains of susceptible animals (Hall *et al.*, 1972). Symptomatic treatment includes rapid termination of the inhalation anaesthetic and the administration of pure oxygen, preferably through a 'clean' anaesthetic system, the administration of i.v. sodium bicarbonate (2 to 4 mEq/kg i.v.) and whole body cooling with cold water applied to the skin. Intravenous dantrolene may be given if available.

SEDATION

The pig's reaction to restraint (struggling accompanied by ear-splitting squeals) is unpleasant for all concerned and, therefore, sedation is widely used to facilitate all handling and minor procedures, as well as for restraint prior to local or general anaesthesia. In pigs, α_2 adrenoceptor agonists seem to be useful in smoothing reactions to ketamine but, for reasons as yet unknown, they are otherwise generally ineffective as sedatives.

SEDATIVE AGENTS EMPLOYED IN PIGS

Azaperone

This extremely safe butyrophenone drug is inexpensive and so effective in pigs that other sedatives are now seldom used in these animals. It is marketed both to the veterinary profession for clinical use and directly to farmers who use it to control fighting when mixing litters in intensive fattening units.

Azaperone must be given by deep i.m. injection, the neck muscles behind the ear usually proving to be the most convenient and best site; s.c. injection is ineffective and i.v. injection results in a phase of violent excitement. Injection into regions likely to be used for human food (e.g. the hams) should always be avoided. The doses used depend on the effects sought and range from 1 to 8 mg/kg, but it is recommended that a dose of 1 mg/kg is not exceeded for adult boars as higher doses cause protrusion of the penis with the risk of subsequent damage to that organ. Following an i.m. injection of 1 to 8mg/kg of azaperone, the pig should be left undisturbed for 20 minutes, as interference before this time may provoke an excitement reaction. Excitement may occur during this induction phase even in the absence of stimulation, but it is usually mild and rarely of clinical significance. After the induction period of some 20 minutes, pigs are deeply sedated and handling for the administration of other drugs or minor procedures is greatly facilitated.

Azaperone causes vasodilatation resulting in a small fall in arterial blood pressure, and some slight respiratory stimulation. Vasodilatation of cutaneous vessels makes sedated pigs particularly likely to develop hypothermia in a cold environment so warm surroundings are essential, but the dilated ear veins are easy to enter for i.v. injection of drugs.

Droperidol

The butyrophenone compound, droperidol, has been used in pigs and doses of 0.1 to 0.4mg/kg give similar sedation to that produced by azaperone. Butyrophenone/analgesic drug mixtures have been used and fentanyl/droperidol produce better sedation than droperidol alone. At the Cambridge School a combination of i.m. droperidol (0.5mg/kg) with midazolam (0.3mg/kg) given separately, or where appropriate, from the same syringe, produces ideal sedation for radiography, lancing of abscesses, etc. (P.G.C. Jackson, personal communication). Dependable sedation of approximately 15min duration follows some 10 minutes from the time of injection, but it is important to leave the pig undisturbed whilst the effects are developing. As with ketamine, sudden awakening without prior warning may occur.

Acepromazine

Phenothiazine derivatives are not as effective in pigs as they are in some other species of animal. However, pigs are more easily restrained for i.v. injection if first given an i.m. dose of 0.03 to 0.10 mg/kg before venepuncture is attempted. Under the influence of acepromazine they squeal

less when handled and are much less likely to dislodge the i.v. needle by head-shaking when injection is made. Acepromazine may be given by i.v. injection but this may be followed by venous thrombosis unless very dilute solutions are used. When given i.v. the drug should be allowed 10 to 20 minutes to produce its full effects. Hyperpnoea lasting for about 15 minutes may follow i.v. injection, but the reason for this is unknown.

Dissociative agents

Phencyclidine was used very successfully as a sedative for pigs for some years until the hallucinatory effects produced in man ingesting the drug led to a ban of the use of the drug in food animals. Phencyclidine has been withdrawn from the market and the dissociative agent in current use, ketamine, is generally used as an anaesthetic rather than as a sedative; low doses are analgesic.

GENERAL ANAESTHESIA

PREPARATION FOR GENERAL ANAESTHESIA

In pigs, 6 to 8 hours fasting and 2 hours deprivation of water is usually adequate to ensure that the stomach is empty. Vomiting at induction or during recovery is rare in pigs (although it used to be seen regularly in pigs recovering from cylcopropane anaesthesia) but a full stomach exerts pressure on the diaphragm and reduces respiratory efficiency. The majority of surgery carried out in pigs, whether clinical or experimental, is elective, and fluid deficits are seldom present before anaesthesia. An i.v. infusion may be needed, however, before anaesthesia for the correction of a strangulated hernia, for example. Details of existing drug therapy such as antibiotic food additives, or anthelminitics, should be noted – especially if neuromuscular blocking drugs whose action they may lengthen are to be used in the anaesthetic technique.

Premedication

During general anaesthesia salivation, even if not excessive, may cause respiratory obstruction.

Atropine, i.v. or i.m. in doses 0.3 to 2.4 mg (total dose), or glycopyrrolate (0.2 to 2.0 mg total dose), depending on the size of the pig, will usually control this salivation.

The degree of sedation required depends on the anaesthetic technique which is to follow. Some anaesthetists prefer to dispense with sedation at this stage while others use it to facilitate the administration of the anaesthetic and to reduce the squealing and struggling which would otherwise occur during inhalation anaesthetic induction. Only rarely is there any need for analgesics to be included in the premedication but if required they may be employed in slightly larger doses than are used in dogs. It is probable that azaperone is the most widely used premedicant drug for porcine anaesthesia. As already mentioned, it is given i.m. in doses of 1 to 8 mg/kg according to the degree of sedation required.

Intravenous technique

Injections are best made into auricular veins on the external aspect of the ear flap. Small pigs are restrained on their side on the table and usually two assistants are needed, one gripping the legs,

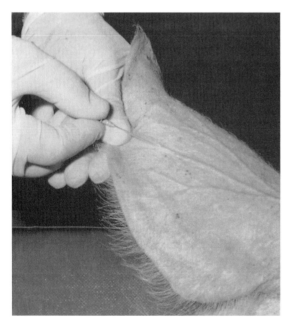

FIG.14.5 Distension of the ear flap veins by the application of a rubber band around the base of the ear.

whilst the second holds the uppermost ear at the base of the conchal cartilage and applies pressure over the vein as near to the base of the ear as possible. If a second assistant is not available a rubber band is applied around the base of the ear flap. In large pigs, a noose is applied around the upper jaw behind the tusks as previously described (see Fig. 14.1). As in small pigs, the ear veins are distended by the application of pressure as near to the base of the ear flap as possible.

Once the skin of the ear flap over the vein has been cleansed, the veins are usually easily visible (Fig.14.5) but if necessary they can be made more obvious by gentle slapping and brisk rubbing of the ear flap with an alcohol-soaked gauze swab.

Venepuncture is then carried out using a needle about 2.5 cm long and depending on the calibre of the vessel to be entered, 21 to 23 gauge (0.6 to 0.65 mm). In large pigs blood can be aspirated into an attached syringe once the needle has been inserted into the lumen of the vein but in small pigs the amount of blood in the vein between the points of pressure and the needle point may be so small that it is impossible to withdraw any into the syringe. In such cases injection must be attempted and if the needle point is not in the vein a subcutaneous bleb will develop. When it is certain that the needle is in the vein the pressure is released (if a rubber band has been applied to the base of the ear flap the band must be cut with scissors) and the injection made. It will be noticed that the injected fluid washes the blood from the vein and this affords further evidence that the needle is correctly placed in the lumen of vessel.

Introduction of a catheter into an ear vein is not difficult (Fig. 14.6) but these veins are not very convenient for the administration of large volumes fluid. Fortunately, infusions of large volumes are seldom needed but if they are anticipated to be necessary it is usually best to implant surgically a catheter into the jugular vein of the anaesthetized pig as the subcutaneous fat makes percutaneous placement difficult. Some workers prefer to catheterize the anterior vena cava by a blind technique. Small pigs are restrained on their backs in a V-shaped trough with the neck fully extended and the head hanging down. The forelegs are drawn back and a 5 to 7.5 cm long 16 s.w.g. (1.65 mm) needle pushed through the skin in the depression

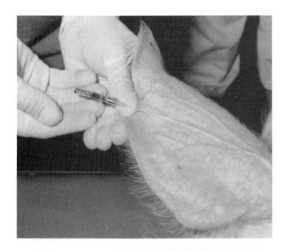

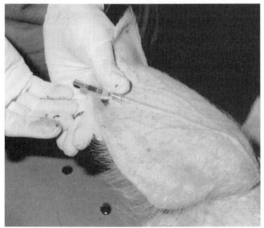

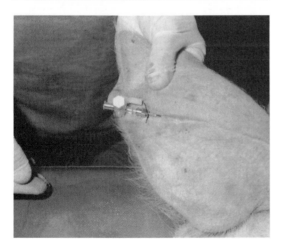

FIG.14.6 Stages in the introduction of a catheter into an ear vein of a pig. The stitch securing the catheter does not penetrate the ear cartilage.'Super-glue' may be used as an alternative to stitching.

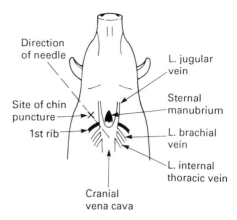

FIG.14.7 Site for the introduction of a needle to penetrate the anterior vena cava. The needle tip is advanced towards an imaginary point midway between the scapulae.

which can be palpated just lateral to the anterior angle of the sternum and formed by the angle between the first rib and trachea. The needle is directed towards an imaginary point midway between the scapulae and advanced until blood can be freely aspirated through it when a syringe is attached. A fine plastic catheter is then threaded through the needle into the anterior vena cava and after its position has been verified by aspiration of blood through it, or by radiography, the needle is completely withdrawn and the catheter secured in position with a skin suture. In large animals the procedure is carried out with the animal standing and hanging back on a nose snare. It is always important to ensure that the head does not deviate from the midline and that the neck is well extended (Fig. 14.7).

Intraperitoneal injection

This method of administration of anaesthetic drugs is very far from ideal, but it is sometimes employed by the laboratory worker and the less skilled veterinarian. Response is variable, and accidental injection into the liver, kidney or gut lumen may follow. The injection of irritant solutions may lead to the subsequent formation of intraperitoneal adhesions. Preferably, pigs should be starved for 24 hours to reduce the gut volume before injection is made. The animal is then restrained on its back or by its hind legs, and an area of skin in the region of the umbilicus is clipped and cleaned. A needle is inserted 2 to 5 cm from the midline at the level of the umbilicus and injection made. A complete absence of resistance to pressure on the plunger of the syringe indicates that the solution is being injected into the peritoneal cavity or, possibly, into the lumen of the gut.

Endotracheal intubation

Endotracheal intubation in the pig is not as easy as in most other domestic animals. It is particularly difficult in the extremely brachycephalic pot-bellied pig. The shape and size of the head and mouth make the use of a laryngoscope difficult. The rima glottis is extremely small and the larynx is set at an angle to the trachea, causing difficulty in passing the tube beyond the cricoid ring (Fig. 14.8). Laryngeal spasm is easily provoked so atraumatic intubation must be carried out under deep general anaesthesia with local analgesic spray of the cords, or with the aid of a neuromuscular blocking agent.

The sizes of endotracheal tubes suitable for pigs are unexpectedly small when compared with those used in dogs of a similar body weight. A 6 mm tube may be the largest which can be passed in a pig weighing about 25 kg; a 9 mm tube is suitable for a 50 kg animal; large boars and sows may accommodate tubes of 14 to 16 mm diameter. Pot-

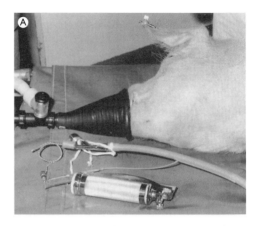

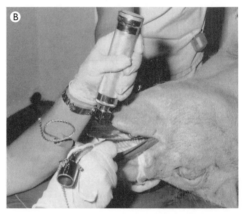

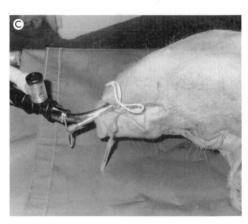

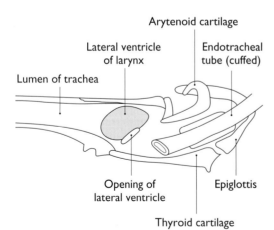

FIG. 14.8 Saggital section of pig's head to show principal structures in relation to the passage of an endotracheal tube. The lumen of the trachea runs at an angle to the line of the glottic opening.

FIG. 14.9 Apparatus needed for endotracheal intubation in the pig. **A** Note the malleable wire stilette inside the tube but not protruding from its bevelled end; **B** the use of the laryngoscope to elevate the lower jaw and displace the tongue to one side; **C** tube tied in position with tape around the lower jaw and cuff inflated.

bellied pigs can only be intubated with smaller diameter tubes – a 90 kg animal can only accommodate a 9 mm diameter tube. Introduction of the tube may be made easier by the use of a malleable stilette such as a copper rod with one end carefully rounded or covered to prevent damage to the mucosa of the larynx or trachea. The stilette is placed inside the endotracheal tube and a moveable side arm adjusted to ensure that the tip does not protrude beyond the end of the tube (Fig. 14.9). Whenever a tube is reinforced in this way care must be taken not to use force in its introduction, as damage to the laryngeal mucosa with subsequent oedema and, after extubation, respiratory obstruction, can easily occur. Laryngoscopes designed for use in man, as used in dogs, are suitable for small pigs, but in large ones the weight of the lower jaw may make its elevation almost impossible and the Rowson laryngoscope may be needed to expose the larynx to view.

The easiest position in which to intubate the anaesthetized pig using a standard laryngoscope blade is with the pig supine and the neck and head fully extended. An assistant pulls on the tongue and fixes the upper jaw while the laryngoscope is introduced and the larynx brought into view by vertical lifting of the tongue and lower jaw, no leverage being exerted (Fig 14.10). Under direct vision the tube is passed between the vocal cords and kept dorsal to the middle ventricle of the larynx. If its progress is arrested at the cricoid ring, the stilette must be partially withdrawn and the head flexed slightly on the neck. The tube may then be advanced gently into the trachea. An alternative is to introduce a stilette about three times the length of the endotracheal tube it is intended to use through the larynx under direct vision and then to 'railroad' the tube over it into the trachea.

Endotracheal intubation in the pig is greatly facilitated by the use of neuromuscular blocking drugs, such as suxamethonium, which relax the jaw muscles and prevent the larynx from going into spasm. The anaesthetized pig is given oxygen to breathe through a face mask and the chosen neuromuscular blocker given i.v. The pig is intubated as soon as the jaw muscles relax and IPPV is carried out until spontaneous respiration is resumed. When suxamethonium is injected, spontaneous respiration returns within 1 to 2 min.

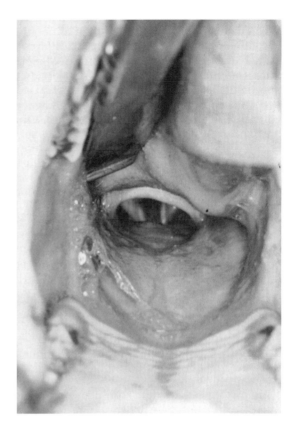

FIG.14.10 View of the pig's larynx when a standard type laryngoscope is used correctly in the supine animal. As can be seen, the laryngoscope blade is used to elevate the base of the tongue and does not come into contact with the epiglottis. The epiglottis is often so soft and flexible that unless due care is taken it folds back into the glottic opening as the tube is passed.

Should an attempt at intubation fail, small pigs may easily be ventilated with pure oxygen by squeezing of the reservoir bag of the anaesthetic apparatus while a face mask is correctly applied (Fig. 14.2). Applying IPPV in this way is more difficult in adult sows and boars, so it is recommended that neuromuscular blocking drugs are only used in these larger animals by anaesthetists experienced at endotracheal intubation and capable of ventilating large individuals through a face-mask.

TECHNIQUES OF GENERAL ANAESTHESIA IN PIGS

Although the pig is a good subject for general anaesthesia the anaesthetist may find problems in maintaining a clear airway and spontaneous breathing in non-intubated animals. When dealing with fat pigs, cessation of breathing is a common complication of deep anaesthesia. A striking feature of this apparent respiratory failure is that it is different from that seen in other species, for expulsion of air from the lungs by pressure on the abdomen is immediately followed by a spontaneous deep inspiration of the type seen when there is some mechanical obstruction to respiration during anaesthesia. It is possible that the position of the head is enough to cause pressure on the larynx sufficient to arrest breathing. The animal's head should be placed at a natural angle to the neck and IPPV applied. In unintubated animals this is performed by applying pressure to the abdomen about every 4 seconds. Unless spontaneous breathing returns within 1 to 2 minutes, endotracheal intubation to facilitate IPPV should be considered. If IPPV is carried out through a closely applied face mask care must be taken to limit the pressures applied to avoid inflation of the stomach.

The prudent anaesthetist avoids trouble by avoiding the need to produce deep anaesthesia in spontaneously breathing animals – if necessary by the simultaneous use of techniques of local analgesia when light general anaesthesia does not suffice on its own.

Intravenous anaesthesia

The i.v. injection of suitable agents into an already sedated animal is an excellent way of inducing general anaesthesia in pigs. Under farm conditions it may be desirable to maintain anaesthesia by use of intravenous drugs but if suitable apparatus is available anaesthesia can be maintained even on farms, with inhalation agents. Numerous agents are available for induction of anaesthesia by the i.v. route and many of them can be used to maintain anaesthesia in situations where this is necessary. In pigs, some of these agents may also be administered by IP injection, but this route is not to be recommended.

Metomidate

This hypnotic drug has been used on the Continent of Europe, usually in combination with azaperone, for the production of deep narcosis (short of general anaesthesia) in pigs both under field conditions and prior to the use of more sophisticated methods in the operating theatre. Ideally, metomidate is given i.v. at dose rates of 3.3 mg/kg about 20 minutes after i.m. injection of 2 mg/kg azaperone. Often the pig moves as the metomidate is injected and this may be a response to pain for the i.v. injection of the related drug, etomidate, is known to cause pain in man. Following i.v. injection of metomidate after azaperone pigs become recumbent and will remain so for some 10 to 20 min. Respiration is well maintained and further doses of metomidate can be given as needed to prolong recumbency. Analgesia is very limited with this combination of drugs and painful stimuli sometimes result in dramatic, even if short-lived, awakening, so it is advisable to utilize some form of analgesia, or even physical restraint, to enable surgery to be carried out. The combination of azaperone and metomidate is compatible with all inhalation and neuromuscular blocking agents used in anaesthesia so they may be used subsequently as needed.

In some centres anaesthesia associated with only minimal analgesia has been maintained by the continuous i.v. infusion of azaperone (2 mg/kg/hour) and metomidate (8 mg/kg/hour). It is claimed that this technique offers a safe alternative when facilities for administration of inhalation agents are not available, although recovery can be prolonged.

It is possible to give azaperone i.p. or i.m. and metomidate i.p. at the same time. Narcosis follows about 20 minutes after injection but this can result in peritonitis and formation of intra-abdominal adhesions.

Thiopental sodium

Anaesthesia can be induced in pigs by the i.v. injection of minimal (5 to 10 mg/kg) quantities of a 2.5% solution of thiopental. As in all other species of animal, larger doses or incremental doses are cumulative and can result in delay in recovery.

The quantity of thiopental taken to induce medium depth surgical anaesthesia and the duration of the anaesthetic period are chiefly governed by the speed at which the i.v. injection is made.

When rapid injection techniques are practised in healthy pigs, the quantity used will be surprisingly small, and the recovery period short. Surgical anaesthesia can be induced in non-premedicated sows weighing about 100 kg by injection of no more than 500 mg of the drug. Moreover, it has been observed that use of a 2.5% solution decreases the total dose required for any operation. Induction of anaesthesia with thiopental sodium is greatly facilitated by azaperone premedication. Provided that the pig is left undisturbed for 20 minutes after injection of the azaperone, controlled injection into an ear vein is easy and complete anaesthesia can be obtained with very low quantities of a 2.5% solution of thiopental. It seems that butyrophenone antagonizes the respiratory depressant effect of thiopental but this clinical impression still awaits controlled investigation.

As with all barbiturate anaesthetics, respiration may fail with the onset of anaesthesia. When rapid injection techniques are used this period of apnoea is short and should not necessitate use of IPPV. Apnoea of more than a few seconds duration must, of course, be treated by IPPV and, provided this is applied efficiently, spontaneous breathing soon returns. Recovery after a very great overdose of thiopental may be expected if efficient IPPV is performed until the concentration of thiopental in the brain has diminished.

Methohexital sodium

Provided the anaesthetist is aware of the special characteristics of methohexital (such as its tendency to produce muscle tremors during induction of anaesthesia) this agent can be used quite safely in pigs. Anaesthesia can be produced in unsedated animals by i.v. injection of 5 to 6 mg/kg as a 2.5% solution and recovery is complete 10 to 15 min after injection of a single dose.

Premedication with azaperone reduces the dose of methohexital required and enables small incremental doses to be used to prolong anaesthesia without delay in recovery.

Pentobarbital sodium

This drug still has a place for surgery carried out on farms and in experimental laboratories. The most satisfactory method of administration of pentobarbital is slow i.v. injection into an ear vein until the desired degree of the central nervous system depression is obtained. However, for non-survival experiments intraperitoneal injection using a computed dose, or for castration intratesticular injection of large doses, may be useful alternatives for the inexperienced anaesthetist.

For healthy, unsedated male and female pigs up to 50 kg (approx 1 cwt) live weight, the average i.v. dose necessary to induce medium depth anaesthesia is about 30 mg/kg. In small pigs there is a considerable margin of safety, but in larger ones great variations in susceptibility may occur. Castrated animals appear to be slightly more susceptible than entires. Provided that injection is made slowly and the onset of muscle relaxation is observed, the method is safe. Induction is not associated with narcotic excitement; in fact, in the case of a squealing animal, the progressive reduction, and finally cessation of squealing, is a good guide to the progress of narcosis. Depths of anaesthesia may be difficult to assess in pigs. The presence of complete relaxation of abdominal muscles and absence of response to pricking of the skin is usually taken as evidence that anaesthesia has been attained. Its duration will be sufficient for the performance of rapid operations such as castration. For very large subjects doses per kg need to be reduced and marked variations in susceptibility will be encountered.

The duration of surgical plane anaesthesia will depend upon the initial depth induced. As a rule it is shorter than in dogs. With light levels of unconsciousness – a brisk corneal reflex and a reflex response to skin pricking – it is of 10 to 15 minutes only; when there is a sluggish corneal reflex and loss of reflex response to pricking – 20 to 25 minutes. Anaesthesia is followed by a period of progressively lightening narcosis which persists for 3 to 8 hours. Recovery is not accompanied by narcotic excitement and the animal usually passes into a state of sleep. For non-survival experiments, after induction with 30 mg/kg pentobarbital, anaesthesia may be maintained by continuous i.v. infusion of pentobarbital at about 2 mg/kg/hour although this rate may need adjustment from time to time.

In very small, unsedated subjects in which intravenous injection may be found to be difficult, the intraperitoneal route may be adopted, although in general, it is not to be recommended. It becomes necessary to compute an anaesthetic dose. For animals up to 20 kg this is put at 30 mg/kg; for those between 20 and 30 kg, at 24 mg/kg. Variations in response are inevitable with such a method. In some cases narcosis only will be obtained and it will be necessary to augment it by inhalation or local analgesic injection, while in others it may become alarmingly deep and even fatal. Provided a careful watch is kept on the breathing pattern and IPPV applied should respiration cease, fatalities should, however, be of rare occurrence. Provided efficient IPPV is used pigs will survive after some three times the anaesthetic dose has been given. In fat subjects there is the possibility that, despite the length of the needle employed, the injection will be made into retroperitoneal fat. In this case absorption will be so slow it is improbable that even light narcosis will develop. When employing this route of administration, the action of the drug will attain its maximum depth in a period of 20 to 30 minutes after injection. The duration of the period of anaesthesia and of narcosis tends to be rather longer than with the i.v. method.

Intratesticular injection of pentobarbital

A concentrated solution of pentobarbital sodium, such as one commercially available for euthanasia of small animals (300 mg/ml) may be administered by intratesticular injection prior to castration. A dose rate of about 45 mg/kg is employed, a very large boar being given 20 ml of solution into each testicle and adequate anaesthesia for castration develops within 10 minutes of injection. Removal of the testicles removes any excess drug so that to prevent overdosage the testicles must be removed as soon as the boar becomes anaesthetized. Care must be taken in disposal of the testicles after their removal since they still contain enough barbiturate to produce fatal poisoning of any animal (e.g. the farm dog) which might eat them.

Saffan

When no premedication is used, i.v. doses of 6 mg/kg produce surgical anaesthesia of 10 to 15 minutes duration followed by smooth recovery.

In larger pigs intravenous doses of 6 mg/kg constitute too large a volume for convenience and it is usual to employ premedication to reduce the dose needed. Following sedation with 4 mg/kg azaperone i.m., i.v. injection of 2 mg/kg of Saffan produces good surgical anaesthesia with adequate muscle relaxation and minimal respiratory depression. Further increments of Saffan can be given to prolong anaesthesia without appreciable increase in recovery time.

Ketamine

Pigs are rapidly immobilized by i.m. injection of 20 mg/kg ketamine, which produces adequate analgesia for the performance of minor operations. Wakening is often abrupt and many pigs seem to remain sensitive to noise throughout the period of 'anaesthesia'. Much better results are obtained by 2 to 5 mg i.v. after pretreatment with 1 mg/kg xylazine, although this latter drug seems to produce no obvious sedation in these animals. Reasonably satisfactory results are also obtained when 10 to 18 mg/kg of ketamine are given after i.v. injection of 1 to 2 mg/kg of diazepam. Pot-bellied pigs generally need about half these doses.

Ketamine (8 mg/kg) and xylazine (2 mg/kg drawn into the same syringe may be injected intratesticularly to provide anaesthesia for castration of large boars. Rapid castration removes the remaining drugs contained in the testicles and recovery is more rapid than after intratesticular pentobarbital.

It must be remembered that ketamine, xylazine and diazepam are all rather expensive for use in farm animals.

Triple drip

The combination of ketamine, xylazine and guaiphenesin in 5% dextrose ('triple drip') given by i.v. infusion, although rather expensive, can be used in pigs as in other species of animal to produce and maintain anaesthesia. The solution is usually prepared immediately before use to contain 2 mg of ketamine, and 1 mg of xylazine per ml of 5% guaiphenesin. Induction of anaesthesia usually needs 0.6 to 1 ml/kg. Following this maintenance of anaesthesia is accomplished by infusion of approximately 2.2 ml/kg/hour but the rate of infusion must, of course, be adjusted to effect as judged by monitoring the usual signs of anaesthesia. Recovery usually takes some 30 to 45 minutes following cessation of administration but can be hastened by the cautious i.v. injection of atipamezole.

Inhalation anaesthesia

Breathing systems designed for use in man, and which are used for dogs, may be employed for all but the largest of boars and sows. In the latter, systems designed for equine anaesthesia are more appropriate.

Endotracheal intubation is essential if IPPV is to be used but otherwise volatile agents may be administered via a face mask. Large Hall-pattern face masks are adequate for small pigs but masks suitable for large pigs are not commercially available. Fortunately, conical or snout-shaped masks are fairly easy to design and construct and although they may not fit tightly around the pig's snout a gas-tight seal can be obtained by wrapping wet towels around the edge of the mask. The pig breathes through the nose, so whatever mask is used it is essential to ensure that it does not block the flow of gas into the nostrils. Luckily, the anterior position of the nostrils makes their obstruction by the mask much less likely than in animals such as cattle where the nares are situated more laterally. If a suitable snout mask is not available the anaesthetic may be administered through a Hall's mask placed over the nostrils, although it is obviously impossible to make this a gas-tight fit and a considerable quantity of anaesthetic escapes to the atmosphere. Whenever the pig is not intubated the tendency towards respiratory obstruction must be overcome by pushing the mandible forward as previously described (Fig. 14.2).

Induction of anaesthesia with inhalation agents is usually free from excitement but, except in small pigs, it is usually more convenient to induce anaesthesia with a parenterally administered drug and use inhalation agents just for maintenance of anaesthesia. Under farm conditions, when methods of administration may lead to considerable wastage of anaesthetic, the older, less expensive agents are usually employed but when more

sophisticated apparatus is available any inhalation agent may be used.

Trichloroethylene

Trichloroethylene – once quite widely used in porcine practice – is no longer commercially available as a preparation for inhalation anaesthesia.

Ether

Inhalation of ether by conscious pigs produces copious salivation and bronchial secretion, even after atropine premedication, so it cannot be regarded as a satisfactory induction agent for this species of animal. Given by semi-closed or low-flow methods following suitable premedication and induction with i.v. agents, it can produce good anaesthesia with marked muscle relaxation.

Non-inflammable inhalation agents

All modern inhalation anaesthetics are safe anaesthetics for pigs other than those susceptible to malignant hyperthermia. Halothane and isoflurane are known to be associated with triggering this condition in susceptible animals but in this respect the position of enflurane, sevoflurane and desflurane is currently uncertain, although it seems likely that they too may act as triggers. Because of the need for suitable equipment for their safe administration use of all these agents is more or less confined to hospital conditions. Desflurane requires a very expensive special vaporizer for its administration and it is likely that at least for the foreseeable future its use will be confined to experimental animals in well equipped laboratories. The physical characteristics of halothane and isoflurane are so similar that they may be administered from the same precision vaporizer designed for either drug provided that it is carefully cleaned before the subsequent use of the other agent.

Because of its potency and relative low cost with an absence of toxicity (except in malignant hyperthermia susceptible pigs), halothane is an excellent anaesthetic for pigs of all ages. Induction of anaesthesia is rapid and provided the animal can be effectively restrained there is seldom any need to use i.m. or i.v. administration of other drugs for this purpose before halothane is given.

Squealing ceases after as few as 4 or 5 breaths and inhalation of the vapour does not provoke salivation or breath holding. Recovery from anaesthesia is equally smooth and rapid.

Isoflurane is similarly effective but tends to cause more respiratory depression in pigs not being subjected to surgical stimulation. Unfortunately, the cost of halothane and isoflurane and the need for accurately calibrated vaporizers limits their use on farms but, where low-flow or semi-closed methods can be used halothane and isoflurane are worthy of consideration for porcine anaesthesia. Their main disadvantages in pigs, as in all species, are those of cardiovascular depression leading to hypotension, respiratory depression and the comparative lack of ability to suppress motor response to surgical stimulation.

Sevoflurane has not been widely used in pigs but there seems no reason to suppose it will not prove to be an effective anaesthetic agent. It solubility characteristics indicate it should produce a rapid induction coupled with prompt recovery from anaesthesia.

Desflurane's solubility in blood is much less than that of the other halogenated volatile agents and thus, induction of anaesthesia and recovery are rapid, while the depth of anaesthesia is readily controllable.

Nitrous oxide (N_2O)

It is impossible to induce anaesthesia in pigs with N_2O but as long as sufficient O_2 is provided it may be supplemented with a volatile anaesthetic agent. In particular, it can be used to speed induction of anaesthesia with the halogenated agents ('second gas' effect).

The sequence of premedication, induction of anaesthesia with thiopental sodium, endotracheal intubation under the influence of a neuromuscular blocker and the maintenance of anaesthesia by endotracheal non-rebreathing administration of N_2O plus an intravenous or inhalational supplement together with a neuromuscular blocker with IPPV has proved to be a very satisfactory method for lengthy experimental surgical procedures in pigs of all ages. By this system N_2O provides valuable analgesia so that very light anaesthesia can be maintained while the neuromuscular blocking drug produces muscle relaxation as needed. Recovery from anaesthesia is rapid and after surgical procedures the administration of analgesics is usually obligatory.

NEUROMUSCULAR BLOCKING AGENTS

Neuromuscular blocking agents are used in pigs to facilitate endotracheal intubation and for thoracic, abdominal, or some experimental procedures. As in all species of animal, two things are essential if these drugs are to be administered:

1. The pig must be unconscious and unaware of its surroundings, i.e. anaesthetized with recognized anaesthetic agents.

2. Means to apply efficient IPPV must be available.

Techniques involving neuromuscular blockers are not designed for use in the field, and can only be properly employed to advantage by a skilled anaesthetist. All those intending to use these drugs in porcine anaesthesia should be thoroughly familiar with the pharmacology (Chapter 7) and with the methods of IPPV (Chapter 8). By providing complete muscular relaxation their use means that the surgeon does not need to apply forcible retraction to tissues to gain access to the surgical site and so avoids tissue bruising which can give rise to post-operative pain.

Suxamethonium

The main use of suxamethonium in pigs is to facilitate endotracheal intubation. Atropine premedication is essential to counter the autonomic stimulating effect of the initial depolarizing process. Following induction of anaesthesia, doses of 2 mg/kg produce complete paralysis of skeletal muscles for about 2 minutes, i.e. long enough to allow unhurried, atraumatic intubation. It is, of course, necessary to perform IPPV until full spontaneous breathing is resumed. When non-depolarizing blockers are to be employed for the remainder of the anaesthetic period many anaesthetists consider recovery from the suxamethonium paralysis should be complete before they are administered but this does not seem to be essential.

Table 14.1 **Neuromuscular blocking drugs which have been used in pigs**

Drug	Dose (mg/kg)	Approximate duration of action (min)
Suxamethonium	2.0	2–3
D-tubocurarine	0.3	25–35
Gallamine	4.0	15–20
Alcuronium	0.1	30–40
Pancuronium	0.12	25–30
Vecuronium	0.1	15–20
Atracurium	0.5	20–60

Non-depolarizing neuromuscular blocking agents

All the non-depolarizing relaxants used in man may be employed in anaesthetized pigs to facilitate surgical or experimental procedures. The choice of drug depends on the duration of action needed, on the route of its elimination, and on the cardiovascular effects it produces. The drugs which have been used are listed in Table 14.1.

The technique most commonly applied is that as described under N$_2$O above. Ventilators designed for use in adult humans are adequate for the majority of pigs, but large boars and sows may have to be ventilated with one of the ventilators designed for use in adult horses and cattle. At the end of the procedure it is usual to give atropine (in doses of up to 0.3 mg/kg) or glycopyrrolate (up to 0.2 mg/kg) followed by neostigmine (up to 2.5 mg total dose) or edrophonium (up to 0.5 mg/kg) to restore adequate spontaneous breathing. In pigs the depth of neuromuscular blockade is best estimated by stimulation of the ulnar nerve as in the dog and cat using 'double-burst' stimulation.

LOCAL ANALGESIA

Caudal nerve block is not employed in pigs and epidural block is usually used simply for economic reasons.

Epidural block

In the pig the spinal cord ends at the junction of the 5th and 6th lumbar vertebrae and the spinal meninges continue, around the phylum terminale, as far as the middle of the sacrum. At the lumbosacral space the sac is comparatively small, and it is improbable that a needle introduced at this point will penetrate into the subarachnoid space. The lumbosacral aperture is large. Its dimensions in the adult are approximately 1.5 cm craniocaudally and 3 cm transversely. The depth of the canal is about 1 cm.

The site for insertion of the needle is located as follows: the cranial border of the ileum on each side is found with the fingers. A line joining them crosses the spinous process of the last lumbar vertebra (Fig. 14.11). The needle is inserted in the midline immediately behind this spinous process and directed downwards and backwards at an angle of 20° with the vertical. The depth to which the needle must penetrate in pigs of from 30 to 70 kg will vary from 5 to 9 cm. The landmarks described are readily detected in animals of smaller size but they may be entirely masked by the overlying tissues in

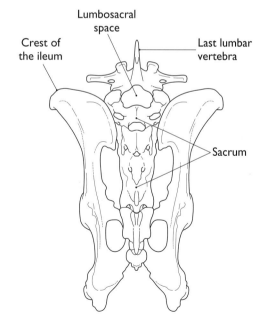

FIG.14.11 Dorsal view of the pig's pelvis. A line connecting the iliac crests crosses the last lumbar vertebra. The lumbosacral space in adult pigs is 2.5 – 3 cm caudal to this point. The patella can be used as a reliable landmark for location of the iliac crest in larger animals; with the hindlegs in a normal standing position, a vertical line through the patella will cross midline on level with the crest of the ileum.

larger ones. In these a point 15 cm cranial to the base of the tail serves as a fairly accurate guide. Provided the needle is introduced in approximately the correct position and direction, the size of the lumbosacral space makes its detection comparatively easy. Eighteen gauge needles are used; for pigs between 30 and 50 kg one 8 cm long, and for animals of 70 kg and above, one 12 cm long are required.

Before inserting the epidural needle an insensitive skin weal should be produced. The animal is restrained either on its breast or side. For small pigs the latter is preferable, as sudden movement can be better controlled. In large sows and boars the injection is made in the standing animal. Owing to difficulties with restraint, it is generally necessary to make the injection comparatively rapidly. Penetration of the canal is often associated with sudden movement, for which attendants must be prepared. Rapid injection seems to cause discomfort, presumably due to transient elevation of CSF pressure. In pigs weighing from 10 to 20 kg the interarcuate ligament is at a depth of about 2 to 3.5 cm from the skin surface while in adult sows and boars it may be at a depth of up to 15 cm.

Epidural analgesia has been used for the castration of pigs of 40 to 50 kg, injecting 10 ml of 2% lignocaine solution with adrenaline. Complete desensitization of the scrotum, testes and spermatic cord was present in 10 minutes, and there was a partial motor paralysis of the hind-limbs. Recovery was complete at the end of the second hour.

It is difficult to know up to what weight of animal this recommendation can be employed, for in larger animals fat often represents a considerable proportion of body weight. It is suggested that for 2% lignocaine the dose should be 1.0 ml per 7.5 kg for pigs weighing up to 50 kg and an additional 1.0 ml for every 10 kg above this in weight. Another suggestion which has proved to be satisfactory is based on occiput–tail base measurement allowing 1.0 ml for the first 40 cm and an additional 1.5 ml for each 10 cm longer length. Certainly, when administered at the lumbosacral space 20 ml of 2% lignocaine is adequate for caesarian section in sows weighing about 300 kg.

Recently the effects of xylazine and detomidine injected at the lumbosacral space have been evaluated (Lumb and Jones, 1996). Epidural xylazine (2 mg/kg in 5 ml 0.9% saline) induces bilateral analgesia extending from the anus to the umbilicus within 5 minutes after completion of the injection and persists for at least 10 minutes. Detomidine (500 μg/kg in 5 ml 0.9% saline) induces recumbency but analgesia caudal to the umbilicus is minimal. In large sows 1 mg/kg of 10% xylazine in 10 ml of 2% lignocaine injected at the lumbosacral space produces analgesia extending from the anus to the umbilicus 5 to 8 minutes after completion of the injection.

Tendillo *et al.* (1995) found that epidural xylazine 0.2 mg/kg diluted in saline to 0.5 ml/kg produced analgesia in isoflurane anaesthetized healthy Landrace–Large White pigs for up to 90 minutes.

Analgesia for castration

Local analgesia is quite suitable for the castration of male pigs up to about 5 months of age but general anaesthesia is probably more satisfactory for older animals.

In the field, intratesticular injection is probably the most practical method of local analgesia. A needle of suitable size is thrust perpendicularly through the tensed scrotal skin and advanced until its point lies in the middle of the testicle. Between 3 and 15 ml, depending on the size the animal, of 2% lignocaine hydrochloride are injected into the middle of the testicle and a further 2 to 5 ml are injected subcutaneously beneath the scrotal skin as the needle is withdrawn. Both sides are treated in the same manner. Operation may commence about 5 minutes after completion of the injections.

POSTOPERATIVE CARE

It is absolutely essential that pigs should be kept in a warm environment until they are completely mobile after sedation or general anaesthesia because, due to their lack of body hair, they are prone to develop hypothermia if left in cold surroundings. Close observation during recovery is necessary so that immediate measures may be taken to relieve any respiratory obstruction which may occur. Postoperative pain relief is essential, particularly following all surgical procedures. Narcotic analgesics may be given as necessary, in doses similar to those used in dogs. Amongst those most commonly employed are morphine (0.1 mg/kg up to a maximum of 20 mg for large pigs) and pethidine (2 mg/kg up to a maximum of 1.0 g in large boars and sows). It is probable that postoperative analgesia is frequently considered as being too uneconomic for use after operations such as castration but, ethically, veterinarians are obliged to give pain relief whenever desirable without undue regard for agricultural economic considerations.

REFERENCES

Hall, L.W., Woolf, V., Bradley, J.W.P. and Jolly, D.W. (1966) Unusual reaction to suxamethonium chloride. *British Medical Journal* **ii**: 1305.

Hall, L.W., Trim, C.M. and Woolf, N. (1972) Further studies of porcine malignant hyperthermia. *British Medical Journal* **ii**: 145–148.

Bradley, W.G., Ward, M., Murchison, D., Hall, L.W. and Woolf, N. (1973) Clinical, electrophysiological and pathological studies on malignant hyperpyrexia. *Proceedings of the Royal Society of Medicine* **66**: 67–68.

Lumb, W. V. and Jones, E.W. (1996) *Veterinary Anesthesia*, 3rd edn. Baltimore: Williams & Wilkins, p. 501.

Tendillo, F.J., Pera, A.M., Mascias, A. *et al.* (1995) Cardiopulmonary and analgesic effects of epidural lidocaine, alfentanil and xylazine in pigs anesthetized with isoflurane. *Veterinary Surgery* **24**: 73–77.

Woolf, N., Hall, L.W., Thorne, C., Down, M. and Walker, R.G. (1970) Serum creatine-phosphokinase levels in pigs reacting abnormally to halogenated anaesthetics. *British Medical Journal* **iii**: 386–387.

Anaesthesia of the dog

15

INTRODUCTION

Within the last 15 years there has been a considerable number of changes in the way anaesthesia is conducted in dogs. Introduction of new drugs has broadened choices for anaesthetic protocols and enabled use of appropriate combinations to meet demands of increasingly sophisticated and more protracted medical and surgical procedures. Monitoring equipment has become available specifically for veterinary medicine and its cost is such as to make its purchase feasible in general veterinary practice. Now, more than ever, it is possible to focus on the individual patient's problems and to design anaesthetic management to provide safe anaesthesia with optimum surgical conditions and minimal adverse impact on postoperative course.

SEDATION AND ANALGESIA

Selection of a drug or drugs for sedation depends on the purpose for which it is intended. Mild tranquilization can be achieved with a phenothiazine such as acepromazine whereas moderate to heavy sedation is better obtained using an α_2 agonist, such as medetomidine, or a neuroleptanalgesic mixture, such as morphine with acepromazine. Dose rates chosen may depend on whether the animal is to be only sedated or whether sedation is to be followed by general anaesthesia. When the drugs are used for premedication to anaesthesia, dose rates are often considerably lower so as to minimize cardiovascular and respiratory depression.

PHENOTHIAZINE DERIVATIVES

Acepromazine is the phenothiazine most commonly used for sedation in dogs. It is best used as a 2 mg/ml solution in dogs as dose administration can be more accurate than when a stronger solution is used. The response to acepromazine is not uniform and depends on the animal's temperament, physical condition, and breed. In general, the giant breeds (e.g. St Bernard and Newfoundland) are exceptionally sensitive to the drug and will become recumbent and reluctant to move following doses of about 0.03 mg/kg. Small breeds, in particular the terrier breeds, are much more resistant and may not show signs of sedation following even large doses.

Dogs of the Boxer breed are renowned for their liability to 'faint' following even small doses of phenothiazine derivatives (e.g. 0.02 mg/kg of i.m. acepromazine). This response may occur quite suddenly, with no prior sedation; the animal becomes flaccid or unconscious and there is severe hypotension with bradycardia. Because this response is similar to a vasovagal reaction which might be blocked by atropine or glycopyrrolate, the authors suggest that not only should minimal doses (0.02 mg/kg) be employed in this breed, but also that they should always be combined with anticholinergics even if being given for purposes other than premedication before anaesthesia.

The actions of acepromazine are potentiated by hypovolaemia, uraemia, and old age. The hypotensive effects of the drug can become particularly serious in the presence of hypovolaemia. Hypotension is best treated by the rapid intravenous infusion of balanced electrolyte solution and, if necessary, by infusion of dobutamine. When an opioid has been administered concurrently, partial reversal of the opioid with naloxone may assist in restoration of blood pressure.

The dose rates for acepromazine decrease with increasing size of the animal; for i.m. administration in small dogs, 0.05–0.10 mg/kg; for dogs 10 to 20 kg, 0.05 mg/kg; for dogs 20 to 40 kg, 0.03–0.05 mg/kg: with a maximum dose of 3 mg for most large dogs, with occasional dogs being given 5 mg acepromazine with an opioid to induce profound sedation (Table 15.1). These dose rates

are usually adequate for sedation of most animals and for premedication. They are lower doses than those recommended on the product data sheets but increasing the dosage rarely increases the sedative effect. The action of acepromazine is primarily anxiolytic and may be negligible in aggressive dogs. In general, there will be better sedation and less cardiovascular depression if an opioid is given concurrently when more pronounced sedation is required.

Acepromazine and atropine solutions may be mixed in the same syringe and injected i.v. (0.03 mg/kg acepromazine) but the drug may still take up to 20 minutes to produce its full effects. Acepromazine is said by some to be poorly absorbed from s.c. sites but has, in fact, been used satisfactorily by this route in dogs for many years. Oral administration is much less reliable and the sedative effect is greatly influenced by whether the drug is administered with food or on an empty stomach.

An advantage to including acepromazine for premedication is that it provides some protec-

TABLE 15.1 Injectable drugs for sedation or premedication in dogs

Drug	Dose (mg/kg)	Comments
Acepromazine	0.05 to 0.20 i.m., i.v. small dogs 0.05 to 0.10 i.m., i.v. 10–30 kg 0.03 to 0.10 i.m., i.v. > 30 kg	Lowest dose for large dogs, max. usually 3 mg, absolute max. 5 mg
Atropine	0.04 i.m., s.c.; 0.02 i.v.	Anticholinergic
Buprenorphine	0.006 to 0.010 i.m., i.v.	Onset time 30–40 min.
Butorphanol	0.2 to 0.4 i.m., i.v.	Premedication
	0.05 to 0.20 i.m., i.v.	Postoperative analgesia
Diazepam	0.2 to 0.5 i.v.	Do not give alone to healthy dogs
Glycopyrrolate	0.010 i.m.; 0.005 i.v.	Anticholinergic
Medetomidine	0.02–0.04 i.m. 0.01–0.02 i.v.	Profound sedation; severely decreases dose of anaesthetic agents
Midazolam	0.1 to 0.2 i.m., i.v.	Do not give alone to healthy dogs
Morphine	0.2 to 1.0 i.m. If using i.v. route, give *slowly* *	Initiates vomiting
Naloxone	0.01 to 0.02 i.m., i.v., s.c.	Opioid antagonist
Oxymorphone	0.05 to 0.20 i.m., i.v.	Max. initial dose 5 mg; highest dose only for induction protocol; initiates vomiting, panting
Pethidine	3.0 to 4.0 i.m.	Premedication
	1.0 to 2.0 i.m. If using i.v. route, give *slowly* *	Postoperative analgesia
Xylazine	0.5 to 2.0 i.m., 0.5 to 1.0 i.v.	Initiates vomiting

* Give slowly over 5 min to avoid hypotension.

tion against catecholamine-induced ventricular irregular rhythms. Acepromazine should be omitted from premedication when severe blood loss or hypotension is anticipated during surgery as the peripheral α blockade complicates treatment of hypotension. Acepromazine decreases the threshold for seizures and it is usual to avoid it in dogs with a history of seizures and when myelography is scheduled.

Other phenothiazine derivatives which are used include propionyl promazine, promazine, promethazine, trimeprazine, and chlorpromazine. The side effects produced by them and the provisions of use are similar to those of acepromazine but methotrimeprazine, which is used as part of the neuroleptanalgesic mixture 'Small Animal Immobilon', is said to have the added advantage of possessing analgesic properties.

α_2 ADRENOCEPTOR AGONISTS

Xylazine

Xylazine was the first α_2 adrenoceptor agonist to be widely used in veterinary medicine. Given i.m. to dogs in doses of 1–3 mg/kg it will produce good sedation and even hypnosis. The drug is classified as a sedative/hypnotic and, as might be expected, increasing the dose leads to greater sedation as well as increased duration of action. Although high doses will apparently produce unconsciousness (absence of visible response to external stimuli) this is associated with severe cardiovascular effects and prolonged recovery, so that high doses cannot be recommended. An obvious side effect in dogs is retching and vomiting as sedation develops.

In dogs, xylazine often causes a rise in arterial blood pressure (ABP) and dose-related respiratory depression. Although atropine may be given to prevent bradycardia its effect is variable, and it is sometimes ineffective.

Even when sedation is not marked, the doses of induction agents are greatly reduced after xylazine premedication. Xylazine slows the circulation, so there is a long delay between i.v. injection of an anaesthetic drug and its effects becoming apparent: unless due allowance is made for this, i.v. anaesthetic agents will be overdosed.

Medetomidine

Medetomidine is a potent α_2 adrenoceptor agonist which produces a dose-dependent decrease in the release and turnover of noradrenaline in the central nervous system which results in sedation, analgesia and bradycardia. In the periphery, medetomidine causes vasoconstriction by activation of postsynaptic receptors in the vascular smooth muscle. Thus, as with xylazine, there is an initial increase in ABP due to an increase in systemic vascular resistance. When administered i.m. at doses which produce deep sedation (40 µg/kg) the rise is minimal and ABP rapidly falls to slightly below the normal resting level. Following medetomidine administration dogs often breathe in an irregular manner, periods of up to 45 seconds of apnoea being followed by several rapid breaths. Although the mucous membranes appear to be cyanotic, PaO_2 is only slightly depressed.

With equisedative doses of xylazine and medetomidine both the type of sedation achieved and the side effects of bradycardia, respiratory depression and mucous membrane colour are similar. Medetomidine provides better sedation and analgesia than xylazine and has a longer duration of action (Tyner *et al.*, 1997). Vomiting occurs in about 20% of dogs receiving medetomidine, but is more frequent and prolonged after xylazine. Both xylazine and medetomidine decrease gut motility. Medetomidine, at 10 and 20 µg/kg i.v., significantly decreases serum insulin concentration but plasma glucose concentration remains within the normal physiologic range (Burton *et al.*, 1997).

Medetomidine has a steep dose–response curve and doses should, ideally, be calculated on a body surface area basis rather than on bodyweight. In practice this means that smaller dogs require relatively higher doses than large dogs. Over the rising phase of the dose–response curve sedation and analgesia are dose-dependent. Although appearing deeply sedated vicious dogs may still be aggressive and must be handled with care. Old age increases the sedative effect of medetomidine and frequently a dose of 20 µg/kg will have the same effect as 40 µg/kg in a younger dog. The effect and duration of medetomidine also depends on the route of administration, i.v. producing a more intense sedation of shorter duration than i.m.

(England & Clarke, 1989). Injection s.c. of medetomidine resulted in poor absorption and unpredictable effect. Following i.v. administration dogs will become recumbent in 2 minutes but maximal effects may take longer to appear. The duration of analgesia may be 45 minutes without further drug administration, and the time to standing will be approximately 90 minutes. After i.m. injection, recumbency may occur within 6 minutes or take 30 minutes and likewise, the time to standing is variable from 1.5 to 2.0 hours.

The drug is also effective when squirted from a syringe into the oral cavity of difficult dogs in doses of 30–80 μg/kg, but in quiet dogs may be administered carefully under the tongue and doses of 5–10 μg/kg are very effective by this sublingual route which avoids a first-pass through the liver. In the UK the data sheet for medetomidine recommends that impervious gloves be worn when handling the drug. Care is necessary to avoid splashing the drug on to mucous membranes when expelling air from syringes.

Investigations relating to the use of anticholinergics with medetomidine have confirmed that incidence of ventricular arrhythmias is higher when atropine and medetomidine are administered at the same time; an effect which is not observed when the atropine is given 10 or more minutes before the medetomidine. Since hypertension is the usual mechanism inducing the bradycardia, administration of an anticholinergic agent will exacerbate the hypertension (Alibhai *et al.*, 1996). Thus, use of an anticholinergic is unnecessary or even contraindicated when medetomidine is to be used only for sedation. However, when medetomidine is to be followed by inhalation anaesthesia there is a valid argument for anticholinergic administration for premedication to avoid a further decrease in cardiac output and blood pressure induced by vasodilation from the inhalation agent.

The use of medetomidine for premedication greatly reduces the doses of subsequent anaesthetic required in a dose-dependent manner, e.g. moderate doses of medetomidine may decrease the subsequent dose of thiopental to 2 mg/kg. Its sedative and hypnotic effects have been shown to be synergistic with those of opioids such as butorphanol and fentanyl (England & Clarke, 1989a) and with other anaesthetic agents.

Romifidine

Romifidine is the most recent α_2 adrenoceptor agonist investigated for use as a sedative in dogs. Similarly to the other agents, romifidine, 40 μg/kg and 80 μg/kg, reduced the subsequent induction dose of thiopental to 6.5 and 4.0 mg/kg, respectively (England & Hammond, 1997).

OPIOID ANALGESICS

Opioids are widely used to provide analgesia, in and outside the operating room (Table 15.1). The choice of opioid for a specific patient will depend on the origin of the noxious stimulus, the required duration of analgesia, the need for sedation or not, assessment of the potential impact of adverse effects on the patient, and the relative cost. The opiates such as morphine, pethidine (meperidine), hydromorphone, and oxymorphone are effective analgesics for orthopaedic pain whereas the partial agonist, butorphanol appears to be less effective. Buprenorphine has been unpredictable in providing postoperative analgesia. Nonetheless, in a clinical study comparing preoperative administration of morphine and buprenorphine for post-arthrotomy analgesia effects, both opioids provided adequate analgesia (Brodbelt *et al.* 1997). The approximate onset of action after i.m. administration for butorphanol and oxymorphone is 10–15 minutes, for pethidine is 20 minutes, and for morphine and buprenorphine is 40 minutes. The degree of sedation induced by opioids depends on the drug, the dose rate, and the individual response. Some sedation is usually obtained with morphine and oxymorphone, although administration of morphine and to a lesser extent oxymorphone to healthy dogs can result in excitement (Robinson *et al.* 1988). Pethidine, butorphanol and buprenorphine may produce little obvious sedation, although dose rates of subsequently administered drugs are decreased. Pethidine and butorphanol have short durations of action of 1–2 h, morphine and oxymorphone may provide analgesia for 3–4 h, and buprenorphine appears to last 4–6 h. Fentanyl is very short lived at 20–40 minutes.

The opioids are renowned for their respiratory depressant effects, particularly when used with inhalation anaesthesia. Hypoventilation (hypercarbia) may increase intracranial pressure and be an undesirable feature for dogs with head trauma, intracranial masses, or spinal cord compression. Hypoventilation may result in inadequate uptake of inhalation agent and an unacceptably light plane of anaesthesia. Panting may be a feature of opioid administration, and this occurs more often with pethidine and oxymorphone. Potent short acting opioids, such as fentanyl, that are injected as supplements during surgery or given as an infusion cause sufficient respiratory depression that controlled ventilation is usually necessary.

Dogs frequently vomit during the onset of action of morphine, hydromorphone and oxymorphone, and this is not a desirable feature for dogs with cervical instability or gastrointestinal foreign bodies or obstruction. Vomiting is less likely to occur if the animal is in pain when the drug is administered. Pethidine and morphine cause severe hypotension when given rapidly intravenously. The hypotension may be the result of histamine release or due to a direct peripheral vasodilation. If given i.v., these drugs must be given slowly over several minutes to avoid severe haemodynamic changes or they may be best given by other routes. The other drugs may be given by i.v. or i.m. routes depending on the need for rapidity of action, but i.m. administration tends to produced a more level, prolonged effect. The cardiovascular effects of i.v. administered opioids are greater when the animal is anaesthetized and decreases in cardiac output and blood pressure should be expected (Martinez *et al.* 1997). Decreases in cardiovascular function may be unexpectedly dramatic when the opioid is given for postoperative analgesia to a patient that has experienced haemorrhage during surgery.

The cardiovascular effects of the opioids are generally minor but there are some differences between the agents. Morphine, 1 mg/kg, given slowly over 5 minutes has only minimal effects on systemic haemodynamics (Priano & Vatner 1981). Similarly, oxymorphone induces minimal cardiovascular depression in healthy dogs although heart rate may decrease (Copland *et al.* 1987).

SEDATIVE/OPIOID COMBINATIONS

The combination of an opioid with a sedative may accomplish one of two goals. On the one hand,

addition of an opioid will increase the degree of sedation and analgesia beyond that achieved by use of the sedative or opioid alone. Conversely, the combination allows a decrease in dose rate of one or both the drugs while still achieving satisfactory sedation. Decreased dose rates may result in less respiratory or cardiovascular depression, less airway obstruction in brachycephalic breeds, and less drug to be metabolized for recovery. Furthermore, at the end of the procedure the opioid component can be antagonized by injection of naloxone. Sedative-opioid combinations (neuroleptanalgesia) are used for procedures such as radiography, examinations, bandage changes and minor orthopaedic manipulations, and for preanaesthetic medication. For some of these combinations dogs remain sensitive to sound and may rouse abruptly in response to a loud noise or sudden movement.

Combinations such as acepromazine, 0.05 mg/kg, with morphine, 0.5–1.0 mg/kg, or oxymorphone, 0.05–0.1 mg/kg (5 mg maximum initial total dose), or the combination of medetomidine, 0.03–0.04 mg/kg, with butorphanol, 0.2 mg/kg, given i.m. will induce profound sedation. The combinations of acepromazine, 0.05 mg/kg, with pethidine, 3–4 mg/kg, or butorphanol, 0.2–0.4 mg/kg, or buprenorphine, 0.01 mg/kg, cause mild to moderate sedation. The route of administration will influence the intensity of sedation. The combination of a benzodiazepine with butorphanol is useful in brachycephalic dogs with low risk for causing airway obstruction. For example, administration of butorphanol, 0.2–0.3 mg/kg, with midazolam, 0.2 mg/kg, i.m. to a Bulldog might induce mild sedation but butorphanol, 0.2 mg/kg, with diazepam, 0.2 mg/kg, given i.v. may produce greater sedation and a tractable animal in lateral recumbency for a short time. Many combinations with different dose rates are used. Other opioids used include methadone, 0.1 mg/kg, and hydromorphone, 0.1–0.2 mg/kg. Omnopon-Scopolamine is a commercially available mixture and 20 mg Omnopon (papaveretum) and 0.4 mg Scopolamine (hyoscine, an anticholinergic) combined with 3 mg of acepromazine provides good sedation in aggressive German Shepherd dogs.

Various premixed combinations of drugs are marketed for sedation in dogs. *Hypnorm* consists of fentanyl with fluanisone. Intramuscular injection produces deep sedation and analgesia of about 20 minutes duration, which is suitable for minor surgical procedures. Dogs sedated with this combination will move in response to noise.

Small Animal Immobilon contains the powerful and long-acting opioid etorphine in combination with methotrimeprazine. Given at the manufacturer's recommended doses to the dog by the i.v., i.m. or s.c. routes, it produces a profound and prolonged state of unconsciousness and analgesia. Intramuscular and s.c. injections are painful. Respiratory depression can be severe and the dog may appear cyanotic. Convulsions following the use of Immobilon have been reported to the Association of Veterinary Anaesthetists Committee concerned with deaths and adverse reactions of drugs used in anaesthesia.

At the end of surgery, the etorphine component of the mixture may be antagonized by the injection of diprenorphine but the patient remains sedated from the effects of methotrimeprazine. It must be remembered that once the antagonist has been given, attempts to provide analgesia with pure agonist opioids will be unsuccessful. Following reversal dogs tend to return to a state of deep sedation, or even unconsciousness, several hours after the antagonist has been given. Instances of post sedation renal failure have occurred after the use of Immobilon which could be a result of hypoxia and/or hypotension during the period of sedation.

Owners have reported that dogs 'appear to be different' after Immobilon. Behavioral changes, including aggression to people within or outside the family have been reported after sedation with acepromazine-oxymorphone (4% of dogs) or fentanyl-droperidol (15% of dogs) (Dohoo *et al.* 1986).

BENZODIAZEPINES

Diazepam or midazolam are not often administered alone to healthy dogs as they may induce excitability. They are frequently used in combination with an opioid for sedation or preanaesthetic medication and within the combination contribute to greater sedation than would be obtained by the opioid alone. Diazepam or midazolam are often injected i.v. just before thiopental, methohexital, or

propofol and will produce a small decrease in the dose rate needed for induction of anaesthesia. These benzodiazepines are often included with ketamine to prevent the central nervous system excitation that may be caused by ketamine.

Diazepam is poorly absorbed from i.m. injection. Midazolam is a water-soluble benzodiazepine that is twice as potent as diazepam and is better suited for i.m. administration. Midazolam, unlike diazepam, is not painful on i.v. injection and does not cause thrombophlebitis. Both agents are commonly used because of their cardiovascular-sparing action. They cause minor changes in cardiac output and mean arterial pressure at the dose rates used clinically (Jones *et al.* 1979). Heart rates may be increased and this may have an adverse influence in dogs with ventricular dysrhythmias. Diazepam is commonly given i.v. at a dose rate of 0.2–0.25 mg/kg but this may be increased to 0.5 mg/kg in some circumstances. Midazolam is administered i.m. or i.v. at 0.1–0.2 mg/kg.

Temazepam does not form active metabolites and has a relatively short duration of action. It may be given to dogs in a soft gelatine capsule in doses of approximately 0.25 mg/kg. Zolazepam is available in a fixed combination with the dissociative anaesthetic, tiletamine.

Flumazenil is a benzodiazepine antagonist that binds competitively, reversibly, and specifically to the same central nervous system sites as benzodiazepines. Agonist-antagonist ratios of flumazenil to rapidly and completely reverse the effects of diazepam and midazolam overdose in dogs is 26:1 for diazepam and 13:1 for midazolam (Tranquilli *et al.* 1992).

NON-STEROIDAL ANTI-INFLAMMATORY DRUGS

Non-steroidal anti-inflammatory drugs (NSAIDs) are frequently used for pain relief in animals before anaesthesia and surgery and can be used to supplement analgesia in the postoperative period. NSAIDs used in dogs include aspirin, phenylbutazone, naproxen, meloxicam, ketoprofen, carprofen, and etodolac. Adverse side effects include gastritis, gastrointestinal haemorrhage, hepatocellular toxicosis, and acute renal failure (Johnston &

Fox, 1997; MacPhail *et al.*, 1998). Gastroduodenal lesions were observed by endoscopy in 71% of healthy dogs receiving carprofen, meloxicam, or ketoprofen for 28 days, although none of the dogs had clinical signs related to the lesions (Forsyth *et al.*, 1998). There is some evidence that the prevalence and severity of adverse side effects are less with carprofen. Dogs undergoing anaesthesia and surgery might be imagined to be at greater risk of adverse effects from NSAIDs because these procedures may produce disturbances of fluid balance and decreased organ blood flow which will slow elimination and result in prolonged blood concentrations of NSAIDs. However, fluid balance disturbances are usually corrected at the time of surgery and for analgesia it is seldom necessary to administer these drugs for more than the first 48 postoperative hours.

A prospective evaluation of carprofen administered at 4 mg/kg preoperatively for a variety of orthopaedic procedures indicated that dogs given carprofen had similar or slightly better pain scores than dogs given pethidine pre- and postoperatively (Lascelles *et al.*, 1994). A later study of the efficiacy of carprofen for analgesia in dogs undergoing ovariohysterectomy confirmed that carprofen provided pain relief and suggested that administration of carprofen preoperatively had advantages over postoperative administration (Lascelles *et al.*, 1998). Immediately after anaesthesia for elective orthopaedic surgery, trials showed that evidence of pain relief was present 4 hours later in dogs given ketoprofen but not in dogs given oxymorphone alone (Pibarot *et al.*, 1997).

PREPARATION FOR ANAESTHESIA

Preparation for anaesthesia includes preanaesthetic evaluation of the ability of the patient to withstand the changes induced by general anaesthesia and of the potential impact of surgery and anaesthesia on the intra- and postoperative course. Choice of anaesthetic agents and management is based on information derived from the dog's history, physical examination, abnormal values detected by laboratory tests, nature of any current illness, and requirements of the proposed medical or surgical procedure. The significance of many

of the conditions which may be discovered during preanaesthetic evaluation are discussed in Chapter 1 and later on in this chapter.

There are, however, some aspects of the preanaesthetic preparation of dogs that deal with routine management and warrant further consideration here.

CONCURRENT DRUG THERAPY

Previous drug therapy can alter the response of dogs to anaesthesia and operation so it is essential that details of drug use should be sought from the case history. A full discussion of all possible drug interactions is beyond the scope of this book and reference should be made to textbooks on pharmacology and drug interactions. Interactions that are encountered fairly commonly in canine anaesthesia are described below.

1. Antibiotics

Chloramphenicol increases the length of action of barbiturate and inhalant agents but this rarely presents a clinical problem. More importantly, antibiotics given rapidly i.v. during anaesthesia can, in some dogs, induce profound hypotension that is unresponsive to treatment (Table 15.2). Antibiotics to be administered i.v. should be given slowly over several minutes with a close watch for effect on the ABP, particularly in dogs with cardiovascular instability. Many antibiotics, including the streptomycin group, the polymixins, and tetracyclines, exert an influence at the neuromuscular junction which enhances the effects of non-depolarizing muscle relaxants. This may induce re-paralysis when these antibiotics are administered at the end of anaesthesia.

2. Corticosteroids

Dogs which have been treated with corticosteroid drugs at any time in the two months preceding anaesthesia may have reduced ability to respond to stress. Additional steroid cover may be advisable in the form of methylprednisolone sodium succinate, 10 to 20 mg/kg i.v., or dexamethasone, 0.5–2.0 mg/kg, or another steroid more appropriate for the individual dog's condition

TABLE 15.2 Impact of concurrent administration of drugs on anaesthetic management

Drug	Significance
Antibiotics	Intravenous administration during anaesthesia causes moderate, occasionally severe, decrease in blood pressure in some dogs. Aminoglycoside antibiotics can cause muscle weakness and potentiate neuromuscular block from non-depolarizing relaxants. Chloramphenicol prolongs sleep time with ketamine and inhalant agents.
Carbonic anhydrase inhibitors	Induce metabolic acidosis
Cardiovascular drugs	Calcium channel blockers and ACE inhibitors may contribute to hypotension during anaesthesia unresponsive to treatment with vasoactive drugs
Corticosteroids	Long term preoperative use may predispose to circulatory collapse
Diuretics	Frusemide (furosemide) decreases serum potassium and may cause muscle weakness and cardiac arrhythmias
Insulin	Risk of hypoglycaemia during and after anaesthesia
Non-steroidal anti-inflammatory drugs	Anaesthesia increases risk for toxic effects; May be prevented by adequate fluid therapy
Organophosphate anthelmintic	Increases toxicity of acepromazine; may decrease anaesthetic requirement; prolongs duration of action of suxamethonium
Phenobarbital	Chronic use for seizure control associated with decreased hepatic function. Hepatic enzyme induction may increase production of metabolites from halothane to toxic level

based on knowledge of the history and previous dosing regime. Further steroid may be needed depending on the severity of the surgical procedure and how the dog recovered from anaesthesia.

3. Barbiturates

Long term barbiturate therapy for epilepsy will lead to enzyme induction and a decrease in duration of action of similar drugs given for anaesthesia. Administration for years leads to hepatic cirrhosis and decreased hepatic function. The effects of acutely administered phenobarbital or pentobarbital for the seizuring animal will be additive to subsequently administered drugs for anaesthesia for collection of cerebrospinal fluid or further diagnostic tests.

4. Other drugs

The number of dogs on cardiac medications has increased in recent years. Calcium channel blocking agents, such as verapamil and diltiazem, may be used to treat dogs with supraventricular tachyarrhythmias. Atrial fibrillation or flutter in dogs with dilated cardiomyopathy or advanced mitral regurgitation may be treated with these drugs, which slow conduction through and prolong the refractory period of the atrioventricular node (Pion & Brown, 1995). The cardiovascular effects of anaesthetic agents may be greater in dogs receiving these drugs. Anaesthesia with halothane or isoflurane may be associated with hypotension and episodes of sinus arrest (Priebe & Skarvan, 1987; Atlee et al., 1990). Treatment with atropine may be necessary to increase sinus rate and atrioventricular conduction. Benzodiazepines may compete for serum binding sites thus increasing free serum levels of verapamil. Lignocaine administration to dogs receiving verapamil results in a change in distribution of verapamil unrelated to protein binding but fortunately has minimal impact on cardiac function (Chelly et al., 1987). In contrast, the combined administration of verapamil and bupivacaine leads to decreased myocardial contractility and to high-grade atrioventricular blocks in conscious dogs. Diltiazem has been found to potentiate the neuromuscular blockade by vecuronium in humans (Takasaki et al., 1995).

TABLE 15.3 **A protocol for anaesthetic management of a regulated diabetic dog**

Sequence of events	Management
Night before surgery	Feed as usual
Morning of the day of surgery	Give one-half of the usual dose of insulin; do not feed
Before anaesthesia	Measure blood glucose; administer dextrose if value is low
During anaesthesia	Administer 5% dextrose in water, 3 to 5 ml/kg/h, in addition to balanced electrolyte solution; measure blood glucose at the end of anaesthesia, or every 1–2 hours, and adjust dextrose infusion rate according to result
After anaesthesia	Measure blood glucose 2 hours after anaesthesia; adjust treatment according to result; feed and return to insulin therapy as soon as appropriate

Angiotensin-converting enzyme (ACE) inhibitors, such as captopril and enalapril, are currently used in the treatment of dogs showing clinical signs of congestive heart failure. These drugs cause vasodilation by blocking the formation of angiotensin II and subsequent administration of anaesthetics that cause vasodilation is often accompanied by profound hypotension. Omitting the dose of drug on the morning of anaesthesia results in fewer treated dogs developing hypotension during anaesthesia.

Diabetic dogs receiving insulin are at risk of developing hypoglycaemia, hypotension and cerebral damage during anaesthesia. An accepted management for the diabetic dog that must be anaesthetized is given in Table 15.3. The blood glucose level should be maintained between 5.5–11.0 mmol/l (100–200 mg/dl) through frequent measurement of blood glucose concentrations and appropriate i.v. administration of 5% dextrose in water. Even dogs with well controlled diabetes can experience wide swings in blood glucose for several hours after anaesthesia, and monitoring should be continued until the following day.

BREED CHARACTERISTICS

The breed, age, and conformation have significant impact on choice of drugs and anticipated complications. Breed predispositions for different diseases and traits are extensive and appear to be constantly changing (Buchanan, 1993). Variable responses to anaesthetic drugs within breeds have also been reported. Some families of the Boxer breed, for example, are very sensitive to the effects of acepromazine. Several other breeds have been suggested as having increased sensitivity to anaesthetic agents, for example, the Belgian Terveurans and the Siberian Husky, and there is no doubt that often an adult St Bernard requires less drug for anaesthesia than an adult Great Dane. It is very likely, and this hypothesis is supported by experience and anecdotal reports, that there are strains of dogs within many breeds that have a very low tolerance for anaesthetic agents. Consequently, safety is increased when balanced anaesthetic techniques are employed and drugs are administered sequentially and 'to effect'.

Brachycephalic breeds

Conformation will have an impact on anaesthetic management. Brachycephalic breeds such as the English bulldog, Pug, Boston Terrier, and Pekingese are at risk of airway obstruction because of elongated soft palates, abnormal narrowing of the larynx, and everted laryngeal ventricles. Prolonged inspiratory stridor contributes to formation of oedema of the soft palate and laryngeal mucosa and tenacious stringy saliva in the oropharynx. These dogs are also more likely to develop cyanosis during induction of anaesthesia and to vomit in the recovery period. Obstruction can occur even during sedation and these dogs should be kept under observation after administration of premedicant drugs. Tracheal intubation is more difficult in these breeds and may involve smaller endotracheal tubes than expected based on the body size. The anatomy of the English Bulldog larynx may be distorted such that only an extremely small lumen tube can be inserted.

'Preoxygenation' is advisable to prevent hypoxaemia during induction of anaesthesia and is accomplished by administration of O_2 by facemask for several minutes before and during induction. Acepromazine should be used cautiously, if at all, and propofol or ketamine are less likely to be associated with prolonged difficulty in breathing than thiopental during recovery from anaesthesia. Opioids are useful agents to provide sedation and analgesia and to decrease the dose of subsequent anaesthetics. One problem with this group is that Bulldogs, Boston Terriers, and Pugs frequently pant during inhalation anaesthesia.

Sighthounds

The lean athletic breeds collectively known as 'sighthounds' include Greyhounds, Afghans, Salukis, Borzois, Whippets, Wolfhounds and Deerhounds. Their significance to the anaesthetist is the prolonged recovery from anaesthesia induced by thiopental because of lack of body fat (and muscle in some breeds), which precludes redistribution and lowering of blood thiopental concentrations. For these dogs, propofol yields vastly improved quality of recovery from anaesthesia. Ketamine is a less satisfactory agent for anaesthesia in these breeds than propofol, unless adequate sedation is provided for recovery, because they may exhibit signs suggestive of dysphoria.

AGE CHARACTERISTICS

Paediatric anaesthesia

Extremes of age have a significant impact on anaesthetic management (Fig. 15.1). Puppies less

Effect of age on anaesthesia

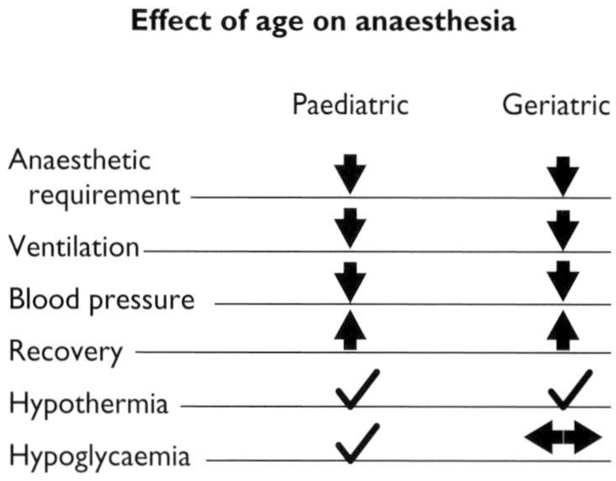

FIG. 15.1 Anaesthetic considerations for paediatric and geriatric animals.

than three months of age are more likely to require small doses of anaesthetic agents and to develop hypoventilation, hypotension, and hypothermia than young adults: O_2 consumption is higher in puppies than in mature animals and respiratory rates are high. Heart rates of around 200 beats/min occur in new-born puppies. Decreased heart rate and decreased preload (blood volume) result in large decreases in cardiac output (Baum & Palmisano, 1997). A small blood loss will cause a greater decrease in cardiac output than in an animal 3 months of age. The MAP is considerably lower in the first month of life than in mature dogs and the problem for the anaesthetist is how low is too low for blood pressure during anaesthesia? MAP of 50–60 mmHg may be satisfactory during anaesthesia in the first two weeks of life provided that peripheral perfusion appears to be adequate as indicated by pink membranes and rapid capillary refill time. Treatment of low pressure can be a problem as the immature heart may not respond satisfactorily to administration of anticholinergics and inotropic agents. The young animal is capable of a significant increase in cardiac output in response to a volume load, but this increase is depressed in the first few weeks of life.

Puppies have a decreased requirement for anaesthetic agents and also immature mechanisms for detoxification. Renal function does not, for example, reach adult function until puppies are 3 months of age (Poffenbarger *et al.*, 1990). Hypoglycaemia may develop during and after anaesthesia. Food should not be withheld for more than a few hours before anaesthesia and the puppy should be fed a few hours after anaesthesia. As prevention against hypoglycaemia, 5% dextrose in water, 3 to 5 ml/kg/h, should be infused intravenously during anaesthesia in addition to balanced electrolyte solution. Hypothermia develops easily in these small patients and will have a significant effect in decreasing ABP and metabolic rate, thus prolonging recovery from anaesthesia.

Geriatric (senior) dogs

Older dogs have a decreased requirement for anaesthetic agents due to a reduction in the number of neurons and neurotransmitter and, because hepatic and renal function are decreased, the dura-

Dog A = healthy   Dog B = overweight

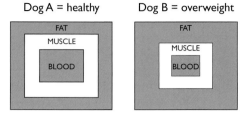

Administration of the same mg/kg dose
in overweight dog = overdosage

FIG. 15.2 Schematic representation of the risk for overdosage of overweight dogs with intravenous anaesthetic agents.

tion of action of drugs may be increased resulting in longer recovery from anaesthesia. The prevalence of hypoventilation is higher in senior dogs because chemoreceptor response to high PCO_2 and low PO_2 is decreased. Hypotension is more likely to develop due to decreased autonomic function with increasing age. Thermoregulation is increasingly impaired and hypothermia develops as a consequence. Pharyngeal and laryngeal reflexes are diminished and aspiration of reflux is more likely to occur than in a younger animal.

OTHER CONSIDERATIONS

Overweight (obese) dogs

Anaesthetic drug dosages for an obese dog should be calculated on its ideal weight since the animal's circulating blood volume is that of a smaller animal and fat contributes little to initial redistribution (Fig. 15.2). Hypoventilation may be severe and controlled ventilation will probably be necessary. An obese animal must not be allowed to breathe only air when anaesthetized as this will result in hypoxaemia.

Auscultation of the thorax

Auscultation of the heart, cardiac rhythm and lung sounds before anaesthesia is essential to identify abnormalities in animals that exhibit no signs of disease to the owner, for example patent ductus arteriosus in the young animal scheduled for castration or ovariohysterectomy. Auscultation of murmurs or abnormal rhythms should be followed up as potential early indicators of car-

diomyopathy (Brownlie, 1991). All dogs that have been injured in a road traffic accident should be auscultated for decreased lung sounds indicating lung collapse, pneumothorax, or diaphragmatic hernia. Abnormal ventricular rhythm in these dogs is an indication of traumatic myocarditis, although this clinical sign may not become apparent until 24 or 36 hours after the trauma. A thoracic radiograph provides valuable information on the integrity of the lungs and diaphragm, and this evaluation is especially important as up to 50% of dogs involved in automobile trauma will have pulmonary contusions.

Preanaesthetic blood tests

Considerable controversy arises concerning blood testing of healthy dogs scheduled for elective surgery. Retrospective studies of the outcomes of anaesthesia of human patients have revealed that in only a very small number of patients are there abnormalities shown by laboratory tests which have an impact on anaesthetic protocol (Pasternak, 1996). In a study of 2000 patients, only 0.22% of tests demonstrated abnormalities that might influence perioperative management (Kaplan *et al.*, 1985) and in another study of 1010 patients involving over 5000 tests, important abnormalities were found relating to only 4 patients (Turnbull & Buck, 1987). Nonetheless, identification of only a few dogs requiring special consideration for anaesthesia may be justification enough for an evaluation including blood tests. There is a rationale for submitting older dogs to blood testing before anaesthesia even when they are thought to be healthy. With increasing age, hepatocyte numbers decrease, pancreatic enzyme secretion diminishes, nephrons decrease, and glomerular filtration rate decreases (Hoskins, 1995). The age at which a dog should be considered geriatric (senior) varies with the breed, but may be said to be 9 years old for small and medium dogs, and 6 years for giant breeds. Many veterinary anaesthetists require that all dogs over 4 or 5 years of age have blood drawn for a complete blood count (CBC), plasma protein, blood urea nitrogen and creatinine, liver enzyme tests such as alkaline phosphatase (ALP), alanine aminotransferease (ALT) and aspartate aminotransferase (AST), the *in vitro* levamisole inhibition test as a screening test for increased serum ALP activity, and glucose. Measurement of electrolytes may also be advisable.

In the UK many veterinary anaesthetists consider that dogs should be blood tested only when, based on the history or physical examination there is an expectation of finding an abnormality, or when the dog is in a high risk population. This may include expanding the list of tests to cover a particular concern, for example, tests for coagulopathy in a Doberman pinscher that may suffer from von Willebrand's disease. Further, patients scheduled for major surgical procedures that are moderately to severely invasive and carry the risk of major blood loss should have blood tests performed to provide baseline values in anticipation of significant changes from surgery. Abnormalities of the results of laboratory tests should be noted for the possible modification of the anaesthetic protocol, e.g. the impact of low plasma protein in altering the amount of free and active anaesthetic drug, or in the ability of the dog to maintain an adequate blood pressure. Abnormalities of hepatic or renal function may dictate an adjustment in the selection of anaesthetic agents based on the dog's decreased ability to eliminate the drugs. Dogs with 30% or less of the normal level of von Willebrand factor tend to bleed and should be treated with 8–D-arginine vasopressin (DDAVP) or an infusion of fresh plasma or cryoprecipitate before anaesthesia and surgery.

It must always be remembered that almost all laboratory tests are costly to perform and the owner is entitled to have these costs justified before they can be expected to agree to procedures which may or may not influence the outcome of their dog's treatment.

Evaluation of the significance of disease

Identification of neurological or cardiac disease, or hepatic or renal malfunction, may have a direct bearing on choice of anaesthetic agents or anaesthetic management as discussed later in this chapter. Some diseases cause derangements of fluid, electrolyte, and metabolic balance and these should be corrected if possible before induction of anaesthesia. Correction of dehydration may not be feasible, but restoration of an adequate circulatory blood volume should be ensured by infusion of crystalloid, plasma or plasma substitute, or blood. The impact of the procedure on anaesthesia should be considered, for example, surgical procedures in the cranial abdomen or performed with the animal in a prone, head-down position will impair ventilation. Orthopaedic procedures require profound analgesia and may be responsible for considerable blood loss. Excision of tumours over the thorax may result in penetration of the pleural cavity. Animals with mast cell tumours should be pretreated with an antihistamine such as diphenhydramine, 2 mg/kg. Anaesthesia for thoracotomy or caesarian section is discussed in detail elsewhere.

Food and water restrictions

Dogs often vomit during induction or recovery from anaesthesia when their stomachs are not empty. Subsequent inhalation of vomit leads to aspiration pneumonia which is frequently fatal. It is usual practice to withhold food from mature dogs for about 12 hours, and water for at least 2 hours, to ensure that a dog will have an empty stomach. Fasting must last at least 16 to 18 hours for dogs eating dry food to ensure a completely empty stomach (Arnbjerg, 1992). A dog that has been involved in a fight or an accident and parturient bitches may have food in the stomach and the anaesthetic technique should be chosen to include a rapid sequence of induction to tracheal intubation. Protective phayngeal and laryngeal reflexes may not be present for several hours after anaesthesia and may not be present when a dog first regains its feet.

PREMEDICATION

Premedication in the dog usually involves administration of anticholinergic, sedative, and opioid drugs, the combination chosen depending on the circumstances and anaesthetic technique which is to follow.

ANTICHOLINERGICS

Anticholinergics are administered to limit bradycardia and to prevent salivation that might obstruct the airway or initiate laryngospasm. Anticholinergics decrease intestinal motility and the benefit observed is less vomiting in the recovery period. Glycopyrrolate decreases gastric acidity and may protect against oesophageal irritation in the case of reflux. Glycopyrrolate results in a smaller increase in heart rate after intramuscular administration than atropine and may be preferable in dogs in which high heart rates may have adverse effects, e.g. geriatric dogs and dogs with myocardial contusions. Atropine may be contraindicated in some animals with cardiac disease as the tachycardia induced may decrease cardiac output, increase the prevalence of ventricular arrhythmias, and increase myocardial ischaemia by increasing O_2 demand. A further contraindication to atropine administration is in dogs with a rectal temperature exceeding 39.7 °C (103.5 °F).

Atropine sulphate may be given i.m., s.c. or i.v. Dose rates commonly used for premedication are 0.04 mg/kg of a 0.5 mg/ml solution s.c. or i.m., or half that dose i.v. Onset of action occurs in about 20 minutes after i.m. injection and lasts about 1.5 hours. Onset of action is within 2 minutes after i.v. injection and the effects on the heart last about 30 minutes. Higher doses may be used where needed and in the antagonism of neuromuscular block and in cardiopulmonary resuscitation. Glycopyrrolate is given at 0.01 mg/kg i.m. and 0.005 mg/kg i.v. Onset of action after i.m. administration is 40 minutes and duration is 2 to 4 hours.

Other anticholinergics are sometimes used as part of neuroleptanalgesic mixtures. Hyoscine is combined with papaveretum in Omnopon/ Scopolamine and when this combination is used atropine is not required.

SEDATIVE AND ANALGESIC PREMEDICATION

Any of the analgesic and sedative drugs already discussed may be used for premedication but in

TABLE 15.4 Drug combinations for anaesthesia with injectable agents*

Premedication	Dose rate (mg/kg i.m.)	Induction	Dose rate (mg/kg i.v.)
Acepromazine	0.03 (large dog) 0.10 (small dog)	Thiopental	12
Acepromazine Pethidine	0.03 to 0.10 3 to 4	Thiopental	10
Acepromazine Butorphanol	0.03 to 0.10 0.3 to 0.4	Thiopental	10
Acepromazine Morphine	0.03 to 0.05 0.5	Thiopental	4 to 6
Medetomidine	0.02	Thiopental	1 to 3
None		Propofol	6 to 8
Acepromazine	0.03 to 0.05	Propofol	4 to 5
Acepromazine Butorphanol	0.03 to 0.05 0.2 to 0.3	Propofol	3 to 4
Acepromazine Morphine	0.03 to 0.05 0.5	Propofol	1 to 2
Medetomidine	0.04	Propofol	1.0 to 1.5
None or acepromazine or butorphanol or buprenorphine		Diazepam (5 mg/ml) Ketamine (100 mg/ml)	0.25 5.0 (=1 ml/10 kg using a 50:50 mixture)
Butorphanol	0.3	Etomidate	0.75 to 1.50
None		Diazepam Oxymorphone	0.2 0.1 to 0.2

* The examples in this table refer to fit healthy dogs. Sick animals may require considerably less while individual dogs may require more or less of the induction agent following premedication.

dogs those most commonly employed for this purpose in are the opioids, the phenothiazines, and the α_2 adrenoceptor agonists (Table 15.4). Opioids will provide analgesia during and after the procedure and when administered with sedatives, will increase the sedation achieved. The choice of agent will depend partly on the dog and the reason for use and partly on availability and cost. When vomiting after premedication is not advisable, such as in dogs with neck pain, gastric or intestinal foreign bodies, decreased ability to protect the airway against aspiration, or with a ruptured cornea, premedication with morphine, oxymorphone, and pethidine should be avoided. Similarly, these agents induce pupillary constriction in dogs and should not be included in protocols for intraocular surgery.

When analgesia is to be supplemented by use of a fentanyl patch or epidural morphine, then use of a partial agonist such as butorphanol for premedication is not advisable as it will decrease the effectiveness of fentanyl or morphine. Opiates that are µ receptor agonists can effectively be used concurrently, such as morphine or oxymorphone for premedication followed by supplementation with i.v. fentanyl during surgery. In the event that butorphanol has been used for premedication and later, during anaesthesia, greater analgesia is required, a higher dose rate of a µ agonist opioid may be necessary if the time elapsed since the initial administration of butorphanol is less than 1.5 hours. One potential use for mixing µ agonists and partial agonists is when an agonist such as morphine or oxymorphone has been used intraoperatively and butorphanol is used postoperatively. The butorphanol will reverse the effects of the previous drug but provide some analgesia with minimal sedation through κ receptors (Dyson *et al.*, 1990).

Neuroleptanalgesia created by concurrent administration of a sedative and an opioid is a popular choice for premedication. Sedation is much improved by the combination and may dramatically decrease the dose rate of drugs used for induction and to enable endotracheal intubation to be carried out. The degree of sedation depends on the drugs used and dose rates, and there is some individual variation. Intramuscular administration of butorphanol, 0.2–0.4 mg/kg, buprenorphine, 0.01 mg/kg, or pethidine, 3–4 mg/kg, alone

may induce very little sedation but when combined with acepromazine, 0.02–0.03 mg/kg they can produce heavier sedation. Sedation is greater from morphine, 0.3–0.5 mg/kg, oxymorphone, 0.07–0.1 mg/kg, or hydromorphone 0.2 mg/kg, but these agents induce profound sedation when combined with acepromazine and may decrease the induction dose of thiopental to 3–4 mg/kg.

Acepromazine alone in i.v. or i.m. doses of 0.02–0.03 mg/kg calms most animals effectively for venepuncture and reduces the induction dose of thiopental or propofol. Active dogs may not be sufficiently sedated and here the addition of an opioid is advisable. Larger doses of acepromazine do not increase sedation but can result in hypotension during anaesthesia. Acepromazine contributes to maintenance of a steady plane of anaesthesia and to a smooth recovery from anaesthesia, while also reducing myocardial irritability.

Xylazine and medetomidine produce profound sedation and greatly reduce the dose of anaesthetics used subsequently. Moderate doses of medetomidine, 10–20 µg/kg, administered with an opioid produce deep sedation that needs only a little of the induction drug for intubation to be possible. Care must be taken during induction of anaesthesia since these drugs slow circulation time, and sufficient time must be allowed to elapse for full effect to be shown before administering more of the drug. Medetomidine, 30–40 µg/kg, given i.m. with butorphanol, 0.2 mg/kg, produces such deep sedation that endotracheal intubation may be accomplished without further drug administration. The cardiovascular effects of this group of drugs are significant and their use in dogs suffering from cardiovascular disease or those with hypovolaemia is inadvisable.

INTRAVENOUS ANAESTHESIA

In dogs, as in other animals, intravenous agents may be used either to induce anaesthesia which is then maintained by inhalation methods, or as sole anaesthetic agents. The use of intravenous drugs as sole anaesthetics does not mean that anaesthetic machines are unnecessary. The i.v. agents commonly produce respiratory depression and endotracheal intubation, administration of oxygen and even controlled ventilation may be necessary if hypoxaemia and hypercapnia are to be avoided. Some i.v. agents may also be given by s.c. or i.m. injection but these routes of administration are not recommended for routine induction of anaesthesia because of variable absorption and difficulty in gauging the dose.

INTRAVENOUS TECHNIQUE

Intravenous injections in dogs are commonly made into the cephalic vein, but other convenient sites include the lateral saphenous vein, the femoral vein, the jugular vein and, in anaesthetized animals, the sublingual veins. Whichever site is used, conscious dogs should be handled quietly and forcible restraint reserved for those occasions when it is essential. Muzzles may be necessary in dogs showing an inclination to bite. The muzzles should be of the type with a quick release catch as delay in removal of a muzzle tangled in facial hair in a dog that has vomited during induction of anaesthesia may lead to inhalation of the vomited material.

Haematoma formation after venepuncture should be prevented by application of pressure to the site for an adequate period – usually about a minute. A haematoma is not only painful for the patient; it may prevent subsequent use of the particular vein for venepuncture for several days. Where a vein has been entered during an unsuccessful attempt at venepuncture, the pressure which was keeping the vein distended should be released and firm pressure applied to the site to stop bleeding before another attempt is made.

If the vein on the right forelimb is to be punctured an assistant stands on the left side of the animal, passes his or her left arm around the animal's neck and raises its head (Fig. 15.3). The assistant's right hand grips the animals right forelimb so that the middle, third and fourth fingers are immediately behind the olecranon and the thumb is around the front side of the limb. The limb is extended by pushing on the olecranon and the vein is raised by applying pressure with the thumb. The hand should be rotated so as to pull the cephalic vein slightly lateral, which straightens it and makes it more visible. Venepuncture must be car-

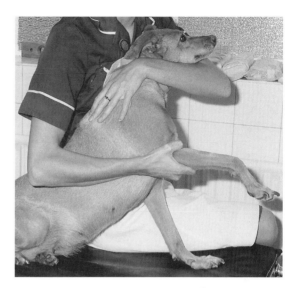

FIG. 15.3 Restraint for injection into the cephalic vein.

ried out with the usual aseptic precautions, so hair over the vein is clipped and the skin is disinfected.

It is an advantage to use syringes of more than 2 ml capacity that have an eccentrically placed nozzle, for this allows the syringe to rest securely on the forearm with the needle more or less flush to the vein. In this way, the angle of entrance, i.e., the angle between the needle and the vein, is small and consequently there is less risk of the needle being pushed right through the vein. Suitable needle sizes depend on the size of the dog and the quantity and viscosity of the fluid to be injected. For most purposes a needle 2.5 cm long and 22 or 23 gauge is satisfactory; a 25 gauge needle can be used for small dogs. The point of the needle should not be cut too acutely, the 'short bevel' being preferred.

Two methods of stabilizing the vein prior to needle puncture are employed. In one, the skin over the vein is tautened without flattening the vein by the anaesthetist's free hand grasping the limb distal to the site of venepuncture and gently pulling the skin down. In this position it is easy for the anaesthetist to adjust the handhold to grip the syringe between thumb and forefinger once the vein has been entered. Usually the skin is penetrated in one move and then the vein entered in a second move. Once blood is observed in the needle hub, the needle should always be threaded deeper into the vein before making any injections.

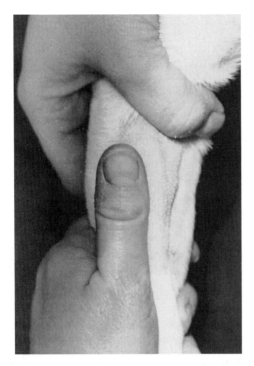

FIG. 15.4 Stabilization of the cephalic vein against the thumb.

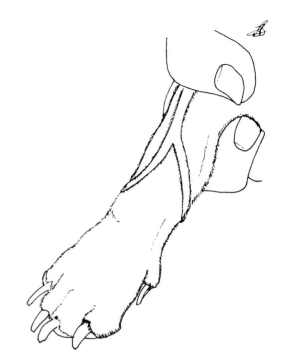

FIG. 15.5 In short-legged dogs such as Dachshunds with very mobile skins the easiest point for venepuncture is at the junction of the veins from the medial and lateral aspects of the carpus where they unite to form the cephalic vein.

In the second method, the thumb of the anaesthetist's free hand is placed just alongside the vein, and the skin is not tensed (Fig. 15.4). The vein is stabilized between the needle and the thumb as the needle is advanced through the skin into the vein. With this method it may be harder to thread the needle up the vein and there is a greater tendency to make contact between the needle point and the branch of the radial nerve running alongside the vein.

The first attempt at needle puncture should be done distally in the limb so that, if a haematoma forms, further attempts can be made more proximally. In Dachshunds and dogs with similar short, bent forelimbs venepuncture is best attempted in the angle where the accessory cephalic and cephalic veins join just cranial to the carpus (Fig. 15.5).

All air should be expressed from the syringe before venepuncture is attempted and there must be sufficient space left in the syringe to allow slight withdrawal of the plunger in order to test whether the needle is within the lumen of the vessel. Blood should enter the syringe when this is done, and no

injection must be made if blood does not appear in the syringe or needle hub. Failure to draw blood usually means that either the vein has not been entered, the needle tip has passed through the opposite wall of the vein, or that the needle has become occluded. Failure to aspirate blood into the syringe is also encountered if the assistant has released occlusion pressure on the vein, if the vein is already thrombosed, or when peripheral perfusion is poor as it may be after administration of an α_2 adrenoceptor sedative.

The lateral saphenous vein may be used for i.v. injection at the point where it passes obliquely on the lateral aspect of the hindlimb just proximal to the tarsus. The dog is usually restrained on its side but two assistants may be required for an alert dog. One restrains the head and forelimbs while the other holds the underneath leg immobilized with one hand and holds the upper limb in full extension by pressure on the stifle while raising the vein as shown in Fig. 15.6. Two hands may be needed to immobilize the limb and raise the vein

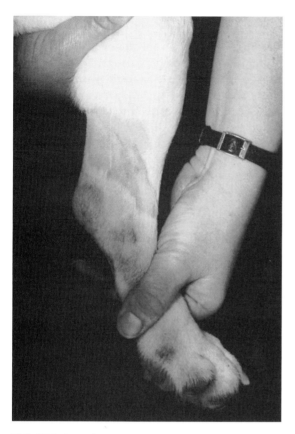

FIG. 15.6 Lateral saphenous vein.

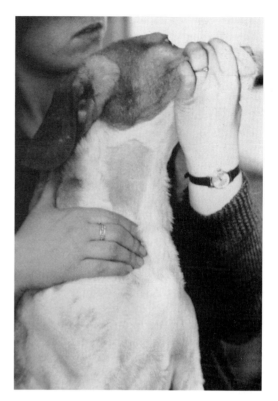

FIG. 15.7 Jugular venepuncture in the conscious sitting dog.

in very large or active dogs. The lateral saphenous vein is usually more prominent than the cephalic vein but it is more mobile and therefore more difficult to puncture. When the needle has been introduced well into the vein the needle is fixed to the leg by pressing on the needle hub with thumb, or thumb and forefinger, while the fingers encircle the limb.

The femoral vein in the middle part of the medial aspect of the thigh may also be used. It is rendered obvious by pressure applied to the inguinal region and is usually more prominent in the cranial part of the thigh. Care should be taken to ensure that injections are not made into the femoral artery which lies directly beneath the vein.

Venepuncture of the jugular vein in the dog can be done with the dog standing or sitting with the head raised (Fig. 15.7). Particularly in smaller or ill patients, it is easier when the animal is restrained on its side and the vein is raised by occlusion near

the sternal inlet. A small foam pad, towel, or sandbag placed under the neck of the dog makes the position of the vein more obvious.

Short catheters (18 gauge and 20 gauge, 5 cm long, or 20 gauge or 22 gauge, 2.5 cm long) are commonly inserted into the cephalic or lateral saphenous veins prior to induction of anaesthesia for administration of anaesthetic drugs, electrolyte solutions and supportive drugs. All of the veins described, cephalic, saphenous, femoral, and jugular, can be used for placement of longer catheters (18 gauge and 22 gauge, 20–30 cm long) when the animal is likely to need several days of treatment with i.v. solutions and drugs after anaesthesia.

Securing a catheter in the jugular vein is more difficult than in a limb. The external end of the catheter is positioned so that it is pointing toward the back of the neck; several folded gauze sponges are placed under the free end of the catheter which is then stabilized by wrapping 2 or 3–inch gauze around the neck and this then secured by white tape and vetwrap or elastic bandage. When a catheter-through-the-needle product is used, the needle usually cannot the removed after the catheter has been inserted in the vein. The needle guard provided should be clipped over the needle and the needle and catheter hubs glued together with a drop of 'superglue'.

The sublingual veins may be used for i.v. injections in anaesthetized dogs. The tongue is pulled over the anaesthetist's finger so that its ventral surface is exposed and injection is made into one of the easily visible veins. It is important to use a small (25 gauge) needle because the vein will bleed very freely after the needle is withdrawn. Pressure should be applied to the site for several minutes to avoid large sublingual haematoma. However, in case of emergency and absence of any other peripheral venous access, an 18 gauge catheter can be inserted in the lingual vein of medium sized dogs for administration of a large volume of electrolyte solution or blood. These veins are also useful for collecting blood to measure the packed cell volume and total protein during anaesthesia and surgery.

Intraosseous injection

Placement of a catheter in a vein is occasionally difficult in dehydrated animals, especially toy breeds and puppies. The intraosseous route is an acceptable alternative for administration of fluids, blood, and drugs. Absorption of drugs is rapid and within one minute for some drugs, such as atropine. Intraosseous injection implies injection into the intramedullary canal of the femur, tibia, or humerus using either a Cooke intraosseous needle, a Jamshidi needle or a spinal needle. A 20 gauge, 2.5 cm spinal needle is satisfactory for the smallest dogs and is inserted aseptically through the trochanteric fossa of the femur and parallel to the long axis of the bone into the medullary cavity. The stilette is removed, the needle flushed with heparinized saline, a T-port is attached and flushed again. Bandaging must be secure to prevent the needle from being dislodged as the animal moves about. Potential complications include infection and exceptional care should be taken in maintaining sterility of injections. The needle should be removed after 72 hours.

Vascular port

The vascular port is a subcutaneously implanted system for i.v. delivery of drugs. It is used when dogs require multiple anaesthesias over a short time, for example for radiotherapy, and the peripheral veins are badly thrombosed. The vascular port consists of two basic parts: an indwelling catheter that is threaded into the jugular vein after surgical dissection in the anaesthetized dog and a rigid puncturable bulb that looks like a volcano and is located subcutaneously in the neck. The bulb has a silicone rubber window that is easily palpated through the skin and allows percutaneous intravenous injections using an appropriate needle.

INTRAVENOUS AGENTS

Intravenous agents may be administered alone but are usually given after preanaesthetic sedation. Induction of anaesthesia will then be calmer, fewer adverse side effects of the induction drugs will be observed, their margin of safety will be increased, and recovery may be faster. Some commonly used drug combinations, with dose rates, are given in Table 15.4.

Thiopental

Solutions of thiopental have a high pH and the drug can only be given i.v. It should always be used in dogs as a 2.5% or weaker solution for more concentrated solutions are unnecessary and dangerous. A 5% solution increases the total quantity of the drug required, causes thrombosis of the vein and, if any is injected perivascularly, produces a serious slough of the overlying tissues and skin. Injection of any quantity of even a 2.5% solution into the tissues outside the vein is an indication for the immediate injection into the area of 2 mg/kg of lignocaine (lidocaine) without adrenaline to precipitate the thiopental into a harmless salt, and up to 20 ml of saline for dilution of the irritant.

The dose of thiopental depends on the condition of the dog, its state of hydration and, particularly, on previous medication. For these reasons the dose rate is often stated to be 'sufficient and no more' but as a rough guide the anaesthetist should expect to have to use up to 12 mg/kg in a dog for induction of anaesthesia. In the healthy but lightly premedicated dog, one half of this, i.e. about 6 mg/kg is given rapidly as a bolus of a 2.5% solution should produce a rapid induction of anaesthesia and a smooth transition to inhalation anaesthesia. If anaesthesia is insufficient to permit endotracheal intubation, additional small increments of the remainder should be given at 20–30 second intervals. The whole dose may be needed in a proportion of dogs and when the drug is given more slowly. Large dogs require relatively less than small, while geriatric dogs have a reduced anaesthetic requirement. A lower dose of 5–6 mg/kg of thiopental may be sufficient in dogs provided with a moderate degree of preanaesthetic sedation from a combination of sedative and opioid, such as acepromazine and butorphanol. The dose of thiopental required for induction will be greatly decreased to 1–3 mg/kg in dogs that are heavily sedated, for example with acepromazine and morphine, xylazine and butorphanol, or medetomidine.

Other drugs may be administered i.v. immediately before thiopental to decrease the dose needed and to enhance the quality of induction. Diazepam or midazolam, 0.1–0.2 mg/kg, may decrease the dose of thiopental required by 15% or more, depending on the physical status of the dog. Potent opioids such as alfentanil may greatly reduce the thiopental dose required to induce anaesthesia. Alfentanil, 5 µg/kg, given over 30 seconds before thiopental may reduce the thiopental dose to about 3 mg/kg. A dilute solution of alfentanil should be used to facilitate slow injection which will minimize the occurrence of apnoea after thiopental injection. Atropine or glycopyrrolate should be given prior to or concurrently with alfentanil administration to prevent bradycardia.

The consequences of reduced thiopental dose rate by prior administration of premedicant or other anaesthetic agents are two-fold. First, overdosage and cardiac arrest are a possibility and always the anaesthetist should assess the dog's need for thiopental based on the degree of central nervous depression and cardiovascular stability. Secondly, low dose administration of thiopental means that the drug will be rapidly redistributed so that the duration and quality of recovery are related to the other agents used. When the other agents are rapidly eliminated or their action can be pharmacologically antagonized, recovery from anaesthesia is more rapid than when a higher dose of thiopental alone has been administered.

In dogs, thiopental is very slowly metabolized and attempts to prolong anaesthesia with multiple or higher doses which saturate the body fat result in very prolonged anaesthesia followed by 'hangover' for 24 or more hours. In thin dogs such as Borzois, Afghans, and Greyhounds (Greyhounds may also be deficient in the liver enzymes necessary for detoxification of thiopental), this level is reached very rapidly, and little more than the minimum induction dose may be given with safety. In fact, recovery will be more satisfactory in these animals if thiopental is omitted and induction achieved by administration of a more rapidly metabolized agent such as propofol.

Thiopental differs from some other intravenous agents in that high doses cause severe respiratory depression so that prolonged anaesthesia cannot be produced by an initial high dose, but must be maintained by incremental doses. Where thiopental is used as the sole anaesthetic, recovery may be violent and noisy. Sedative premedication can prevent this, so should always be employed, but if it is omitted, a sedative or analgesic should be given at the end of anaesthesia.

The maximum total dose of thiopental for a healthy dog is about 25 mg/kg – and this would represent a gross overdose in a sick animal. Recovery is prolonged after a dose of this magnitude. Because of its lack of analgesic properties, attempts to use thiopental for painful procedures, even short ones, tend to result in overdosage. It is far preferable to provide a base of sedation and analgesia with other drugs so that only small doses of thiopental must be injected to produce the minimum of respiratory depression while only just abolishing or modifying the response to stimulation.

In the absence of surgical stimulation the first indication that thiopental anaesthesia is passing off is that stiffening of the jaws and curling of the tongue occur when the mouth is opened. There may be licking of the nose and from this point recovery is rapid. The time taken to assuming sternal position will then depend on the lingering effects of premedication or provision for postoperative analgesia. After light preanaesthetic sedation, when no other anaesthetic agent has been given to prolong anaesthesia, the dog is obviously quite conscious and aware of its environment about half an hour after induction . Limb coordination, especially the hind, is delayed, and the dog may stagger in a drunken manner for about an hour.

Methohexital

Although recovery from a single bolus dose of methohexital is due mainly to redistribution to the muscles and body fat, the drug is rapidly eliminated from the body by metabolism and excretion so that dogs recover from even large doses quickly. In general it is advisable to use sedative premedication to smooth induction and recovery, because without such sedation both periods may be violent. Doses of 4 to 6 mg/kg i.v. in a 1 or 2% solution are suitable for the induction of anaesthesia in dogs premedicated with acepromazine, and further small increments given as required may be used to prolong anaesthesia. The method of injection is similar to that for thiopental, although a slightly slower rate of initial injection is less likely to result in apnoea. Because of its rapid elimination from the body, recovery after prolonged methohexital anaesthesia usually occurs within half an hour of the last dose being given. Overdose produces severe respiratory depression, and even anaesthetic doses produce more respiratory depression than equipotent doses of thiopental. Depression of cardiac output with low anaesthetic doses is also greater than after equipotent doses of thiopental (Clarke & Hall, 1975). Cumulation and, therefore, delayed recovery occurs in doses in excess of 10–12 mg/kg.

Because recovery is so rapid and complete, methohexital is most useful for outpatient anaesthesia and induction of anaesthesia in brachycephalic dogs, thin dogs, young dogs, and for caesarian section. Even in these animals, however, methohexital has largely been replaced by propofol.

Pentobarbital

Pentobarbital was formerly widely used in canine anaesthesia and there can be no doubt that at the time of its introduction in the early 1930s it caused a revolution in small animal practice. By the end of 1938 the slow intravenous injection of pentobarbital had been used to produce anaesthesia in more than 2000 operation cases at the Beaumont Hospital of the Royal Veterinary College, London, by J. G. Wright and his colleagues. Pentobarbital soon became the standard agent for producing anaesthesia of about an hour's duration. Although pentobarbital is not often used now, it is occasionally used in the intensive care unit to produce deep sedation in dogs with neurological disease and it is still widely employed in experimental laboratories.

After weighing the dog the approximate dose is estimated on a basis of about 30 mg/kg body weight. In healthy unpremedicated animals, about a half to two-thirds of the computed probable dose is injected rapidly intravenously in order to ensure that the dog passes quickly through the excitement phase of induction of anaesthesia. Because the onset of action of pentobarbital is much slower than that of thiopental, the remainder of the dose is administered in increments over 3–5 minutes, pausing after the injection of each increment and assessing its effect. When complete relaxation of the head and neck is obtained, relaxation of the jaws is assessed. Opening the mouth provokes movement of the tongue and jaws varying from a complete yawn to a slight curling of the tip of the tongue. A little more of the anaesthetic is injected and after an appropriate wait the jaws are again opened. The aim is to reach the point at which the jaws are completely relaxed and the tongue, when drawn out, hangs limply.

When this is attained, a light level of unconsciousness can be assumed. The corneal reflex is present, the pupil reacts to light and the pedal reflex is brisk. Respirations are regular and deep. This is the degree of anaesthesia to be induced for superficial operations. If it is decided to induce deeper unconsciousness with pentobarbital, the so-called 'pedal reflex' is then used as the index of depth. If the web between the digits, or the nail bed, is pinched firmly with the finger and thumb nails, it will be found that the pedal reflex comprises a definite upward and backward jerking of the limb. Often the response continues for several seconds after the stimulus has ceased. Administration is slowly continued until the reflex is just lost and then the depth of unconsciousness is adequate for the performance of intra-abdominal procedures.

When used to control seizures in a patient with neurological disease, pentobarbital must be given over several minutes in small increments to avoid overdosage, as the dose in these patients may be as low as 4 mg/kg.

Propofol

Propofol, as the free-flowing oil-in-water emulsion which does not give rise to histamine release, is commonly used in dogs (Hall, 1984; Watkins *et al.*, 1987). The dose for induction of anaesthesia in unpremedicated dogs is 6 mg/kg and premedication with 0.02–0.05 mg/kg of acepromazine reduces this to about 4 mg/kg. Females are more susceptible than males, the induction dose in unpremedicated females being 5.23 mg/kg (SD 1.58, n = 68) and in males 5.74 mg/kg (SD 1.53, *n* = 39) (Watkins *et al.*, 1987). Administration of propofol for induction of anaesthesia is similar to thiopental in that one-half of the anticipated dose is administered initially as a bolus but the initial administration should be slower to avoid or minimize apnoea. Recommendations for the rate of the initial bolus vary from rapid to up to 3 minutes. However, administration of half the anticipated dose over 30 seconds seems to be satisfactory. Administration of O_2 by facemask during induction to prevent cyanosis is advisable, particularly in geriatric and sick dogs. The cyanosis occurring at induction of anaesthesia with propofol in some dogs has been attributed to apnoea, a transient decrease in arterial blood pressure, or opening of pulmonary shunts.

After induction, propofol may be given in incremental doses as needed to maintain anaesthesia. In dogs premedicated with an anticholinergic and acepromazine (0.03 mg/kg) or butorphanol (0.2–0.3 mg/kg) anaesthesia can be maintained by continuous infusion of propofol at a rate of 0.3–0.4 mg/kg/min (Fig. 15.8). Anaesthesia may be light for surgical procedures and muscle rigidity may be present in some animals. Retching and vomiting have been encountered in the recovery period in 16% of dogs after continuous infusion of the agent. Dogs left unstimulated in the recovery

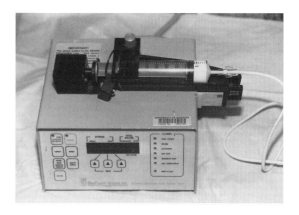

FIG. 15.8 Syringe driver (Medex Inc., Duluth, Georgia, USA) for continuous administration of propofol or other anaesthetic agents or fluids.

period appear to sleep – arousal during this stage can result in immediate awakening with an ability to walk without ataxia. Dogs given one dose of propofol recover completely in about 18 minutes from the time of injection and those given intermittent injections recover in about 22 minutes from the time of injection of the final increment. Preanaesthetic sedation will prolong recovery according to the drugs used.

Propofol has been used for induction of anaesthesia in dogs after a variety of medications. Medetomidine, 20–40 µg/kg, decreases the induction of dose of propofol to 2–4 mg/kg (2 mg/kg after the high dose of medetomidine) and the dose rate for maintenance of anaesthesia to 0.15–0.2 mg/kg/min (Vanio, 1991; Hall *et al.*, 1997; Hellebrekers *et al.*, 1998). Alfentanil, 10 µg/kg i.v. mixed with 0.3 mg atropine, given one minute before induction of anaesthesia also decreased the dose of propofol for intubation to 2 mg/kg (Chambers, 1989) but apnoea of more than 3 minutes duration occurred in 11% of dogs and 6% showed twitching or paddling, usually of the forelimbs. Later trials (Hall, unpublished observations) demonstrated that a dose of 5 µg/kg of alfentanil, mixed with atropine, given over 30 seconds resulted in less apnoea without significantly increasing the subsequent dose of propofol needed. Recovery from injection to full awakening (no ataxia) is of the order of 7 minutes – a very fast recovery.

The effect on respiratory rate is variable but dogs which are panting before the induction of anaesthesia are likely to continue to do so throughout anaesthesia. Induction of anaesthesia in healthy dogs with propofol produces dose-dependent respiratory depression. Respiratory rate and minute ventilation decrease with a transient mild increase in $PaCO_2$ (Quandt *et al.*, 1998). No significant changes in HR, MAP or CO were measured. Others have concluded that although propofol may preserve MAP and CO if the preload is maintained, propofol may decrease MAP and CO secondary to a reduction in preload by a direct venodilator effect. Administration of propofol in dogs made hypovolaemic by withdrawal of 37% of their estimated blood volume resulted in a serious decrease in MAP (Ilkiw *et al.*, 1992). Premedication with different agents alter the cardiovascular response to propofol. Medetomidine, for example, results in increased MAP such that arterial pressure is maintained after administration of propofol. Like thiopental and halothane, myocardial sensitivity to the effects of catecholamines is increased by propofol and propofol should be used cautiously in patients at risk for ventricular arrhythmias, such as occur in cardiomyopathy and myocardial ischaemia or contusions.

Propofol may be a good choice for induction of anaesthesia in dogs with seizures, meningitis, brain tumours, or spinal cord disease as it decreases intracranial pressure. Likewise, propofol decreases intraocular pressure and may be used satisfactorily for induction of anaesthesia in dogs with severe corneal ulcers or those scheduled for intraocular procedures.

Ketamine

The dose of ketamine which produces anaesthesia in dogs produces excessive muscle tone and spontaneous muscle activity and is near to that which causes convulsions. Thus, ketamine cannot be recommended as a sole agent for canine anaesthesia. It can be used in combination with various sedative agents to induce anaesthesia for short term procedures or for maintenance with halothane, isoflurane, or sevoflurane. Unless specifically contraindicated anticholinergics may be administered for premedication to reduce the salivation induced by ketamine, or to prevent the decrease in heart rate induced by xylazine or medetomidine.

A common combination used for induction of anaesthesia is 0.25 mg/kg of diazepam and 5 mg/kg of ketamine given intravenously at the same time (equivalent to combining 5 mg/ml of diazepam and 100 mg/ml of ketamine in the same syringe as a 50:50 mixture and dosing at a rate of 1 ml of the mixture per 10 kg of body weight). Premedication may also include acepromazine, or an opioid, or a tranquillizer-opioid combination. Frequently one half to two-thirds of the calculated dose is administered rapidly initially and the remainder administered in increments as needed. The onset of action is much slower than thiopental and the signs of anaesthesia differ. Up to one minute may elapse after injection of ketamine before endotracheal intubation can be accomplished and even then there is little relaxation of the jaws; the eyelids will be wide open and a brisk palpebral reflex should be present.

Ketamine, 10 mg/kg i.v., to dogs results in increased HR, MAP, CO and systemic vascular resistance that is attributed to a centrally mediated, generalized increase in sympathetic tone (Haskins *et al.*, 1985). The combination of diazepam and ketamine produces similar effects (Haskins *et al.*, 1986). Although the preservation of cardiovascular function is useful in ill dogs, the significant increase in heart rate may induce rhythm problems in dogs with an ischaemic or damaged myocardium. Administration of ketamine to experimental dogs with haemorrhagic hypovolaemia revealed that ketamine supported cardiovascular function well (Haskins & Patz, 1990). However, induction of anaesthesia in critically ill dogs with ketamine in combination with diazepam or an opioid may usually be accomplished safely but using reduced dose rates.

In the past, the combination of xylazine, 1 mg/kg, and ketamine, 10 mg/kg, given either i.v. or i.m. has been used for short term anaesthesia. However, severe cardiopulmonary changes have been measured during anaesthesia with this drug combination such that there is concern about the safety of its use in old and sick dogs. CO is significantly decreased, and HR and ABP are increased, for 30 minutes following i.v. xylazine and ketamine (Kolata & Rawlings, 1982). The combination also produces moderate hypercapnia, acidaemia, and hypoxaemia for 20 minutes. Respiratory arrest is occasionally noted in clinical dogs anaesthetized with xylazine-ketamine. The more recent introduction of medetomidine has revived interest in the use of an α_2 agonist sedative-ketamine combination for injectable anaesthesia. The clinical features of anaesthesia in healthy dogs with medetomidine, $1000\mu g/m_2$ body surface area (approximately $40\mu g/kg$ in a 25 kg dog), administered intramuscularly 10–15 minutes before i.v. ketamine, 3–4 mg/kg, have recently been reported (Hellebrekers & Sap, 1997; Hellebrekers *et al.*, 1998). The duration of anaesthesia from single dosing was 54 ± 31 minutes (mean ± SD). Administration of ketamine reversed the medetomidine-induced bradycardia and caused hypertension with MAPs at 150 mmHg (Hellebrekers & Sap, 1997). Recovery from anaesthesia with ketamine is often associated with restlessness or hyperactivity and indeed, only 63% of recoveries from medetomidine-ketamine were judged to be smooth; this is in contrast to 89% of anaesthetics utilizing medetomidine-propofol (Hellebrekers *et al.*, 1998).

Tiletamine-zolazepam

In those countries where tiletamine is available it is obtained in a premixed combination with the benzodiazepine, zolazepam, under the trade names of Telazol and Zoletil. The drug preparation consists of 500 mg of lyophilized tiletamine-zolazepam (250 mg of tiletamine and 250 mg of zolazepam) which is reconstituted with sterile water. The doses reported are the sum of tiletamine and zolazepam doses so that 4 mg/kg of Telazol is equivalent to 2 mg/kg of tiletamine and 2 mg/kg of zolazepam. Initial studies of this drug combination were with higher dose rates than are now used commonly. Tiletamine-zolazepam, 4 mg/kg, i.m. with an anticholinergic provides effective sedation for aggressive or dangerous dogs. Sedation is profound but ranges from the dog being just capable of walking to the dog that is almost unconscious and ready for tracheal intubation. Onset of adequate sedation may be within minutes or up to 10 minutes. An alternative technique is to use lower doses of tiletamine-zolazepam i.v. to achieve anaesthesia for tracheal intubation prior to inhalation anaesthesia.

HR, MAP, and CO are increased by tiletamine-zolazepam but larger i.v. doses result in a transient and severe decrease in MAP (Hellyer *et al.*, 1989).

Etomidate

Etomidate is a short acting non-barbiturate i.v. anaesthetic. Its main feature is that induction of anaesthesia with etomidate is accompanied by little or no change in cardiovascular function and with less myocardial depression than thiopental, and etomidate does not predispose the heart to arrhythmias. Even in experimental dogs made hypotensive and hypovolaemic by haemorrhage, little cardiovascular change was measured during anaesthesia with etomidate (Pascoe *et al.*, 1992). Etomidate decreases intracranial pressure. Thus, the main indication for use is for dogs with cardiovascular compromise, such as cardiomyopathy, pericardial tamponade, sick sinus syndrome, or for dogs that are in haemorrhagic shock. Etomidate i.v. can be associated with undesirable side effects such as excitement, myoclonus, pain on injection, vomiting, and apnoea (Muir III & Mason, 1989). These effects should not be observed if etomidate, 0.75–1.5 mg/kg, is given after premedication with an opioid or diazepam. The technique of administration of etomidate is similar to that of thiopental, with half of the calculated dose (the dose used is modified by the evaluation of the individual dog's clinical condition) being given as a bolus injection and additional drug given in increments.

An important additional side effect of etomidate is that it interferes directly with adrenocortical production of corticosteroids and aldosterone. Reduced cortisol response to the stress of surgery in comparison to thiopental was measured for up to 6 hours after induction with etomidate, 2 mg/kg (Dodam *et al.*, 1990). For this reason, anaesthesia should not be maintained by additional injections of etomidate beyond the calculated dose. Exogenous steroid can be administered if necessary.

Neuroleptanalgesia

Some combinations of neuroleptanalgesia are sufficiently potent to induce anaesthesia that is adequate for endotracheal intubation in old or sick dogs. The dogs initially may be responsive to noise and endotracheal intubation must be performed quietly and gently followed by administration of sufficient inhalation agent to deepen anaesthesia. The administration of this type of induction is slightly more prolonged (over 2–3 minutes) than bolus injections of thiopental or propofol, however, the main advantage is preservation of haemodynamic stability (Haskins *et al.*, 1988). The drugs used for induction of anaesthesia may also be continued during surgery either as sole agents or to provide a substantial base of sedation and analgesia such that a very low concentration of inhalation agent is required. Large doses of opioids frequently induce bradycardia and administration of an anticholinergic may be advisable. In old and sick dogs given opioids IPPV may be necessary to correct hypoventilation. Preoxygenation is recommended.

Diazepam or midazolam, 0.2 mg/kg, with oxymorphone, 0.1–0.2 mg/kg, can be injected i.v. in alternate increments, flushing the catheter between injections, until all the benzodiazepine and as much of the oxymorphone as necessary for induction has been administered. A similar technique involves administration of diazepam, 0.2 mg/kg, and fentanyl, 2–5 µg/kg. Another combination recommended for cardiovascularly compromized dogs, including those with gastric dilatation/volvulus is sufentanil-midazolam (Hellebrekers & Sap, 1992). Mean doses for induction are 3 µg/kg sufentanil and 0.9 mg/kg midazolam. This combination has been continued for maintenance of anaesthesia without additional inhalation agent and the mean dose per hour was the same as the induction dose, namely 3 µg/kg/h sufentanil and 0.9 mg/kg/h midazolam (Hellebrekers & Sap, 1992); IPPV was applied throughout anaesthesia. A combination of metdetomidine, 1500 µg/m² body surface area, with fentanyl, 2 µg/kg, resulted in satisfactory induction of anaesthesia in healthy dogs but attempts to maintain anaesthesia with fentanyl were unsatisfactory, producing severe respiratory depression and the need for O_2 (Hellebrekers & Sap, 1997).

Alphaxalone-alphadalone

Saffan is marketed for use in cats but it is specifically contraindicated by the manufacturers for use in dogs, as it is solubilized in Cremophor EL – a compound which may cause massive release of histamine in all *Canidae*. Although it has been claimed that following heavy premedication with potent antihistamines Saffan can be used safely in dogs, reports to the Association of Veterinary Anaesthetists of Great Britain and Ireland indicate that even after this premedication Saffan administration can be followed by anaphylaxis. It is the authors' view that, given that safer alternatives exist, Saffan should not be administered to dogs.

INHALATION ANAESTHESIA

A wide variety of inhalation agents has been used in the past for canine anaesthesia. The choice of agent or agents in any particular case is largely governed by the limitations of each agent and relative contraindications imposed by the abnormalities of the dog. The properties of the gaseous and volatile agents currently employed in dogs which impact on the agent selection are summarized in Table 15.5.

The inhalation agents may be used in dogs both to induce or maintain anaesthesia or, more commonly, to maintain anaesthesia which has been induced with an i.v. agent. Induction of anaesthesia with i.v. agents is rapid and pleasant for the animal. Induction of anaesthesia with the inhalant agent using a facemask is usually only done in lightly sedated puppies or old dogs,

TABLE 15.5 Properties of inhalation agents currently used in dogs

Agent	Rapidity of action	Analgesic activity	Other properties
Halothane	++	Poor	Hypotension, respiratory depression
Isoflurane	+++	Poor	Hypotension, respiratory depression
Nitrous oxide	++++	Good	Inadequate on its own
Sevoflurane	++++	Poor	Hypotension, respiratory depression

and in other dogs that are moderately or heavily sedated.

INDUCTION USING A FACEMASK

Facemask induction is slower than induction with injectable agents and pollution of the room with anaesthetic gases usually occurs. The dog should be placed on a table at a convenient height and gently restrained by an assistant. The facemask is lightly placed over the dog's nostrils with only O_2 flowing to accustom the animal to the feel of the procedure. When the dog is quiet, the inhalation agent can be introduced and vaporizer setting should be increased by 0.5% increments after every three or four breaths. The face mask should be applied closely to the dog's face only when consciousness is lost. Attempts to introduce a high concentration of anaesthetic immediately through a closely fitted mask to a conscious dog will result in struggling, breath holding and excitement. When a non-rebreathing system is used for anaesthetic delivery, the inspired anaesthetic concentration will change within seconds of a change in the vaporizer setting. The increase in inspired concentration will be more gradual and, therefore, induction slower when a rebreathing system such as a circle is used. The O_2 flowmeter setting will be governed by the type of system in use, with moderate to high O_2 flows used during mask induction with a rebreathing circuit and an out-of-circle vaporizer. The maximum vaporizer setting used during induction should depend on the degree of preanaesthetic sedation, the type of delivery system, and the health of the dog. When a halothane vaporizer is set to above 2.5%, or the isoflurane vaporizer to above 4%, the anaesthetist must closely observe the progression of anaesthesia to avoid overdosage. Inclusion of 50–66% nitrous oxide from the start of administration will increase the speed of induction of anaesthesia by utilizing the 'second gas' effect (Chapter 6). Induction will also be rapid with sevoflurane. When a rebreathing system is to be used for maintenance of anaesthesia in a small dog, induction may be facilitated by use of a non-rebreathing system during induction and connecting the dog to the rebreathing system after tracheal intubation. When a rebreathing system is used for induction, it

may be advisable to express the low anaesthetic concentrations from the rebreathing bag periodically during the induction phase and then to express the highest anaesthetic concentration from the rebreathing bag before connecting the dog to the anaesthetic system after endotracheal intubation. In all cases the anaesthetist must remember to decrease the vaporizer setting to a safe level before connecting the endotracheal tube to the breathing system.

In circuits such as the Stephens machine, where the vaporizer is incorporated within the breathing circuit, each breath of the dog serves to vaporize more anaesthetic and the effect is maximal when the O_2 inflow rate is low. The rebreathing bag should also be emptied several times during induction to minimize accumulation of exhaled N_2 within the circuit.

SYSTEMS OF ADMINISTRATION

The different types of breathing systems which are available are described in Chapter 9 and the choice of system will depend on the size of the dog. Resistance to breathing in the circuit and apparatus deadspace should be low for small dogs. Suitable circuits include the T-piece, Norman elbow, Magill circuit, and the coaxial circuits such as the Bain or Lack systems. An advantage to use of these systems is that the inspired anaesthetic concentration is the same as that leaving the vaporizer, so that it is easier to maintain a stable level of anesthesia or to quickly change the depth of anaesthesia. The inspired concentration of anaesthetic agent changes within seconds of changing the vaporizer setting. Disadvantages compared with rebreathing systems are the greater decrease in body temperature that may occur because the inspired gases are dry, and the increased cost of anaesthesia because high gas flows are required and more anaesthetic agent is vaporized and wasted. Inclusion of a disposable humidifier between the endotracheal tube and the circuit will help to retain exhaled water vapor and, by moistening inspired gas, slow the rate of fall in body temperature.

Rebreathing systems used to administer inhalation anaesthesia include the circle and to-and-fro systems which contain carbon dioxide absorbers.

Their main advantage over non-rebreathing systems is that they are economical in use because low O_2 flows are used and less anaesthetic agent is vaporized. Furthermore, heat is generated by the action of the exhaled CO_2 on the soda lime in the absorber, water vapour is conserved in the circuit and the dog consequently breathes warm, moist gases. Dogs with a heavy hair coat, anaesthetized in a warm room using a rebreathing circuit can develop hyperthermia.

The resistance to breathing offered by the CO_2 absorbent may contribute to hypoventilation in small dogs. The smallest size of animal that should be connected to a circle circuit usually used for human adults (internal diameter 22 mm) is controversial. Paediatric hoses (internal diameter 15 mm) where available may be substituted for animals between 3 and 8 kg bodyweight. Resistance to breathing in these small sized dogs may result in failure to move gases through the absorber and result in rebreathing of CO_2. This inability to overcome the resistance of the soda lime may be countered by maintaining an oxygen flow of 1 l/min which will facilitate movement of gases around the circle and using IPPV.

The to-and-fro rebreathing system with a soda lime canister capacity of 0.5 kg is usually used in dogs weighing more than 10 kg and has the disadvantage of increasing dead space with use. The presence of the soda lime canister close to the dog's head is physically awkward.

Low-flow administration of inhalation anaesthetics

A low-flow system can be defined as one in which there is substantial rebreathing of previously expired gas which has passed through a CO_2 absorber (usually in a circle system). The minimum O_2 flow that can be delivered safely to a circle circuit is a flow equal to the animal's metabolic oxygen consumption (approximately 6 ml/kg/min). This is called a closed system of administration because there is no excess oxygen to be discharged through the 'pop-off' valve. A closed system does not require that the 'pop-off' valve be shut closed because the valve is designed to remain closed until a pressure builds within the circuit. During low-flow administration, the O_2 inflow exceeds metabolic needs and a small amount of waste gases will enter the scavenging system after each exhalation. An O_2 flow of less than 15 ml/kg/min is usually considered to be low-flow anaesthesia.

When low-flow administration is employed with an out-of-the-circuit vaporizer, the number of molecules of inhalation agent delivered to the circle per unit time is low in proportion to the uptake of agent into the patient's body. Consequently, exhaled gas low in agent exerts a significant diluting effect on the percent concentration of fresh agent entering the circle. The circle anaesthetic concentration may be lower than (down to one-half) the vaporizer setting. Thus, the vaporizer setting may have to be higher than 1.5–2.0 MAC in order to achieve a sufficiently high inspired anaesthetic concentration to maintain anaesthesia. Changes in circuit anaesthetic concentration will develop only slowly after the vaporizer setting is changed. When the concentration must be increased quickly, such as when the dog is too lightly anaesthetized for surgery, the vaporizer setting must be increased for a few minutes and then decreased to a value just above the original. Alternatively, the circle anaesthetic concentration can be increased rapidly by increasing the O_2 flow to 1 l/min. It must be realised that excessive anaesthetic administration can occur if the O_2 flow is increased from an established low-flow system. The circle concentration will have been low and if the vaporizer setting is at a percentage greater than 2 MAC, increasing the oxygen flow will bring the circle concentration up to deliver an excessive concentration.

To ensure that there is enough anaesthetic agent in the circle in the early part of anaesthesia, it is common to use a high oxygen flow (1 l/min) in the first 15 minutes of anaesthesia to wash-out expired nitrogen and wash-in sufficient anaesthetic agent. The oxygen flow rate is then decreased when the transition from injectable anaesthesia to inhalation anaesthesia has occurred. The vaporizer setting will be determined not only by whether high or low-flow administration is employed but also by which anaesthetic agents have been used for premedication and induction of anaesthesia. For healthy dogs, the vaporizer must be high after diazepam-ketamine induction but low after tiletamine-zolazepam induction or high dose medetomidine premedication.

Low-flow administration must never be used with N_2O unless the inspired concentration of O_2 is measured with an O_2 monitor. The concern is that N_2O will accumulate in a low-flow system, reducing the O_2 concentration to a value resulting

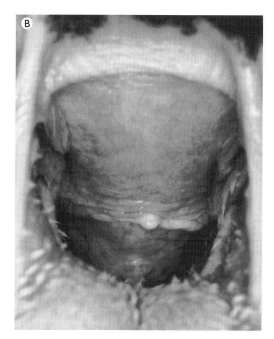

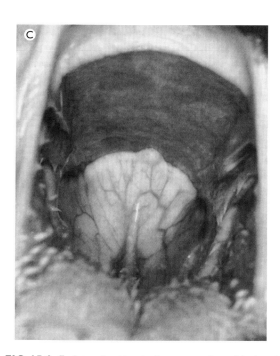

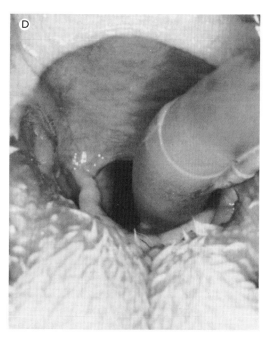

FIG. 15.9 Endotracheal intubation as seen by a right handed anaesthetist. **A** The assistant is holding the upper lips and the anaesthetist is drawing the tongue out of the mouth, protecting its undersurface by placing a finger over the dog's incisor teeth. **B** The epiglottis is almost completely obscured by the soft palate. **C** The soft palate has been lifted by the tip of the tube to allow the tip of the epiglottis to come forward. **D** The tip has been passed over the epiglottis, through the vocal cords and on towards the sternum.

in hypoxia. For practical purposes, the ratio of O_2 to N_2O will not be distorted if the O_2 and N_2O flow rates are each set at 30 ml/kg/min; at least 750 ml/min of each (total flow 1.5 l/min) for a 25 kg dog. Higher flows should be used if the ratio of N_2O to O_2 is increased to 2:1.

Circle circuits which incorporate the vaporizer within the breathing circuit are designed for the low-flow system of administration. It is the dog's own ventilation that draws oxygen through the vaporizer and vaporizes the inhalation agent. The lower the oxygen flow rate the more quickly the circle anaesthetic concentration increases. If the vaporizer was not initially intended for use with the highly volatile anaesthetic agents, only the low and middle settings on the vaporizer are needed for adequate anaesthetic delivery.

Endotracheal intubation

Cuffed endotracheal tubes for dogs vary from 2.5 mm to 16.0 mm internal diameter (ID). The diameter of the largest tube which can be introduced into the trachea is related to both the size and the breed of the dog with the requirement that the tube selected should be a good approximation of the tracheal lumen diameter but not a 'push' fit. For example, a 14 mm tube can usually be inserted in the trachea of an adult German Shepherd and an 11 or 12 mm tube used for most 25 kg dogs. In contrast, the Bulldog often has an exceptionally small-diameter laryngeal lumen and trachea for its body weight and a selection of smaller tubes should be available at anaesthetic induction of this breed.

The tubes should be checked for length alongside the dog because the tip of the tube should not extend beyond the thoracic inlet into the chest. Excess tube extending outside the incisors contributes to deadspace and CO_2 breathing and, therefore, some tubes may have to be shortened by cutting off 2 to 6 cm length with scissors. Thin-walled endotracheal tubes (e.g. ID to OD difference of mm) with small volume cuffs should be purchased for use in puppies and very small dogs to allow the largest lumen size possible in their small tracheas. Alternatively, uncuffed or Cole pattern tubes can be used to eliminate the space occupied by the cuff. IPPV and aspiration of foreign material are potential problems with use of uncuffed tubes and should be prevented by packing the pharynx with moistened gauze.

A good light source is needed in the form of bright overhead lighting or a laryngoscope since intubation in dogs is accomplished under direct viewing of the epiglottis and the position of the tube in relation to it. A laryngoscope is advisable for intubation of brachycephalic dogs. It is usual to induce anaesthesia in the dog to a level which is just adequate to allow the dog's mouth to be held open without initiating chewing movements, yawning, or tongue curling. When thiopental or propofol have been used for induction of anaesthesia and the dog is swallowing when intubation is attempted, the depth of anaesthesia is too light and more drug should be administered. Swallowing during intubation is normal during ketamine anaesthesia.

The dog may be positioned in either sternal or lateral recumbency. In either case, the assistant must hold the dog's head and neck in a straight line with one hand holding the top jaw, thumb and forefinger either side of the jaw behind the canine teeth and holding the upper lips up and away from the teeth to facilitate the anaesthetist's view. The dog's tongue is pulled rostrally to spread open the larynx and is held either by the assistant or by the anaesthetist in such a way as to protect it from laceration by the teeth (Fig. 15.9A). The blade of the laryngoscope is placed flat on the tongue with the tip of the blade depressing the tongue at the base of the epiglottis. In some dogs the epiglottis may be trapped behind the soft palate and must be released by using the tip of the endotracheal tube to push the soft palate dorsally (Fig. 15.9 B,C). The lubricated tube should be used to depress the epiglottis on to the tongue and to keep it here while the tube itself is advanced in front of the arytenoid cartilages into the trachea (Fig. 15.9D). Frequently, rotating the tube 90° about its longitudinal axis as the tip passes through the larynx allows the tube to be advanced more easily into the trachea. A strip of gauze should be tied tightly to the tube within the mouth just behind the canine teeth and then either around the jaw or behind the dog's head (Fig. 15.10). The knot around the tube must be tight to avoid slipping and accidental extubation. The endotracheal tube cuff should be inflated with just enough air to prevent a leak that

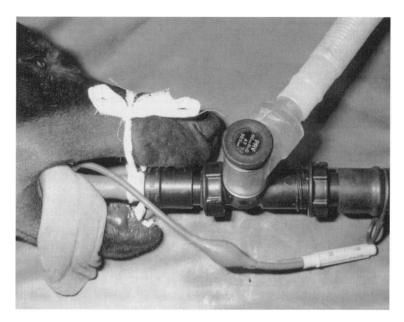

FIG. 15.10 Endotracheal tube secured in place by a tie placed tightly around the connector and then tied around the upper jaw behind the canine teeth. Note that the tube has been shortened so that the expiratory valve is at the nostrils, ensuring minimum dead-space. The inflating tube for the cuff has been doubled over and sealed by a disposable needle case (alternatively a 3-way tap can be used).

can be detected when listening for air escaping around the tube during inflation of the lungs by squeezing the reservoir bag to a pressure of 20–25 cm H_2O with any 'pop-off' valve screwed down. The anaesthetist must remember to release the valve after this procedure.

The process of intubation should be performed gently to avoid trauma to the pharynx and larynx which can cause tissue swelling and may result in airway obstruction during recovery from anaesthesia (even necessitating tracheotomy). Furthermore, any time that the dog's position or location is changed, the endotracheal tube should be briefly disconnected from the breathing circuit to avoid twisting the tube within the trachea and tearing tracheal mucosa.

HALOTHANE, ISOFLURANE, SEVOFLURANE

Cardiovascular effects

Increasing doses of all three agents cause significant decreases in cardiac index, MAP, and mean pulmonary arterial pressure, a significant increase in CVP, and a slight decrease or increase in HR (Hoffman *et al.*, 1991; Hysing *et al.*, 1992). Responses in MAP, mean pulmonary arterial pressure, and CVP vary considerably between individual dogs. In some studies the decrease in CO is less during deep isoflurane anaesthesia than at equipotent concentrations of halothane (Hysing *et al.*, 1992). Changes in cardiovascular parameters induced by sevoflurane anaesthesia are most similar to those produced by isoflurane (Mutoh *et al.*, 1997). Nonetheless, since all three agents decrease cardiovascular function, excessively low MAP will occur during inhalation anaesthesia in hypovolaemic dogs (Pascoe *et al.*, 1994).

Halothane increases the sensitivity of the myocardium to catecholamines and premature ventricular depolarizations may develop in the presence of hypercapnia. The prevalence of abnormal ventricular rhythms may increase in animals with myocardial ischaemia caused by thoracic contusions and gastric dilatation/volvulus. In contrast, sensitivity of the myocardium is not increased by isoflurane or sevoflurane. Occasionally, conscious dogs with ventricular premature depolarizations maintain a more stable cardiac rhythm when anaesthetized with isoflurane.

Isoflurane, but not halothane, has antifibrillatory effects in atrial tissue (Freeman *et al.*, 1990).

In healthy dogs without significant cardiovascular disease, the effects of the inhalation agents on cardiovascular function are relatively unimportant until deep anaesthesia is produced. The impact of inhalation anaesthesia must be considered in animals with ischaemic heart disease and cardiomyopathy. Myocardial blood flow is increased during isoflurane anaesthesia (despite decreased CO and MAP) and decreased during halothane anaesthesia (Gelman *et al.*, 1984). The myocardial depressant effects in dogs are comparable between isoflurane and sevoflurane, however, isoflurane causes coronary vasodilation whereas sevoflurane decreases coronary blood flow with no change in coronary vascular resistance (Tomiyasu *et al.*, 1999). Thus isoflurane is a coronary vasodilator with potential beneficial (increased myocardial blood flow) and hazardous ('coronary steal') effects. 'Coronary steal' occurs when blood flow is redirected away from ischaemic myocardium. This may occur during isoflurane anaesthesia since this agent causes dilation of normal myocardial arteries, preferentially the smaller coronary resistance vessels than the larger conductive vessels, and this may divert blood from stenotic or damaged arteries that are unable to dilate (Merin & Johns, 1994). The significance of the differences between the agents on myocardial blood flow is not as yet resolved. Many dogs with cardiovascular disease are anaesthetized satisfactorily with isoflurane with no untoward postoperative consequences. It may be a wise precaution to use an anaesthetic protocol that relies heavily on opioids for analgesia and only low doses of isoflurane in dogs with serious cardiac disease.

Both halothane and isoflurane increase cerebral blood flow, decrease portal blood flow, and preserve renal blood flow (Gelman *et al.*, 1984; Bernard *et al.*, 1991). Isoflurane increases hepatic blood flow whereas halothane decreases it during deep anaesthesia.

Ventilation

The decrease in ventilation during inhalation anaesthesia in healthy dogs is unpredictable. In some dogs, particularly small dogs and brachy-cephalic breeds, breathing may be fast and shallow (panting). This rapid rate must not be mistaken for a light plane of anaesthesia, although sometimes the tidal volume is so inadequate that uptake of halothane is insufficient to maintain anaesthesia. Hypoventilation will occur during deep inhalation anaesthesia and is very likely to occur in old dogs, obese dogs, and dogs receiving opioids.

Sevoflurane and compound A

Sevoflurane reacts with soda lime and generates several degradation products, of which compound A is reported to be nephrotoxic. Since the concentration of compound A is greater in circle circuits using low oxygen flows there has been concern for patient safety when using sevoflurane in closed circuit or low flow systems. In a clinical trial of sevoflurane in dogs involving three University Teaching Hospitals no evidence of impaired renal function was detected when the O_2 inflow was maintained at 500 ml/min (Branson *et al.*, 1997). Concentrations of compound A measured in circle circuits administering low-flow (< 15 ml/kg/min) sevoflurane to dogs were substantially lower than the concentrations reported to cause renal toxicoses in rats (Muir & Gadawski, 1998).

Administration

Halothane, isoflurane, and sevoflurane are potent inhalation agents that can be used to change the depth of anaesthesia rapidly. Anaesthesia can be induced with these agents through a facemask following preanaesthetic sedation with a sedative or sedative/opioid combination or they can be used for maintenance of anaesthesia after induction with an injectable anaesthetic agent. Induction of anaesthesia by facemask is faster and smoother with sevoflurane than isoflurane and, unlike isoflurane, sevoflurane does not cause airway irritation. The concentration of agent required to maintain anaesthesia is usually between 1.0 and 1.5 MAC values. Values reported for MAC vary slightly but are approximately 0.9% for halothane, 1.4% for isoflurane, and 2.1% for sevoflurane.

Occasionally, the anaesthetic agent for maintenance may be changed from halothane to isoflurane, for example, in the face of increasing frequency of ventricular arrhythmias or when the surgical procedure is unexpectedly prolonged and the anaesthetist wishes to take advantage of the shorter recovery time of isoflurane. Elimination of halothane takes longer than uptake of isoflurane because up to 20% of an inhaled dose of halothane is retained for metabolism in the liver. However, isoflurane is less potent than halothane and a higher vaporizer setting is required for the same depth of anaesthesia. A compromise is achieved by turning off the halothane vaporizer and turning on the isoflurane vaporizer to the identical setting for about 20 minutes, after which the vaporizer may have to be increased slightly to maintain the same depth of anaesthesia.

Recovery

In contrast to halothane, almost none of the inhaled isoflurane or sevoflurane is retained for metabolism. Consequently, recovery from anaesthesia can be very fast and complete unless underlying sedation is present or an opioid is administered for postanaesthetic analgesia.

NITROUS OXIDE

It is generally agreed that dogs cannot be anaesthetized with unsupplemented mixtures of N_2O and O_2. N_2O is used in non-rebreathing or circle circuits either:

1. As a vehicle for the vaporization and delivery of volatile anaesthetic agents and as a mild analgesic supplement to inhalation anaesthesia. The proportion of O_2 in the mixture must be at least 30%;

[or:]

2. In conjunction with injectable agents and analgesic supplements, such as fentanyl, and with muscle relaxants, for maintaining a light plane of anaesthesia. The percent of N_2O should be approaching 70% since it plays an important part in maintaining unconsciousness. Gas flow into a circle must be sufficiently high to wash out N_2 and allow N_2O concentration to increase. The cuff on the endotracheal tube must be inflated to achieve an airtight seal and prevent dilution of the inspired gases with air. As stated earlier, N_2O

should not be utilized in a low-flow system unless an O_2 analyser is incorporated in the breathing system.

N_2O is a useful adjunct to anaesthesia with halothane, isoflurane, or sevoflurane, providing sufficient analgesia is given to maintain an uninterrupted course of anaesthesia. N_2O will block patient response to intermittent intense surgical stimulation such as traction on the ovaries, clamping of the spermatic cord, or the manipulation involved in reducing a long bone fracture. Inclusion of N_2O allows a reduction in the concentration of volatile anaesthetic agent and, therefore, MAP remains at an acceptable value.

ARTIFICIAL VENTILATION OF THE LUNGS

Controlled ventilation (IPPV) may be needed to correct hypoventilation especially in overweight or geriatric dogs, dogs with depressed ventilation from administration of opioids or high concentrations of inhalant anaesthetics, or for dogs with impaired ventilation from positioning for perineal, back, or upper abdominal surgery. Sometimes IPPV is indicated in treatment of a moderate degree of anaesthetic-induced hypoventilation that is resulting in an inadequate uptake of inhalational anaesthetic and a depth of anaesthesia that is too light for the medical or surgical procedure to be performed. IPPV will be required in dogs for intrathoracic surgery, during neuromuscular paralysis, in neurological procedures that either include muscle weakness or dictate the need for decreased intracranial pressure, and for respiratory or cardiac resuscitation.

O_2 or O_2/N_2O gas flow rates do not need to be changed at the onset of IPPV. When IPPV is needed to decrease hypercapnia but no change in the depth of anaesthesia is desired, the vaporizer setting should be decreased by 20–25% at the onset of IPPV to adjust for the increase in alveolar ventilation and anaesthetic uptake. When a circle circuit with a vaporizer inside the circle is being used, the vaporizer setting should be decreased to almost off, as the positive pressure generated in the circuit and the increase in gas flow through the vaporizer can result in a dramatic increase in inspired anaesthetic concentration, with potentially fatal consequences.

Regardless of the spontaneous respiratory rate of the dog, satisfactory arterial carbon dioxide tension ($PaCO_2$) can be achieved in dogs with IPPV incorporating a respiratory rate of 12 breaths/min with a tidal volume of 15 ml/kg body weight, or 20 breaths/min with a tidal volume of 10 ml/kg. A tidal volume of 15 ml/kg can be achieved in healthy dogs with a peak inspiratory pressure of 18 to 20 cmH$_2$O, as observed on the pressure gauge of the Bain or circle circuits. Inspiratory time should be kept short and less than 2 s. These values may have to be adjusted for the individual patient so that for an overweight dog, for example, the tidal volume should be calculated on the dog's ideal weight since the contribution of fat to CO_2 production is minimal. In contrast, the tidal volume for an athletic or lean dog with a large frame and minimal fat should be increased from 15 to 20 ml/kg. The inspiratory pressure may be as low as 15 cm H$_2$O in tiny, thin dogs or may have to be increased up to 35 or 40 cm H$_2$O to achieve an adequate tidal volume in dogs with pressure on the diaphragm, such as from increased intra-abdominal fat or positioned in a prone head-down position. Inspiratory pressure should be limited to 25 cm H$_2$O in dogs with pulmonary disease or contusions to decrease the risk of barotrauma and pneumothorax. The chest of the dog should always be observed to confirm inflation of the lungs in the inspiratory phase of the IPPV cycle.

Assessment of the adequacy of IPPV can be precise with arterial blood gas measurement and reasonably so with end-tidal CO_2 measurement. Without these, an approximate guide can be obtained from observation of the inspiratory pressure on a pressure gauge in the breathing circuit and from the amplitude of chest excursion. Observation of mucous membrane colour provides no information about $PaCO_2$. The occurrence of spontaneous respiratory movements during the application of IPPV in a dog with pink mucous membranes usually, although not invariably, indicates that hypoventilation is still present. Other causes that should be considered are failure to expand the lungs owing to a leak at the level of the endotracheal tube or to pneumothorax, hypoxaemia, hyperthermia, or inadequate analgesia.

General considerations applying to IPPV in all animals are given in Chapter 8.

NEUROMUSCULAR BLOCKING AGENTS

Muscle relaxation can be achieved during anaesthesia by inducing deep general anaesthesia, by incorporation of agents that induce central relaxation, such as medetomidine, diazepam, or midazolam, or by use of agents that induce neuromuscular blockade. Use of neuromuscular blocking agents provides profound relaxation while permitting a reduction in dose rate of general anaesthetic agents and consequently the anaesthetic protocol results in less cardiovascular depression. Neuromuscular blockers are commonly used for ocular surgery, ensuring a central eye position to facilitate the surgical procedure. Further, relaxation of the extraocular muscles decreases intraocular pressure – a prerequisite for intraocular surgery to avoid prolapse of the vitreous. These drugs are also used during anaesthesia for thoracotomy to control the respiratory movements and for abdominal surgery to fully relax the abdominal muscles and increase surgical exposure to the organs. The relaxation induced by neuromuscular blocking agents means that the surgeon needs to use much less forcible retraction of muscles to gain access to the body cavities and so causes far less bruising of muscles, greatly contributing to reduction in postoperative pain. These drugs may occasionally be necessary to facilitate surgical reduction of a fractured long bone or a dislocated hip. The use of neuromuscular blocking agents and their general pharmacology has been considered in Chapter 7.

When neuromuscular blocking agents are used, facilities for IPPV must be available because effective spontaneous respiratory movements are abolished. Monitoring depth of anaesthesia may be difficult when breathing and palpebral reflex are abolished. When excessive anaesthetic administration occurs, there is increased risk of hypotension and prolonged recovery from anaesthesia. Insufficient anaesthesia results in awareness, increased sympathetic nervous system stimulation and increased intraocular pressure. One approach is to anaesthetize the patient and to achieve a stable plane of anaesthesia before administration of the relaxant. Subsequently, vaporizer settings and oxygen flow rates are used that in the anaesthetist's experience result in an adequate depth of anaesthesia. In dogs, signs of autonomic stimulation listed below may be observed in response to inadequate anaesthesia or analgesia:

1. Pupillary dilation
2. Salivation
3. Tongue twitch
4. Increased heart rate and blood pressure.

Agents used

The agents most commonly used at present to produce neuromuscular block in dogs are listed in Table 15.6. Other agents used less frequently are suxamethonium (succinylcholine), cisatracurium, doxacurium, and rocuronium. The dose rates given have been found to be clinically effective but individuals may vary in the dose required to induce a complete block. Further, a dose one-fifth of the dose used to produce total paralysis may be used for intraocular surgery because the extraocular muscles are paralysed earlier (at lower dosage) than muscles of the abdomen or thorax. At these low dose rates some respiratory movements may continue but alveolar ventilation is inadequate and IPPV should still be employed (Lee *et al.*, 1998).

TABLE 15.6 **Neuromuscular blocking agents in dogs. Approximate doses and indications for use**			
Agent	**Dose (mg/kg)**	**Effective duration (min.); halothane**	**Indication for use**
Pancuronium	0.06	40	Abdominal and thoracic surgery
Pancuronium	0.01	60	Central eye position for ocular surgery
Atracurium	0.5	40	Abdominal and thoracic surgery
Atracurium	0.1	25	Central eye position for ocular surgery
Vecuronium	0.1	25	Abdominal and thoracic surgery

When the duration of neuromuscular block must be extended beyond one dose, subsequent injections for top-up should be one-half of the initial dose approximately every 20 minutes. Continuous infusion of agent will produce a more consistent blockade. Maintenance of block with atracurium requires 0.5 mg/kg/h after an initial bolus dose of 0.5 mg/kg with halothane anaesthesia (Jones & Brearley, 1987). Two infusion rates for vecuronium have been recommended: an initial bolus of vecuronium 0.1 mg/kg followed by an infusion of 0.1 mg/kg/h (Jones & Young, 1991) and an initial bolus of 0.05 mg/kg with an infusion of 0.054 mg/kg/h (Clutton, 1992). The higher dose rate was antagonized with intravenous injections of atropine and neostigmine, 0.05 mg/kg, and the lower infusion rate was reversed with atropine and edrophonium, 0.5 mg/kg.

As described in Chapter 7, other factors influence the duration of neuromuscular block. Pancuronium and vecuronium will have a prolonged duration of action in dogs with hepatic or renal disease. Atracurium is spontaneously destroyed in plasma (Hofmann elimination) and is detoxified independently of hepatic or renal function. Atracurium, but not pancuronium or vecuronium, may occasionally result in histamine release and a decrease in arterial blood pressure.

Suxamethonium (succinylcholine) is a depolarizing neuromuscular blocking agent that causes initial muscle fasciculation after injection and before the onset of paralysis. Suxamethonium, 0.3–0.4 mg/kg, will produce about 20 minutes of paralysis in dogs. Salivation and bradycardia may be induced such that prior administration of an anticholinergic is advisable. There is no reversal agent for suxamethonium available but its action usually terminates rapidly and completely.

Termination of neuromuscular block

As the effects of neuromuscular block wear off, assuming the anaesthetic depth to be that of light surgical anaesthesia, the dog's eyes, which have been central, start to rotate downwards and spontaneous respiration returns. It can usually be safely assumed that once spontaneous breathing becomes adequate that neuromuscular block will not become re-established unless a further dose of relaxant is given. Administration of an aminogly-coside antibiotic during recovery from anaesthesia may potentiate residual neuromuscular blockade and result in re-paralysis.

Neostigmine and edrophonium are commonly used anticholinesterase antagonists of non-depolarizing neuromuscular block in dogs. The response to a reversal agent varies considerably with the degree of block present and should only be attempted when the block begins to wane. When full paralysing doses are given, the time lapse from last administration of vecuronium should be 10–15 minutes or 25–40 minutes for pancuronium and atracurium. When the train-of-four twitches are being monitored with a peripheral nerve stimulator, at least two twitches should be present before attempting to reverse the block. In the absence of this monitoring, decreasing chest compliance, attempts at spontaneous breathing or response to stimuli afforded by movement of the endotracheal tube in the trachea should be observed before attempts are made to restore normal neuromuscular transmission. It should be remembered that respiratory acidosis prolongs the action of most non-depolarizing relaxants and will impair reversal by neostigmine. IPPV should, therefore, be continued during the reversal process. Monitoring of neuromuscular block should be continued until all four twitches of the train-of-four are of equal strength. Inhalation anaesthesia is usually continued through the reversal process so that the patient is still lightly anaesthetized when neuromuscular function is restored.

An anticholinergic drug such as atropine, 0.02 mg/kg, or glycopyrrolate , 0.005 mg/kg, should be given i.v. 1–2 minutes before administering the anticholinesterase to block the adverse effects of bradycardia, salivation and increased intestinal motility. HR should be monitored and a repeat dose of anticholinergic given if necessary. Alternatively, the anticholinergic can be mixed with neostigmine in the same syringe (1.2 mg atropine or 0.5 mg glycopyrrolate to 2.5 mg neostigmine) and the mixture injected i.v. in small increments until satisfactory reversal is achieved. The dose of neostigmine varies from 0.01 to 0.10 mg/kg, with a maximum total dose of 0.1 mg/kg. The dose of edrophonium is 0.05 to 0.10 mg/kg. Onset of action of neostigmine is slower than edrophonium and may take several minutes.

Residual neuromuscular block may remain even after restoration of apparently normal breathing. In the dog, this is shown by the eyes remaining central with an absence of palpebral reflexes whatever the depth of anaesthesia. Pharyngeal and laryngeal reflexes may remain weak and airway obstruction may develop after tracheal extubation. The dog must be closely observed for evidence of residual block and inability to raise its head and protect the airway during recovery from anaesthesia.

When the low doses of relaxant are employed for ocular surgery, administration of an anti-cholinesterase may be unnecessary when only one or two doses are given and the duration of surgery exceeds an hour after last administration.

ANAESTHETIC MANAGEMENT

MAIN CONSIDERATIONS

Positioning

Care should be taken when positioning the animal to pad parts of the body that might be subject to pressure ischaemia. Limbs should not be allowed to hang off the side of the table. Some positions will compromise abdominal movement and contribute to hypoventilation. Access to the head for monitoring may be facilitated by placing a drape stand in front of the animal. A drape stand can be easily created by bending a metal rod into a semi-circle, with the diameter of the circle as wide as the operating table, and 15 cm at each end bent at right angles and parallel to the table edges for taping the stand to the operating table.

Fluid therapy

All paediatric, geriatric, and sick dogs, and all that will be anaesthetized for more than an hour, should receive balanced electrolyte solution intravenously during anaesthesia. Indeed, it may be preferable for *all* anaesthetized animals to be given fluid to maintain blood volume and transport of anaesthetic agents to detoxification sites, thereby facilitating recovery from anaesthesia. An appropriate rate of infusion for most patients is 10 ml/kg bodyweight/hour. The infusion rate should be halved after 3 hours for patients that do not have a body cavity open or when blood loss is minimal because from this point haemodilution will develop. Accurate infusion of the volume of fluid in very small patients is essential and may be accomplished by using a paediatric administration set delivering 60 drops/ml, or by using a drop counting pump or a syringe driver (Fig. 15.8), or simply by hand delivery of small boluses of fluid from a syringe. Patients with low blood glucose or who are at risk for hypoglycaemia should in addition be given 5% dextrose in water at 3 to 5 ml/kg/h.

Monitoring

Routine monitoring techniques have been described in Chapter 2. It should be remembered that both respiratory rate and depth of breathing must be observed during evaluation of ventilation and that mucous membrane colour is not an indicator of adequacy of ventilation. A serious potential consequence of an anaesthetized animal breathing air is hypoxaemia. Monitoring blood O_2 saturation with a pulse oximeter increases the safety of anaesthesia induced and maintained with injectable agents. Halothane and isoflurane significantly depress cardiovascular function and measurement of arterial blood pressure increases the safety of inhalation anaesthesia.

Analgesia supplements

Supplementation with additional opioid may become necessary during anaesthesia as the effects of premedication wane. A rough rule of thumb is to administer the supplemental dose at one-third to one-half of the initial premedication dose. An alternative is to add a short acting opioid to the protocol, such as fentanyl or alfentanil. Fentanyl can be administered as a bolus of 2 µg/kg every 20 minutes or as a continuous infusion of 0.2–0.7 µg/kg/min. Fentanyl may cause bradycardia, for which an anticholinergic may be given, and hypoventilation necessitating IPPV. An alternative is to use supplements of alfentanil, 2–5 µg/kg. The addition of N_2O to the inspired gases,

TABLE 15.7 **Causes of hypotension during anaesthesia**	
Decreased venous return	**Decreased myocardial contractility**
• Airway obstruction • Blood loss • Mechanical compression of caudal vena cava by surgeon or enlarged organ • Pancreatic enzymes released during surgery for pancreatitis • Tension pneumothorax	• Anaesthetic drugs • Adjunct drugs, e.g. antibiotics • Arrhythmias, e.g. ventricular premature depolarization and atrial fibrillation • Hypercapnia • Mediators of sepsis and endotoxaemia

with or without an opioid, will often supply sufficient analgesia to abolish the dog's response to the procedure.

Complications

Hypoventilation commonly occurs in dogs that are overweight, old, sick, deeply anaesthetized, and those which have increased intra-abdominal pressure. Treatment is IPPV.

Hypotension is a common complication that develops during anaesthesia caused by decreased venous return and decreased cardiac contractility (Table 15.7). Initial treatment of hypotension during anaesthesia involves decreasing anaesthetic administration and expansion of blood volume with balanced electrolyte solution as a 10 to 20 ml/kg i.v. bolus. Mechanical causes of decreased venous return, such as a closed 'pop-off' valve on a circle circuit or compression of the caudal vena cava by an enlarged organ such as the spleen, should be eliminated. Expansion of plasma volume by infusion of hydroxyethylstarch (hetastarch) or plasma at 20 ml/kg over 30 min may be effective in restoring ABP, especially in the patient with low plasma protein concentration (Table 15.8). Blood loss of up to 20% of blood volume may be replaced by infusion of balanced electrolyte at three times the volume of blood lost. In the event of rapid blood loss, treatment with hypertonic (7.5%) saline at 4 ml/kg over 10 minutes should sustain cardiac output and blood pressure at

TABLE 15.8 **Drug to increase cardiovascular performance**

Drug	Indication	Dose rate
Dopamine	Hypotension, advanced atrioventricular heart block, cardiac arrest, to increase renal blood flow	2–7 μg/kg/min of a 100 μg/ml solution in 0.9% saline; 10–15 μg/kg/min for cardiac arrest
Dobutamine	Hypotension	2–7 μg/kg/min of a 100 μg/ml solution in 0.9% saline; increase to 10 μg/kg/min in emergency
Hetastarch	Low plasma protein	10–20 ml/kg over at least 30 minutes
Hypertonic (7.5%) saline	Hypotension from haemorrhage or endotoxaemia, for precautions see text	4–5 ml/kg over 10 minutes
Lignocaine	Premature ventricular contractions, ventricular tachycardia	1–2 mg/kg up to 10 mg/kg over 10 minutes; infusion 0.02–0.02 mg/kg/min of a 1 mg/ml solution
Sodium bicarbonate	Metabolic acidosis	1–1.5 mEq/kg, repeated once; use formula mEq to be infused = Base deficit × 0.3 × kg bodyweight given over 60 minutes

acceptable values for about 1.5 hours. Meanwhile, additional therapy in the form of crystalloid solution, whole blood, packed red blood cells, or oxyglobin can be initiated. Hypertonic saline probably should not be given when the source of the bleeding cannot be controlled. An antihistamine, diphenhydramine, 2 mg/kg, is given before plasma or blood transfusion to minimize the risk of an anaphylactic reaction, and transfusion should be started slowly to allow an early detection of a transfusion reaction. Although hemodilution occurs during fluid administration in the face of haemorrhage, measurement of haematocrit and total protein should be performed periodically during anaesthesia in patients with considerable blood loss.

Catecholamines used to improve cardiovascular function include dopamine, 2 to 7 μg/kg/min (100 μg/kg solution made by adding 50 mg of drug to 500 ml of 0.9% saline solution), or dobutamine, 2 to 7 μg/kg/min (100 μg/100 ml solution) delivered using a paediatric administration set (60 drops/ml) for most dogs (Table 15.8). Dopamine is most effective in conditions of cardiac arrest or advanced atrioventricular heart block, and can be used to improve urine production. Dobutamine is best used for patients with cardiomyopathy, congestive heart failure, or who are at risk for ventricular arrhythmias. Both dopamine and dobutamine can be responsible for the appearance of premature ventricular depolarizations, however, dopamine is metabolized to noradrenaline and this may increase the risk of abnormal cardiac rhythm. Ephedrine, 0.02 mg/kg, can be used to increase ABP in dogs with excessive venodilation. An anticholinergic is only effective in increasing blood pressure when the heart rate is low.

Ventricular arrhythmias not infrequently develop during anaesthesia as a consequence of myocardial ischaemia following automobile trauma, or abdominal distension from gastric dilatation/volvulus, or from myocarditis or vasoactive mediators of sepsis. Management should include ruling out or treating hypoxia and hypercapnia. Treatment should be intravenous lignocaine when the ventricular premature depolarizations are multifocal or sufficiently frequent to decrease cardiac output and blood pressure (Fig. 15. 11). Lignocaine 2% or 4% can be injected as an i.v. bolus at 1 mg/kg and repeated if ineffective. Additional lignocaine up to 8 mg/kg over 10 minutes can be given to dogs if a lower dose is ineffective. Lignocaine can be given as a continuous infusion at 0.02 to 0.08 mg/kg/min. A 1 mg/ml solution of lignocaine can be prepared by adding 500 mg of lignocaine (25 ml of 2% or 12.5 ml of 4%) to 500 ml of 0.9% saline.

POSTOPERATIVE MANAGEMENT

Care of the dog in the immediate postanaesthetic period should include allowing it to breathe 100% O_2 for about 10 minutes, or as long as seems appropriate, after discontinuing anaesthetic administration. Inhalation agents can severely depress

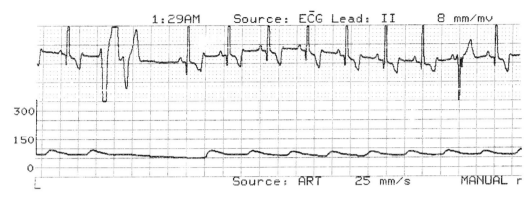

FIG. 15.11 This ECG was recorded from a Hound anaesthetized for surgical repair of intestinal rupture and abdominal herniation as a result of trauma. The trace shows two consecutive premature ventricular depolarizations that resulted in a pulse deficit. The dog's blood pressure progressively deteriorated and was sustained by treatment with hetastarch, plasma, dobutamine and lignocaine. The dog survived to go home.

ventilation and this is masked when the animal is attached to high concentrations of O_2 in the anaesthesia system. Hypoxaemia may develop if the animal is disconnected and made to breathe room air when still deeply anaesthetized. O_2 should be supplied for at least 5 minutes after N_2O is discontinued to avoid diffusion hypoxia.

Gastric reflux into the pharynx may occur anytime during anaesthesia but when it has occurred the mouth must be cleaned before extubation and suction of the nasal passages may be advisable. Gastric reflux into the oesophagus occurs more commonly than is usually recognized (Raptopoulos & Galatos, 1995). In a series of 510 dogs the incidence of oesophageal reflux was 17% but the gastric contents reached the mouth only in 0.6% (3 dogs). Many factors may contribute to gastro-oesophageal reflux. Intra-abdominal surgery is associated with an increased frequency of reflux and oesophageal sphincter pressure is significantly decreased at the end of surgery during isoflurane anaesthesia at the time of suturing of the skin (Hashim *et al.*, 1995). The incidence of gastro-oesophageal reflux is significantly higher when anaesthesia has been induced with propofol than with thiopental (Raptopoulos & Galatos, 1997). The information concerning the influence of pre-operative fasting on the volume and acidity of gastric fluid and the impact of anaesthetic combinations on lower oesophageal sphincter tone is not sufficiently definitive to make specific recommendations to minimize gastric reflux.

Before the dog regains consciousness, the urinary bladder should be expressed by abdominal palpation or catheterized to avoid soiling of bandages from urination in the cage during recovery. The volume of urine collected should be measured or estimated to assess the adequacy of urine flow during anaesthesia. Approximately 1 ml/kg/h of urine should have been produced. When the volume is less, consideration should be given to continuation of fluid therapy after anaesthesia. Blood should be collected from dogs that have suffered blood loss for measurement of haematocrit and total protein concentration. Blood glucose should be measured in diabetic dogs, and those that are less than 3 months of age or are thin.

Rectal temperature should be measured and heat applied when the temperature is low. The temperature of animals frequently decreases further after the end of surgery when the covering drapes are removed. Warming is highly effective when using a device blowing hot air into pads placed over the animal (Bair Hugger, Augustine Medical Inc., Eden Prairie, Minnesota, USA).

Oxygen supplementation

O_2 therapy should be considered for dogs that have trouble adequately oxygenating. An O_2 chamber or baby incubator, if available, can be used to supply an inspired concentration of

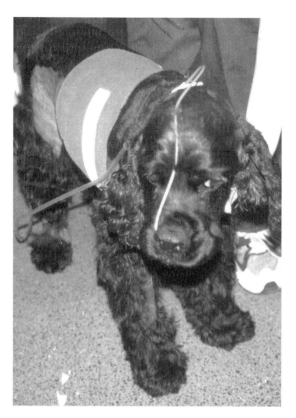

FIG. 15.12 Nasal tube for O₂ insufflation.

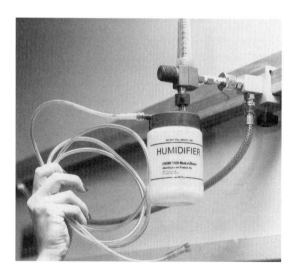

FIG. 15.13 Oxygen flowmeter and humidifier for nasal insufflation.

40–60% O₂ and warm the animal at the same time. Nasal administration of O₂ may achieve

TABLE 15.9 **Placement of a nasal O₂ tube**	
Supplies	**Placement**
• **Polyvinyl or rubber feeding 5F or 8F**	• Measure tube from medial canthus to nostril
• **Permanent pen marker**	• Mark distance with pen
• **Lignocaine 2%**	• Lubricate tube
• **Lubricant gel**	• Push nose dorsally, introduce tube dorsally for a few mm, then medially and ventrally
• **Haemostat forceps**	
• **Suture± 'Superglue'**	• Suture at the nares, between the eyes, and on the forehead ± glue tube to hair

a 40% inspired O₂ concentration and can be a more economical method of administration (Fig 15.12). A bleb of lignocaine can be injected subcutaneously at the site for suture placement but is not needed when the nasal tube is inserted and secured before the animal regains consciousness (Table 15.9). O₂ is humidified by bubbling through sterile water and insufflated into the patient at 100 ml/kg/min (Fig. 15.13). The oxygen delivery tubing should be secured to a collar or tape around the neck.

Analgesia

Display of pain during recovery from surgery may be obvious or subtle and veterinarians differ widely in their assessment of the degree of pain and in their interpretation for the need for analgesia. The signs of pain in dogs may vary from excitement, vocalization, and mutilation of the painful area to shivering, reluctance to move, excessive salivation and pupillary dilation. Dogs may become aggressive, guard the painful site and avoid human touch. There are individual and breed differences in tolerance for pain and it is possible that sporting or working dogs are less likely to exhibit behaviour changes to a noxious stimulus. Various types of pain scoring scales have been described in an attempt to accurately detect severity of pain. To complete a visual analogue scale, the patient is observed for a specific behaviour and the

TABLE 15.10 **Examples of intramuscular dose rates of opioids for analgesia in the early recovery period**

Opioid	Dose rate (mg/kg)	Dosing interval (h)
Morphine	0.3–0.5	4
Pethidine	2–3	2
Oxymorphone	0.05–0.10	4
Butorphanol	0.2–0.3	2
Buprenorphine	0.006–0.010	4–6

observer places a mark on a line on which the left end represents no pain and the right end represents the most pain possible. Use of a numerical rating scale is similar except that a number is assigned to the behaviour where 0 represents normal or preprocedural behaviour and 2 or 3 represents abnormal behaviour (Conzemius *et al.*, 1997; Holton *et al.*, 1998; Firth & Haldane, 1999). Evaluations of pain scoring techniques have discovered that measurements of some clinical signs, such as heart rates and respiratory rates, do not accurately reflect the severity of postoperative pain. Although combining scores from a variety of observations including activity, mental status, posture, vocalization, etc., can provide a reliable assessment of pain (Firth & Haldane, 1999), scores from different observers may vary considerably (Holton *et al.*, 1998).

Plans for provision of analgesia should have been made before anaesthesia and whenever possible a multimodal approach should be employed that includes local nerve blocks with opioid or local anaesthetic solution. Parenterally administered opioids should be given before consciousness returns. Examples of opioids for postoperative analgesia and dose rates are given in Table 15.10 but adjustments should be made for the individual dog. A small dose of sedative or tranquillizer may be needed to potentiate the effect of the opioid, for example, acepromazine 0.025 mg/kg i.v., or medetomidine 1–2 µg/kg. Disadvantages of the i.m. or i.v. routes of administration for opioids include a variable degree of respiratory depression, even hypoxaemia, potential decrease in ABP, and decreased effectiveness of the pharyngeal and laryngeal reflexes, with increased risk for aspiration.

Transdermal fentanyl patch

A method of postoperative pain control that is gaining popularity in North America is the transdermal fentanyl patch (Chapter 4, p.97). Delivery of fentanyl is proportional to the patch surface area and delivered fentanyl doses are 25, 50, 75, and 100 µg/hour. Appropriate dose rates in veterinary patients are under investigation but current usage is 25 µg/h for small dogs > 2 kg, 50 µg/h for 10–20 kg dog, 75 µg/h for 20–30 kg dog, and 100 µg/h patches for dogs >; 30 kg. The patches should be placed and covered so that the animals cannot remove them and ingest the contents. Measurement of plasma fentanyl concentrations has determined that steady state plasma concentrations are not achieved for 24 hours after patch application (Kyles *et al.*, 1996; Egger *et al.*, 1998). Consequently, the patch must be applied the day before surgery to provide some intraoperative analgesia. If the patch is applied at the end of surgery, another form of analgesia must be provided for the first 12–24 postoperative hours. There is considerable individual variation in the analgesia provided by a fentanyl patch, and even when the patch is applied sufficiently early, the analgesia is not enough to prevent the dog experiencing the acute pain in the immediate postoperative period. Plasma fentanyl concentrations are sustained for 72 hours but decline rapidly after the patch is removed. Respiratory depression has not been a notable problem. The patch should be removed if signs of overdosage such as a restlessness, drowsiness, or inappetence are observed.

SPECIFIC PATIENT PROBLEMS

CARDIAC DISEASE

General recommendations for anaesthesia of dogs with cardiac disease include premedication to present a calm, unstressed animal for induction of anaesthesia and sufficient analgesia during and after surgery. Management of cardiovascular function must include maintenance of an adequate blood volume without overload, preoxygenation and provision of O_2 during anaesthesia to avoid hypoxaemia, and adequate monitoring of the cardiovascular system during anaesthesia to detect

TABLE 15.11 Significance of cardiac disease to anaesthesia

Patient problem	Anaesthetic considerations
Mitral valve insufficiency	Increased risk for hypotension. Consider increasing cardiac preload (i.v. fluids to maintain blood volume), avoid decreasing cardiac contractility, avoid bradycardia, and consider slightly decreasing cardiac afterload (some vasodilation preferable to vasoconstriction)
Cardiomyopathy	Increased risk for hypotension and death. Careful choice of anaesthetic agents to avoid decreased cardiac contractility
Ventricular arrhythmias e.g. automobile trauma, gastric dilatation volvulus	Increased risk for hypotension or ventricular fibrillation and death. Consider use of agents that do not sensitize the myocardium to catecholamines, e.g. benzodiazepines, opioids, ketamine, isoflurane
Patent ductus arteriosus	Increased risk for hypotension before ligation and for pulmonary oedema after ligation. Minimize dose of agents that cause vasodilation and limit baseline intraoperative fluid rate to 6 ml/kg/h

unacceptable abnormalities. Different forms of cardiac disease require specific management (Table 15.11). Knowledge of the physiology of the disease can be used to define the pharmacological requirements of the anaesthetic drugs.

Mitral insufficiency

Anaesthesia for the old dog with mitral insufficiency must take into consideration the impact of old age on anaesthetic requirements and that mitral insufficiency decreases cardiac output in the presence of bradycardia, decreased venous return, and increased systemic vascular resistance.

Consequently, premedication with glycopyrrolate is indicated and agents that should be avoided include xylazine, medetomidine, large doses of acepromazine, and thiopental.

Patent ductus arteriosus

A dog with a patent ductus arteriosus has low diastolic and MAP pressure and care should be taken with anaesthetic agents that cause vasodilation. Infusion of balanced electrolyte solution to these patients should be restricted to 6 ml/kg/h, unless individual evaluation indicates need for a modified rate, to avoid pulmonary oedema after ligation of the ductus. ABP may be increased by infusion of dobutamine, although a dramatic increase in diastolic and mean pressures usually occurs when the ductus is ligated. Other requirements for management relate to the thoracotomy which is discussed later and in Chapter 19.

ENDOSCOPY

Gastrointestinal endoscopy

Gastroduodenoscopy and proctoscopy may be performed in relatively healthy dogs or in dogs with a history of chronic weight loss. In the latter case, decreased serum total protein concentration may result in decreased anaesthetic requirement for thiopental or propofol and serious loss of fat and muscle will result in prolonged recovery from thiopental. Although the ease of introduction of the endoscope into the duodenum is directly related to the experience of the veterinarian in this procedure, premedication with atropine and morphine has been documented to significantly increase the number of attempts to successfully pass the endoscope (Donaldson *et al.*, 1993). Complications of endoscopy include excessive distension of the stomach and intestines resulting in hypoventilation and gastric reflux into the pharynx. The cardiovascular changes caused by gastrointestinal distension depend on the severity of distension. Changes in ABP and CO are small during gastrointestinal endosopy in the majority of healthy dogs (Jergens *et al.*, 1995) but the anaesthetist must be alert for bradycardia and hypotension that develop in individuals. Biopsy of the intestines carries the risk of perforation and tension pneumoperitoneum resulting in hypotension and the need for an emergency exploratory laparotomy. Endoscopy for removal of an oesophageal foreign body or for dilation of an oesophageal stricture also introduces the potential for pneumothorax.

Bronchoscopy

Bronchoscopy and bronchoalveolar lavage (BAL) are most difficult to manage in smaller dogs. The ability to cough should be retained during BAL and this requires a light plane of anaesthesia with either thiopental or propofol. Anticholinergics should be omitted to preserve the volume of secretions and should not be used in dogs with pneumonia to avoid consolidating secretions. Butorphanol is marketed as an antitussive, however, it has proven to be a useful agent for premedication in these dogs provided that the dose of induction drug is kept to a minimum. The drug for induction should be administered in small increments to retain the coughing response to introduction of the sterile endotracheal tube and to instillation of sterile saline for bronchial wash. Hypoxaemia is a common complication, especially during bronchoscopy in a small dog where the diameter of the endoscope may be large in comparison with the lumen of the trachea. Preoxygenation is essential and use of a pulse oximeter is advisable during the procedure. O_2 may be supplied intermittently by facemask when the endoscope is removed or insufflated around or down the endocope. When the procedure is expected to last for more than a few minutes, anaesthesia may have to be continued with an injectable drug such as propofol.

GASTRIC DILATATION/VOLVULUS SYNDROME

Abdominal distension resulting from gastric dilatation and volvulus (GDV) decreases CO and ABP. Experimental investigations of GDV have documented a 64% decrease in CO (Orton & Muir III, 1983) or as much as an 89% decrease associated with 50% decrease in coronary blood flow (Horne et al., 1985). Even when the stomach has been decompressed before anaesthesia, myocar-

dial ischaemia increases the risk of hypotension and poor organ perfusion during anaesthesia. Overt clinical signs of myocardial ischaemia such as cardiac arrythmias may not appear until after anaesthesia has been induced or even after surgery has been completed. Forty percent of dogs with GDV or gastric dilatation develop cardiac arrhythmias, mainly ventricular premature depolarizations or ventricular tachycardia, between 12 and 36 hours after the onset of the problem (Muir, 1982; Brockman et al., 1995).

Gastric decompression should be accomplished before induction of anaesthesia by passage of a stomach tube. Blood volume should be expanded with crystalloid solution administered intravenously up to 90 ml/kg in the first hour. Hypertonic (7.5% saline solution) saline, 4 ml/kg i.v. over 10 minutes, will induce a more rapid improvement in cardiovascular function. Hypertonic saline in 6% Dextran 70, 5 ml/kg, has also proven to be effective (Allen et al., 1991; Schertel et al., 1997). Further volume expansion can be achieved by administration of hetastarch, 20 ml/kg. Reperfusion injury may occur after decompression of the stomach. Deferoxamine 30 mg/kg i.m. (Desferal, Novartis, East Hanover, New Jersey, USA), which inhibits production of hydroxyl radicals, given before anaesthesia may increase survival rate (Lantz et al., 1992).

Routine administration of sodium bicarbonate is not recommended because of uncertainty of the dog's metabolic status. Gastric sequestration may result in metabolic alkalosis, however, hypotension and decreased peripheral perfusion may result in metabolic acidosis. Treatment of suspected metabolic derangements are best reserved until pH and blood gas analysis can be performed. Dogs with gastric necrosis are likely to have abnormal hemostatic function, most frequently thrombocytopenia and decreased antithrombin III activity, and a proportion will develop disseminated intravascular coagulation (DIC) (Millis et al., 1993).

Anaesthetic management of GDV

The clinical status of these dogs before anaesthesia varies from relatively healthy to moribund. Anaesthetic agents, dose rates and additional

TABLE 15.12 **Significance of hepatic disease to anaesthesia**	
Patient problem	**Anaesthetic considerations**
Decreased hepatic function	Increased risk for excessive bleeding, hypoglycaemia, prolonged recovery from anaesthesia. Consider checking coagulation profile before anaesthesia (may need fresh plasma), monitoring blood glucose and giving 5% dextrose in water 3 ml/kg/h as part of fluid therapy, using anaesthetic agents that are easily eliminated or antagonized. During anaesthesia, avoid further hepatic damage by preventing hypotension and hypercarbia
Portosystemic shunt	Increased risk for hypotension, hypoglycaemia, and hypothermia. Benzodiazepines contraindicated with encephalopathy; use agents with minimal cardiovascular depressant effects and that can be antagonized or do not depend on hepatic function for elimination. During anaesthesia, give 5% dextrose in water 3 ml/kg/h as part of fluid therapy and treat hypotension with dopamine or dobutamine
Bile duct calculi	Increased risk for surgical procedure to cause hypoventilation and hypotension (mechanical obstruction of venous return). Contraction of bile ducts may be initiated by opiates. Impact of partial agonists under debate

management will have to be adjusted to the individual dog and administered bearing in mind that the dog may have severely decreased anaesthetic requirements.

Cardiovascular monitoring should begin before induction of anaesthesia by attaching ECG leads or a form of indirect or direct blood pressure measurement. Preoxygenation is advisable by administration of O_2 by facemask for several minutes before induction. Two induction techniques that are preferable for dogs with GDV are diazepam/ketamine and neuroleptanalgesia. A suitable alternative technique (except for the high expense) is to use etomidate which preserves cardiovascular function. Thiopental and propofol are less appropriate as these agents decrease CO to a greater extent. Because of the risk of regurgitation and aspiration mask induction is inadvisable .

Induction of anaesthesia with i.v. diazepam, 0.25 mg/kg, and ketamine, 5 mg/kg, preserves cardiovascular function. Tachycardia caused by these drugs may potentiate ventricular arrhythmias and i.v. lignocaine, 2 mg/kg, can be given before or after ketamine to control abnormal rhythms. After the airway is secured analgesia can be supplemented with an opioid. An alternative induction technique is neuroleptanalgesia. The combination of diazepam and fentanyl, or diazepam and oxymorphone will provide anaesthesia with minimal cardiovascular depression. Disadvantages of these techniques are vomiting and probable hypoventilation necessitating IPPV. Anaesthesia can be maintained with an inhalation agent or by continuous infusion of an opioid.

HEPATIC DISEASE

Administration of anaesthesia to dogs with decreased hepatic function presents two difficulties. First, recovery from anaesthesia will be slow if the anaesthetic agents used must be detoxified by the liver. Secondly, further hepatic damage can occur during anaesthesia from hepatic hypoxia as a consequence of hypotension, splanchnic vasoconstriction from hypercapnia, or arterial hypoxaemia. Dogs with moderate to severe hepatic disease may have disorders of clotting and tests of coagulation should be performed before surgery. Hypoglycaemia is also a potential complication and 5% dextrose in water should be infused during anaesthesia. Surgical problems relating to the liver, such as portosystemic shunt and bile duct calculi, have specific anaesthetic considerations (Table 15.12).

TABLE 15.13 **Significance of neurological disease to anaesthesia (ICP = intracranial pressure)**	
Patient problem	Anaesthetic considerations
Seizures	Avoid acepromazine. Use agents that decrease ICP e.g. thiopental, propofol, etomidate, diazepam
Depression, decreased mentation, meningitis	Adjust dose rates for decreased anaesthetic requirement
Increased ICP, e.g. brain tumour, hydrocephalus head trauma	Use agents that decrease ICP. Use controlled ventilation to prevent hypercarbia

NEUROLOGIC DISEASE

Dogs with neurologic disease range from being essentially healthy to comatose. Anaesthesia may be straightforward, or the dog may be at risk of anaesthetic overdose or serious neurologic consequences from increased intracranial pressure (Table 15.13). Diagnostic procedures, such as collection of cerebrospinal fluid (CSF), myelography, or magnetic resonance imaging (MRI) have specific considerations relating to anaesthesia.

Increased intracranial pressure

Dogs with increased intracranial pressure (ICP) before anaesthesia can be treated with methylprednisolone sodium succinate and mannitol. Anaesthesia may be induced with a combination of agents known to decrease ICP and cerebral metabolic O_2 demand, such as diazepam, midazolam, thiopental and propofol. Halothane and isoflurane are usually used to maintain anaesthesia even though they increase ICP by increasing cerebral blood flow and causing hypercapnia. Hypercapnia has a direct effect on cerebral vasculature causing increased cerebral blood flow that increases ICP. Consequently, IPPV should be used throughout anaesthesia in dogs with increased ICP (e.g those suffering from hydrocephalus, brain tumours, or head trauma). IPPV should also be instituted during collection of cerebrospinal fluid, as increased ICP during this procedure may result in cerebellar herniation. Hypertension must be avoided as it also increases ICP. Acepromazine is usually avoided in dogs at risk for seizures as it decreases the seizure threshold.

Myelography

Dogs must be observed closely for mild to serious adverse side effects during injection of iohexol for myelography. Respiratory arrest should be treated by IPPV and hypotension by decreasing anaesthetic administration. Severe decreases in ABP may be treated with dopamine or dobutamine. Occasionally cardiac arrest ensues. Balanced electrolyte solution should be infused during anaesthesia at a rate of 10 ml/kg/hour to promote excretion of the contrast agent. The dog's head must be supported in an elevated position after the myelogram to encourage flow of contrast agent from the brain. Recovery from anaesthesia for myelography may be complicated by seizures requiring specific treatment.

ORTHOPAEDIC SURGERY

General considerations for anaesthesia for orthopaedic surgery include awareness of the specific problems created by a traumatic accident. Prolonged anaesthesia, significant blood loss, provision of analgesia, and hypothermia are common problems for anaesthetic management. Analgesia for surgery on the forelimb can include, in addition to parenteral administration of opioid and NSAID, epidural block with morphine and, for surgery distal to the elbow, brachial plexus nerve block with bupivacaine. Analgesia for surgery of the hindlimbs and pelvis can include parenteral opioid and NSAID, and epidural nerve block with morphine alone or with bupivacaine. An alternative to epidural block for elective surgery of the stifle is intra-articular morphine or bupivacaine.

Repair of a fractured jaw introduces the risk of aspiration of blood and debris and care must be taken to ensure that the endotracheal tube cuff is sufficiently inflated and that the mouth is cleaned before recovery from anaesthesia. Surgical repair may require that the endotracheal tube be removed from the oropharynx to increase exposure to the fracture and to enable the surgeon to judge correct alignment and avoid malocclusion of the teeth. Anaesthesia is induced and orotracheal

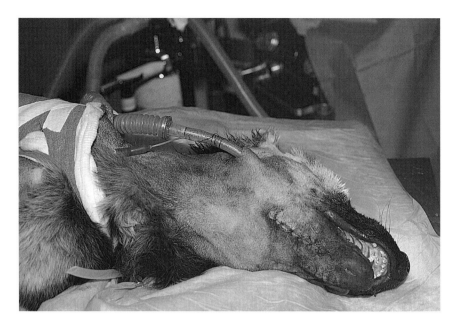

FIG. 15.14 The endotracheal tube has been inserted through a pharyngostomy incision to provide better surgical access for repair of the fractured mandible. A reinforced metal spiral endotracheal tube has been used to avoid kinking of the tube as it turns 180° within the pharynx.

intubation is performed as usual. The site for a pharyngostomy tube is clipped, the skin prepared for surgery, and the pharyngostomy made with appropriate surgical technique. The endotracheal tube cuff is deflated and the tube is disconnected from the anaesthetic system and tube adapter. First, the pilot balloon is grasped with the tip of forceps introduced through the pharyngostomy and pulled through to the outside, and then the oral end of the endotracheal tube is exteriorized. The endotracheal tube is reconnected to the adapter and anaesthetic system, the cuff inflated, and anaesthesia proceeds (Fig. 15.14). Use of an endotracheal tube with a metal spiral embedded in its wall will ensure that the tube does not become kinked during placement or the surgical procedure. An alternative technique for pharyngostomy intubation is to introduce the endotracheal tube from the outside and to use forceps to grasp the end of the endotracheal tube inside the mouth to direct the tube into the larynx.

RENAL DISEASE

Anaesthesia and surgery decrease urine formation by decreasing renal blood flow through decreased CO and ABP, and by causing sympathetic nervous system stimulation. Thus, dogs with chronic renal disease are at risk for acute renal failure after anaesthesia. Adverse effects of anaesthesia can usually be prevented by adequate fluid therapy during anaesthesia and choice of an anaesthetic technique providing a rapid recovery from anaesthesia. For some dogs, adequate fluid therapy should include starting infusion before anaesthesia and continuing fluid administration at a reduced rate for some hours after anaesthesia.

Acute renal failure from urethral obstruction or urinary bladder or ureter rupture includes problems of hypovolaemia, azotemia, and metabolic acidosis, all of which result in decreased anaesthetic requirement and increased risk of hypotension and arrhythmias. Intensive care before anaesthesia will decrease complications occurring during anaesthesia. Anaesthetic agents should be administered at markedly decreased dose rates.

THORACOTOMY

Consideration of the appropriate choice of anaesthetic agents for the dog's problems is essential to minimize complications of thoracotomy. Victims of car accidents often have myocardial contusions. Agents that do not sensitize the myocardium to catecholamines, such as diazepam, ketamine and isoflurane, may be selected over agents that increase the risk of arrhythmias, such as xylazine, thiopental, propofol, and halothane. Patients with low PaO_2 before anaesthesia (e.g. those with chylothorax and some cases of diaphragmatic hernia), will benefit from a rapid i.v. induction sequence rather than a slower mask induction. If possible, monitoring should include use of a pulse oximeter as hypoxaemia may develop soon after induction of anaesthesia. Adequate oxygenation may be restored by institution of IPPV or by changing the dog's body position to remove the weight of abdominal organs or collapsed lung on normal lung.

IPPV will be necessary during anaesthesia and appropriate procedures have been described in a previous chapter. Inspiratory pressure needs to be less when the chest is open. When a lung is packed off during surgery, the respiratory rate should be increased to 20/min and the tidal volume decreased to 11 ml/kg. Lobes of lung that have been collapsed for many hours should not be forcefully reinflated or reperfusion injury may result. This may result in pulmonary oedema that

---

TABLE 15.14 Significance of renal disease to anaesthesia

Patient problem	Anaesthetic considerations
Chronic renal disease	Increased risk for prolonged recovery from anaesthesia and further deterioration of renal function after anaesthesia. Use a combination of anaesthetic agents to facilitate low dose rates and rapid elimination. Consider initiating diuresis with i.v. balanced electrolyte infusion 10 ml/kg/h for 60 min before induction of anaesthesia, prevent hypotension during anaesthesia, monitor urine production, continue i.v. fluids into recovery period
Urethral obstruction, ruptured ureter, urinary bladder or urethra	Increased risk for anaesthetic overdose, hypoventilation, hypotension, and prolonged recovery from anaesthesia. Provide medical treatment before anaesthesia to expand blood volume and decrease serum potassium to <6.5 mmol/l. Administer anaesthetic agents in small increments to avoid overdosage and monitor cardiac rhythm and blood pressure during anaesthesia

---

TABLE 15.15 Planning for thoracotomy

Problem	Management
Pain control during and after surgery	Use multimodal analgesia involving more than one method of analgesia: morphine epidural, intercostal nerve block, interpleural analgesia, systemic opioid, non-steroidal agent
Inadequate ventilation	IPPV via endotracheal tube will be required
Pneumothorax	Do not use N_2O when the chest is closed. Limit peak inspired pressure to 25 cm H_2O in trauma patients to minimize risk of further alveolar rupture
Cardiac rhythm disturbances originating from myocardial damage or surgical manipulation	Lignocaine i.v. bolus and infusion to treat ventricular arrhythmias; lignocaine, 2 mg/kg, without adrenaline, can be applied topically to the heart; avoid hypercapnia
Collapsed lung	Do not attempt to reinflate lung that has been collapsed for more than a few hours as this may cause pulmonary oedema
Hypoxaemia after anaesthesia	Supplement PiO_2 by nasal tube insufflation or O_2 chamber
Anticipated complications with specific surgical procedures	*Diaphragmatic hernia*: may develop hypoxaemia after induction and may develop hypotension when abdominal organs are removed from thorax *Lung lobe torsion*: decreased anaesthetic requirement; may develop hypoxaemia and hypotension after induction

spreads throughout the lungs resulting in hypoxaemia. The changes may be severe and progress to a fatal outcome.

Monitoring ABP, HR and cardiac rhythm are of prime importance during thoracotomy. The dog's problems, the anaesthetic agents, and surgical manipulation can all cause hypotension and arrhythmias. Cardiovascular performance may have to be improved as previously described in the section on anaesthetic management. Premature ventricular contractions or ventricular tachycardia may need to be treated by i.v. lignocaine.

Analgesia can be provided by systemic administration of opioids, by regional analgesia from intercostal nerve blocks with bupivacaine, interpleural instillation of bupivacaine (up to a total dose of 2.5 mg/kg), and epidural analgesia with morphine (0.1 mg/kg). Postanaesthetic ventilation and oxygenation should be monitored closely and administration of O_2 by O_2 chamber or nasal insufflation (100 ml O_2/kg/min) may be required for several hours.

The extent of postoperative care needed after thoracotomy varies from case to case. Minimal care may be necessary after repair of a patent ductus arteriosus, unless a complication occurred or the dog has heart failure, and similarly, for many ruptured diaphragm repairs. However, intensive care will be needed for dogs with complications, such as sepsis, persistent pneumothorax, continual fluid accumulation, or after complicated surgery. Chest tubes not connected to an underwater drain or Heimlich valve should be sucked avoiding excessive pressures, every 1–2 hours initially, decreasing to every 4 hours, depending on the progress of recovery. Lavage will be necessary when bacterial contamination is present.

LOCAL ANALGESIA

Local analgesia is frequently used as an adjunct to general anaesthesia or in the treatment of pre- or postoperative pain and less frequently employed as the sole method of analgesia for surgical procedures in dogs. The techniques for these blocks, listed alphabetically, are described in this section.

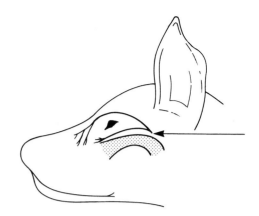

FIG. 15.15 Auriculopalpebral nerve block. The nerve is blocked just where the zygomatic ridge dips medially.

SPECIFIC APPLICATIONS

Auriculopalpebral nerve block

The nerve runs caudal to the mandibular joint at the base of the ear and, after giving off the cranial auricular branch, proceeds as the temporal branch along the dorsal border of the zygomatic arch towards the orbit. Before reaching the orbit the nerve divides into two branches, which pass medially and laterally to supply the orbicularis muscle.

The needle is introduced through the skin and fascia over the midpoint of the caudal third of the zygomatic arch (just where the arch can be felt to dip sharply medially) and up to 1 ml of 2% lignocaine is injected (Fig. 15.15). The blocking of this branch of the facial nerve does not produce any analgesia. By paralysing the orbicularis muscle it facilitates examination of, and operations on, the eyeball. It is of particular value in preventing squeezing of the eyeball after intraocular operations.

Brachial plexus block

Block of the brachial plexus will provide analgesia below the elbow. Injection can be made with the anaesthetized dog in lateral recumbency using a 22 gauge 3.75 cm, 6.25 cm, or 8.75 cm long spinal needle, according to the size of the dog. Bupivacaine, 2.0–2.5 mg/kg, should provide at least 6 hours of analgesia with an onset time of 10 to 40 minutes. Alternatively, lignocaine, 6 mg/kg, can be used for a shorter duration of action – approxi-

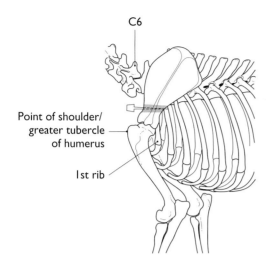

C6

Point of shoulder/
greater tubercle
of humerus

1st rib

FIG. 15.16 Landmarks for brachial plexus nerve block.

mately 2 hours. The brachial plexus originates from the ventral branches the 6th, 7th and 8th cervical and the 1st and 2nd thoracic spinal nerves which form three cords which run for a short distance before segregating into the nerves of the thoracic limb. Local anaesthetic solution must be spread over a wide area to block all the nerves. Commercially available solutions can be diluted with saline by 25% to produce a larger volume for injection and increase the spread of anaesthetic.

An area rostral to the cranial border of the scapula, between the point of the shoulder and the cervical vertebrae should be clipped and the skin prepared as for surgery. The point of the needle should be inserted halfway between the point of the shoulder and the transverse process of the 6th cervical vertebra. It is then advanced medial to the scapula and parallel to the vertebral column to the 1st or 2nd rib (Fig. 15.16). Aspiration before injection of local anaesthetic is essential to ensure that the needle is not in a blood vessel. Part of the total volume is injected and the remainder injected as the needle is withdrawn, aspirating before each subsequent injection.

Some complications may occur as a consequence of this procedure. Large blood vessels pass through the area for injection and needle puncture may create a large haematoma. Further, the local analgesic solution may be injected intravascularly, the needle may enter the thorax and permit the entry of air into the pleural cavity, the brachial plexus may be damaged, causing neuritis or permanent paralysis, or infection may be introduced into the axilla. However, if due care is exercised, the technique may be regarded as a relatively safe procedure, of particular value for intraoperative and postoperative analgesia or even one that can be used as the sole anaesthetic agent for surgery.

EPIDURAL BLOCK

Epidural block with lignocaine or bupivacaine can provide analgesia for major surgery of the hindlimbs and pelvis. Opioids, morphine, oxymorphone, fentanyl, sufentanil, and butorphanol have been used in the epidural space to provide analgesia during and after surgery, although other methods of analgesia may be needed to manage acute pain in the immediate recovery period. Combinations of an opioid with bupivacaine or xylazine or medetomidine have been used to extend the duration of analgesia. Epidural block is contraindicated if the dog has a coagulopathy or skin infection over the lumbosacral area.

Technique

The technique of epidural block has already been discussed in Chapters 10 and 13. The spinal cord ends in the dog at the junction of the sixth and seventh lumbar vertebrae, and the meninges continue to the middle of the sacrum. Not infrequently, a needle inserted at the lumbosacral space penetrates the dura and cerebrospinal fluid (CSF) is aspirated.

The epidural injection may be performed with a conscious dog in the sternal or lateral positions but is usually performed with the anaesthetized dog in lateral recumbency. Sudden forceful movement in the conscious dog in sternal position cannot effectively be prevented when the animal's limbs are beneath it. Better control is achieved by the assistant restraining the dog holding the hocks forward so that the hind limbs are in extension. The hair should be clipped over a sufficient area to observe the landmarks for injection and to maintain sterility. The site for needle insertion is located by identifying the cranial dorsal iliac spines of the pelvis (Fig. 15.17). An imaginary line joining these crosses midline over the dorsal spinous process of the last lumbar vertebra. The lumbosacral junction is pal-

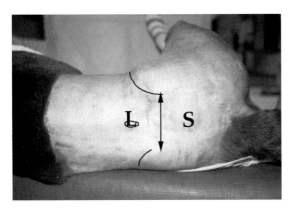

FIG. 15.17 Site for epidural injection. This dog is anaesthetized and clipped for orthopaedic surgery. An imaginary line between the caudal dorsal iliac spines crosses the midline at the lumbosacral space. An imaginary line between the cranial edges of the cranial dorsal iliac spines crosses the midline at the dorsal spinous process of the last lumbar vertebra.

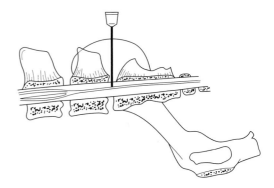

FIG. 15.18 Epidural analgesia. The site and direction for insertion of the needle.

pated as a depression immediately caudal to this midline prominence, adjacent to the caudal dorsal iliac spines, which in thin dogs can be seen as the most dorsal bumps of the pelvis. In heavily muscled or fat dogs and dogs with rounded hindquarters, the caudal dorsal iliac spines are difficult to palpate and heavy reliance is placed on identifying the spinous process of the last lumbar vertebra. Palpation of the spinous process of the previous lumbar vertebra can be used as a guide. The needle should be inserted caudal to the last spinous process at a distance that is half of the distance between the two spinous processes.

In conscious dogs an insensitive skin weal is made with a fine needle and a bleb of local anaesthetic. A 21 or 22 gauge spinal needle, 3.75 cm for small dogs and 6.25 cm for large dogs, is inserted midline perpendicular to the skin and to the curvature of the rump (Fig. 15.18). Penetration of the interarcuate ligament imparts a distinct 'popping' sensation to the fingers. Should bone rather than ligament be encountered, it indicates that the direction of the needle has been wrong and that its point has struck an articular process or the roof of the first sacral segment. If this occurs the needle is slightly withdrawn and a search made for the space by redirecting it a little caudally, cranially or laterally. The hub of the needle should be held securely as the stilette is removed. A 3 ml syringe containing 0.5 ml air should be attached

and, after aspiration has not drawn cerebrospinal fluid (CSF) or blood into the syringe, injection of air should offer no resistance. Confirmation of correct placement is made by ensuring that the needle is midline, that it is sufficiently deep (needle should be supported securely by surrounding tissues when the tip is in the epidural space), that a slight resistance then penetration 'pop' is appreciated during traverse of the interarcuate ligament, and there is no resistance to injection of the air. If CSF or blood are aspirated into the syringe, the syringe should be disconnected, the stilette reinserted and the tip of the spinal needle repositioned. Injection of the anaesthetic solution should be made over 30 seconds to avoid an increase in intracranial pressure. The injectate should be warmed before performing epidural analgesia in the conscious dog to avoid movement in response to the cold solution.

A catheter can be introduced easily some 2–3 cm into the epidural space through a correctly placed Tuohy needle (Fig. 15.19). This technique is useful for continuous postoperative analgesia.

Drugs used in the epidural space

Lignocaine 2% with 1:200 000 adrenaline will produce analgesia in 15 minutes and last 1.5–2.0 hours. Bupivacaine 0.50% or 0.75% has a slower onset of action at 20–40 minutes and a longer duration of at least 6 hours. To produce analgesia up to L1 a dose of approximately 1 ml per 4.5 kg body weight is required and for cranial laparotomies where analgesia is needed to the 4th or 5th thoracic segment this dose is usually increased to about 1

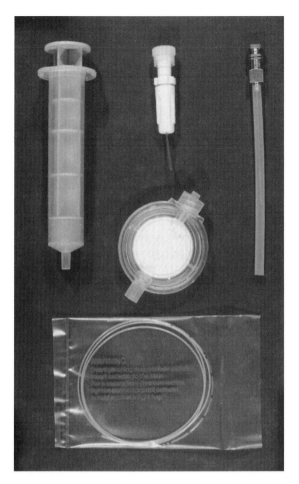

FIG. 15.19 Epidural 'Minipack' set (Portex Ltd) which is ideal for the introduction of a catheter into a dog's epidural space. The set contains a 10 ml syringe, 19 G Tuohy needle graduated 10–45 mm × 5 mm, open-ended catheter marked at 20–100 mm × 10 mm from tip, loss-of-resistance device, flat filter and Luer Lock connector.

ml per 3.5 kg. The dose should be decreased about 25% in pregnant animals. In contrast, epidural block may not extend as far cranially as expected in dogs that have experienced serious weight loss.

Morphine, 0.1 mg/kg in a total volume of 0.10–0.25 ml/kg (a preservative-free solution contains 1 mg/ml), is the opioid used most frequently for epidural injection in veterinary medicine. Morphine preparations containing phenol or formaldehyde should not be used whereas the preservative chlorbutanol has not been shown to be neurotoxic (Du Pen *et al.* 1987). The onset of analgesia is about 45 minutes and lasts from 6–12 hours

(Branson *et al.*, 1993), or even as long as 23 hours (Bonath & Saleh, 1985). Analgesia may extend as far forward as the forelimb and provides a significant decrease in anaesthetic requirement for surgery (MAC value for halothane decreased by 30–40%) (Valverde *et al.*, 1989; Valverde *et al.*, 1991). The duration of analgesia after epidural injection of oxymorphone, 0.05 mg/kg, was measured at 7.6 hours after hindlimb orthopaedic surgery (Vesal *et al.*, 1996) and 10 hours after thoracotomy (Popilskis *et al.*, 1991). The anaesthetic requirement for halothane is reported to be significantly decreased after epidural administration of oxymorphone, 0.1 mg/kg, and further by oxymorphone with bupivacaine, 1 mg/kg (Torske *et al.*, 1998). Epidural fentanyl and butorphanol have also been used, but the duration of analgesia is short.

Potential complications

In dogs, temporary interference with hindlimb motor power is of no clinical consequence. Analgesia caused by local anaesthetic solution that diffuses into the thoracic segments may be accompanied by hypotension that can be minimized by infusion of balanced electrolyte solution, 10–20 ml/kg, as the block develops. ABP and peripheral perfusion should be monitored throughout and a catheter for infusion of fluid and vasoactive drugs should they be needed must be placed in a vein before epidural block is induced.

In man, respiratory depression has been reported to occur several hours after epidural morphine injection, but this does not appear to be a problem in dogs. Oxymorphone is absorbed into the systemic circulation rapidly with peak values attained within 15 minutes after administration, similar to absorption after intramuscular injection (Torske *et al.*, 1999). Serum values of morphine peak 30 minutes after epidural administration. Epidural oxymorphone results in significant decreases in HR and CO (Vesal *et al.*, 1996; Torske *et al.*, 1999). These effects can be satisfactorily improved by administration of glycopyrrolate. ABP, HR and CO are not depressed after administration of morphine in anesthetized dogs (Valverde *et al.*, 1991). A case of postoperative urinary retention was reported in a dog following epidural analgesia with morphine and bupivacaine (Herperger, 1998).

A clinically insignificant complication that may be regarded most adversely by the owners of show dogs is inability of hair over the lumbosacral region to grow back at the same rate as expected for other parts of the body and to be darker than the original hair.

Infiltration of the dental nerves

Nerve block of the infraorbital nerve will provide analgesia of the upper teeth and block of the inferior alveolar nerve will desensitize the lower teeth. The infraorbital nerve is blocked within the infraorbital canal located by palpation between the dorsal border of the zygomatic arch and the canine tooth. The inferior alveolar nerve is blocked by insertion of a needle through the mental foramen adjacent to the second premolar tooth. A recent report of chloroprocaine, 1 ml of 2% at each site, for dental blocks in anesthetized dogs described the onset of analgesia occurring within 10 minutes (Gross *et al.*, 1997). The duration of analgesia lasted less than 90 minutes in the majority of dogs but persisted in isolated teeth for up to 96 hours. Use of bupivacaine results in a slow onset of action but should provide analgesia postoperatively.

Infiltration of the digital nerves

The digital nerves are approached laterally and medially to the first phalanx of the digit to be rendered analgesic. A fine needle is introduced subcutaneously on each side of the digit (Fig. 15.20) and 0.5–1.0 ml of local analgesic solution is injected on each aspect to block the dorsal and palmar or plantar branches of the digital nerves. Alternatively, the common dorsal and palmar (or plantar) digital nerves can be blocked by injections dorsally and ventrally at the distal end(s) of the main metacarpal (metatarsal) space(s).

Intercostal nerve block

This block is commonly used to provide analgesia after thoracotomy and is usually performed by the surgeon before starting closure of the thoracic wall. The intercostal nerve should be blocked where it lies on the caudal surface of the rib.

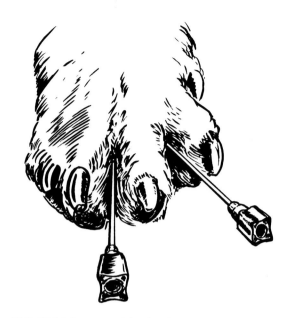

FIG. 15.20 Injection of the digital nerves.

Injection of 0.25 to 1.00 ml of 0.5% bupivacaine (1 mg/kg) should be made as close to the head of the rib as possible before the nerve begins to send off branches. The block should include two nerves immediately cranial to the thoracotomy incision and two nerves caudal. Analgesia may be produced in this way in at least 3 out of 4 dogs and will persist for the critical first 12 hours after surgery (Pascoe & Dyson, 1993).

Interpleural analgesia

Injection of bupivacaine, 1.5–2.5 mg/kg, into the interpleural space will provide analgesia after thoracotomy. The bupivacaine can be instilled into the pleural cavity at the end of surgery before starting wound closure or instilled down a chest tube, flushed in by several ml of sterile saline. Analgesia develops most effectively when the dog is in dorsal recumbency so that the bupivacaine collects near the vertebral column and blocks the nerves at that point. Injection with the dog in sternal position may only result in ventral analgesia.

Injection of 1.5 mg/kg after lateral thoracotomy was found to produce a significant improvement in PaO_2 and some measures of pulmonary function for several hours after anaesthesia when compared to systemic administration of morphine, 1 mg/kg (Stobie *et al.*, 1995) or buprenorphine (Conzemius *et al.*, 1994). Furthermore, analgesia was at least as good from interpleural bupivacaine as morphine (pain scores were lower after bupivacaine for 10 hours) and better than buprenorphine. A larger dose of bupivacaine will be needed for analgesia after median sternotomy, however it should be noted that a dose rate of 3 mg/kg 0.5% bupivacaine caused hypotension in some anaesthetized dogs (Kushner *et al.*, 1995). This occurred 15 minutes after injection and was coincident with peak bupivacaine blood concentrations.

Supplemental injections of bupivacaine can be made down the chest drain tube as analgesia fades. Transient 30 second discomfort may be observed after injection in the conscious dog.

Intra-articular analgesia

Postoperative analgesia after arthrotomy may be provided by injection of 0.5% bupivacaine (0.5 ml/kg) or preservative-free morphine (0.1 mg/kg diluted with saline to 0.5 ml/kg). A prospective blinded study comparing the analgesic effects of these drugs after stifle surgery in dogs confirmed that less supplemental analgesia was needed in dogs receiving intra-articular morphine or bupivacaine compared with dogs receiving a placebo (Sammarco *et al.*, 1996). Injections were made after the joint capsule was closed, extra-articular stabilization was performed, and subcutaneous tissues were closed. Intra-articular bupivacaine provided the greatest analgesia with consistently lower values postoperatively for HR, MAP, respiratory rates, and cumulative pain scores (Sammarco *et al.*, 1996). The duration of beneficial effects of bupivacaine seemed to be up to 24 hours.

The advantage of local analgesia after joint surgery lies in the provision of analgesia and comfort for the dog without systemic side effects. The peripheral antinociceptive effects of opioids are dependent on the presence of inflammation at the site. The effect of morphine is most likely at a μ opioid receptor at the site of injection and mediated in part by a direct reduction in terminal excitability (Nagasaka *et al.*, 1996).

Intravenous regional analgesia

This method provides a very safe and simple way of obtaining analgesia in tractable or sedated dogs of the distal part of the limb for suturing lacerations, excision of tissue masses, and surgery of the toes.

The dog should be restrained on its side and the appropriate limb held above heart level for 2–3 minutes to partially exanguinate it prior to application of a tourniquet. Thin rubber tourniquets can be painful and the least likely to cause the dog distress is a blood pressure cuff inflated to a pressure above systolic arterial pressure. On the forelimb the tourniquet is placed either high on the forearm or above the elbow and on the hind limb above the hock. Lignocaine, 4 mg/kg, is injected with a 25 gauge needle into any vein distal to the occluding cuff, with the direction of injection being made towards the toes. The lignocaine should not include adrenaline which will cause vasoconstriction, impair diffusion of lignocaine and possibly result in tissue ischaemia. Onset of analgesia will be in about 15 minutes and this will persist as long as the tourniquet is in place. Failure of analgesia will occur if the tourniquet does not effectively occlude arterial or venous blood flow. Sensation will return to the limb within a few minutes of removal of the tourniquet.

Intravenous injection may be difficult in thick skinned dogs and this problem can be circumvented by preplacement of a small indwelling catheter prior to exanguination and application of the tourniquet.

The dog can be sedated with any drug combination appropriate for the dog. If the sedatives are to be reversed at the end of the procedure, it must be remembered that intravenous regional analgesia confers no lasting analgesia after the tourniquet is removed.

REFERENCES

Alibhai, H.I., Clarke, K.W., Lee, Y.H. and Thompson, J. (1996) Cardiopulmonary effects of combinations of medetomidine hydrochloride and atropine sulphate in dogs. *Veterinary Record* **138**, 11–13.

Allen, D.A., Schertel, E.R., Muir, W.W. and Valentine, A.K. (1991) Hypertonic saline/dextran resuscitation of dogs with experimentally induced gastric dilatation-volvulus shock. *American Journal of Veterinary Research* **52**: 92–96.

Arnbjerg, J. (1992) Gastric emptying time in the dog and cat. *Journal of the American Animal Hospital Association* **28**: 77–81.

Atlee, J.L., Bosnjak, Z.J. and Yeager, T.S. (1990) Effects of diltiazem, verapamil, and inhalation anesthetics on electrophysiologic properties affecting re-entrant supraventricular tachycardia in chronically instrumented dogs. *Anesthesiology* **72**: 889–901.

Baum, V.C. and Palmisano, B.W. (1997) The immature heart and anesthesia. *Anesthesiology* **87**: 1529–1548.

Bernard, J.-M., Doursout, M.-F., Wouters, P., Hartley, C., Cohen, M., Merin, R.G. and Chelly, J.E. (1991) Effects of enflurane and isoflurane on hepatic and renal circulations in chronically instrumented dogs. *Anesthesiology* **74**, 298–302.

Bonath, K. and Saleh, A. (1985) Long term treatment in the dog by peridural morphines. *Proceedings of the 2nd International Congress of Veterinary Anesthesia*, Sacramento, California p. 161.

Branson, K., Ko, J., Tranquilli, W., Benson, J. and Thurmon, J. (1993) Duration of analgesia induced by epidurally administered morphine and medetomidine in dogs. *Journal of Veterinary Pharmacology and Therapeutics* **16**: 369–372.

Branson, K.R., Quandt, J.E., Martinez, E.A., *et al.* (1997) Multi-site clinical trial of sevoflurane. *Veterinary Surgery* **26**, 156 abstract.

Brockman, D.J., Washabau, R.J. and Drobatz, K.J. (1995) Canine gastric dilatation/volvulus syndrome in a veterinary critical care unit: 295 cases (1986–1992). *Journal of the American Veterinary Medical Association* **207**: 460–464.

Brodbelt, D.C., Taylor, P.M. and Stanway, G.W. (1997) A comparison of preoperative morphine and buprenorphine for postoperative analgesia for arthrotomy in dogs. *Journal of Veterinary Pharmacology and Therapeutics* **20**, 284–289.

Brownlie, S.E. (1991) An electrocardiographic survey of cardiac rhythm in Irish wolfhounds. *Veterinary Record* **129**: 470–471.

Buchanan, J.W. (1993) Changing breed predispositions in canine heart disease. *Canine Practice* **18**: 12–14.

Burton, S.A., Lemke, K.A., Ihle, S.L. and Mackenzie, A.L. (1997) Effects of medetomidine on serum insulin and plasma glucose concentrations in clinically normal dogs. *American Journal of Veterinary Research* **58**: 1440–1442.

Chambers, J.P. (1989) Induction of anaesthesia in dogs with alfentanil and propofol. *Journal of Veterinary Anaesthesia* **16**: 14–17.

Chelly, J.E., Hill, D.C., Abernethy, D.R., Dlewati, A., Doursout, M.-F. and Merin, R.G. (1987) Pharmacodynamic and pharmacokinetic interactions between lidocaine and verapamil. *Journal of Pharmacology and Experimental Therapeutics* **243**: 211–216.

Clarke, K. and Hall, L. (1975) In: *World Veterinary Congress*, p. 1688 (Thessaloniki, 1975).

Clutton, R.E. (1992) Combined bolus and infusion of vecuronium in dogs. *Journal of Veterinary Anaesthesia* **19**, 74–77.

Copland, V.S., Haskins, S.C. and Patz, J.D. (1987) Oxymorphone: Cardiovascular, pulmonary, and behavioral effects in dogs. *American Journal of Veterinary Research* **48**, 1626–1630.

Conzemius, M.G., Brockman, D.J., King, L.G. and Perkowski, S.Z. (1994) Analgesia in dogs after intercostal thoracotomy: A clinical trial comparing intravenous buprenorphine and interpleural bupivacaine. *Veterinary Surgery* **23**: 291–298.

Conzemius, M.G., Hill, C.M., Sammarco, J.L. and Perkowski, S.Z. (1997) Correlation between subjective and objective measures used to determine severity of postoperative pain in dogs. *Journal of the American Veterinary Medical Association* **210**: 1619–1622.

Dodam, J.R., Kruse-Elliot, K.T., Aucoin, D.P. and Swanson, C.R. (1990) Duration of etomidate-induced adrenocortical suppression during surgery in dogs. *American Journal of Veterinary Research* **51**: 786–788.

Dohoo, S.E., O'Connor, M.K., McDonell, W.N. and Dohoo, I.R. (1986) A clinical comparison of oxymorphone/acepromazine and fentanyl/droperidol sedation in dogs. *Journal of the American Animal Hospital Association* **22**, 313–317.

Donaldson, L.L., Leib, M.S., Boyd, C., Burkholder, W. and Sheridan, M. (1993) Effect of preanesthetic medication on ease of endoscopic intubation of the duodenum in anesthetized dogs. *American Journal of Veterinary Research* **54**: 1489–1495.

Du Pen, S.L., Ramsey, D. and Chin, S. (1987) Chronic epidural morphine and preservative-induced injury. *Anesthesiology* **67**, 987–988.

Dyson, D.H., Doherty, T., Anderson, G.I. and McDonell, W.N. (1990) Reversal of oxymorphone sedation by naloxone, nalmefene, and butorphanol. *Veterinary Surgery* **19**: 398–403.

Egger, C., Duke, T. and Cribb, P. (1998) Comparison of plasma fentanyl concentrations by using three transdermal fentanyl patch sizes in dogs. *Veterinary Surgery* **27**: 159–166.

England, G.C.W. and Clarke, K.W. (1989) The effect of route of administration upon the efficacy of medetomidine. *Journal of the Association of Veterinary Anaesthetists* **16**: 32–34.

England, G.C. and Clarke, K.W. (1989a) The use of medetomidine/fentanyl combinations in dogs. *Acta Veterinaria Scandinavia Supplement* **85**, 179–186.

England, G.C. and Hammond, R. (1997) Dose-sparing effects of romifidine premedication for thiopentone and halothane anaesthesia in the dog. *Journal of Small Animal Practice* **38**, 141–146.

Firth, A. and Haldane, S.L. (1999) Development of a scale to evaluate postoperative pain in dogs. *Journal of the American Veterinary Medical Association* **214**: 651–660.

Freeman, L.C., Ack, J.A., Fligner, M.A. and Muir III, W.W. (1990) Atrial fibrillation in halothane-and isoflurane-anesthetized dogs. *American Journal of Veterinary Research* **51**, 174–177.

Forsyth, S.F., Guilford, W.G., Haslett, S.J. and Godfrey, J. (1998) Endoscopy of the gastroduodenal mucosa after carprofen, meloxicam and ketoprofen administration in dogs. *Journal of Small Animal Practice* **39**: 421–424.

Gelman, S., Fowler, K.C. and Smith, L.R. (1984) Regional blood flow during isoflurane and halothane anesthesia. *Anesthesia & Analgesia* **63**, 557–565.

Gross, M.E., Pope, E.R., O'Brien, D., Dodam, J.R. and Polkow-Haight, J. (1997) Regional anesthesia of the infraorbital and inferior alveolar nerves during noninvasive tooth pulp stimulation in halothane-anesthetized dogs. *Journal of the American Veterinary Medical Association* **211**: 1403–1405.

Hall, L.W. (1984) A clinical study of a new intravenous agent in dogs and cats. *Journal of the Association of Veterinary Anaesthetists* **12**: 115–121.

Hall, L.W., Nolan, A.M. and Sear, J.W. (1997) Disposition of propofol after medetomidine premedication in beagle dogs. *Journal of Veterinary Anaesthesia* **24**: 23–30.

Hashim, M.A., Waterman, A.E. and Pearson, H. (1995) A comparison of the effects of halothane and isoflurane in combination with nitrous oxide on lower oesophageal sphincter pressure and barrier pressure in anaesthetised dogs. *Veterinary Record* **137**: 658–661.

Haskins, S.C., Farver, T.B. and Patz, J.D. (1985) Ketamine in dogs. *American Journal of Veterinary Research* **46**: 1855–1985.

Haskins, S.C., Farver, T.B. and Patz, J.D. (1986) Cardiovascular changes in dogs given diazepam and diazepam-ketamine. *American Journal of Veterinary Research* **47**: 795–798.

Haskins, S.C., Patz, J.D., Copland, S.V., Yamamoto, Y. and Orima, H. (1988) A comparison of the cardiopulmonary effects of oxymorphone and ketamine in hypovolemic dogs. *Veterinary Surgery* **17**: 170–172.

Haskins, S.C. and Patz, J.D. (1990) Ketamine in hypovolemic dogs. *Critical Care Medicine* **18**: 625–629.

Hellebrekers, L.J. and Sap, R. (1992) Sufentanil-midazolam anaesthesia in the dog. *Journal of Veterinary Anaesthesia* **19**: 69–71.

Hellebrekers, L.J. and Sap, R. (1997) Medetomidine as a premedicant for ketamine, propofol or fentanyl anaesthesia in dogs. *Veterinary Record* **140**: 545–548.

Hellebrekers, L.J., vanHerpen, H., Hird, J.F.R., Rosenhagen, C.U., Sap, R. and Vainio, O. (1998) Clinical efficacy and safety of propofol or ketamine anaesthesia in dogs premedicated with medetomidine. *Veterinary Record* **142**: 631–634.

Hellyer, P., Muir III, W.W., Hubbell, J.A.E. and Sally, J. (1989) Cardiorespiratory effects of the intravenous administration of tiletamine-zolazepam to dogs. *Veterinary Surgery* **18**: 160–165.

Herperger, L. (1998) Postoperative urinary retention in a dog following morphine with bupivacaine epidural analgesia. *Canadian Veterinary Journal* **39**: 650–652.

Hoffman, W.D., Banks, S.M., Alling, D.W., Eichenholz, P.W., Eichacker, P.Q., Parillo, J.E. and Natanson, C. (1991) Factors that determine the hemodynamic response to inhalation anesthetics. *Journal of Applied Physiology* **70**, 2155–2163.

Holton, L.L., Scott, E.M., Nolan, A.M., Reid, J. and Welsh, E. (1998) Relationship between physiological factors and clinical pain in dogs scored using a numerical rating scale. *Journal of Small Animal Practice* **39**: 469–474.

Holton, L.L., Scott, E.M., Nolan, A.M., Reid, J., Welsh, E. and Flaherty, D. (1998) Comparison of three methods used for assessment of pain in dogs. *Journal of the American Veterinary Medical Association* **212**: 61–66.

Horne, W.A., Gilmore, D.R., Dietze, A.E., Freden, G.O. and Short, C.E. (1985) Effects of gastric distention-volvulus on coronary blood flow and myocardial O_2 consumption in the dog. *American Journal of Veterinary Research* **46**: 98–104.

Hoskins, J.D. (1995) The geriatric dog. *Perspectives* May/June, 39–46.

Hysing, E.S., Chelly, J.E., Doursout, M.-F. and Merin, R.G. (1992) Comparative effects of halothane, enflurane, and isoflurane at equihypotensive doses on cardiac performance and coronary and renal blood flows in chronically instrumented dogs. *Anesthesiology* **76**, 979–984.

Ilkiw, J.E., Pascoe, P.J., Haskins, S.C. and Patz, J.D. (1992) Cardiovascular and respiratory effects of propofol administration in hypovolemic dogs. *American Journal of Veterinary Research* **53**: 2323–2327.

Jergens, A.E., Riedesel, D.H., Ries, P.A., Miles, K.G. and Bailey, T.B. (1995) Cardiopulmonary responses in healthy dogs during endoscopic examination of the gastrointestinal tract. *American Journal of Veterinary Research* **56**: 215–220.

Johnston, S.A. and Fox, S.M. (1997) Mechanisms of action of anti-inflammatory medications used for the treatment of osteoarthritis. *Journal of the American Veterinary Medical Association* **210**: 1486–1492.

Jones, D.J., Stehling, L.C. and Zauder, H.L. (1979) Cardiovascular responses to diazepam and midazolam maleate in the dog. *Anesthesiology* **51**, 430–434.

Jones, R.S. and Brearley, J.C. (1987) Atracurium infusion in the dog. *Journal of Small Animal Practice* **28**: 197–201.

Jones, R.S. and Young, L.E. (1991) Vecuronium infusion in the dog. *Journal of Small Animal Practice* **32**: 509–512.

Kaplan, E.B., Sheiner, L.B., Boeckmann, A.J., Roizen, M.F., Beal, S.L., Cohen, S.N. and Nicoll, C.D. (1985) The usefulness of preoperative laboratory screening. *Journal of the American Medical Association* **253**: 3576–3581.

Kolata, R.J. and Rawlings, C.A. (1982) Cardiopulmonary effects of intravenous xylazine, ketamine, and atropine in the dog. *American Journal of Veterinary Research* **43**: 2196–2198.

Kushner, L.I., Trim, C.M., Madhusudhan, S. and Boyle, C.R. (1995) Evaluation of hemodynamic effects of interpleural bupivacaine in dogs. *Veterinary Surgery* **24**: 180–187.

Kyles, A., Papich, M. and Hardie, E. (1996) Disposition of transdermally administered fentanyl in dogs. *American Journal of Veterinary Research* **57**: 715–719.

Lantz, G.C., Badylak, S.F., Hiles, M.C. and Arkin, T.E. (1992) Treatment of reperfusion injury in dogs with experimentally induced gastric dilatation-volvulus. *American Journal of Veterinary Research* **53**: 1594–1598.

Lascelles, B.D., Butterworth, S.J. and Waterman, A.E. (1994) Postoperative analgesic and sedative effects of carprofen and pethidine in dogs. *Veterinary Record* **134**(8): 187–191.

Lascelles, B.D., Cripps, P.J., Jones, A. and Waterman-Pearson, A. (1998) Efficacy and kinetics of carprofen, administered preoperatively or postoperatively, for the prevention of pain in dogs undergoing ovariohysterectomy. *Veterinary Surgery* **27**: 568–582.

Lee, D.D., Mayer, R.E., Sullivan, T.C., Davidson, M.G., Swanson, C.R. and Hellyer, P.W. (1998) Respiratory depressant and skeletal muscle relaxant effects of low-dose pancuronium bromide in spontaneously breathing, isoflurane-anesthetized dogs. *Veterinary Surgery* **27**: 473–479.

MacPhail, C.M., Lappin, M.R., Meyer, D.J., Smith, S.G., Webster, C.R. and Armstrong, P.J. (1998) Hepatocellular toxicosis associated with administration of carprofen in 21 dogs. *Journal of the American Veterinary Medical Association* **212**: 1895–1901.

Martinez, E.A., Hartsfield, S.M., Melendez, L.D., Matthews, N.S. and Slater, M.R. (1997) Cardiovascular effects of buprenorphine in anesthetized dogs. *American Journal of Veterinary Research* **58**, 1280–1284.

Merin, R.G. and Johns, R.A. (1994) Does isoflurane produce coronary vasoconstriction? *Anesthesiology* **81**: 1093–1096.

Millis, D.L., Hauptman, J.G. and Fulton, R.B. (1993) Abnormal hemostatic profiles and gastric necrosis in canine gastric dilatation-volvulus. *Veterinary Surgery* **22**: 93–97.

Muir, W.W. (1982) Gastric dilatation-volvulus in the dog, with emphasis on cardiac arrhythmias. *Journal of the American Veterinary Medical Association* **180**: 739–742.

Muir III, W.W. and Mason, D.E. (1989) Side effects of etomidate in dogs. *Journal of the American Veterinary Medical Association* **194**: 1430–1434.

Muir, W.W. and Gadawski, J. (1998) Cardiorespiratory effects of low-flow and closed circuit inhalation anesthesia, using sevoflurane delivered with an in-circuit vaporizer and concentrations of compound A. *American Journal of Veterinary Research* **59**: 603–608.

Mutoh, T., Nishumura, R., Kim, H.-Y., Matsunaga, S. and Sasaki, N. (1997) Cardiopulmonary effects of sevoflurane, compared with halothane, enflurane, and isoflurane, in dogs. *American Journal of Veterinary Research* **58**: 885–890.

Nagasaka, H., Awad, H. and Yaksh, T.L. (1996) Peripheral and spinal actions of opioids in the blockade of the autonomic response evoked by compression of the inflamed knee joint. *Anesthesiology* **85**: 808–816.

Orton, E.C. and Muir III, W.W. (1983) Hemodynamics during experimental gastric dilatation-volvulus in dogs. *American Journal of Veterinary Research* **44**: 1512–1515.

Pascoe, P.J., Ilkiw, J.E., Haskins, S.C. and Patz, J.D. (1992) Cardiopulmonary effects of etomidate in hypovolemic dogs. *American Journal of Veterinary Research* **53**: 2178–2182.

Pascoe, P.J., Haskins, S.C., Ilkiw, J.E. and Patz, J.D. (1994) Cardiopulmonary effects of halothane in hypovolemic dogs. *American Journal of Veterinary Research* **55**, 121–126.

Pascoe, P.J. and Dyson, D.H. (1993) Analgesia after lateral thoracotomy in dogs. Epidural morphine vs. intercostal bupivacaine. *Veterinary Surgery* **22**: 141–147.

Pasternak, L.R. (1996) Preanesthesia evaluation of the surgical dog. *Refresher Courses in Anesthesiology* **24**: 205–220.

Pibarot, P., Dupuis, J., Grisneaux, E. *et al.* (1997) Comparison of ketoprofen, oxymorphone hydrochloride, and butorphanol in the treatment of postoperative pain in dogs. *Journal of the American Veterinary Medical Association* **211**: 438–444.

Pion, P.D. and Brown, W.A. (1995) Calcium channel blocking agents. *Compendium of Continuing Education* **17**: 691–706.

Poffenbarger, E.M., Ralston, S.L., Chandler, M.J. and Olsen, P.N. (1990) Canine neonatology. Part I. Physiologic differences between puppies and adults. *Compendium of Continuing Education* **12**: 1601–1609.

Popilskis, S., Kohn, D., Sanchez, J. and Gorman, P. (1991) Epidural vs intramuscular oxymorphone analgesia after thoracotomy in dogs. *Veterinary Surgery* **20**: 462–467.

Priano, L.L. and Vatner, S.F. (1981) Morphine effects on cardiac output and regional blood flow distribution in conscious dogs. *Anesthesiology* **55**, 236–243.

Priebe, H.-J. and Skarvan, K. (1987) Cardiovascular and electrophysiologic interactions between diltiazem and isoflurane in the dog. *Anesthesiology* **66**: 114–121.

Quandt, J.E., Robinson, E.P., Rivers, W.J. and Raffe, M.R. (1998) Cardiorespiratory and anesthetic effects of propofol and thiopental in dogs. *American Journal of Veterinary Research* **59**: 1137–1143.

Raptopoulos, D. and Galatos, A.D. (1995) Post anaesthetic reflux oesophagitis in dogs and cats. *Journal of Veterinary Anaesthesia* **22**: 6–8.

Raptopoulos, D. and Galatos, A.D. (1997) Gastro-oesophageal reflux during anaesthesia induced with either thiopentone or propofol in the dog. *Journal of Veterinary Anaesthesia* **24**: 20–22.

Robinson, E.P., Faggella, A.M., Henry, D.P. and Russell, W.L. (1988) Comparison of histamine release induced by morphine and oxymorphone administration in dogs. *American Journal of Veterinary Research* **49**, 1699–1701.

Sammarco, J.L., Conzemius, M.G., Perkowski, S.Z., Weinstein, M.J., Gregor, T.P. and Smith, G.K. (1996) Postoperative analgesia for stifle surgery: a comparison of intra-articular bupivacaine, morphine, or saline. *Veterinary Surgery* **25**: 59–69.

Schertel, E.R., Allen, D.A., Muir, W.W., Brourman, J.D. and DeHoff, W.D. (1997) Evaluation of a hypertonic saline-dextran solution for treatment of dogs with shock induced by gastric dilatation-volvulus. *Journal of the American Veterinary Medical Association* **210**: 226–230.

Stobie, D., Caywood, D.D., Rozanski, E.A. *et al*. (1995) Evaluation of pulmonary function and analgesia in dogs after intercostal thoracotomy and use of morphine administered intramuscularly or intrapleurally and bupivacaine administered intrapleurally. *American Journal of Veterinary Research* **56**: 1098–1109.

Takasaki, Y., Naruoka, Y., Shimizu, C., Ochi, G., Nagaro, T. and Arai, T. (1995) Diltiazem potentiates the neuromuscular blockade by vecuronium in humans. *Masui* **44**: 503–507.

Tomiyasu, S., Hara, T., Ureshino, H. and Sumikawa, K. (1999) Comparative analysis of systemic and coronary hemodynamics during sevoflurane- and isoflurane-induced hypotension in dogs. *Journal of Cardiovascular Pharmacology* **33**: 741–747.

Torske, K.E., Dyson, D.H. and Pettifer, G. (1998) End tidal halothane concentration and postoperative analgesia requirements in dogs: a comparison between intravenous oxymorphone and epidural bupivacaine alone and in combination with oxymorphone. *Canadian Veterinary Journal* **39**: 361–368.

Torske, K.E., Dyson, D.H. and Conlon, P.D. (1999) Cardiovascular effects of epidurally administered oxymorphone and an oxymorphone-bupivacaine combination in halothane-anesthetized dogs. *American Journal of Veterinary Research* **60**: 194–200.

Turnbull, J.M. and Buck, C. (1987) The value of preoperative screening investigations in otherwise healthy individuals. *Archives of Internal Medicine* **147**, 1101–1105.

Tyner, C.L., Woody, B.J., Reid, J.S. *et al*. (1997) Multicenter clinical comparison of sedative and analgesic effects of medetomidine and xylazine in dogs. *Journal of the American Veterinary Medical Association* **211**: 1413–1417.

Valverde, A., Dyson, D. and McDonell, W. (1989) Epidural morphine reduces halothane MAC in the dog. *Canadian Journal of Anaesthesia* **36**: 629–632.

Valverde, A., Dyson, D., Cockshutt, J., McDonell, W. and Valliant, A. (1991) Comparison of the hemodynamic effects of halothane alone and halothane combined with epidurally administered morphine for anesthesia in ventilated dogs. *American Journal of Veterinary Research* **52**: 505–509.

Vanio, O. (1991) Propofol infusion anaesthesia in dogs pre-medicated with medetomidine. *Journal of Veterinary Anaesthesia* **18**: 35–37.

Vesal, N., Cribb, P. and Frketic, M. (1996) Postoperative analgesic and cardiopulmonary effects in dogs of oxymorphone administered epidurally and intramuscularly, and medetomidine administered epidurally: A comparative clinical study. *Veterinary Surgery* **25**: 361–369.

Watkins, S., Hall, L. and Clarke, K. (1987) Propofol as an intravenous anaesthetic agent for dogs. *Veterinary Record* **120**: 326–329.

Anaesthesia of the cat

16

INTRODUCTION

So often in the past domestic cats have been regarded as being simply small dogs, but this attitude has gradually changed and it is now recognized that cats are unique among domestic animals (Hall & Taylor, 1994). Despite the cat's reputation for having nine lives, anaesthetic fatalities are not unknown in apparently fit, healthy animals. Indeed, in veterinary general practice in the UK the Association of Veterinary Anaesthetists survey in 1990 indicated a death rate of 1 in 550 for fit, healthy cats (Clarke & Hall, 1990). A study of deaths associated with the perianaesthetic period in a University Teaching Hospital (Gaynor *et al*, 1994) estimated the occurrence to be less than 1%, while anaesthetic related complications occurred in approximately 10.5% of cases. It may be that ignorance of the wealth of information relating to feline physiology and pharmacology appearing in journals and other texts not readily available to veterinary clinicians has contributed to these quite unacceptably high mortality and morbidity rates. Now that the peculiarities of the species have been recognized so that due allowance can be made for them it is to be hoped that great improvements will follow.

Cats object to being restrained and even friendly cats may prove difficult to inject intravenously; unhandled cats may be impossible to anaesthetize using this route. For this reason it may be necessary to give parenteral drugs by other routes, or to induce anaesthesia using inhalation agents. Cats are small in size and this means that the margin of error is small; using large syringes and needles can compromise accurate dosage so that anaesthetic overdoses are easy. For inhalation anaesthesia special apparatus is necessary if asphyxia is to be avoided. Respiratory obstruction can occur from even a small blob of mucus in the airway due to the small diameter of the cat's trachea and the tendency for laryngeal spasm to develop. Endotracheal intubation may not reduce this danger, as trauma to the larynx from inexpert intubation may result in obstruction from mucosal oedema postoperatively. Adrenaline release during a stormy induction or recovery can cause ventricular fibrillation and this is especially likely to happen if the heart is suffering from the insults of hypoxia or hypercapnia due to partial respiratory obstruction, or to the use of inappropriate anaesthetic apparatus. In the cat, vagal reflexes are very active during light anaesthesia, they are triggered by surgery of the head and neck, particularly of the eyes, nose and larynx, and give rise to laryngeal spasm or, occasionally, to cardiac arrest.

Suitable premedication, a quiet induction of anaesthesia, careful monitoring, the maintenance of a clear airway, adequate oxygenation, the efficient removal of carbon dioxide, and appropriate attention to fluid and electrolyte balance, should ensure an extremely low mortality rate.

ANALGESIA

OPIOIDS

The cat usually only vocalizes when pain is acute and the tone of vocalization is higher than when the animal is merely resenting being handled or restrained. 'Swearing' or hissing indicates that the animal resents interference but purring does not necessarily mean that all is well. Cats in pain will often purr when stroked or petted. Chronic pain is often manifested by the animal hiding in dark corners of the cage, together with loss of appetite and self-grooming activity. In severe acute pain cats may pant or mouth breathe.

Cats have often been denied adequate analgesia on the mistaken grounds that the use of opioids causes maniacal excitement in *Felidae*. Certainly, the use of high doses as employed by pharmacologists studying pharmacological effects can do so, and violent excitement may be seen after intravenous injection of these drugs, as this method of administration may expose the brain to a (temporary) overdose. Thus, i.v. administration of potent opioids such as fentanyl or alfentanil to conscious cats can only be recommended if injection is made extremely slowly. In the correct doses, and by appropriate routes of administration, opioids will not induce excitement even in fit, healthy animals (Davis & Donelly, 1968) and if the cat is in pain when the analgesic is given higher doses are tolerated without problems. Any of the opioids of moderate potency, which have been recommended for use in other species of animal may be used to provide pre- or postoperative analgesia in cats (Table 16.1).

TABLE 16.1 Opioid analgesics suitable for use in cats; s.c. = subcutaneous injection; i.m. = intramuscular injection; i.v. = intravenous injection

Drug	Dose	Route of administration
Buprenorphine	0.006–0.010 mg/kg	s.c., i.m., i.v.
Butorphanol	0.2–0.5 mg/kg	i.m.
Methadone	0.10–0.2 mg/kg	s.c., i.v.
Morphine	0.10–0.15 mg/kg	s.c., i.m., i.v.
Pethidine (meperidine)	2–5 mg/kg	i.m.
Oxymorphone	0.05–0.10 mg/kg	i.m.

Pethidine and buprenorphine

It is probable that pethidine (meperidine), i.m. at total doses of 10 to 20 mg to average sized animals has been the opioid most widely used, but cats in severe pain may safely be given i.m. morphine at doses of 0.10–0.15 mg/kg. Of the partial agonist drugs, butorphanol 0.2–0.5 mg/kg i.m. has been recommended by Short (1987) and i.m. buprenorphine (0.006 mg/kg) given at the end of surgery provides excellent analgesia although at the expense of considerably delayed recovery from anaesthesia.

Neuroleptanalgesia

Neuroleptanalgesic techniques which employ large doses of opioid analgesics may cause cats to respond with violent excitement. They are, therefore, contra-indicated in domestic cats and, indeed, in all other *Felidae*. Low doses of opioids such as pethidine (1–2 mg/kg) may be used together with acepromazine but the improvement in sedation over that provided by acepromazine is minimal. However, acepromazine (0.05 mg/kg i.m.) is often used with 0.1 mg/kg morphine i.m. to produce sedation, and oxymorphone, buprenorphine, butorphanol, papaveretum and methadone can also be used, although doses of these opioid drugs need to be kept to a minimum (e.g. butorphanol 0.2–0.4 mg/kg, oxymorphone 0.05 mg/kg i.m.). Geriatric or sick cats may be premedicated with butorphanol 0.3 mg/kg i.m. and midazolam 0.1–0.2 mg/kg i.m. prior to facemask induction of anaesthesia.

NON-STEROIDAL ANTI-INFLAMMATORY DRUGS (NSAIDs)

Table 16.2 gives recommended dosages for various NSAIDs used in cats. Phenylbutazone is quite toxic to cats, even in moderate doses, but aspirin

TABLE 16.2 NSAID dosages in cats

Drug	Dose
Aspirin	5 mg/kg/ 24 hours orally for < 2 days
Carprofen	1–4 mg/kg i.v. or s.c.
Ketoprofen	1 mg/kg/24 hours s.c. for <3 days
Phenylbutazone	10 mg/kg/24 hours orally

may be given in small doses by mouth. When indicated 10–20 mg of aspirin should be given in divided doses over a period of 48 hours. Given over one or two days this dose is generally both safe and effective and allows for the fact that the rate of hepatic drug metabolism is slow due to a deficiency of bilirubin-glucuronoside glucuronosyltransferase. Long term aspirin administration can lead to aplastic anaemia or thrombocytopaenia.

Carprofen, which does not appear to act by inhibition of cyclo-oxygenase or lipoxygenase, as the older NSAIDs do, may have fewer side effects. However, experience has shown that *all* NSAIDs must be used with caution in cats and only in the recommended doses for periods not in excess of 2 to 3 days at a time. Other drugs such as acetaminophen (paracetamol), ibuprofen, indomethacin and naproxen are contraindicated in cats because of their hepatoxicity.

LOCAL ANALGESIA

Infiltration of fracture sites or wounds with local analgesics can be very effective means of relieving pain in cats, but the total dose of drug administered must be carefully regulated. If lignocaine is used the total dose should not exceed 10 mg/kg – this means a maximum of about 8 ml of a 0.5 % solution or 16 ml of a 0.25 % solution in an average sized, conscious cat. Doses of 0.125 % or 0.070% bupivacaine are correspondingly smaller but the use of this drug for longer duration analgesia in cats has not been widely explored. Gross distension of the tissues with local analgesic solution must be avoided for this interferes with blood flow and may result in delayed wound healing.

Epidural blocks are sometimes difficult to produce and in cats nearly always need to be combined with heavy sedation or light general anaesthesia so their use is limited. If the block is induced during preparation of the surgical site it is an effective analgesic long before the end of surgery.

Ancillary aids to analgesia

The importance of good nursing care in alleviating pain must never be overlooked. Provision of warmth and appetizing food should always be a priority. Grooming and wiping around the mouth and eyes with moist cotton wool can do much to increase the animals' comfort and they seem to feel much better for this attention.

SEDATION

PHENOTHIAZINE DERIVATIVES

Acepromazine

Acepromazine may be given at dose rates of 0.03 to 0.10 mg/kg and by the routes described for dogs (p. 394) but in cats the sedation produced is very variable and is seldom adequate to assist in control of an animal. The pharmacokinetics of orally administered acepromazine in cats was poorly documented until the studies of Verstegen *et al.* (1994). These workers found the apparent elimination half life to be about 3 hours but the determination of the elimination constant was hampered by imprecise estimation of the detectable concentrations using specific HPLC.

Premedication with phenothiazine derivatives such as acepromazine results in a smoother recovery from anaesthesia and reduces excitement side effects of certain anaesthetic agents. Promethazine, a potent antihistamine, is sometimes used before Saffan anaesthesia to reduce the risk of allergic-type reactions.

α_2 ADRENOCEPTOR AGONISTS

Xylazine

Xylazine has been widely used, but it may produce variable results. Its action is that of a sedative/hypnotic so that increasing the dose increases the depth and duration of sedation produced, and doses of 1 to 3 mg/kg by the i.m. route may be used to give mild to fairly profound sedation; s.c. injection may be used but gives less reliable results. Vomiting and retching occur as the drug starts to exert its effect and are most commonly seen after the lower dose rates are employed. Cardiovascular effects are dose-dependent and although there may be an initial period of hypertension, doses of more than 3 mg/kg result in cardiac depression and hypotension. Dunkle *et al.*(1986), using echocardiography, found xylazine to have a marked depressive effect on cardiac performance and showed that glycopyrrolate may not completely alleviate the bradycardia due to this α_2 adrenoceptor agonist. Very high doses of xylazine have been used to anaesthetize cats but they are associated with respiratory depression, cardiovascular depression and a very protracted recovery. They represent overdosage and such misuse cannot be condoned.

When xylazine is used for premedication, its effects summate with those of all other central nervous depressant drugs, so that doses of all parenterally administered anaesthetics have to be greatly reduced. This additive effect seems to depend on the dose of xylazine rather than the effect which it has produced, so that great care is necessary in even apparently lightly sedated cats. Following xylazine premedication doses of barbiturate drugs are at least halved, and doses of Saffan have to be reduced even more than this. Xylazine has often been used with ketamine and use of these two drugs will be discussed later.

Medetomidine

Medetomidine has almost completely replaced xylazine and a dose of $80\,\mu g/kg$ appears to give sedation similar in type and depth to that produced by $3\,mg/kg$ of i.m. xylazine. Duration of effect is dose related, but after an i.m. dose of $80\,\mu g/kg$ clinically useful effects last for approximately 1 hour and recovery appears to be complete in about 2.5–3.0 hours. Side effects are as expected for an α_2 adrenoceptor agonist, there being marked bradycardia and transient arterial hypertension followed by hypotension, depression of respiratory rate, pallor of mucous membranes and vomiting early on as sedation develops. Prolonged sedation with high doses of medetomidine may cause hypothermia.

Dexmedetomidene

Dexmedetomidine is the active sterioisomer of the racemic medetomidine preparations currently available for veterinary use. If this pure isomer becomes available there should be no problems for its actions are those of the mixed veterinary preparation. All that will need to be remembered is that the effective dose of dexmedetomidine is half that of the current commercial preparation of medetomidine employed in veterinary medicine.

Considerations when using α_2 adrenoceptor agonists

Should there be any worries about the condition of an animal sedated with these drugs bradycardia may be treated with atropine or glycopyrrolate, although this may not be altogether beneficial (Dunkle *et al.*, 1986). Their sedative effects may be antagonized with atipamezole. However, the ideal dose of atipamezole is uncertain. Doses of one to four times the original dose of medetomidine have been recommended and there is no consensus of the dose to be used to antagonize the effects of xylazine. High doses, or doses given at a time when sedation is already waning, have led to some cats being over-alert. The over-alert state did not progress to obvious excitement and, when left quiet in a cage, the animals resumed normal behaviour over the course of the next hour. As there are times when it may be desirable for a cat to remain very slightly sedated (e.g for the journey home) the decision as to the most suitable dose for any individual case should be adjusted according to the time lapsed since the administration of the agonist drug and degree of reversal required. It should be noted that in the authors' experience under-reversal using lower doses of atipamezole still leaves the cat liable to hypothermia.

BENZODIAZEPINES

Diazepam

Diazepam and other benzodiazepine drugs produce no obvious sedation when given to domestic cats. They are sometimes used in premedication for their muscle-relaxing properties and their use is associated with an increased duration of action of other drugs used in anaesthesia. Diazepam is given in doses of up to $0.5\,mg/kg$ i.m.; its injection appears to give rise to pain no matter what preparation is used.

Other benzodiazepines

Midazolam (0.1–0.2 mg/kg) is sometimes used i.m. mixed in the syringe with ketamine 6 mg/kg to produce a state of good sedation for the performance of minor procedures such as skin biopsy or radiography.

There are currently no reports of the use of climazolam or zolazepam given on their own to cats, but zolazepam is available in Australia, North America and on the Continent of Europe in a fixed ratio combination with the dissociative agent tiletamine ('Telazol', containing 50 mg tiletamine plus 50 mg zolazepam per ml) for the induction of a state resembling general anaesthesia. Telazol is not available in the UK. Muscle relaxation is poor, there is usually profuse salivation and many cats show respiratory depression as well as tachyarrhythmias. The author's experience agrees with that of Short (1987) that recovery from this combination can be prolonged and excited.

GENERAL ANAESTHESIA

PREANAESTHETIC PREPARATION

Preanaesthetic examination should be carried out in a manner similar to that described in Chapter 1, and any pathological conditions found, together with any pre-existing drug therapy, taken into account during subsequent anaesthesia. In clinical practice it is common to find that cats have been exposed to organophosphorus insecticides from flea collars or sprays and this may increase the duration of action of suxamethonium given for intubation. Corticosteroids are frequently used in cats to control allergies to external parasites and corticosteroid cover should be given over the anaesthetic and operating periods if the cat has received such therapy in the 2 months preceding anaesthesia.

About 12 hours of fasting will usually ensure that cats have an empty stomach and water need only be withheld for 2 hours prior to anaesthesia, or the water bowl removed at the time premedication is given. If surgery is to be carried out on the day of admission, enquiry should be made as to whether the cat was closely confined throughout the previous night for a roaming, hunting cat may have filled its stomach by eating its prey.

ANAESTHETIC TECHNIQUES

Intravenous injection

The minimum of forcible restraint should be used to enable injection to be carried out. Cats object strongly to restraint and respond to its imposition by trying to escape from it, thus inviting more forcible measures which only too often result in scratched and bitten assistants and a very frightened, excited cat. Such stormy conditions during induction of anaesthesia can lead to cats dying from ventricular fibrillation.

In conscious cats, i.v. injections are best made into the cephalic vein. The animal is placed in a sitting position on a table of convenient height and for injection into the right cephalic vein the assistant stands to the cat's left side, raising and supporting its head between the thumb and fingers of the left hand (Fig. 16.1). In this position the assistant can usually help to keep the cat calm by tickling it below the ears (Fig. 16.2). The assistant's right hand is placed so that the middle, third and fourth fingers are behind the olecranon, and the thumb is around the front of the cat's right forelimb. The limb is extended by pushing on the olecranon and the vein is raised by applying gentle pressure with the thumb. The limb must not be held in a vice-like grip because this cuts off the arterial blood supply and distresses the cat.

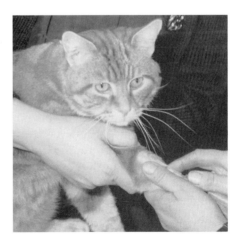

Fig. 16.1 Injection into the cephalic vein. Note that only the minimum of restraint is being used and as can be seen from this cat's expression it is not frightened or otherwise upset by the procedure.

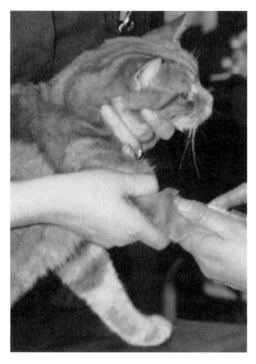

FIG. 16.2 The 'ear-tickling' position for restraint during venepuncture. This is the position to be used for animals not as calm as the one illustrated in Fig. 16.1.

Most friendly household cats will allow venepuncture to be carried out easily as long as the needle is sharp (and modern disposable ones are) and no thrust is made with the needle. The needle must be introduced steadily and gently through the skin and into the lumen of the vein without stabbing. Should it become obvious that more restraint is needed the assistant can provide this rapidly by holding the cat between his or her body and right arm while preventing movement from the hind limbs by pressing the cat firmly on to the table surface. The cat's head can easily be controlled when held firmly in the left hand as described. Sometimes, for the protection of the handler, it is necessary to wrap the cat in a towel held around the neck, leaving only the head and the limb to be used for injection exposed. If it is clear that greater restraint than this is needed, it is probably preferable to abandon attempts at i.v. injection until an appropriate premedication has had time to take effect, or to induce anaesthesia by other means.

A short needle with a fine bore is suitable for injections into the cephalic vein and, in general, a 25 gauge needle (0.5 mm external diameter), 15 mm long is ideal as long as venepuncture is free from difficulties and the limb is unlikely to be moved excessively during positioning for operation, but it is probably always preferable to use either a 'Butterfly' set or an over-the-needle catheter which can be taped securely in position.

Introduction of an i.v. needle or catheter may be helped in nervous or 'needle-shy' cats by the prior use of a local analgesic cream (e.g. EMLA, Astra, or amethocaine ointment). The site for venepuncture is shaved and a 2–3 mm thick layer of cream applied to the skin before covering it with an occlusive dressing for 40 to 45 min. This procedure produces full thickness skin analgesia and after removing the dressing, the skin is wiped clean, disinfected and venepuncture carried out.

Although in theory any of the methods of venepuncture described for use in dogs may be applied in cats, the problems of restraint make them difficult to use in conscious animals. In moribund or anaesthetized animals, the jugular vein can be used. The cat is placed in lateral recumbency with its neck over a small pad or sandbag, its forelimbs are stretched backwards towards its tail, and the uppermost jugular vein occluded in the jugular groove near to the sternal inlet by the assistant's thumb. Jugular venepuncture is particularly useful for the administration of intravenous fluid therapy. When relatively large blood samples are required for diagnostic or other purposes the jugular vein is commonly the only practicable site for cannulation, although alternatively, the easily visible saphenous medial vein on the medial aspect of the thigh can be used.

Endotracheal intubation

Cats generally maintain a good airway under general anaesthesia so endotracheal intubation is often unnecessary for short periods of anaesthesia when a mask can be used to administer oxygen and any volatile anaesthetic. The mask may be kept in position by the application of a simple elastic harness passing from hooks on the mask (or a wire frame applied over the mask) to around the back of the head (Fig. 16.3). However, there are many instances where intubation is essential and the cat's larynx is a small and delicate structure

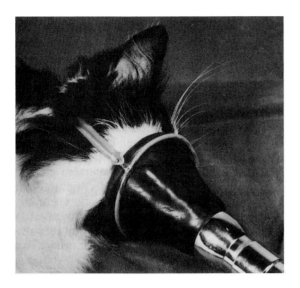

FIG. 16.3 'Hall mask' secured in position with a simple harness.

easily damaged by rough attempts at intubation. Atraumatic intubation is essential and may be made difficult by laryngospasm. Endotracheal intubation carried out when there is no strict indication for it ensures that the technique can be carried out quickly when it is essential to do so. Moreover, endotracheal intubation with an appropriate breathing system can be used to limit atmospheric pollution which might otherwise be serious during long operations.

Laryngospasm

Laryngospasm means the intrinsic muscles of the larynx contracting to occlude the glottis, preventing ventilation and resulting in hypoxaemia. It is very easily provoked in cats, and when it occurs, atraumatic intubation can only be carried out after the laryngeal reflexes responsible for the spasm have been suppressed by adopting one of the following methods:

1. The laryngeal mucous membrane of the anaesthetized cat can be desensitized by spraying it with a solution of a local analgesic drug such as 4% lignocaine hydrochloride. The larynx usually goes into a spasm when the spray is applied and attempts of intubation should be delayed for about 30 seconds or until it is seen to relax. Pure

lignocaine solutions (2–4 %) should be used since some of the additives in medical preparations cause chemical irritation of the mucous membrane (Watson, 1992; Taylor, 1992, 1993) giving rise to oedema-related airway problems after extubation. Relaxation of the jaw muscles is not produced by spraying of the larynx and must be ensured by an adequate depth of anaesthesia. Following intubation after local analgesic spray it must be remembered that the larynx will be insensitive and the normal protective reflexes absent until the effects of the local analgesic have worn off. The amount of lignocaine used is critical since the drug is readily absorbed from mucous membranes. Care must be taken not to exceed the safe dose (approximately 1–2 mg/kg per laryngeal spray) to avoid systemic effects.

In cases where quick intubation is essential this technique is not suitable since spraying the larynx with local analgesic solution does not produce immediate desensitization and paralysis of the vocal cords. Attempts should not be made to force a tube through the non-relaxed, active larynx, for this can cause serious injury. On more than one occasion attempts to force a tube through a larynx showing spasm have resulted in penetration of the pharyngeal wall and passage of the tube down the neck between the oesophagus and trachea, with fatal results.

2. When rapid intubation is essential the anaesthetized cat may be paralysed by the administration of a neuromuscular blocker after inhaling pure oxygen from a face-mask for 30 to 60 seconds to prevent hypoxaemia during the subsequent intubation procedure. Paralysis is produced most rapidly by i.v. 3–5 mg of suxamethonium (for an adult cat), and oxygen administration is continued during the fasciculations caused by the initial depolarizing action of this agent. When relaxation is complete the cat is intubated through completely flaccid vocal cords (Fig 16.4).

Rapid intubation made possible in this way minimizes the risk of inhalation of regurgitated stomach contents. Artificial ventilation of the lungs is continued through the endotracheal tube until spontaneous respiration returns

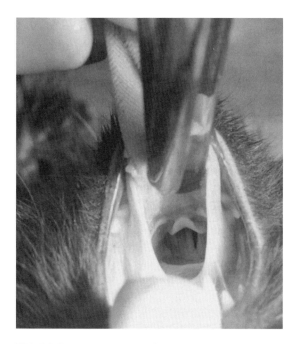

FIG. 16.4 Exposure of the larynx by simple lifting of the laryngoscope blade when the cat is supine.

some 3–5 minutes later. Should intubation prove difficult the cat is prevented from becoming hypoxic while further efforts are made by manual ventilation of the lungs using a face-mask. The mask is applied and the lungs inflated several times with pure oxygen whenever (but preferably before) the mucous membranes take on a dusky, cyanotic appearance, and a further attempt is made to intubate as soon as the colour is a normal pink. Manual ventilation of the lungs through a face-mask is not difficult. Cats' faces are reasonably uniform in shape and it is easy to get a gas-tight seal between a properly designed mask (e.g. modified 'Hall' mask) and face, although difficult to achieve with the transparent plastic-rubber diaphragm type of mask. The lower jaw must be pushed forward to ensure the airway is clear and only gentle pressure applied to ventilate the lungs or gas will be forced down the oesophagus into the stomach. It is possible to ventilate the lungs of almost all cats with open airways with pure oxygen at any time and well oxygenated cats can be intubated under the influence of a neuromuscular blocker such as suxamethonium without the need for undue haste.

Ventilation of the lungs using a face-mask is only impossible in cats with upper airway obstruction (usually an abscess or tumour) and in these a tracheostomy may be the only way in which patency of the airway can be assured so that the wisdom of using suxamethonium in such cases is debatable. Particular care should be taken to exert only minimal pressure on the bag in cats with ruptured diaphragms, for in them it is very easy to inflate the stomach.

Obviously, techniques of introducing an endotracheal tube should be practised when intubation of the cat is not strictly needed so that it can be performed competently and quickly when essential.

3. Laryngeal spasm does not occur during deep anaesthesia but deep anaesthesia cannot be recommended as the depth necessary to prevent laryngospasm is only achieved after considerable overdose. However, where emergency intubation is required following an accidental overdose of anaesthetic, it is never necessary to employ either of methods 1 or 2 above to secure relaxation of the jaw muscles and vocal cords.

Attempts to carry out forcible intubation through tightly opposed vocal cords, even if initially successful, will result in damage to the mucous membrane with oedema and danger of obstruction after extubation. The cat's larynx may also go into a spasm after extubation, especially if there is any mucus on the cords, so endotracheal tubes should, if there are no surgical contraindications, be removed without any previous deliberate lightening of anaesthesia and after careful aspiration of mucus from the airway.

Performance of endotracheal intubation

Intubation is performed under direct vision as soon as the jaw muscles are relaxed by general anaesthesia or the effects of the neuromuscular blocker, and intubation is, of course, possible at much lighter levels of anaesthesia when neuromuscular blockers are used. Although the expert should be able to intubate regardless of the position of the cat, the procedure is best learned if one standard position is employed until the technique is mastered. Two positions are used for teaching intubation; the cat is either prone or supine.

In the supine position the head and neck of the cat are extended by placing a small sandbag under the neck, or by an assistant supporting the head with a hand placed beneath the neck, and the tongue is pulled out of the mouth, care being taken not to injure it on the teeth. A standard laryngoscope with an infant-sized blade is introduced and the tip of the blade placed so that it is over the dorsum of the tongue and resting just in front of the epiglottis. The blade is then lifted to expose the glottic opening and give a good view of the vocal cords (Fig.16.4). The blade is not used as a lever but simply as a means of lifting the tongue and lower jaw while the mouth is kept open by use of the little finger of the hand which holds the laryngoscope against the upper canine tooth.

The endotracheal tube may then be passed between the cords without any difficulty. If a laryngoscope is not available, a lighted tongue depressor can be used in much the same way but tongue depressors are not so easy to control and it may be found easier to expose the larynx if the cat is lying on its side as described for the dog.

In the prone position endotracheal intubation is facilitated by an assistant raising the head and extending the neck. Careful positioning by the assistant ensures that the path for the introduction of the tube is a relatively straight line. Ease of intubation of the cat in the prone position depends on the assistant being properly trained, whereas in the supine position the anaesthetist can be in complete control of the whole operation.

Whatever position is adopted it is important that the laryngoscope blade does not come into contact with the dorsal surface of the epiglottis for this is likely to be followed by oedema. It is possible to intubate cats under direct vision but the use of a laryngoscope greatly facilitates the procedure and by displaying the glottic opening enables estimation of the appropriate size of tube to be made. There is often a temptation to use a tube that is too small because it is easier introduce, but this should be resisted for a small tube constitutes a partial airway obstruction. For most adult cats non-cuffed tubes of 4.0 to 5.5 mm internal diameter are suitable; cuffed tubes have to be smaller and the cuff may cause laryngeal trauma. A tight seal, such as

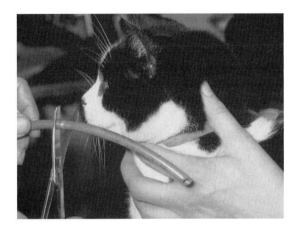

FIG. 16.5 New endotracheal tubes must be cut to the correct length before use. This is measured from the nostrils to the point of the shoulder.

may be needed to prevent inhalation of foreign materials, can be ensured by a pharyngeal pack of moistened ribbon gauze although relatively small, thin walled, cuffed portex tubes are commonly used for this purpose in North America. Endotracheal tubes should be long enough to pass well beyond the larynx but not so long that they will enter a main bronchus. The correct length may be assessed as being from the nostrils to the point of the shoulder, and all new tubes should be cut to this measurement before use (Fig. 16.5).

An excess of tube between the mouth and anaesthetic breathing system should not be tolerated because this, in small animals such as cats, adds significantly to the respiratory deadspace. A tape tied tightly around the tube over the endotracheal tube connector can be secured behind the cat's ears to anchor the tube in position once it has been introduced (Fig.16.6).

PREMEDICATION

Anticholinergic drugs should generally be included in the premedication given to cats to prevent saliva and bronchial secretions from obstructing the small-diameter airway; they should be given whenever it is proposed to use suxamethonium for endotracheal intubation, and to block vagal reflexes. The only contraindications to their use are the general ones of pre-existing tachycardia or glaucoma. Analgesics should be given whenever it

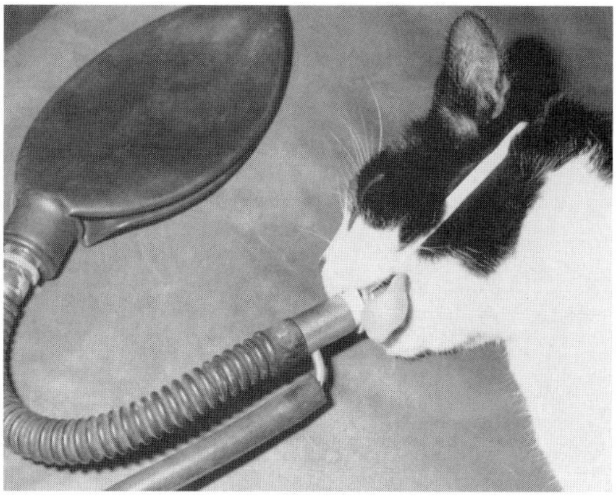

FIG. 16.6 A correctly intubated cat with no excess length of tube protruding from the mouth and the tube securely anchored in place with a tape. Apparatus deadspace is minimal.

is necessary to relieve pain, for cats in pain may not be easy to handle. Sedative use is governed by the temperament of the cat and by the anaesthetic technique to follow. Phenothiazines do little to calm a wild cat, but are useful in quieter animals to counteract excitement caused by some drugs, and to improve the quality of recovery. Xylazine and medetomidine markedly reduce the dose of all other agents used for anaesthesia and need to be used with very great care. In the survey of anaesthetic problems promoted by the Association of Veterinary Anaesthetists of Great Britain and Ireland, xylazine was associated with particularly high number of fatalities (1 per 117 cats given the drug), that were primarily due to overdosage with agents given later to produce anaesthesia. However, xylazine and medetomidine appear to be useful in reducing the side effects of ketamine, as indeed are the benzodiazepines.

Anticholinergic agents

In the UK atropine, at a total dose of 0.3 mg i.m., i.v. or s.c. for an adult cat and 0.125 or 0.060 mg for smaller or younger animals, is commonly used without any attempt being made to calculate the dose on a mg/kg basis. This is because atropine is available in ampoules which still contain 0.6 mg of atropine sulphate per ml (a relic of the days when the standard dose of atropine for an adult human

patient in the UK was 1/100th of a grain!). Elsewhere in the world ampoules generally contain 0.5 mg of atropine simplifying the calculation of a dose of 0.02 to 0.10 mg/kg. Atropine interferes with vision and cats which have received this drug should be handled particularly carefully to avoid inducing panic reactions.

Glycopyrronium bromide 0.010 mg/kg i.m. or 0.005 mg/kg i.v. may be preferred. It does not cause as marked an increase in heart rate as does atropine, nor does it cross the blood-brain barrier and so results in less visual disturbance. It may be the anticholinergic of choice for caesarian section or in accident cases which may have a contused myocardium.

Sedatives and analgesics

Phenothiazines such as acepromazine and propionylpromazine produce a variable degree of sedation. Some cats become deeply sedated on doses of 0.05 mg/kg i.m. of acepromazine, whereas others show no appreciable effect. There is a ceiling effect and usually there is no more sedation produced by increasing doses but they will increase undesirable effects such as extrapyramidal signs and duration of action. All the phenothiazines directly depress the temperature regulating mechanisms and cats are prone to develop hypothermia when sedated with them. Premedication with acepromazine does not significantly reduce the induction dose of propofol (Brearley *et al.*, 1988) but the dose of thiopental needed to induce anaesthesia is reduced after acepromazine premedication by about 30%.

Acepromazine is often used in combination with opioids to increase sedation without increasing the side effects of either drug. Most commonly, morphine is the drug used (0.1 mg/kg morphine with 0.03 mg/kg acepromazine i.m.) but in equivalent doses other opioids such as papaveretum, butorphanol, methadone and buprenorphine can be used with acepromazine.

Xylazine (0.2–0.4 mg/kg i.m.) and medetomidine (80μg/kg i.m.) may be used prophylactically when there is any likelihood of the presence of a full stomach, for both these drugs induce vomiting in some 60 % of cats. This very property indicates that these drugs should be avoided in cats with open eye or head injuries and those suffering from eosophageal or intestinal obstruction. Xylazine (0.55–1.00 mg/kg i.m. or s.c.) may be used prior to ketamine administration to counteract the side effects of this dissociative agent. It should be noted that increasing doses of both xylazine and medetomidine cause increased duration of sedation rather than increased depth. They also, by slowing the circulation, delay the onset of action of injected anaesthetic agents. Medetomidine 15–30 μ/kg sprayed under the tongue is a useful way of sedating unmanageable cats prior to anaesthesia.

The prime role of benzodiazepines in feline premedication is before ketamine administration to counteract the rigidity and convulsions produced by this agent, and in animals that may be liable to convulsions (e.g. epileptics or animals undergoing myeolography with some of the older contrast agents). They may be considered suitable premedicants for cats with cardiorespiratory disease for at normal doses they have little influence on the respiratory or cardiovascular systems. Diazepam may be given i.m. or i.v. at doses of 0.1–0.5 mg/kg i.v. or 0.3–1.0 mg/kg i.m., and midazolam (0.2 mg/kg i.m.) has been used before ketamine (6 mg/kg i.m.). Before propofol anaesthesia the dose of midazolam should not exceed 0.3 mg/kg i.v.

PARENTERALLY ADMINISTERED ANAESTHETICS

Intravenous injection is relatively easy in dogs but in cats problems of restraint may make i.v. injections more difficult or even impossible, so that agents which can be given by other routes (e.g. i.m.) tend to have a greater part to play in feline than in canine anaesthesia. The disadvantages of such administration – slow induction, variable absorption, variable effects, prolonged recovery, and inability to dose to effect, – must be weighed against the temperament of the cat, skill and experience of the anaesthetist and the likelihood of being able to carry out a controlled injection. Table 16.3 compares the properties of parenteral anaesthetic agents commonly used in cats.

Thiopental sodium

Thiopental may only be given i.v. and in cats it should be used as a 1.25 % or even more dilute solution. Induction doses are up to 10 mg/kg and if the cat has not been given sedative premedication it is probable that the full dose will be required. Very small doses (e.g. 2 mg/kg) will be needed after heavy premedication with α_2 adrenoceptor agonists. If thiopental is to be used as the sole agent, incremental doses up to a maximum of 20 mg/kg may be used, but at these high doses, saturation of the fat depots may mean that recovery will take several hours and the effects will still be observable the next day. If recovery is prolonged, the cat must be kept warm, for the development of hypothermia (more marked when acepromazine premedication is used) will delay recovery still more.

Methohexital sodium

Methohexital may be given only i.v., and is used at a concentration of 0.5% for feline anaesthesia.

TABLE 16.3 **Injectable anaesthetics in the cat. Dose rates, duration of action and recovery times must be regarded as only approximate and the use of other agents concurrently can prolong or reduce these doses and times. Moderate or heavy preanaesthetic sedation will decrease these doses and prolong the times for anaestheia and recovery**

Agent	Dose rate (mg/kg)	Route	Approx. duration of anaesthesia (min)	Approx. time to standing /walking (h)
Ketamine	10–35	i.m.	30–45	3–4
Ketamine	2–10	i.v.	20–40	1–4
Methohexital	5–12	i.v.	5–10	1.0–1.5
Pentobarbital	20–30	i.v.	60–90	4–8
Propofol	5–8	i.v.	3–6	0.5
Saffan	4–12	i.v.	5–15	0.75–2.00
Saffan	Up to 18	i.m.	5–20	Average 1.0
Thiopental	15–25	i.v.	5–15	1–2

Although it can be used for induction of anaesthesia at a dose of about 5 mg/kg, and given in incremental doses to maintain anaesthesia, in cats its tendency for causing excitement means that recovery is often far from uneventful. The use of sedative premedication helps to reduce the incidence of excitatory phenomena but in general, is only employed in cats when very rapid recovery is needed (e.g. after caesarian section).

Pentobarbital sodium

Until some 30 years ago pentobarbital was widely used in general practice and experimental laboratories as an anaesthetic for cats. Doses of 25 mg/kg i.v., half given fast to avoid induction excitement and the rest given slowly over 2–3 minutes to effect, give about 2 hours of surgical anaesthesia. Recovery from such doses is very prolonged, the cat not becoming fully conscious until the next day. Despite the long-acting nature of the drug and the respiratory depression it causes, pentobarbital anaesthesia has, over the years, been successfully and safely administered clinically to many thousands of cats. Most deaths following pentobarbital anaesthesia probably result from hypothermia and it is essential that cats are kept warm in the recovery period.

Pentobarbital can also be given by intraperitoneal injection but the results are variable, depending on its absorption from the peritoneal cavity. Induction of anaesthesia is slow and cats frequently show a stage of marked excitement so that if released from a cage at this stage they may literally run around the walls of the room. Today, this route of pentobarbital administration should, if used at all, be restricted to those laboratory workers untrained in more acceptable anaesthetic methods. Some veterinarians have in the past administered pentobarbital to cats by intrapleural injection and although absorption from this cavity is better than from the peritoneum, injection is very painful and the potential complications are such that the intrapleural route must be regarded as quite unacceptable. Today there is little to recommend the use of pentobarbital even i.v. in veterinary clinical practice.

Alphaxalone-alphadolone ('Saffan')

Since its introduction into clinical feline anaesthesia this steroid mixture has become an extremely popular anaesthetic agent, especially in general practice in the UK. Doses are commonly expressed as mg/kg of the total 12 mg/ml steroid content of the solution. This solution is non-irritant and is given to cats i.v. or i.m. Doses of 3 mg/kg i.v. produce unconsciousness for a few minutes, whilst doses of 9 mg/kg give 10–15 minutes of anaesthesia with very little increase in the initial depth of unconsciousness or respiratory depression. The increased duration of action with initial higher doses reaches a plateau at about 18 mg/kg i.v. and giving higher i.v. doses is pointless and may be dangerous. If it is necessary to prolong anaesthesia further increments may be given later on, or an inhalation agent employed.

Both steroids are rapidly broken down in the liver so that an incremental dose regimen does not result in undue delay in recovery and cats are usually completely conscious within 2 hours of administration of the last increment. The rapid breakdown of the steroids is undoubtedly responsible for the wide safety margin as far as dose is concerned.

Induction of anaesthesia is usually smooth and rapid, but occasionally it is complicated by retching, vomiting and laryngeal spasm. Although in the majority of healthy, unpremedicated cats the i.v. dose needed to produce some 15 minutes of anaesthesia (9 mg/kg) may be given as a single injection, in a few it may be an overdose. It certainly causes a significant depression of cardiac output, stroke volume and peripheral vascular resistance (Dyson et al., 1987).

The authors much prefer to give an initial i.v. injection of 2 to 3 mg/kg and administer the rest of the dose after gauging the response to the initial injection. Where sedative premedication is given the dose of Saffan has to be reduced and if xylazine is employed a reduction of more than 50% may be necessary. The use of other i.v. agents with Saffan may result in severe respiratory and cardiovascular depression and the manufacturers state that Saffan should not at any time be combined with any other i.v. anaesthetic.

There is normally little respiratory depression during Saffan anaesthesia although high doses i.v.

(more than 12 mg/kg) may give rise to some depression and a period of apnoea. Hypothermia may occur but is rarely clinically significant unless the operation involves wide opening of the body cavities for more than 15 minutes, or the cat is fluid depleted. Recovery from Saffan anaesthesia is often rather restless and if the animal is stimulated in some way recovery may be violent, the cat becoming rigid, twitching, convulsing and even showing opisthotonus. The smoothness of recovery can be improved by ensuring that the animal is pain-free and left undisturbed in a quiet, warm, comfortable cage. Acepromazine premedication is also claimed by many to improve the quality of recovery from Saffan anaesthesia.

When Saffan is used as an induction agent before inhalation anaesthesia it is often necessary to increase the concentration of any volatile agent to above what might be expected in order to suppress the twitching associated with recovery from Saffan. Laryngeal spasm may be provoked by head and neck surgery under light Saffan anaesthesia (reports to the Association of Veterinary Anaesthetists) and for this type of surgery cats must be premedicated with atropine and intubated.

Saffan may also be given i.m. and doses of 18 mg/kg are followed in about 10 minutes by anaesthesia which lasts some 10 to 20 minutes. These doses represent a rather large volume (4.5 ml for a 3 kg cat) but the injection appears painless and cats do not resent administration. Lower doses can be used for minor procedures such as dematting the coat. As the anaesthetic is eliminated so rapidly from the body, it is ineffective if given either s.c. or into the fascial planes between muscles so to ensure its proper effect it should be given deep into the vastus group of muscles. An i.m. administration is never as reliable as i.v. and it is, therefore, generally employed either where deep sedation rather than anaesthesia is needed or where it is possible to supplement by an i.v. injection once the cat is unconscious.

Hyperaemia and swollen paws, ears and noses are common following Saffan and there are reports of laryngeal and pulmonary oedema. Other side effects include sneezing, retching, vomiting and laryngeal spasm, but provided a clear airway is maintained and respiration and cardiac function are not depressed by other agents, Saffan is undoubtedly a reasonably safe induction and maintenance agent for use in general practice. Evans estimated from the quantities sold by the manufacturers coupled with the deaths reported to them, that the mortality rate was less than 1 in 10 000, but it seems more likely that the true mortality rate for Saffan in cats is nearly 10 times greater than this at about 1 in 900 (Clarke & Hall, 1990).

Propofol

Propofol has been used quite extensively in cats as an i.v. anaesthetic. The dose needed to induce anaesthesia is 6 to 7 mg/kg in both unpremedicated animals and in animals premedicated with 0.03 mg/kg acepromazine. The dose following medetomidine premedication has yet to be established but is likely to be very low. Induction is smooth and blood pressure and heart rate are well maintained, but there is some significant respiratory depression. Maintenance of anaesthesia with propofol requires about 0.4 mg/kg per min by continuous infusion but may be less when intermittent doses are administered as needed to simply obtund responses to particularly painful stimuli. Recovery is generally smooth but retching, sneezing or pawing of the face may occur in about 15% of cases.

The cat's liver does not metabolize phenols as rapidly as does the dog's liver and although considerable first pass extraction of propofol is said to occur in the cat's lungs (Matot et al., 1993), rapid recovery is not a marked feature of propofol anaesthesia. Also, some cats have disturbed recoveries, pawing at their noses in a manner reminiscent of that seen after the use of Saffan. Acepromazine premedication appears to improve the quality of recovery. Propofol seems less likely than Saffan to produce anaphylactoid reactions but, in the vast majority of cats these reactions with Saffan are relatively mild, so this is not a reason to prefer the use of propofol. It is doubtful whether propofol offers any major advantage over other i.v. agents and, indeed, many cats have very prolonged recoveries, while the mortality rate, although not yet reliably established, may prove to be quite unacceptable.

Ketamine

Ketamine is available as the water soluble racemic mixture of two isomers and the standard for veterinary use is a solution containing 100 mg/ml ketamine hydrochloride with benzethonium chloride 0.01% as preservative. Lower strength solutions (10 mg/ml and 50 mg/ml) are available for use in man. As well as by i.v. injection ketamine can be administered i.m. or s.c. and this has encouraged its use in cats that are difficult or impossible to handle. The volume of solution which has to be injected is small and the i.m. or s.c. injection can, when deemed to be essential, be made by a dart projectile fired from a blowpipe. It should be noted, however that i.m. or s.c. injection of ketamine appears to be painful, in that it is often violently resented by the animal. Application to the mucous membranes of the mouth (squirting from a syringe) can also be an effective route of administration in cats which are difficult to handle. When given i.v. there is usually a delay of 1–2 minutes before its effects become apparent, but this is the best route of administration. Ketamine has become a drug of abuse in man and care must be taken in its safe storage and disposal. In the USA it is now a scheduled drug.

Cats become recumbent 3–5 minutes following either 10 mg/kg or 20 mg/kg i.m. Sternal recumbency is usually regained 30 minutes after the lower dose and 50 minutes following the higher one, but standing and behaving normally takes considerably longer. Higher doses are seldom more reliable and result in very long recovery periods associated with ataxia, increased motor activity and increased sensitivity to external stimuli. In man, ketamine emergence reactions are coupled with a range of hallucinations and mood alterations but, of course, it is impossible to establish whether similar phenomena occur in cats. The manufacturers recommend i.m. doses 11–33 mg/kg, the lower doses to be used for minor restraint, and the larger doses for minor surgery and restraint of fractious cats. Very small kittens of less than 4 weeks of age appear to need still higher doses of up to 35 mg/kg. Doses of up to the lower end of the range are recommended when the drug is given i.v. Today, however, for the reasons given below, ketamine is seldom used on its own and these doses are greatly excessive when many of the current drug combinations are employed.

Ketamine induces a state of catalepsy with some degree of analgesia. It appears to abolish responses to superficial, painful stimuli, but not to abdominal pain (Sawyer *et al.*, 1991). Ketamine dosed cats exhibit marked muscle tone, their eyes remain open and spontaneous movement quite unrelated to any stimulation may occur. Such movements may lead an anaesthetist unaccustomed to the effects of the drug to assume that anaesthesia is lightening, but this is not the case and further doses given in attempts to suppress them result in overdosage. Laryngeal and pharyngeal reflexes are often said to be retained, but no reliance can be placed on this protection and all normal precautions to protect the airway must be taken. Salivation is often profuse, so atropine or glycopyrrolate premedication is advisable. Although ketamine is claimed to produce minimal respiratory depression, relative or absolute overdoses cause apnoea (Clarke & Hall, 1990). It is essential that cats should be kept under continuous observation from the time ketamine is given until it is obvious that recovery is complete.

Ketamine produces sympathomimetic effects but has a negative inotropic on the myocardium so that the overall effect on the circulatory system may vary according to the clinical state of the animal. In healthy, normovolaemic cats the stimulatory action appears to predominate and the ABP and heart rate increase. The drug normally causes some depression of respiratory function but in cats these effects are complex and dose-dependent. When ketamine is used in healthy individuals the degree of respiratory depression is usually insignificant.

Ketamine combinations

A wide range of sedative agents have been used in order to reduce side effects, in particular those of emergence excitement and increased muscle tone. Where premedication enables a reduction in the dose of ketamine, speed of recovery may be enhanced. Atropine is generally recommended at doses of 0.03 to 0.05 mg/kg to reduce salivation. Inhalation anaesthesia may be used after ketamine injection and may be maintained by suitable combinations of O_2 with N_2O or halothane, or isoflurane.

Acepromazine

Acepromazine (0.01–0.03 mg/kg i.m.), although widely used, has little influence on the dose of ketamine subsequently required. It reduces the muscle rigidity associated with ketamine alone and appears to produce a state resembling more conventional general anaesthesia, although the eyes remain open with a dilated pupil. Better conditions result when butorphanol (0.4 mg/kg i.m.) is added to increase analgesia (Tranquilli *et al.*, 1988).

Diazepam and midazolam

Diazepam (1 mg/kg) is also disappointing but midazolam with ketamine (0.2 mg/kg midazolam with 10 mg/kg ketamine) mixed in the same syringe and administered i.m. produces heavy sedation with good muscle relaxation (Chambers & Dobson, 1989) suitable for radiotherapy or radiography. Useful sedation lasts about 30 minutes (some cats become cyanosed when breathing air) and recovery is usually complete within 2–3 hours.

Xylazine

Xylazine has been used for some years to prevent ketamine-induced emergence excitement but its use is also associated with the side effects of bradycardia (unless anticholinergics have been used for premedication) and vomiting. Earlier high doses have been replaced by much safer ones and the recommendation now is that 1 mg/kg of i.m. xylazine is followed by 5 mg/kg of i.m. ketamine. This yields a reasonably rapid recovery. The dose of i.m. xylazine has been reduced to 0.5 mg/kg and the i.m. dose of ketamine increased to 20–25 mg/kg by Arnbjerg (1979) with a recorded death rate of 3 in over 7000 cats. Thus even these dosage rates are comparatively safe but the prolonged recovery period of 3–5 hours may present problems in busy practice conditions.

Medetomidine

The relatively recently introduced α_2 adrenoceptor agonist, medetomidine, provides more analgesia than does xylazine and hence the dose of ketamine needed to produce surgical anaesthesia can be reduced to 5–7 mg/kg i.m. when preceded by 80 μg/kg i.m. medetomidine. These doses produce a mild bradycardia and no apnoeic periods but increasing the ketamine dose to 10 mg/kg results in tachycardia (? from hypotension) and brief periods of apnoea. The data sheet for ketamine suggests a dose of 80 μg/kg i.m. medetomidine followed by a 2.5–7.5 mg i.m. ketamine and that these may be combined in the same syringe, although the vials should have separate needles inserted for withdrawal to minimize the likelihood of cross contamination. Accurate measurement of the dose is best assured by the use of a tuberculin syringe. Surgical anaesthesia of 30 to 60 minutes duration follows after an interval of some 3–4 minutes.

Except for heart and respiratory rate records, published data concerning the cardiovascular and respiratory effects of these drug combinations is lacking. In view of the similar actions of xylazine and medetomidine it seems reasonable to assume that medetomidine/ketamine combinations will cause some degree of arterial hypotension. The cardiovascular depressant effects of medetomidine / ketamine combinations can be countered by the administration of 200 μg/kg i.m. atipamezole (Verstegen *et al.*, 1991a). In clinical practice it is unwise to administer atipamezole until the effects of ketamine have waned – probably about one hour after a dose of 5 mg/kg – because of the likelihood of ketamine emergence excitement.

Tiletamine

Tiletamine, a dissociative agent related to ketamine is seldom if ever used as the sole sedative or immobilizing agent in cats. Investigations by

TABLE 16.4 **Composition of Zoletil (marketed by Virbac) according to the direction sheet**

One vial contains:	Zoletil 20	Zoletil 50	Zoletil 100
Tiletamine	50 mg	125 mg	250 mg
Zolazepam	50 mg	125 mg	250 mg
Dissolved in 5 ml water, each ml contains	20 mg/ml	50 mg/ml	100 mg/ml

Garmer (1969) showed that i.m. it was painful, high doses were required to abolish response to stimulation and recovery was prolonged and excited. Recently it has been combined with zolazepam, a member of the benzodiazepine group of drugs, as 'Telazol' or, in Australia, 'Zoletil' (Table 16.4).

Injection produces profuse salivation that can be controlled by atropine, the degree of muscle relaxation is poor in comparison to medetomidine/ketamine and ketamine/xylazine and respiratory depression is equal to that produced by tiletamine alone (Verstegen *et al.*, 1991b). Recovery takes 2–6 hours and if the cat is stimulated in any way there may be periods of excitement. If more than the one initial dose has been administered recovery can be very prolonged.

INHALATION ANAESTHESIA

Inhalation agents may be used in cats to induce and maintain anaesthesia but because of the small size of the animals it is relatively easy to administer an overdose of volatile agents. The fit, unsedated cat strongly resents attempts to force it to breathe volatile agents from a face-mask and it is seldom possible to avoid struggling or fighting with the animal at some time during attempts to induce anaesthesia in this way. For this reason many anaesthetists prefer to induce inhalation

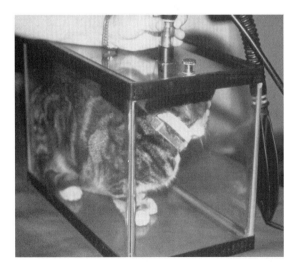

FIG. 16.7 A cat box with transparent sides for the induction of inhalation anaesthesia. Scavenging of gases issuing from the box is to be recommended.

anaesthesia by placing the cat in a rectangular glass or clear plastic chamber and piping the gases and vapours into the chamber (Fig. 16.7). Scavenging is recommended to avoid pollution of the room air. The cat usually accepts this quite calmly provided it can see out of the container and the transparent walls of the chamber enable the behaviour of the cat to be observed. It must be removed from the chamber as soon as it loses consciousness and collapses in a state of light anaesthesia.

Restraining a fully conscious, unsedated cat and applying a face-mask to force it to inhale any anaesthetic mixture, although often done in the past with apparent safety, must be regarded as being inhumane. It results in adrenaline release, which in the frightened animal may occasionally result in ventricular fibrillation and death, but the method has been applied without fatalities for very many years. The animal is usually restrained in lateral recumbency with all four legs held by an assistant while the anaesthetist controls the head with one hand and uses the other to apply the face-mask. Cats seldom object to breathing a nitrous oxide/oxygen mixture and the volatile agents may be added in gradually increasing concentrations. The normal rule is to increase the concentration of the volatile agent every three breaths until the safe maximum is obtained. This technique avoids the prolonged breath-holding which occurs if the animal is suddenly introduced to high induction concentrations of the anaesthetic. If the cat struggles it usually breathes rapidly and deeply so the induction of anaesthesia is more rapid; if breath-holding is encountered care must be taken not to release the restraint as the cat may be in the stage of narcotic excitement. In heavily premedicated or very sick cats, induction of anaesthesia by volatile agents (e.g. 2.5 % for halothane or 3.5 % for isoflurane) given by face-mask can usually be carried out without provoking excitement or struggling and is often the method of choice.

Breathing circuits

Any breathing system used to administer inhalation anaesthetics to cats must have a very low resistance and small deadspace. In practice, this limits the possible systems to non-rebreathing ones because the soda lime canister and connect-

TABLE 16.5 **Average cardiovascular data for anaesthetized normal adult cats of all domestic breeds (measurements made at the Cambridge School between 1952 and 1990)**

Respiratory rate	24–28 breaths/min
Tidal volume	12–24 ml
Minute volume	280–760 ml/min
Heart rate	160 beats/min
Arterial blood pressure:	
systolic	120–140 mmHg
diastolic	70–80 mmHg
Arterial blood pH	7.34
PaO_2	9/(95) 5 mmHg (12–13.9 kPa)
PaO_2	35 mmHg (4.7 kPa)

ing tubes of rebreathing systems create too much resistance to respiration.

The Ayre's T-piece system

This is the circuit of choice when the cat is intubated but it may also be used with a face-mask. It has minimal resistance and deadspace and IPPV can be carried out very efficiently by squeezing the partially filled bag of the Jackson-Rees modification of the T-piece system. Fresh gas flows of twice the minute volume of respiration (Table 16.5) are sufficient to prevent rebreathing.

Co-axial systems

In practice the Bain system does not behave like a T-piece system and appears to offer too much resistance for spontaneously breathing cats, but it seems that the performance of the modified Bain system is improved if the 'tail' of the bag is amputated! The Lack system behaves rather like a Magill system but the weight of the tubing tends to drag the face-mask away from the face or endotracheal tube out of the trachea. The expiratory valve needs to be removed from the Lack circuit. The parallel circuits in these configurations offer no advantage in feline anaesthesia.

The Magill system

Although the expiratory valve of the Magill system creates too much resistance for cats, the system is frequently used with a face-mask to administer inhalation anaesthetics. If the mask is applied tightly to the cat's face most anaesthetists lift the valve plate by introducing a needle or pin beneath the plate. Other anaesthetists use a large face-mask which is not applied tightly to the cat's face so that expiration can take place freely between the face and mask. These modifications of the system can result in considerable pollution of the atmosphere of the room by the anaesthetic agents.

In the USA circle systems with their paediatric hoses designed for use in small human infants are commonly used with a fresh gas inflow of 1 l/min for cats weighing more than 3 kg. Circuits designed for adult human patients can be satisfactorily used in cats, but gentle IPPV is essential.

Inhalation agents used

All the inhalation anaesthetics may be used in cats in a similar way to that in which they are used in dogs (Chapter 15). Chloroform has no place today in feline anaesthesia.

Nitrous oxide

Nitrous oxide/oxygen mixtures (3/2 in the Ayre's T-piece and 50/50 in circle rebreathing systems) are useful after anaesthesia has been induced with Saffan, especially when it has been given i.m., as they seem to suppress the muscle twitching often seen when the effects of Saffan are waning. However, nitrous oxide/oxygen mixtures are usually used in feline anaesthesia simply as a vehicle for the delivery of volatile agents.

Ether

For well over 100 years ether was used as a particularly safe anaesthetic for cats. Today, however, because of its inflammable nature it is largely discarded in most developed countries in favour of more recently introduced non-inflammable agents. Nevertheless, although induction is slower, the margin for error is much greater than it is for more potent agents such as halothane and isoflurane. Many thousands of cats have been anaesthetized with ether and the number of deaths which can be attributed to its proper use is small. It appears that anaesthetization is often followed by nausea for many cats are reluctant to eat for the first 24–48 hours after ether anaesthesia. This is, perhaps, a small price to pay for safety and the only real objection to the use of ether in feline anaesthesia is the risk of fires or explosions when it is mixed with air or oxygen. Anticholinergics are essential to reduce the copious secretions induced by the irritant nature of its vapour.

Halothane

Cardiac arrhythmias occur quite frequently in cats under halothane anaesthesia. When they occur they can usually be abolished and normal rhythm restored by the performance of IPPV to increase the gaseous exchange in the lungs. It appears that the respiratory depressant activity of halothane allows CO_2 to accumulate in the body and once the $PaCO_2$ exceeds a certain threshold value arrhythmias appear. Lowering the $PaCO_2$ by IPPV is followed by a prompt return to normal cardiac rhythm. Very satisfactory anaesthesia results when an accurately calibrated vaporizer is used and halothane is administered in oxygen or a nitrous oxide/oxygen mixture through a non-rebreathing system. For cats, the total fresh gas flow to a T-piece system need not exceed 1.5 to 2.0 l/min, little halothane is used and consequently, the method is not expensive. Provided ducting of waste gases from the open end of the T-piece is practised, there is no justification for attempting to use closed methods of administration

Methoxyflurane

In cats methoxyflurane has been used to reinforce the effects of nitrous oxide/oxygen mixtures but this agent is no longer generally available for veterinary use.

Enflurane

Although as yet there is little published information relating to the use of enflurane in cats it has been used quite successfully to produce anaesthesia with short induction and recovery periods. It may be volatilized, preferably from any calibrated vaporizer in a stream of oxygen or nitrous oxide/oxygen and delivered to the cat by any of the methods usually employed in feline anaesthesia. Evidence of seizures from central nervous irritation has not been observed, but myotonia is common during recovery from anaesthesia.

Isoflurane

Isoflurane is a quite satisfactory agent for feline anaesthesia although in cats not subjected to surgical or other stimuli it produces marked dose-dependent respiratory depression. Dose-dependent arterial hypotension is of the same order as that produced by halothane but results from reduction in peripheral resistance rather than the cardiac depression associated with halothane. Unlike its isomer, enflurane, it has not been linked to cerebral irritation in cats.

Sevoflurane

There seems to be nothing exceptional in relation to the use of sevoflurane in cats. With the possible exception of a higher heart rate with sevoflurane, its respiratory and circulatory effects are similar to those of isoflurane and halothane (Hikasa *et al.*, 1996).

Desflurane

The cardiopulmonary effects of desflurane in cats during spontaneous and controlled ventilation were recorded by McMurphy and Hodgson (1994) who in 1995 reported the MAC to be 9.79 ± 0.70 vol%. They noted that 1.7 MAC of desflurane caused a profound depression of respiration which they suggested resulted in high pulmonary artery pressures. Desflurane apparently had a sparing effect on cardiac output similar to isoflurane.

Because a newly designed, special temperature-controlled, pressurized vaporizer is needed to deliver the agent in a predictable fashion, this with the associated costs makes it likely that the development of desflurane anaesthesia in cats will be slow.

Intermittent positive-pressure ventilation (IPPV)

In the intubated cat, IPPV can be carried out by manual compression of the reservoir bag of the

Jackson-Rees modification of the T-piece system. It is possible to apply IPPV when an uncuffed endotracheal tube is in place and indeed the absence of a cuff acts as a safety device by preventing the application of too high a pressure and over-inflation of the small feline lungs. When the cat is not intubated, IPPV can be applied through a tightly fitting face-mask attached to either an Ayre's T-piece or Magill system, but care must be taken to ensure that the airway is clear and that too much pressure is not applied or the stomach will be inflated. A clear airway is produced by avoiding over-flexion or extension of the head and applying forward pressure behind the vertical ramus of the mandible as the face is pushed into the mask. The Magill system is only used for emergencies because when IPPV is performed it gives rise to almost total rebreathing so that the mask must be removed from the patient's face every few breaths to allow exhalation to the atmosphere and the mask to refill with fresh gas.

Most mechanical ventilators used in canine surgery produce tidal volumes which are too large for cats and if they are used in these animals a controlled leak has to be introduced into the circuit. Ventilators such as the Drager, the Halliwell and the Columbus are quite suitable for use in feline anaesthesia but they are needed too infrequently to justify their purchase unless their routine use is necessary.

Neuromuscular blocking agents

In cats there is seldom any indication for the use of competitive neuromuscular blocking agents as muscle tone is insufficient to interfere with most feline surgery. However, when they are indicated (e.g. for intraocular surgery) they may be used at the same dose rates, and their action antagonized in the same way, as described for the dog. The depolarizing agent, suxamethonium, is used to aid endotracheal intubation or endoscopy and in cats total doses of 3–5 mg i.v. will, after the initial muscle fasciculation, give complete relaxation for some 4 – 6 minutes. During the period of apnoea IPPV is, of course, necessary, and no difficulty is experienced in continuing this IPPV for much longer than the paralysis due to the neuromuscular blocker lasts.

Special problems in feline anaesthesia

The small size of neonatal kittens renders them particularly prone to develop hypothermia and respiratory obstruction. Kittens should always be premedicated with an anticholinergic (0.005 mg of atropine is appropriate) and anaesthesia is best induced and maintained with volatile anaesthetics.

Endotracheal intubation should be avoided unless absolutely essential – as it is if IPPV is needed. Very careful attention should be given to the maintenance of body temperature and to the replacement of blood or fluid losses.

POSTOPERATIVE CARE

Endotracheal tubes should be removed from cats when anaesthesia is still reasonably deep as their removal during light anaesthesia can give rise to troublesome laryngeal spasm. The quality of recovery in cats depends to a great extent on the anaesthetic agents that have been employed. It is usually smooth and uneventful after inhalation anaesthesia but cats may be hypersensitive to noise and other stimulation after Saffan or ketamine. Whatever anaesthetic agents have been used, recovery will be improved by keeping the cat in a quiet environment. It is particularly important for the cage to be of adequate size, as many of the 'seizures' seen during recovery are provoked by the cat being unable to stretch out fully without touching the sides of the cage. Cats are prone to develop hypothermia and the recovery area should be kept warm or the cage should be heated. It is difficult to keep cats warm with heated water pads or hot water bottles because their claws cause punctures if the animal moves vigorously as it regains consciousness.

Adequate pain relief is as essential in cats as in all other animals. Narcotic analgesics may be given i.m. as long as excessive doses are not employed. Morphine in doses of 0.1 mg/kg does not cause excitement even in fit, healthy cats, and post trauma it gives postoperative pain relief for 3 to 4 hours. Pethidine, given at a dose of 4 mg/kg gives analgesia for 2 hours but no effect is apparent after 4 hours and the use of this agent should probably be restricted to preoperative use. In the authors' experience doses of 10 to 25 mg (depending on the size of the cat) given i.m. at 3 – 4 hourly intervals produce excellent pain relief in the postoperative period for the majority of animals. Buprenorphine (0.006 mg/kg i.m.) can also be very effective.

As cats start to regain consciousness they may react to the presence of such things as chest drains and occasionally it is necessary to give drugs to control the animal at this time, even if they delay return to full consciousness. In such circumstances, provided that barbiturates have not been employed during anaesthesia, small incremental doses of i.v. Saffan given into an intravenous infusion by the nursing staff as required to produce the necessary control, may be prescribed quite safely and the cat still awakens rapidly after the last dose.

It is often claimed that if local analgesics have been sprayed on the laryngeal mucous membranes to permit endotracheal intubation, the cat should not be allowed access to food or water for 4 hours afterwards in case laryngeal protective reflexes are still blocked. In practice, the local analgesic is absorbed so rapidly from the laryngeal mucous membrane that it becomes ineffective about 15 minutes after application. Cats may always be encouraged to eat and drink, provided that there are no surgical contraindications, as soon as they have fully regained consciousness.

LOCAL ANALGESIA

Local analgesia is seldom used in cats because of the problems involved in adequate restraint and in restricting the dose of drug to non-toxic levels in these small, active animals. However, it can be valuable in very sick or moribund cats or when the animal is controlled by deep sedation or light anaesthesia. Whatever method of local analgesia is employed care must be taken that the total dose of the agent does not constitute a toxic dose of about 0.12 g, i.e. 12 ml of 1% lignocaine, or its equivalent, in an 4 kg adult cat. In cats local analgesia usually involves local infiltration of the operation site, but techniques such as IVRA or specific nerve blocks can be employed if restraint is adequate.

Epidural analgesia

The technique is identical to that used in dogs and using 2% lignocaine doses of 1 ml/ 4.5 kg administered at the lumbosacral space will block cranially to the level of L1, while doses of 1 ml/3.4 kg extend the block to the fifth thoracic vertebral level.

Most practical anaesthetists consider that in view of the heavy sedation needed to control the cat during operation, properly administered general anaesthesia is safer and preferable in all circumstances where lumbar epidural block might be used in other species of animal.

WILD *FELIDAE*

Large zoological *Felidae* can usually be trapped in 'squeeze' or transport cages and when properly placed in a 'squeeze' cage, a limb can usually be roped and pulled through the bars so that an intravenous injection can be made. They may then be treated as large domestic cats and procedures are not as difficult or hazardous as might be anticipated. If thiopental is used the dose should be kept to a minimum since recovery from its effects can take up to 2 days in the larger animals such as lions and tigers. Many lions and tigers in zoological collections and circuses can be enticed up to the bars to have their backs scratched and, although some caution is needed, s.c. injections can often be made while they are apparently enjoying the scratching.

If the animal cannot be approached closely, xylazine/ketamine or medetomidine/ketamine can be administered i.m. by pole or projectile syringe, taking care to use the shortest needle commensurate with penetration of the skin. Needles should be large bore and have holes on the side of the shaft, for ordinary open-ended needles may block with a core of skin. It is advisable to have atipamezole readily available because it is easy to over-estimate the weight of animals that cannot be weighed and it may be found that doses of xylazine or medetomidine used were excessive. Antagonism of ketamine is seldom needed because the safe dose range is wide.

REFERENCES

Arnberg, J. (1979) Clinical manifestations of overdose of ketamine-xylazine in the cat. *Nordiske Veterinary Medicine* **31**: 155–161.

Brearley, J.C., Kellagher, R.E.B. and Hall, L.W. (1988) Propofol anaesthesia in cats. *Journal of Small Animal Practice* **29**: 315–322.

Chambers, J.P. and Dobson, J.M. (1989) A midazolam and ketamine combination as a sedative in cats. *Journal of the Association of Veterinary Anaesthetists* **16**: 53–54.

Clarke, K.W. and Hall, L.W. (1990) A survey of anaesthesia in small animal practice: AVA/BSAVA report. *Journal of the Association of Veterinary Anaesthetists* **17**: 4–10.

Davis, L.E. and Donelly, E.J. (1968) Analgesic drugs in the cat. *Journal of the American Veterinary Medical Association* **53**: 1611–1667.

Dunkle, N., Moise, N.S., Scarlett, K.J. and Short, C.E. (1986) Cardiac performance in cats after administration of xylazine or xylazine and glycopyrrolate: echocardiographic evaluations. *American Journal of Veterinary Research* **47**: 2212–2216.

Dyson, D.H., Allen, D.G., Ingwersen, W., Pascoe, P.J. and O'Grady, M. (1987) Effects of Saffan on cardiopulmonary function in healthy cats. *Canadian Journal of Veterinary Research* **51**: 236–239.

Evans, J. (1979) Steroid anaesthesia five years on. *Proceedings of the Association of Veterinary Anaesthetists of Great Britain and Ireland* **8**: 73–83.

Garmer, L. N. (1969) Efects of 2-ethylamino- 2′-(2′phenyl) cyclohexanone HCl (CI-634) in cats. *Research in Veterinary Science* **10**: 382–388.

Gaynor, J.S., Dunlop, C.I., Wagner, A.E., Wertz, E.M., Golden, A. and Demme, W. (1994) Morbidity and mortality associated with small animal anesthesia. *Proceedings of the 5th International Congress of Veterinary Anesthesia, Guelph,* p. 173.

Hall, L.W. and Taylor, P.M. (eds) (1994) *Anaesthesia of the Cat.* London: Baillière Tindall.

Hikasa, Y., Kawanabe, H., Takase, K. and Ogoasawara, S. (1996) Comparisons of sevoflurane, isoflurane and halothane anaesthesia in spontaneously breathing cats. *Veterinary Surgery* **25**: 234–243.

Matot, I., Neely, C.F., Ray, M.D., Latz, R.Y. and Neufield, G.R. (1993) Pulmonary uptake of propofol in cats, effect of fentanyl and halothane. *Anesthesiology* **78**: 1157–1165.

McMurphy, R.M. and Hodgson, D.S. (1994) Cardiopulmonary effects of desflurane in cats. *Proceedings of the 5th International Congress of Veterinary Anesthesia, Guelph,* p. 191.

McMurphy, R.M. and Hodgson, D.S. (1995) The minimum alveolar concentration of desflurane in cats. *Veterinary Surgery* **24**: 453–455.

Sawyer, D.C., Rech, R.H. and Durham, R.A. (1991). Does ketamine provide adequate visceral analgesia when used alone or in combination with acepromazine, diazepam, or butorphanol in cats *Proceedings of the 4th International Congress of Veterinary Anaesthesia,* Utrecht p. 381. Special Supplement to *Journal of Veterinary Anaesthesia* 1993.

Short, C.E. (1987) '*Principles and Practice of Veterinary Anesthesia.* Baltimore: Williams and Wilkins, p. 550.

Taylor, P.M. (1992) Use of Xylocaine pump spray for intubation in cats. *Veterinary Record* **130**: 583.

Taylor, P. M. (1993) Veterinary use of Xylocaine spray. *British Journal of Anaesthesia* **70**: 113.

Tranquilli, W.J., Thurmon, J.C., Speiser, J.R. Benson, G.J. and Olson, W.A. (1988) Butorphanol as a preanesthetic in cats: its effects on two common intramuscular regimens. *Veterinary Medicine* **83**: 848–854.

Verstegen, J., Fargetton, X., Zanker, S., Donnay, I. and Ectors, F. (1991a) Antagonistic activities of atipamezole, 4-aminopyridine and yohimbine against medetomidine/ketamine induced anaesthesia in cats. *Veterinary Record* **128**: 57–60.

Verstegen, J., Fargetton, X., Donnay, I. and Ectors, F. (1991b) An evaluation of medetomidine/ketamine and other drug combinations for anaesthesia in cats. *Veterinary Record* **128**: 32–35.

Verstegen, J., Deleforge, J. and Rossillon, D. (1994) Pharmacokinetics of ACP after single oral administration in dogs and cats. *Proceedings of the 5th International Congress of Veterinary Anesthesia, Guelph,* p. 171.

Watson, A.K. (1992) Use of Xylocaine pump spray for intubation in cats. *Veterinary Record* **130**: 455.

Anaesthesia of birds, laboratory animals and wild animals

17

INTRODUCTION

The problems involved in anaesthetizing birds, laboratory animals and wild animals for clinical procedures are usually much less complicated than those encountered when these animals are anaesthetized for experimental purposes where it is important that the method of anaesthesia should have little or no influence on the result of the experiment. The techniques to be described in this chapter are those which the authors have found to be satisfactory in general practice for most clinical purposes in the various species of animal presented to them and, except in fish, do not require drugs not generally found in most veterinary general practices.

RODENTS AND OTHER SMALL MAMMALS

Although rodents and other small mammals are anaesthetized in large numbers for laboratory procedures with apparently few serious problems, when similar species are anaesthetized for clinical purposes the mortality is high. (In a survey by the Association of Anaesthetists of Great Britain and Ireland, 1 in 32 small mammals or birds anaesthetized in small animal practices died.) The cause of the high clinical mortality probably results from unfamiliarity with the species and the generally less healthy state of the animals.

Many small mammals become very distressed by handling, increasing the risk of physical damage and of adrenaline release leading to problems under subsequent anaesthesia. The risk of physical damage is considerably reduced by proper handling and animals may be weighed with minimal distress by placing them in a bag or small box hung from a suitable spring balance. Adequate preanaesthetic examination is often difficult but many have respiratory disease so oxygen should be available even if only injectable agents are to be used. The high metabolic rate of these small mammals means that they require an almost constant supply of food, so preanaesthetic fasting should not exceed 3 hours. There is no need to curtail the water supply up to the time of induction of anaesthesia. During anaesthesia small mammals are particularly prone to hypothermia and precautions to avoid this should be taken. Removal of hair and wetting (particularly with alcohol based preparations) should be kept to a minimum; the animal should be placed on a heating pad during anaesthesia and recovery. Heat loss can be considerably reduced by wrapping the animal in foil or bubble paper, although this reduces the access of both surgeon and anaesthetist to the patient. When inhalation agents are used, carrier gases also contribute to cooling effects, thus gas flows should be adequate but not excessive. Adequate monitoring of the animal's condition, including cardiac and respiratory function and ensuring it is not hypothermic, is essential until recovery is complete (Table 17.1).

TABLE 17.1 Some physiological measurements in guinea pigs, hamsters, hens, mice, rabbits and rats. Values from various sources including Green, C.J. (1979) Animal Anaesthesia. London: Laboratory Animals Ltd, and measurements made at Cambridge Veterinary School

	Weight (kg)	Heart rate (beats/min)	Arterial BP (mmHg syst/diast)	Functional residual capacity (ml)	Tidal volume (ml)	Minute volume (l/min)	Breaths/ min
Guinea pig	0.69	150	90/55	4.75	3.5	0.13	100
range	0.43–1.05	130–190		4.1–5.1	1.0–4.0	0.08–0.40	90–150
Hamster	0.1	350	150/110		0.8	0.06	90
range	0.90–0.12	250–450			0.65–0.85		30–140
Domestic hen	1.6	300	140/85		35	0.7	33
Mouse	0.02	570	110/80		0.15	0.025	190
range		500–600					100–250
Rabbit	2.4	220	110/80	11.3	15.8	0.62	40
range	2.05–3.00	205–235		7.2–15.8	11.5–24.4	0.37–0.89	32–53
Rat	0.25	350	115/90		1.6	0.22	90
range	0.2–0.3	260–450			1.40–1.75	0.21–0.30	70–150

The commonest cause of death is respiratory failure. Ideally, O_2 and the ability to administer artificial ventilation of the lungs should always be available. However, intubation of rodents requires considerable practice as the narrow mouth makes visualization of the larynx difficult. Suitable antagonists should be at hand and there may be a place for analeptic agents such as doxapram in circumstances where intubation is difficult. The other common cause of mortality is surgical blood loss so that care must be taken to minimize this and, whenever possible, to replace that which does occur, with plasma volume expanders (colloids) or Ringer's lactate solution.

The use of anticholinergic premedication is controversial as in other species but as small airways are easily blocked by saliva or mucus, its use is often desirable. Doses of 0.04–0.05 mg/kg of atropine are suitable for most rodents but rabbits need much higher doses (e.g. 1–2 mg/kg).

Small mammals are generally poor subjects for local analgesia since even if this is effective they still require restraint. If used, local analgesic drugs should be diluted and care taken to avoid overdose. General anaesthesia is preferred for most purposes and may be induced and maintained with volatile agents, induced with injectabable drugs and maintained with volatile agents, or maintained with injectable drugs alone.

ANAESTHESIA WITH VOLATILE AGENTS

The most popular agents are halothane and isoflurane. Ether, often used in the past, is not recommended as the excessive bronchial secretions it provokes may cause respiratory obstruction even if an anticholinergic premedication has been given.

Mask induction can lead to handling stress and the use of an induction chamber is to be preferred. Several such chambers are commercially available but they are relatively easy to improvize and there is no reason why they should not be available in most general veterinary practices.

Once induced, anaesthesia should be maintained by volatilizing the volatile agent in a stream of oxygen and administering the mixture through a T-piece or similar low-resistance breathing system, taking care not cause hypothermia by excessive flow rates. Suitable face masks for small rodents can be made from plastic syringe barrels and should not be a tight fit around the muzzle, for allowing gas to escape reduces resistance to breathing. Such a leak of gas does, however, constitute problems of atmospheric pollution and some form of active scavenging of gases should be used.

ANAESTHESIA WITH INJECTABLE DRUGS

Theoretically, any injectable anaesthetic can be used in small mammals and usually the necessary doses for healthy animals are well known from the original developmental work in laboratory animals carried out by the company concerned with marketing the drug. However, practical limitations are set by the possible methods of administration. In some animals with easily accessible veins (e.g. in rabbits) drugs such as propofol or thiopental can be used as in cats and dogs (although the duration of effect may be shorter). Where i.v. injection is more difficult, drugs which can be given by i.p., i.m. or s.c. injection are generally used. The most popular combinations of drugs are the neuroleptanalgesics or mixtures incorporating ketamine. There are marked differences between species responses and even within one species of animal many drug actions may be unreliable, a given drug producing deep anaesthesia in one animal whilst only providing some sedation in another of the same species.

Ketamine

Ketamine has the advantage that it is effective no matter what the route of administration. Doses required and efficacy vary greatly between the various species of animal. Lower doses may be used for sedation and immobilization for non-surgical procedures. As in other species of animal, ketamine is used in combination with drugs such as the benzodiazepines (diazepam or midazolam) and/or α_2 adrenoceptor agonists (xylazine or medetomidine) in order to reduce the dose of ketamine, improve muscle relaxation and to increase the effectiveness of the dissociative agent as an anaesthetic. It is worth noting that the formulations of ketamine at lower concentrations, which are available for use in children, can prove more convenient for use in very small animals than the standard veterinary preparation which needs to be further diluted before use.

Neuroleptanalgesia

Although most commercially available neuroleptanalgesic combinations can be used, the mixture of fentanyl and fluanisone ('Hypnorm') has proved to be the most popular in the UK; it can be administered by any route. The dose of fentanyl in Hypnorm is high, resulting in a prolonged length of action and, occasionally, in respiratory arrest. Combinations of Hypnorm with diazepam or midazolam give better muscle relaxation and allow a reduction of some 50% in the dose of Hypnorm. If anaesthesia becomes too deep the fentanyl component may be antagonized with naloxone (0.1 mg/kg). Flecknell (1988) has reported on the use of buprenorphine to antagonize the fentanyl in the drug combination – the technique of sequential analgesia.

Other agents

A mixture that is often used, although unlicensed, is known as the 'Hellabrunn Mixture'. It was developed primarily for administration to zoo animals and is prepared by adding 4 ml of ketamine (100 mg/ml) to a vial of dry xylazine (500 mg). This yields a stable injectable solution containing xylazine 125 mg/ml together with ketamine 100 mg/ml. Its stability means that it is immediately available and it is relatively safe for the administrator.

Alphaxalone/alphadolone (Saffan) has proved to be useful in some species of animal when given i.v., and it may also be given i.m.

Pentobarbital and thiopental may be used by i.p. injection in some animals but give prolonged sedation and respiratory depression; they cannot be recommended for clinical use.

Analgesia

Postoperative analgesia must not be neglected. Some opioid drugs are suitable and other methods utilizing local analgesics should be considered. It is regrettable that the rat, which has probably contributed more than most animals to advances in medical and veterinary sciences, still seems in many laboratories to be ignored in circumstances where postoperative analgesia would be regarded as essential for other animals.

LAGOMORPHS

Rabbits (*Oryctolagus cuniculus*) and hares (*Lepus europaeus*)

Rabbits and hares need to be handled carefully; they tend to panic if placed on slippery surfaces

TABLE 17.2 Recommended doses of a variety of agents for use in rabbits. These are in accordance with the majority of recommendations in the literature

Drug	Dosage	Route of injection	Reference
Xylazine	3 mg/kg	i.v.	Flecknell (1988)
+	+		
ketamine (3 min. later)	3 mg/kg	i.v.	
Thiopental	10–12 mg/kg to effect	i.v.	Sedgwick (1986)
Medetomidine	300 µkg	s.c.	Mero et al. (1989)
Ketamine	20 mg/kg		
+	+		
diazepan	0.75–1.00 mg/kg		
Methohexital	5–10 mg/kg to effect	i.v.	Green (1975)
Saffan	2–8 mg/kg to effect	i.v. for induction of anaesthesia only	
	12 mg/kg	i.m. (sedation only)	
Ketamine	20–60 mg/kg	i.m.	Clifford (1984)

and are best held for injection wrapped in a towel in the arms of an assistant or placed in a restraining box. A rabbit or hare struggling against forcible restraint may fracture a vertebra, so any restraint technique used should only entail the minimum of force. They should be caught by grasping the scruff of the neck firmly and pressing down on a flat surface until they relax; they may then be lifted by supplementing the neck grip with support for the hindquarters. Rabbits, especially when kept as pets, can be calmed by scratching behind the ears and stroking the back. Respiratory problems, usually due to pasteurella infections, are common in rabbits which may appear to be healthy, and auscultation of the lungs for diagnosis is not easy; many authorities advise thoracic radiography prior to anaesthesia so that owners may be warned of the anaesthetic risks associated with the presence of lung disease.

Intramuscular injections are made into the quadriceps or triceps or lumbar muscles. Intravenous injections are given into the marginal vein of the ear and i.v. injection is greatly facilitated by the use of a restraining box which leaves the ears accessible.

Endotracheal intubation is relatively difficult because of the long, narrow oropharynx and long incisor teeth limiting access through the mouth. The tongue is thick, fleshy, friable and easily torn. The soft palate is long and the epiglottis is large. Endotracheal intubation is either accom-

plished by direct visualization of the larynx using a straight, premature human infant blade, or blindly. For blind intubation the the head should be held in extension on the neck to provide a straight line of passage for the tube. A semi-rigid stilette can be used as a guide to aid in the passage of the endotracheal tube. Tubes of 2.5 to 4.0 mm internal diameter are suitable for use in rabbits.

Rabbits produce atropinase, which rapidly inactivates atropine, so to be effective doses of this agent must be high (1–2 mg/kg) and repeated every 15 to 20 min. Alternatively, glycopyrrolate (0.01–0.02 mg/kg) may be used as an anticholinergic.

Although i.v. anaesthetic agents can be used to induce anaesthesia in rabbits (Table 17.2), they are not good for maintaining anaesthesia for even very small incremental doses may cause death through respiratory arrest. Similarly, unexpected deaths may occur following ketamine or fentanyl combinations, but Scandinavian workers (Mero et al., 1989) have reported no deaths in a series of 340 rabbits undergoing experimental surgery and anaesthetized by a s.c. mixture of medetomidine (300 µg/kg), ketamine (20 mg/kg) and diazepam (0.75 to 1.50 mg/kg).

Induction of anaesthesia with thiopental (10 to 12 mg/kg), methohexital (5 to 10 mg/kg) or Saffan (2 to 8 mg/kg) given i.v. to effect, is satisfactory but it is doubtful whether methohexital or Saffan have any real advantages over thiopental. These agents are best given i.v. through a 21 swg or 23 swg butterfly needle strapped into an ear vein.

For an inhalation induction a 1:1 mixture of N_2O/O_2 should be administered through a face-mask from a T-piece system at a flow rate of about 2 litres/min for 1 to 2 minutes before halothane or isoflurane is cautiously added in small step increments up to 2 to 3 %. Induction of anaesthesia is usually quiet when the volatile agents are vaporized in the N_2O/O_2 mixture in this way. Once anaesthetized the rabbit may be intubated. An alternative method which is probably better if N_2O is not available is to place the rabbit in a box and introduce a stream of halothane or isoflurane volatilized in O_2 into the box until the animal is unconscious. Anaesthesia is usually maintained with 1.5 to 2.0% halothane or 2 to 3 % isoflurane given by face mask or through an endotracheal tube and, as always in rabbits, O_2 administration is essential since anaesthetized rabbits rapidly develop hypoxaemia.

The depth of anaesthesia is assessed by tickling the inside of the ear pinnae, since with many anaesthetic methods the pedal withdrawal reflex may remain strong until the animal is very close to death. Loss of the corneal reflex is a sign of dangerously deep anaesthesia.

Postoperative analgesia may be provided by buprenorphine (0.02–0.05 mg/kg s.c.) every 8–12 hours, or pethidine (10 mg/kg s.c. or i.m.) every 2–3 hours. Postoperatively, rabbits should be kept warm, e.g. in a baby incubator at 95 °F (35 °C).

RODENTIA

Rats (*Rattus norvegicus*)

Rats that are not tame can be very difficult to handle; they cannot be restrained by the tail for any long time for they will turn and climb up their own tails to bite the restraining hand. They can be restrained in a towel which is folded over the rat and rolled, making sure that the legs are secure. Experienced handlers often grasp the rat with the palm of the hand over the animal's back and restrain the forelegs by folding them across each other under the chin so that the chin cannot be depressed enough to bite.

There are very many ways of anaesthetizing rats but simple halothane or isoflurane anaesthesia is very satisfactory for all clinical purposes.

TABLE 17.3 Injectable drugs for use in rats			
Drug	**Dose**	**Route**	**Reference**
Ketamine	50–100 mg/kg	i.m.	Green et al. (1981)
Ketamine +	70–80 mg/kg +	i.m.	Flecknell (1988)
acepromazine	2.5 mg/kg	i.m.	
Ketamine +	60–75 mg/kg +	i.p.	Nevalainen et al.
medetomidine	0.25–0.5 µg/kg	s.c.	(1989)
Ketamine +	40–87 mg/kg +	i.p., i.m.	Green et al. (1981)
Xylazine	5–13 mg/kg	i.p., i.m.	
Hypnorm	0.4–0.5 ml/kg	i.m. or i.p.	Green (1975)

Anaesthesia may be induced in a box used as an induction chamber, or by face-mask, with the agent volatilized in a stream of O_2. Injectable agents may be given i.v. into the dorsal metatarsal vein or a tail vein, or i.p.

Ketamine is generally unsatisfactory in rats in that i.m. doses of 60 mg/kg usually only produce sedation. There are age and sex differences in the response of rats to ketamine. Duration of effect decreases as young rats mature from 1 to 3 weeks of age. After 3 weeks females sleep longer than males. To produce anaesthesia in rats ketamine should always be combined with other drugs such as xylazine (Table 17.3).

In inexperienced hands inhalation anaesthesia is safer and anaesthesia is best induced in a chamber although if contamination of the room air is ignored it can be done by blowing the anaesthetic gas mixture over the face through a face mask. Rats should be kept warm until full recovery is apparent and postoperative analgesia can be obtained from buprenorphine 0.1–0.2 mg/kg s.c. at 8 to 12 hourly intervals or pethidine 20 mg/kg s.c. at intervals of 2–3 hours.

Mice (*Mus musculus*)

Mice should be lifted by holding the base of the tail between the thumb and forefinger and immediately transferred to a horizontal cloth surface (e.g. the coat of the handler). As it attempts to escape, it is grasped by the loose scruff of the neck and the tail

TABLE 17.4 **Drugs for use in mice**			
Drug	**Dose**	**Route**	**Duration**
Ketamine	100 mg/kg	s.c.	Sedation only
Ketamine + **xylazine**	100–200 mg/kg + 5–15 mg/kg 100–200 mg/kg	i.m. i.p.	60–100 min. Sedation to compete anaesthesia
Hypnorm	0.01 ml/30g	i.p.	Approx. 60 min.
Hypnorm + **diazepam**	0.01–0.02 mg/30g + 5 mg/kg	i.p. i.p.	60–90 min.

is gripped, turning the animal so that its abdominal wall is presented for i.p. injections given 2–3 mm from the mid-abdominal line. With skill, i.v. injections can be made into a lateral vein of the tail using a 10 mm long 27 to 28 gauge needle. The margin of safety is generally considered to be too small for the routine use of inhalation anaesthetics such as halothane and isoflurane to induce and maintain anaesthesia but methoxyflurane, where it is still available, can be used with greater safety (Green, 1979). Assessment of anaesthetic depth is based on the respiratory rate and depth, corneal, tail-pinch and pedal reflexes.

As in rats, ketamine on its own is generally unsatisfactory but it may be used with other drugs (Table 17.4). It is most important to keep mice warm whilst they are anaesthetized and in the recovery period.

Guinea pigs (*Cavia porcellus*)

Guinea pigs are best restrained by grasping around their pectoral and pelvic structures. They are not good subjects for anaesthesia with injectable agents whether given by i.v. injection or other parenteral routes. Visible veins are fragile and venepuncture is often difficult, while the use of other routes necessitates an accurate estimation of body weight for computation of the dose. Since the gastrointestinal tract can contribute anything from 20 to 40% of the total weight of the animal, depending on its content of ingesta, it is not surprising that variable results follow

from i.p. or i.m. injections of computed doses of injectable drugs. Moreover, respiratory disease is common.

Fortunately, halothane or isoflurane anaesthesia meets most of the needs of clinical practice. A mixture of the volatile agent with O_2 is supplied to an induction chamber (box) or face-mask at 1 to 2 l/min, starting with a minimal concentration and gradually increasing it until the animal loses consciousness. Anaesthesia is usually produced in about 2 to 3 min and can be maintained with concentrations of halothane (0.5 to 1.5%) or isoflurane (1 to 2%), given through a face-mask from a T-piece system. Full recovery follows in less than 20 to 30 min after termination of administration of the anaesthetic.

Maintenance of a clear airway is not always easy in guinea-pigs since nasal and oropharyngeal secretions tend to become viscid during anaesthesia and are liable to give rise to obstruction. The risk may be countered by frequent aspiration of the mouth and oropharynx using a fine rubber catheter attached to a 60 ml syringe. Endotracheal intubation is virtually impossible unless a semi-rigid stilette is used as an introducer and a small endotracheal tube (1.5 mm i.d) is threaded over it once it is in the trachea. As with all small mammals, conservation of body heat is important and a warm environment should be provided.

Ketamine, whether used alone or in combination with α_2 adrenoceptor agonists, immobilizes and produces anaesthesia in these animals (Table 17.5).

TABLE 17.5 **Drugs used in guinea pigs**			
Drug	**Dose**	**Route**	**Duration**
Saffan	16–20 mg/kg	i.v.	10–20 min.
Saffan	40–45 mg/kg	i.p. or i.m.	40–90 min. sedation only
Pentobarbital	30 mg/kg	i.p.	60 min.
Ketamine + **xylazine**	30–44 mg/kg + 0.1–5.0 mg/kg	i.m. i.m.	75 min. sedation
Ketamine + **xylazine**	40–100 mg/kg + 4–5 mg/kg	i.m. i.m.	60 min. anaesthesia

TABLE 17.6 Drugs recommended for use in hamsters and gerbils

Drug	Dose	Route	Duration of effect	Reference
Hamsters				
Pentobarbital	70–80 mg/kg	i.p.	60–75 min.	Orland & Orland (1946)
Ketamine	40–80 mg/kg	i.m.	Sedation only	Green et al. (1981)
Hypnorm	0.1 ml/kg	i.p.	60 min.	Green (1975)
Gerbils				
Pentobarbital	30–100 mg/kg	i.p.	Approx. 60 min.	
Saffan	80–120 mg/kg	i.p.	Approx. 75 min.	

Hamsters and gerbils (*Mesocricetus auratus* and *Gerbillidae*)

It should be remembered that hamsters are nocturnal and often greatly resent being disturbed during daytime, making them liable to bite. The hamster's scruff is quite loose so restraint by grasping the scruff needs to be quite vigorous.

Hamsters and gerbils are best anaesthetized by inhalation methods. They should be placed in an induction chamber such as a small cardboard box with a perforated lid and anaesthetized with isoflurane or halothane introduced into the box in a stream of O_2, using scavenging of emergent gases whenever possible. The animal is removed from the box as soon as it becomes unconscious. Unconsciousness is usually equated with loss of the righting reflex when the box is tilted; anaesthesia is then maintained using a face-mask. If the use of injectable agents is obligatory, neuroleptanalgesic combinations appear to give the most reliable results. Ketamine is very variable in effect (Table 17.6).

Mink (*Mustela vison*)

Mink are not domestic animals – they are nervous, fast and vicious. All mink are best handled by persuading them to enter a clear sided induction box. Mink dislike a human blowing into their face and will retreat from such an onslaught. Moreover, mink are very inquisitive and will investigate the source of gentle scratching noises such as can be made on the side of a box. Once in the box they can be anaesthetized with a volatile anaesthetic such as isoflurane or halothane. If necessary the box may be covered with transparent plastic sheeting to make it more gas-tight, and until it is unconscious the animal is not removed from the box.

Ferrets and skunks (*Mustela putorius furo; Mephitis mephitis*)

Ferrets are tractable and are usually easily tamed. They readily vomit when anaesthetized so they should be fasted for about 6 hours before induction of anaesthesia. Skunks can spray the anaesthetist with musk unless precautions are taken to avoid this. The scent glands can be emptied by holding the skunk up with its hindquarters away from the handler and pulling the tail up and forwards towards the head.

Ferrets and skunks can be anaesthetized with isoflurane or halothane passed into an induction box until they are unconscious, following on with the administration of the agent through a face-mask from a T-piece system. Skunks are probably best anaesthetized in a disposable clear plastic bag, surgery being performed through a hole cut in the bag At the end of the procedure the bag is discarded, eliminating the problem of persistent odour otherwise probable when a box is used. Inhalation anaesthesia presents no special features in these animals.

Stoats and weasels (*Mustela erminae; Mustela nivalis*)

Stoats and weasels can be dealt with in a similar manner, using an induction box, but it should be remembered that they are much more vicious than ferrets or skunks. Preferred injectable agents are i.m. ketamine 20–30 mg/kg or ketamine (25 mg/kg i.m.) with diazepam (2 mg/kg i.m.) or Saffan (10–15 mg/kg i.m.).

OTHER SMALL MAMMALS

Badgers (*Meles meles*)

Badgers resist handling by biting and scratching. The safest procedure for handling them is to immobilize them with ketamine (10–20 mg/kg i.m.) prior to maintenance of anaesthesia with conventional inhalation techniques.

Hedgehogs (*Erinaceus europaeus*)

Hedgehogs are usually given drugs i.p. or anaesthesia is induced in a chamber with a volatile agent. Hypnorm, the fentanyl-fluanisone mixture (0.2 ml/kg) together with diazepam 2.5 mg/kg, both given i.p. are said to be the most useful agents in this species of animal. However, to give an i.p. injection the animal must first be made to unroll by prodding it on the rump or back of the neck. As it unrolls the strong spines on the crown of the head are grasped with stout artery forceps and used to gently rock the animal up and down until it uncurls. Keeping the hind limbs pinioned then prevents it rolling itself up.

CHELONIA

In tortoises, terrapins and turtles anaesthetic problems are posed by the very low metabolic rate which varies with environmental temperature and the ability to retract the head into the protective shell. Some species present further problems due to their adaptation to a semi-aquatic or aquatic mode of life. It should be remembered that some species of soft shelled turtles can move quickly and handlers can be bitten or scratched.

The lungs are well developed and the respiratory movements are produced chiefly by muscles at each leg pocket beneath the viscera. Although these muscles have been described as diaphragms, they are too weak to drive gases around any anaesthetic system. Most chelonians have the ability to survive on a single respiratory movement per hour, making attempts to induce anaesthesia with inhalation agents rather unsuccessful.

Ketamine is probably the anaesthetic agent of choice although it does not produce muscle relaxation. It may be given in doses of 60 to 80 mg/kg

into gluteal muscles and if the sedation produced is not sufficient for surgery it may be deepened by administration of isoflurane or halothane because the head will protrude from the shell and breathing will be reasonably rapid. Saffan may be used instead in i.m. doses of 12 to 18 mg/kg. Loss of muscle tone in the neck is the best guide to the depth of central nervous depression. Chelonia are easily intubated.

Recovery from a dose of 60 mg/kg of ketamine takes up to 24 hours. Tortoises should be allowed to recover at normal room temperature, preferably in a straw filled box. Terrapins and turtles should be kept at a slightly lower environmental temperature and have their bodies kept damp by the application of cold water at frequent intervals.

REPTILIA

Snakes are difficult subjects for the anaesthetist. They have a low basal metabolic rate which is directly related to the environmental temperature so that if parenteral agents are used the induction and recovery times are very variable. Moreover, they are relatively resistant to hypoxia and can hold their breath for several minutes so that the induction of inhalation anaesthesia may be very prolonged.

Snakes have peculiar anatomical features. The absence of an epiglottis and the position of the glottis makes it possible to intubate non-venomous snakes under simple physical restraint and inhalation anaesthesia may then be induced by the use of IPPV (Fig. 17.1). (Even so, non-venomous snakes can still inflict bite wounds which often become septic!) Most snakes have only one functional lung which consists of a thin walled tube terminating in an air sac extending to the level of the cloaca, the trachea being open along one side within the lung. There is no diaphragm and the three chambered heart yields a slushing noise instead of the clear 'lub-dub' of the mammalian heart on auscultation.

Snakes appear to be extremely sensitive to painful stimuli and strike or contract violently when an injection needle is inserted through the skin. It is, therefore, essential to have snakes properly restrained before attempting any injection. A

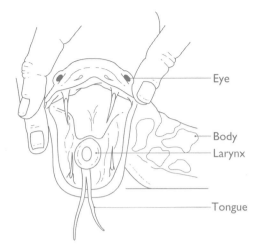

FIG. 17.1 Intubation of snakes. Once the mouth is opened widely the larynx is visible and endotracheal intubation presents no problems.

Eye

Body

Larynx

Tongue

simple aid to handling is to reduce the environmental temperature to below 10 °C for this makes the poikilothermic snake very sluggish. If injectable agents are to be used only the lightest level of narcosis compatible with safe handling should be used, for deeper levels which require larger doses of drug may be followed by a recovery period extending over several days.

Of the injectable central nervous depressants only ketamine is really useful and initial i.m. doses of the order of 50 mg/kg produce moderate sedation which facilitates handling but muscle relaxation is poor and serpentine movements may occur. Ketamine anaesthesia can be supplemented by infiltration of the surgical site with 0.5 to 1.0% lignocaine, or by the administration of isoflurane or halothane after endotracheal intubation.

Snakes may also be anaesthetized with inhalation anaesthetics when a rapid recovery is important. Induction is best achieved by placing the snake in a clear plastic box, strong plastic bag or an aquarium tank into which 7 to 10% halothane or isoflurane vapour in oxygen or nitrous oxide/oxygen is piped. Induction may take as long as 15 minutes and the snake should not be removed until agitation or turning of the container demonstrates that righting reflexes have been lost. It is then removed, intubated and anaesthesia maintained with about 3% of halothane or 4% of isoflurane vapour given with IPPV. Lung ventilation should

be at the rate observed in the previously conscious individual and fluid balance should be maintained by giving 5 ml of isotonic saline every 1–2 hours. Most snakes may be kept at normal ambient temperatures of around 20 °C unless it is desired to cool them for restraint purposes.

Induction of anaesthesia in a tank has the advantage that venomous snakes can be anaesthetized with the minimum of handling, but because anaesthetic vapours are heavier than air they sink towards the bottom of the tank and snakes can raise their heads above the anaesthetic layer so delaying the onset of anaesthesia. It is always wise to ascertain the righting reflexes really have been abolished before removing the snake from the tank.

Most snakes exhibit a short period of excitement or agitation when first exposed to an anaesthetic vapour but they quieten down and it is not always easy to ascertain the depth of anaesthesia. The first indication that the snake can be safely removed from the tank is certainly loss of righting reflexes but the tail withdrawal reflex is also valuable. Absence of response to pricking of the tail indicates that surgical anaesthesia is present. If the tip of the tongue is gently grasped with forceps there is a marked resistance to its withdrawal until the stage of surgical anaesthesia is reached.

FISH

Fish are usually anaesthetized by allowing them to swim in a solution of the anaesthetic agent. The solution should be made up in some of the water in which they are normally maintained (NOT in tap water which is often heavily chlorinated) and various drugs are used:

1. Carbon dioxide may be used at a concentration of 200 ppm.

2. Diethylether 10–15 ml per litre of water is usual but 50 ml per litre of water has been used for large fish. In goldfish anaesthesia is induced in about 3–5 minutes; recovery once placed in anaesthetic-free water takes 5–15 minutes.

3. Tricaine methanesulphonate is probably the best agent to use. It is a white powder which dissolves in both fresh and sea water.

Concentrations of 1:30 000 up to 1:1000 are employed, the more concentrated solutions being used for larger fish. Anaesthesia is induced in 1–2 minutes and fish recover once placed in non-medicated water in about 15 minutes.

4. Propoxate hydrochloride (R7464) is very soluble in both fresh and sea water. It is used in concentrations of 0.5 to 10.0 ppm to obtain varying degrees of depth of central nervous depression. Unfortunately, propoxate is difficult to obtain.

5. Benzocaine in an immersion solution at concentrations of 20–30 ppm is an excellent anaesthetic for tagging, marking and measuring fish (Laird & Oswald, 1975). For surgical anaesthesia 50 ppm solutions are used. It is dissolved in acetone at 40 mg/ml giving a stable solution which, if protected from light, will keep for up to 3 months. For use, this concentrated solution is diluted in fresh or sea water as required.

When a fish is immersed in the anaesthetic solution there is initial excited swimming, becoming increasingly erratic. The fish then becomes inactive, sinking to the bottom of the container to rest on its back. For surgery, the fish is removed from the tank and placed on a moist cloth. Complete recovery from the effects of the anaesthetic ensues when the fish is place in clean, aerated water (fresh or sea water but NOT tap water).

BIRDS

In recent years interest in conservation of wild life has led to an increased demand for anaesthesia for surgical purposes in wild or semi-wild birds as well as the more domesticated chicken, duck or goose. Cage birds have also become popular as companions, especially for elderly people living in urban districts, and as a result of these trends it is now commonplace for the veterinary anaesthetist to be confronted with avian patients requiring anaesthesia for a wide variety of conditions. It is well known that birds do not react in the same way as mammals to stimuli which in man cause pain. For example, after a slight reaction to the skin incision, conscious birds do not show any response to the manipulations involved in caponization. Many operations on hens, such as the suturing of a torn crop or the removal of superficial neoplasms, cause little response and the heart rate, which might be expected to increase if pain was experienced, remains normal. In spite of these differences humane considerations seem to dictate that anaesthesia should be used for birds as it is for mammals.

The special problems presented by birds, especially wild ones, are related to their physiological, anatomical and metabolic differences from mammals. The problems of handling wild birds are often greatly exaggerated. Provided they are handled quietly and that the normal precautions are taken (such as the wearing of gauntlets when dealing with birds of prey), few difficulties or dangers are encountered.

The high metabolic rate has several implications for the anaesthetist. It implies a higher rate of utilization of foods so that starvation of 6 to 8 hours is often sufficient to produce fatal hypoglycaemia and ketosis. Metabolism of parenterally administered agents is also rapid. The high avian body temperature means that excessive cooling occurs when the bird is exposed to a cool environment during or after anaesthesia, especially if many feathers are plucked around the operation site. Small birds such as budgerigars have very high, labile heart rates and heart failure is frequently encountered when these birds are frightened by handling. The blood volume of birds is such that small surgical haemorrhages may be sufficient to cause death from shock.

The avian respiratory tract is very different from that of mammals, one obvious difference being that inspiration in birds is normally passive whilst expiration is active. The respiratory system is constructed around a central 'core' of relatively fixed lung volume and its anatomy has been well described by Dunker (1972), Piiper (1972) and Piiper and Schneid (1973). The trachea divides into two mesobronchi which in turn divide to give secondary bronchi, one group of which, the ventrobronchi, communicates with the cranial air sacs (cervical and interclavicular). The dorsal and lateral secondary bronchi arise from each mesobronchus before these terminate in caudal air sacs (abdominal and posterior thoracic air sacs). The dorsal and ventral bronchi are joined by narrow tubes, the parabronchi, which form the analogue to mammalian lungs and are where gaseous exchange takes place between the air and the blood. Air passing through the parabronchi moves in one direction only during both inspiration and expiration: blood flows across the direction of gas flow. Thus, the gas composition must change from the inspiratory to expiratory ends of the parabronchi so that capillary blood must equilibrate with parabronchial gas at widely different PO_2 and $PaCO_2$. The arrangement is such that gas exchange takes place during both inspiration and expiration and its efficiency is dependent on an uninterrupted flow of air through the lungs. Tidal exchange is generated through the air sacs and fluid such as blood or injected solutions will interfere with ventilation. Even short periods of apnoea are serious and will produce marked hypoxia.

Anaesthetic gases and vapours are rapidly absorbed into the blood stream so that induction of anaesthesia is rapid when inhalation anaesthesia is used and, equally recovery is also rapid. Most inhalation anaesthetics are less soluble in in avian than in mammalian blood so that brain tensions equilibrate more rapidly with lung tensions and the clinical anaesthetist will often find induction and recovery disconcertingly abrupt.

After anaesthesia birds must be kept warm in a darkened, padded box and they should be supported in sternal recumbency. During recovery vigorous flapping of the wings may occur and this should be prevented by wrapping the bird in a towel because a wing bone may be fractured if the wing beats against the cage or box wall.

ANAESTHETIC TECHNIQUES

Local analgesia

Because birds such as budgerigars are so small it is very easy to give a gross overdose of a local analgesic agent, but in larger birds local analgesia can be used quite safely. Even so, in large birds it is wise to watch the total dose which is administered and to use very dilute solutions (e.g. 0.25–0.50% lignocaine) for injection because there is some evidence that birds are more sensitive to local analgesics than are mammals of the same body weight. Many workers consider that local analgesia has no place in avian anaesthesia because even when correctly used the bird still requires restraint and this may produce undue distress.

Injectable agents

Whenever possible birds should be weighed before any drug is given by injection. This is usually possible if the bird can be confined to a plastic box. Physical restraint should be kept to a minimum because small birds such as budgerigars and canaries are prone to become very distressed and large birds may fracture bones whilst trying to escape. Poultry should be grasped so that the wings are held back along the abdomen to quieten them. Budgerigars and the like should be cradled in the palm of the hand with the neck between the index and middle fingers, taking care not to apply pressure to the neck. Hawks usually present no problem after being hooded and parrots may be gripped around the neck and wings with a hand wrapped in thick towelling.

Intramuscular injection is made into the pectoral muscles on either side of the cariniform sternum or into the thigh muscles. Intravenous injections are made into the brachial vein where is passes over the ventral aspect of the elbow joint. Although very many injectable agents have been used in birds of all kinds it is probable that ketamine is the one of choice in every case (Table 17.7). When an injectable agent has to be used ketamine may be given i.m. in doses of 15 mg/kg. The bird should be confined in a warm, darkened box

TABLE 17.7 **Doses of ketamine and 'Hellabrunn Mixture' for various birds. (Data from several sources but mainly from published data sheets, Bayer UK Ltd and Parke-Davis Veterinary)**

Bird	Adult BW (g)	Ketamine dose (mg)	'Hellabrunn Mixture' (ml/kg)
African Grey parrots	350–450	10–14	0.02
Budgerigars	30–50	2	–
Geese	5000–7000	60–85	0.03–0.08
Gulls	500–800	12–15	0.030–0.035
Kestrels	150–250	6–8	0.03–0.06
Macaws	750–850	15–18	0.020–0.025
Muscovy ducks	3500–5000	35–50	0.02
Parakeets	80–100	3	0.03
Penguins	3200–6000	70–175	0.06
Mute swans	6000–7000	70–85	0.03–0.06

as soon as the injection has been made and the depth of anaesthesia produced is assessed by noting response to pinching the wattle or skin of the neck and although the eyelids often close the corneal reflex should persist throughout. Increments can be given to produce the desired degree of unconsciousness. There is a wide safety margin and doses of 25 mg/kg of ketamine may safely be given to all species of birds, although recovery may sometimes be prolonged.

Inhalation anaesthesia

Whenever possible it is probably desirable to induce and maintain anaesthesia with an inhalation agent. Birds may be restrained so that anaesthesia can be induced using a face-mask or they can be confined in a box made of transparent plastic material while anaesthetic gases or vapours are introduced into the box. Probably the best method is to induce anaesthesia by passing halothane or isoflurane into the box in which the bird is confined and then to maintain anaesthesia by administering the same agent through a face-mask or endotracheal tube.

Endotracheal intubation is not difficult in birds (Fig. 17.2) and suitable tubes may be constructed from silicone rubber or PVC tubing. Tubes should be long enough to reach the syrinx but deadspace must be kept to a minimum and their ends should be be cut at a bevel to facilitate passage into the trachea. Airway secretions may block the flow of gas in both intubated and non-intubated birds so it is always wise to have suction available for their removal by aspiration. Adequate suction can be provided from a 60 ml syringe fitted with a short length of fine catheter.

Most birds can be anaesthetized with 0.5–1.0 % halothane or 1.0–1.5% isoflurane vapour in oxygen delivered to the endotracheal tube or facemask from a T-piece system. The air sacs should be flushed at about 5 minute intervals by occlusion of the open arm of the T-piece system, their overdistension being prevented by escape of gas around the loose-fitting endotracheal tube or by partial lifting of the facemask away from the face. Total gas flow rates should be about two to three times the estimated minute volume of respiration of the bird, e.g. about 750 ml in an adult domestic hen,

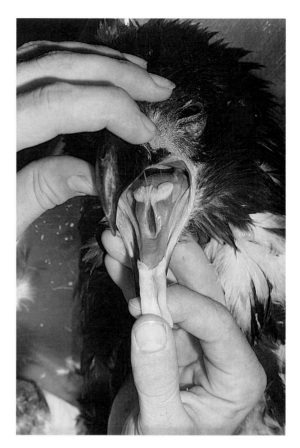

FIG. 17.2 Larynx of a raptor – to demonstrate the accessibility for endotracheal intubation.

250 ml in a pigeon and 25 ml in a budgerigar. Inhalation anaesthetics may also be administered through a needle introduced directly into an air sac, but this has litle to commend it.

Recovery from anaesthesia is accelerated by administering oxygen and flushing the air sacs from time to time until the bird has regained its righting reflexes. Unless this is done the anaesthetic which passes into the air sacs may not be cleared by the depressed respiratory activity so that it will be taken up again by the parabronchial capillary blood and recovery will be prolonged.

Combinations of inhalation and injectable agents

Very satisfactory results are obtained by the combination of injectable and inhalation agents.

Although many combinations have been used, the induction of unconsciousness with ketamine (10–15 mg/kg i.m.) followed by the inhalation of isoflurane/O_2 or halothane/O_2 is probably the simplest and safest.

Measurement of ketamine doses for small birds such as canaries and budgerigars which may weigh from 30 to 60 g is not easy and these birds may be dosed with 1 to 2 mg per bird. The standard solution of ketamine for veterinary use contains 100 mg/ml and if 0.1 ml is diluted to 1 ml birds may be given 0.1–0.2 ml of the diluted solution i.m. into the pectoral muscles. The larger dose (0.2 ml of the diluted solution) will usually produce light anaesthesia in 2–3 minutes from the time of injection.

It has been claimed, often anecdotally, that certain species of birds including moorhens, coots, doves and vultures are unsuitable for anaesthesia with ketamine on its own or in combination with other drugs. Saffan can be used in place of ketamine for most birds but when given i.m. it produces more variable results, probably due to the difficulty of ensuring that the dose is correctly administered into a muscle mass. The aim should always be to give just enough of the injectable agent to make the bird unconscious and to use only as much isoflurane or halothane as is necessary for the maintenance of anaesthesia.

RATITES

Ostriches and emus pose challenging problems for restraint. Adult birds can move very quickly, peck with great accuracy and have large-toed feet which they use to strike forwards. Handling can be facilitated by hooding and it is always wise, whenever possible to work with attendant(s) familiar with these flightless birds. Ketamine (15 mg/kg i.m.)appears to produce the most reliable and smoothest induction of anaesthesia, especially when combined with diazepam (0.5 mg/kg i.m.) or xylazine (3.5 mg/kg i.m.). Inhalation anaesthesia can be maintained in emus and ostriches weighing less than 130 kg using small animal breathing systems, but a large animal breathing system is needed for larger birds.

BEARS

Bears can inflict severe injuries; their faces are curiously expressionless and it is difficult to detect their mood. Even a playful blow from a paw can inflict a severe injury. Grizzly and polar bears may deliberately attack human beings.

In zoos and circuses, they can be confined in squeeze cages or airtight boxes where injected or inhalation agents can be administered, but if these facilities are not available, ketamine can be administered from a projectile syringe (see below). Doses are not well established but various doses from 15–25 mg/kg have been administered safely, with atropine to control salivation. Suggested optimal doses are i.m. xylazine (2.9 mg/kg) plus i.m. ketamine (2–9 mg/kg) but it should be noted that young bears seem notably sensitive to sedation and should have reduced doses.

Venepuncture is not easy, even in sedated bears, because the limb veins are small and embedded in fat so that if sedation produced by ketamine does not allow surgery an inhalation agent such as halothane or isoflurane should be given. Endotracheal intubation is not difficult in the unconscious animal.

NON-HUMAN PRIMATES

Not only can monkeys inflict bites and scratches, they are also carriers of viruses which are extremely pathogenic to man as well as diseases such as tuberculosis, salmonellosis and shigellosis. For these reasons it is always undesirable to handle conscious monkeys, and even domestic pets should be viewed with suspicion. Handling of any pet monkey should, preferably, be left to its owners.

If the owner of a small pet monkey can be induced to hold its arms behind its back the anaesthetist can usually make an intravenous injection of an anaesthetic such as thiopental or Saffan into the recurrent tarsal vein on the dorsal surface of the gastrocnemius muscle. Caution is necessary for these monkeys often weigh much less than is estimated and it is seldom necessary to exceed 5 mg/kg of thiopental or 2 mg/kg of Saffan. Once unconscious the monkey may be given a small dose of suxamethonium (e.g. 1 mg/kg) and intubated with an uncuffed tube. Anaesthesia may then be maintained by the administration of halothane or isoflurane in N_2O/O_2, or O_2 alone, from a T-piece system. When suxamethonium is to be given it is wise to inject atropine (0.15–0.30 mg i.v.) as soon as the induction agent has been given.

Alternatively, if the owner or an assistant can hold the monkey, again with its arms held behind its back, an inhalation agent can be used for both induction and maintenance of anaesthesia. The use of N_2O is a distinct advantage in these circumstances and halothane is probably the volatile agent of choice for, in the authors' experience, isoflurane often provokes breath holding. A suitable face-mask is held over, but not touching, the face and N_2O/O_2 (3:1) is administered at a flow rate of 4 l/min for 1–2 minutes. Halothane is then introduced into the gas mixture, increasing the concentration of the vapour every 3 to 4 breaths to a maximum of about 3%. The mask is applied to the face as soon as it is judged that the monkey is unconscious and induction is usually free from excitement and struggling. Scavenging of waste gases is usually not possible during the induction of anaesthesia. Anaesthesia is maintained with 1.2– 1.5% of halothane vapour in the N_2O/O_2 mixture.

Larger or less co-operative monkeys may need sedating by i.m. injection before an attempt is made to induce anaesthesia (Green, 1979). The use of projectile syringes is not to be recommended for monkeys are adept at dodging or even deflecting the projectile with their hands, and they usually pull the needle out before the injection is complete even when a hit is obtained! In the case of the smaller varieties it is usually possible to catch the monkey's arm through the bars of the cage so that injection can be made into the deltoid muscle, but a squeeze cage may be needed for the larger, strong animals such as adult chimpanzees.

Ketamine is probably the agent of choice in all except squirrel monkeys and marmosets for chemical restraint or preanaesthetic sedation. At dose rates of 10–25 mg/kg the volume of the veterinary preparation 'Vetalar' injected is small so that the drug can be given rapidly into the thigh muscles of even struggling animals. The peak effect is obtained 5 to 10 minutes after injection and the period of sedation is from 30 to 60 minutes. Recovery is complete in 1.5 to 4.5 hours depending on the dose and species of the monkey. When the desired degree of sedation is not produced by ketamine further depression of the central nervous system is probably best produced by administration of N_2O/O_2 supplemented with 0.5 to 1.0% halothane delivered through a face-mask from a T-piece system.

For squirrel monkeys and marmosets Saffan is the sedative of choice and this preparation is also useful in other species of non-human primates. In squirrel monkeys and marmosets doses of 15–18 mg/kg produce light general anaesthesia some 5 minutes after injection into the thigh muscles. Anaesthesia lasts about 45 minutes and is followed by recovery to full consciousness 1–3 hours later. In baboons, i.m. doses of 12–18 mg/kg make the animal safe to handle about 10 minutes after injection and recovery is much quicker than in squirrel monkeys. In all monkeys anaesthesia may be deepened by giving i.v. increments of Saffan until the desired depth is obtained. Animals can then be intubated and maintained unconscious with inhalation agents such as halothane, or sequential incremental i.v. doses of Saffan can be given over several hours if need be. The main disadvantage of Saffan is the large volume which has to be given i.m., although these volumes do not appear to result in pain at the injection site.

When it is impossible to give an i.m. injection to a large monkey or ape the simplest thing is to entice it into a cage which can be made airtight by covering with a sheet of plastic material so that anaesthetic gases and vapours can be piped in. The animal must be observed carefully and removed from the cage as soon as it is unconscious and relaxed.

It is important to conserve body heat and the anaesthetized monkey should be placed on a warm water blanket maintained at 38 °C; this is especially important for small monkeys. If sedation or anaesthesia is to last for more than about an hour, an intravenous drip infusion of N/5 saline or Hartmann's solution (Ringer's lactate) should be started as soon as the animal is anaesthetized or sufficiently sedated. The fluid should be given at the rate of 10 ml/kg per hour and, for the smaller monkeys it should be warmed to 38 °C by passing it through a blood warmer before it reaches the animal. The use of atropine is somewhat controversial but it is probable that it should be given as soon as the monkey becomes anaesthetized, in a dose of 0.15 to 1.20 mg depending on the size of the animal.

Recovery from anaesthesia should take place in a warm environment and endotracheal tubes and i.v. cannulae must be removed while it is still safe to handle the animal. Postsurgical analgesia should be provided by the i.m. injection of a suitable analgesic (e.g. pethidine at 2 mg/kg or morphine at 0.1 mg/kg).

WILD ANIMALS

Only species of wild animal which are likely to be encountered by those in general veterinary practice in the UK will be considered here, but as a general rule the principles of anaesthesia as applied to domesticated or captive pet animals apply equally well in all wild animals and the main differences arise from the need to protect the anaesthetist and any assistants from injury by unanaesthetized subjects.

Difficulty in getting close to the subject, either because of its timidity or aversion to mankind, and the obvious need to avoid being attacked, have led to two approaches to the problems. The first is the use of squeeze cages, the animal being enticed into the cage then squeezed between a fixed and movable wall so that cannot turn around or move very far whilst being given an injection of a sedative or anaesthetic agent. These cages should be standard equipment at zoos, some research centres and similar establishments and they have a definite role in the capture of farmed deer, but they are unlikely to be available to the veterinarian in general practice. The second which is, perhaps, more generally applicable, is the administration of agents from projectile syringes. These syringes may be projected from rifles, crossbows, or blow-pipes so that the administrator can remain a safe distance from the subject (Fig. 17.3). They were originally developed for the capture of wild game animals but they are now finding a use in ordinary veterinary practice where, for example, current methods of farming (particularly of some European breeds of cattle) are producing virtually unhandled beasts which are often aggressive, especially if frightened.

The use of projectile syringes for the capture and restraint of wild game animals was well reviewed by Harthoorn (1971). The problems related to the use of projectile syringes in general veterinary practice are somewhat different. The projectile syringe is designed to inject its contents after the needle has penetrated the skin of the animal and its impact with the tissues can result in serious bruising. They should empty within seconds of penetration and the force of the injection should be adequate to push the plunger fully home even if the needle is partially obstructed by a skin plug. To minimise tissue damage the syringe should strike the beast towards the end of the firing trajectory, although obviously this is less important when the projectile is propelled from a blowpipe. When fired from a gun or cross-bow at too close range the syringe needle may enter body cavities, and often when striking too hard, syringes bounce off without penetrating effectively in spite of barbs and collars on the needles. Extensive and fatal trauma may be caused by injection into the thoracic or abdominal cavities.

In all cases the shortest needle commensurate with penetration of the skin should be used and large bore needles should terminate in a cone, with holes on the side of the shaft, for the ordinary open-ended needle may block with a core of skin. Collared needles are seldom satisfactory and tend to allow fluids to flow back out of the hole caused by penetration of the collar. To remove a barbed needle a small incision is made over the site of the barb.

Irritant solutions may not be used since their administration under the non-sterile conditions associated with the use of dart-guns may produce an abscess, but when simple precautions are routinely taken, untoward reactions at the site of injection are surprisingly rare. Valuable animals may be given a precautionary dose of antimicrobial substances and in summer the wounds should be dressed with fly repellents.

There are now many patterns of projectile syringes designed for use with rifles, pistols and cross-bows but, in general, they usually inject their contents through the agency of an explosive cap and striker mechanisms, or by gas evolved from a chemical reaction initiated in a capsule by a similar striker mechanism, incorporated behind the syringe plunger. The projectiles used with blow-pipes have needles with side holes which are covered by a short plastic sleeve and displacement of this sleeve as the needle penetrates the skin and its displacement allows the pressure of air or gas previously injected behind the plunger to inject the syringe contents. In projectiles fired from crossbows, rifles or pistols detonation of an explosive cap produces such a force that the ejected fluid penetrates far into the tissues and haematoma formation is common so that the slow-er injection due to gas propulsion is usually to be preferred.

Projectile syringes usually have a capacity of up to 4–5 ml so that only relatively soluble drugs can be administered. If they are to be used on common land or in dense undergrowth any temptation to use Immobilon or etorphine should be resisted for should the projectile bounce off the animal or the animal be missed completely, these projectiles are surprisingly difficult to locate in spite of their bright silver barrels and coloured flights, and their subsequent discovery by a child or even an adult could have fatal consequences for that individual. It must be appreciated that projection is very far from accurate. The weight of the projectile accord-ing to its capacity and degree of filling has a great influence at all but the shortest of ranges which can, in any case, only be estimated. Experience has shown that the best results are obtained by getting as close to the animal as is possible or safe, and aiming for the neck or shoulder region.

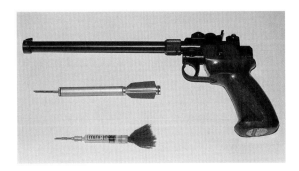

FIG. 17.3 'Dist-Inject' dart pistol with projectile syringe. The lower illustration is of the 'Miniject' projectile syringe for use with a blowpipe.

It is always advisable to use doses of injectable agent which allow the animal to be approached with safety and so allow general anaesthesia to be produced with i.v. or inhalation agents. Although a quick recovery is essential in the wild, as partially sedated animals are at risk from predators, it is not so important in captive animals. To date, the tech-niques most frequently used for immobilizing a wide variety of species have been based on use of opioids such as etorphine or carfentanil coupled with sedatives, anaesthesia being terminated with antagonists such as diprenorphine or ati-pamezole. Ketamine and ketamine combinations are now being employed much more commonly in ruminants.

The doses of drugs required by various species of animal and breeds within a species varies enor-mously so that an extensive literature on the sub-ject is now available. Anyone wishing to make use of agents to be administered by projectile syringe is strongly recommended before doing so to con-sult suitable literature available from commercial sources.

REFERENCES

Cooper, J.E. (1989) Anaesthesia of exotic species. In: Hilbery, A.D.R. (ed.) *Manual of Anaesthesia for Small Animal Practice.* Cheltenham: British Small Animal Veterinary Association, ch. 17, pp. 139–151.

Dunker, H.R. (1972) Structure of avian lungs. *Respiratory Physiology,* **14**: 44–63.

Flecknell, P.A. (1988) *Laboratory Animal Anaesthesia.* London: Academic Press.

Green, C.J. (1975) Neuroleptic drug combinations in the anaesthetic management of small laboratory animals. *Laboratory Animals* **9**: 161–178.

Green, C.J. (1979) *Animal Anaesthesia.* London: Laboratory Animals

Green, C.J., Knight, J., Precious, S. and Simpkin, S. (1981) Ketamine alone and combined with diazepam or xylazine in laboratory animals. London: *Laboratory Animals Ltd*

Harthoorn, A.M. (1971) *Chemical Capture of Animals.* London: Baillière Tindall.

Mero, M., Vainionpaa, S., Vasensius, J., Vihkonen, K. and Rockkanen, P. (1989) Medetomidine-ketamine-diazepam anaesthesia in the rabbit. *Acta Veterinaria Scandinavica,* **85** (Suppl): 135–137.

Nevalainen, T., Pyhala, L., Hanna-Maija, V. *et al.* (1989) Evaluation of anaesthetic potency of medetomidine-ketamine combination in rats, guinea pigs and rabbits. *Acta Veterinaria Scandinavica* **85**: 139–143.

Orland F.J. and Orland, P.M. (1946) Pentobarbital sodium anesthesia in the Syrian hamster. *Journal of the American Pharmaceutical Association* **35**: 263–265.

Piiper, J. (1972) In: Bolis, L., Schmidt-Nielsen, K. and Maddrell, S.H.P. (eds) *Comparative Physiology*. Amsterdam: North Holland Veterinary Medicine Reviews, ch. 3, p. 204.

Piiper, J. and Scheid, P. (1973) Gas exchange in avian lungs: models and experimental evidence. In: Bolis, L., Schmidt-Nielsen, K. and Maddrell, S.H.P. (eds) *Comparative Physiology*. Amsterdam: North Holland Veterinary Medicine Reviews, pp. 616–618.

Sedgewick, C.J. (1986) Anesthesia for rabbits. *Veterinary Clinics of North America. Food Animal Practice* **2**: 731–736.

Special Anaesthesia

Anaesthesia for obstetrics

18

INTRODUCTION

There is no one anaesthetic agent or technique that is ideal for all parturient animals. In veterinary practice the choice of anaesthetic methods and drugs is often influenced by whether the offspring are alive and wanted, unwanted, or dead due to obstetrical problems. In any case the choice must be such as to ensure the safety of the mother and any living foetus(es), comfort of the mother during parturition or hysterotomy and convenience of the obstetrician/surgeon. To make a rational choice the anaesthetist must be familiar with physiological alterations induced by pregnancy and labour, the pharmacology of the agents used, and significance of obstetric complications necessitating assisted delivery of the offspring. Most studies have been carried out in ewes, but physiological alterations are broadly comparable in other species of animal even if their magnitude differs. The following brief account of changes in physiology and in actions of drugs administered during pregnancy and parturition is a summary of many published papers and accounts in standard textbooks and should apply to all species of domestic animals.

THE STATE OF PREGNANCY

PHYSIOLOGICAL AND ANATOMICAL ALTERATIONS

Physiological and anatomical alterations occur in many organ systems during pregnancy and delivery of the foetuses. Early in pregnancy changes are due, at least in part, to metabolic demands of the foetus(es), placenta and uterus, due largely to increasing levels of progesterone and oestrogen. Later changes starting around mid-pregnancy are anatomical in nature and are caused by mechanical pressure from the enlarging uterus.

Circulatory changes

Circulatory changes develop primarily to meet increased metabolic demands of the mother and foetus(es). Blood volume increases progressively, most of the added volume being accommodated in the increased capacity of vessels in the uterus, mammary glands, renal, striated muscle and cutaneous tissues so that there is no evidence of circulatory overload in healthy pregnant animals. Increase in plasma volume is relatively greater than that of red cells, resulting in haemodilution with decreased haemoglobin content and haematocrit. The purpose of this increase in blood volume is usually assumed to be twofold. First, it increases placental exchanges of respiratory gases, nutrients and waste metabolites. Secondly, it acts as a reserve if there is any abnormal maternal blood loss at parturition so that increased autotransfusion of blood can occur from the involuting uterus. Cardiac output increases in pregnancy to a similar degree as blood volume and there is an additional increase in cardiac output during all stages of labour. In 3rd stage labour it probably results from blood being expelled from the involuting uterus into the general circulation. Peripheral vascular resistance usually decreases during pregnancy so that ABP does not change. A serious decrease in venous return due to compression of the vena cava and aorta by the enlarged uterus and its contents can occur if the animal is restrained or positioned in the supine position This decrease in venous return will, of course, cause a fall in cardiac output for the heart cannot pump more blood than is being returned to it. Cardiac work is increased during pregnancy so that at parturition cardiac reserve is reduced and pulmonary congestion and heart failure may occur in animals that had previously well compensated cardiac disease.

Respiratory system changes

During pregnancy the sensitivity of the respiratory centre to carbon dioxide is increased, presumably due to changes in hormone levels, so that $PaCO_2$ and serum bicarbonate decrease although arterial pH is maintained due to long term renal compensation. Oxygen consumption is increased by the demands of the developing foetus(es), placenta, uterine muscle and mammary glands. During labour, ventilation may be further increased by apprehension or anxiety. Airway conductance is increased and total pulmonary resistance is decreased, apparently from hormone-induced relaxation of bronchial smooth muscle. Cranial displacement of the diaphragm results from increasing volume of the gravid uterus leading to a decrease in FRC, so that it is possible for airway closure to occur at end-expiration. Reduction in oxygen storage capacity from reduced FRC leads to an unusually rapid decline in PaO_2 during apnoea. Some compensation for the tendency of the FRC to decrease is achieved by increases in the transverse and antero-posterior diameters of the chest cavity and flaring of the ribs.

Other systems

Liver function is generally well maintained during pregnancy. Plasma protein concentration is decreased but total plasma protein is increased due to increase in blood volume.

Renal plasma flow (RPF) and glomerular filtration rate (GFR) increase progressively, paralleling the increases in blood volume and cardiac output. Due to increases in renal clearances blood urea and creatinine levels are lower than in non-pregnant animals.

Uterine blood flow is directly proportional to perfusion pressure and inversely proportional to uterine vascular resistance, so that it can be compromized from vasoconstriction due to catecholamine release from fright or anxiety.

PHARMACOLOGY OF DRUGS ADMINISTERED DURING PREGNANCY

The effects of pregnancy on drug disposition, biotransformation and excretion are largely unknown in domestic animals. The MAC of inhalation agents is decreased due to unknown mechanisms. The increase in RBF and GFR favours renal excretion of drugs. Any drug administered to the mother is liable to cross the placenta to the foetus(es) and induce effects similar to those observed in the mother.

Placental transfer of drugs is governed by the physiochemical properties of the drug and anatomical features of the placenta. Transfer of drugs can occur by simple diffusion, facilitated diffusion via transport systems, active transport and pinocytosis. Of these simple diffusion is by far the most important and this will be affected by the surface area and thickness of the placenta. The larger farm animals have thick epitheliochorial placentae with relatively small areas for diffusion due to their cotyledonary or patchy diffuse distribution, whereas dogs and cats have thinner endotheliochorial placenta with larger zonular areas of implantation. Thus, the placental diffusion barrier is greatest in ruminants, pigs and horses and least in dogs and cats. However, the diffusion barrier does not appear to be of great clinical significance in the transfer of drugs from mother to foetus(es) in any species of animal.

More important is the diffusion constant which is unique to each drug and determined by molecular weight, degree of protein binding in maternal blood, lipid solubility and degree of ionization in the plasma. Most drugs used in anaesthesia have large diffusion constants – low molecular weights, high lipid solubility and poor ionization – and diffuse rapidly across the placenta. The exceptions are the neuromuscular blocking drugs, which are highly ionized and of low lipid solubility.

Maternal blood concentrations of drug depend on total dose administered, site or route of administration, rate of distribution and uptake of it by maternal tissues and maternal detoxification and excretion. Thus drugs with rapidly declining plasma concentration after administration of a fixed dose (e.g. thiopental) result in a short exposure of the placenta and hence foetus(es) to high maternal concentrations, whereas drugs administered continuously (e.g. inhalation anaesthetics, infused agents during TIVA) are associated with a continuous placental transfer to the foetus(es).

The concentration of drug in the umbilical vein of a foetus is not that to which the foetal target organs such as the heart and brain are exposed, for most of the umbilical blood passes initially through the liver, where the drug may be metabolized or sequestrated. The remainder of the umbilical blood passes through the ductus venous to the vena cava where it is diluted by drug-free blood from the hind end of the foetus. Thus, the foetal circulation protects vital tissues and organs from exposure to sudden high drug concentrations.

CLINICAL SIGNIFICANCE OF CHANGES DURING PREGNANCY AND PARTURITION

Circulatory changes of pregnancy and parturition can put a mother suffering from even normally well compensated heart disease at risk unless care is taken to ensure a minimum cardiac depression from anaesthetic drugs. Ecbolics used early on in labour can have an adverse effect on cardiovascular function. Oxytocin will induce vasodilatation and hypotension that will have an adverse effect on both mother and foetus(es) due to decreased tissue and placental perfusion. Ergometrine causes vasoconstriction and may give rise to an increase in systemic vascular resistance sufficient to produce heart failure in the immediate postpartum period when cardiac output is high from the increased circulating blood volume. Venous engorgement of the epidural space decreases the volume of solutions needed to produce block to any given level.

Reduction in FRC means that any respiratory depression caused by drugs is more significant in pregnant than in non-pregnant animals and hypoventilation will lead to hypercapnia and hypoxaemia; the hypoxaemia is particularly undesirable during labour when oxygen consumption is increased. In small animals induction of anaesthesia with inhalational agents will be more rapid than in non-pregnant animals due to decrease in FRC and increased alveolar ventilation as well as the decrease in MAC, but in recumbent large animals shunting of pulmonary blood may make the induction and maintenance of inhalation anaesthesia more difficult.

In monogastric animals there is an increased risk of both vomiting and silent aspiration of gastric contents in parturient animals for frequently the time of last feeding is unknown, and intragastric pressure is increased in the stomach displaced by the gravid uterus. Risk of regurgitation of ruminal contents when general anaesthesia is induced seems to be great in cattle, but perhaps not in sheep and goats which normally have less fluid rumen contents.

DRUG ACTIONS

Opioids

Opioids rapidly cross the placenta from mother to foetus(es) and can cause marked respiratory and central nervous depression in neonate(s) with sleepiness and reluctance to feed. Opioid antagonists also readily cross the placenta and it has been suggested that they should be given to the mother immediately before delivery to counter neonatal respiratory and central nervous depression, but this deprives the mother of analgesia at the time when it is most needed and may result in her regaining consciousness on the operating table. If used, the opioid antagonists such as naloxone should be given to the neonate(s). Because the action of naloxone is shorter than that of some opioids, depression may return when naloxone is metabolized and careful observation is indicated to allow this to be detected and treated by the injection of more naloxone.

α_2 adrenoceptor agonists; ketamine

All α_2 adrenoceptor agonists rapidly cross the placenta and can cause respiratory and cardiovascular depression in both mother and babies, although this can be counteracted by antagonists. The use of acepromazine/ketamine combinations is theoretically unwise but, in practice, provided only minimal doses are used little harm appears to result.

Intravenous anaesthetics; neuromuscular blockers

Low doses of thiopental, methohexital, propofol and Saffan produce minimal respiratory or central nervous depression in neonates. Neuromuscular blocking drugs do not cross the placenta but are seldom needed in obstetrical anaesthesia. No muscle relaxation is required for vaginal delivery and in caesarian section the only time it might be needed is for suture of the abdominal wall, but this is usually very relaxed following removal of the bulky uterine contents. Use of neuromuscular blockers to decrease the quantity of more depressant anaesthetic agents needed is, however, a legitimate indication for their use in balanced anaesthesia techniques.

Inhalation anaesthetics

Inhalation anaesthetics readily cross the placental barrier with rapid equilibration between the mother and foetus(es). The degree of depression they cause in the neonate is directly proportional to the depth of unconsciousness induced in the mother. Deep levels of maternal depression will cause maternal hypotension, decreased uterine blood flow and foetal acidosis. There is a reduction in anaesthetic requirements with a fall in MAC. When measured in ewes, MAC is 25 to 40% lower in gravid as compared with non-pregnant animals. Use of the less soluble agents enflurane, isoflurane, sevoflurane and desflurane will lead to more rapid recovery of the newly delivered animals than when more soluble agents such as halothane are employed. Nitrous oxide will often enable concentration of more potent soluble anaesthetic agent to be reduced and its use does not add to depression of the newborn.

Foetal haemoglobin can carry more O_2 for a given PO_2 due to the low concentration of 2,3-diphosphoglycerate (2,3-DPG) in foetal red cells. This ensures a higher level of haemoglobin saturation at the normally low PO_2 of umbilical venous blood. Administration of O_2 to the mother results in a most significant increase in foetal oxygenation and maternal inspired O_2 concentrations of over 50% during general anaesthesia are associated with delivery of more vigorous newborn. However, it must be remembered that administration of high concentrations of oxygen for any prolonged time to spontaneously breathing animals may lead to unrecognized, but fatal, hypercapnia.

Local analgesics

Local analgesics are not as harmless as sometimes supposed. Amide derivatives (e.g. lignocaine, mepivacaine, bupivacaine) are broken down by hepatic microsomal enzymes. After absorption from the site of injection maternal blood levels decrease slowly and blood levels can reach a significant level in the foetus(es) causing depression in the neonate. Sufficiently high concentrations seldom occur after epidural or paravertebral administration, but can be found after the indiscriminate local infiltration of large volumes of local analgesic solutions. Epidural block may produce hypotension and this may be treated by infusing fluid to fill the dilated vascular bed, or better, by injection of ephedrine. Ephedrine acts centrally to increase venous tone and thus cardiac preload; it has minimal vasoconstrictor effect on the arterial system.

Anticholinergics

Because glycopyrrolate does not readily cross the placental barrier it is probably the anticholinergic of choice if anticholinergics are to be used to minimize the effects of traction on the uterus and broad ligaments by the surgeon.

HORSES

In horses, obstructed labour quickly leads to exhaustion of the mare and death of the foal.

Prompt relief is necessary and anaesthesia may have to be provided for vaginal delivery or caesarian section. The viability of the foal will depend on its state at the time of anaesthesia but the mare will invariably have a distended abdomen and may show signs of weakness or be in shock. The anaesthetic problems presented by the mare are very similar to those encountered in horses with bowel obstruction, although the degree of dehydration is generally much less severe. When the foal is alive, the effects of any drugs to be given to the mare on uterine blood flow and foetal oxygenation, as well as on the respiratory centre of the foal after delivery, must also be taken into account.

It can be assumed that any drug given to the mare will cross the placenta to the foal, but its actual concentration in the foal will depend on such factors as fat solubility, degree of protein binding and ionization, dose given to the mare and time interval between its administration and delivery of the foal, and the neonatal foal's ability to eliminate the drug from its body. Thus, opioids such as pethidine given to the mare will produce respiratory depression in the foal, but low doses of thiobarbiturates will be tolerated because recovery from central nervous depression is more dependent on redistribution than on metabolism. The more insoluble inhalation anaesthetics given to the mare are readily excreted by the foal if it breathes properly after delivery. Although neuromuscular blocking drugs such as vecuronium, atracurium and pancuronium do not cross the placenta in significant amounts guaiphenesin does, so for obstetrical anaesthesia it is best avoided or used in much reduced dose if the foal is alive when anaesthesia is induced. Respiratory and central nervous depression in the foal resulting from administration of opioids to the mare can be antagonized by giving naloxone to the foal but, in general, stimulant drugs have only a minor role in the management of problems in newborns. Doxapram (0.5 mg/kg i.v.) may be effective in provoking the first breath and aiding lung expansion. However, instead of relying on stimulant drugs to resuscitate foals, resuscitation should normally involve clearing of the airway, endotracheal intubation, O_2 administration, and IPPV.

Abdominal distension of the mare will probably be the problem which gives rise to most concern because many mares have great difficulty in breathing once they are recumbent under general anaesthesia. Due to intrapulmonary shunting of blood they may also be difficult to keep unconscious with inhalation anaesthetics. In the supine position which some surgeons prefer for caesarian section, the weight of the gravid uterus will compress the vena cava and aorta, reducing venous return and causing a marked decrease in ABP. Once the foal is delivered, the condition of the mare shows immediate improvement – pulmonary ventilation increases and ABP rises towards normal levels. Attempts by the surgeon to remove the placenta should be discouraged since this provokes hypotension and, occasionally, considerable blood loss requiring the infusion of 20 to 30 ml/kg of lactated or acetated Ringer's solution. To minimize difficulties before delivery of the foal, the mare should be positioned so that she is lying inclined towards her left side and respiration may need to be controlled. As always in equine anaesthesia, the magnitude of the problems encountered is related to size; small pony mares present only relatively minor problems. It is important to remember this for techniques successful for elective caesarian section in small experimental pony mares operated on in lateral decubitus are often inadequate for the large mares of the heavy breeds requiring emergency obstetric procedures while in the supine position.

In practice, vaginal repositioning and delivery of the foal can often be carried out in the sedated mare, using one of the drug combinations discussed earlier in this book. If general anaesthesia is essential the α_2 adrenoceptor agonist/ketamine combination, in spite of some theoretical objections, can be recommended, for it has been used without giving rise to problems in either the parturient mare or the foal. Should longer periods of light general anaesthesia be required small i.v. doses of thiopental (or after delivery of the foal, guaiphenesin), may be given to prolong the effects of this drug combination.

Caudal epidural block is not as useful as it is in cattle because in mares there is a rather long delay between injection and onset of full analgesia. A 450 kg mare requires 6 to 8 ml of 2% lignocaine or 2% mepivacaine (or 0.17 mg/kg xylazine or 60 µg/kg detomidine diluted in 10 ml of 0.9% NaCl) for effective analgesia whilst remaining standing with no apparent side effects. The development of maximum analgesia can be delayed for 10 to 30 minutes.

For caesarean section, if the foal is alive, induction with an α_2 adrenoceptor agonist before i.v. thiopental or methohexital followed by endotracheal halothane/oxygen or isoflurane/oxygen seems to be quite satisfactory, but ketamine is undoubtedly better than either of the barbiturates as the induction agent. Only the minimal amounts of halothane or isoflurane should be used and IPPV may be necessary until the foal is delivered. Involution of the uterus is hastened when xylazine has been used and may be assisted by 2.5 to 10 units i.v. of oxytocin. Bleeding from the uterus is best controlled by i.v. injections of 3 to 5 mg of ergometrine tartrate, but this may give rise to cardiac arrhythmias in hypercapnic or hypertensive animals. Vigorous supportive therapy with i.v. fluids may be necessary. If the foal is dead any technique of general anaesthesia suitable for laparotomy in horses may be used.

CATTLE

In cattle, caudal block is nearly always used for vaginal delivery of the calf. The substitution of xylazine for lignocaine (0.05 mg/kg xylazine in 10 ml 0.9% saline for 5 to 10 ml 2% lignocaine) confers no obvious advantages. Whenever possible sedation should be avoided but, if needed for control, xylazine (0.05 mg/kg i.v.) will, in most cases, provide adequate maternal tranquillization to enable the block and obstetrical manoeuvres to be undertaken with minimal trouble. Lumbar segmental epidural block may be used for caesarian section carried out through the left flank of the standing animal but it is not easily performed and most veterinarians prefer to use paravertebral block of the 13th thoracic, 1st, 2nd and 3rd lumbar nerves on that side. Local infiltration techniques can be employed but they do not relax the abdominal muscles and, if the foetus is alive, the injection of large volumes of the amide-type local analgesics may result in cardiopulmonary depression in the neonatal calf.

Caesarian section via a ventral abdominal incision is usually carried out under general anaesthesia with endotracheal intubation. Anaesthesia may be induced by the i.v. injection of minimal doses of xylazine (0.1 mg/kg)/ketamine (2.2 mg/kg), thiopentone (5–10 mg/kg), or even propofol (0.2 mg/kg) and, after endotracheal intubation maintained with an inhalation agent (usually halothane or isoflurane). Alternatively, after xylazine (0.1 to 0.15 mg/kg i.v.) or detomidine (10 to 20 µg/kg i.v.) has been given to produce deep sedation, the animal may be intubated and anaesthesia completed by the administration of the inhalation agent.

Involution of the uterus after delivery may be assisted by the use of ecbolic drugs provided the cow is not hypercapnic or hypertensive. All cows subjected to caesarian section under general anaesthesia should be given calcium borogluconate s.c. to prevent the occurrence of hypocalcaemia which is otherwise frequently seen in the postoperative period. Postoperative analgesia is also important and 0.5 to 1.0 g pethidine (meperidine) depending on the size of the cow, repeated at 4 to 6 hourly intervals for the first 24 hours, has proved to provide analgesia as shown by the cow looking comfortable and cudding or eating.

Removal of a dead, putrefying normal-sized calf by hysterotomy should only be attempted after resuscitation of the toxaemic or shocked cow with intravenous fluids; antimicrobial cover is essential and the cow should be closely observed for adverse reactions to the antimicrobial drug used.

SHEEP AND GOATS

Sheep are seldom given any analgesia or anaesthesia for the vaginal delivery of lambs but, in difficult cases requiring extensive repositioning of the lamb in the birth canal, caudal block is very satisfactory, using 1 ml/4.5 kg of 2% lignocaine hydrochloride. For caesarian section, which is usually carried out through the left flank, epidural or paravertebral blocks, local infiltration and general anaesthesia are all suitable. Sedation, when indicated by the behaviour of the ewe, may be obtained with i.v. diazepam (0.25 to 1.0 mg/kg). The ewe is usually easily restrained for operation and hence techniques of local analgesia are popular. Probably the technique of choice is paravertebral block of the 13th thoracic, 1st, 2nd and 3rd lumbar nerves, for the ewe is then able to stand and suckle her lambs immediately the operation is completed and the wound area remains analgesic for one or more hours depending on the local analgesic drug used. If local infiltration is used care must be taken to restrict the total dose of any amide-type local analgesic to below 5 mg/kg to minimize toxicity in the ewe and the likelihood of depression of the lambs.

Ewes carrying dead lambs or suffering from pregnancy toxaemia are often very toxic, dehydrated and dull or collapsed. Hysterotomy should be preceded by resuscitation with intravenous fluids.

Postoperative analgesia is all too often neglected. The ewe, like any other animal, is entitled to adequate pain relief in the postoperative period and 4 hourly morphine (up to 10 mg i.m.), pethidine (meperidine) up to 250 mg i.m., or epidural opioid drugs should be used as freely as may be required to keep the animal comfortable. Obviously, epidural block will have minimal effects on the suckling lambs.

Goats do not seem to be as robust as sheep, require more careful handling and have a greater need for effective postoperative analgesia to ensure rapid recovery from operation. Postoperative analgesia can be obtained with doses of morphine and pethidine (meperidine), butorphanol or buprenorphine as used in sheep. Many individual goats are much more used to human company than are sheep and seem to derive comfort from the presence of sympathetic people.

PIGS

Anaesthesia for obstetrical procedures in sows is almost completely limited to provision of anaesthesia for caesarean section. The general principles are similar to those in all other species of animal – it is necessary to provide adequate surgical conditions to prevent the sow from experiencing pain and to use a method which produces minimal depression of the piglets. Ideally, both the sow and

piglets should recover from the effects of the anaesthetic in the minimum of time.

Caesarian section may be carried out under conditions which vary from those encountered on the farm to those provided in an operating theatre. Elective caesarian section is carried out more commonly for the production of minimal disease herds of pigs, or gnotobiotic animals for research purposes, than in ordinary farm sows, but is usually performed in well equipped operating theatres.

On the farm, caesarean section is probably best carried out under local or regional analgesia. Although paravertebral blocks are theoretically possible, they are difficult to perform because the thick layer of subcutaneous fat makes palpation of landmarks almost impossible, and infiltration of the line of incision is the method usually employed. Epidural block may also be used (see later).

The major problem is the restraint of the sow and today sedation with azaperone is usually used for this although the drug does cross the placental barrier and the piglets are sleepy when delivered. However, respiratory depression in the offspring seems minimal and if kept warm they usually survive. The sedative effects of azaperone on the sow are rather prolonged and she may not be able to suckle the piglets for some hours; if left unattended with the neonatal piglets she may suffocate some by lying on them. If the sedation produced by azaperone is inadequate, i.v. thiopental or metomidate may be given to effect. This does not appear to add to the depression of the piglets and is preferable to increasing the dose of azaperone. If thiopental or metomidate is used the sow loses control of her airway, so that care must be taken to ensure that respiratory obstruction does not develop. In most animals it is as well to limit the total dose of the i.v. agent to that which just produces immobility and to supplement with some form of local analgesia.

Under conditions encountered in hospitals, techniques are not usually limited by availability and a wide variety of techniques can be employed. The piglets are not always returned to the dam and in these circumstances speed of recovery of the sow is less important than under farm conditions. Surgical sterility is usually vital and the main task of the anaesthetist is to ensure unconsciousness and immobility so that asepsis is not broken by movement of the sow during the operation. The staff and equipment needed for resuscitation of the piglets are usually available but in elective caesarian sections there is always the risk of the delivery of premature young and the resuscitation of these is not always easy.

Probably the most viable piglets are obtained when anaesthesia is induced and maintained with an inhalation anaesthetic and maintained with a high concentration of inspired oxygen. In the majority of sows anaesthesia is rapidly attained with agents such as halothane, isoflurane or enflurane, but if the sow is very large or difficult to handle, a minimal dose of thiopental or propofol can be employed.

Satisfactory results are also achieved by the use of ketamine, usually in combination with diazepam (2 mg/kg i.v.) and atropine (0.03 mg/kg i.v.) followed by i.v. injection of ketamine given to effect. Usually about 5 to 10 mg/kg of ketamine is needed to produce a peculiar state in which the sow appears to be aware of the environment yet does not react to skin incision or other surgical stimulation. If necessary nitrous oxide with or without a more potent inhalation anaesthetic can be used to control any slight restlessness which may occur towards the end of the operation.

Sedative premedication with azaperone followed by induction of anaesthesia with inhalation or intravenous agents (such as medetomidate) has been widely used for elective caesarean section with generally satisfactory results. However, in the authors' experience, there can be no doubt that piglets delivered after the use of this sedative drug are, for some hours, sleepier than if no sedation is employed.

Methods of anaesthesia involving the use of neuromuscular blocking agents result in the delivery of lively piglets and rapid recovery of the sow; they can be used whenever endotracheal intubation and IPPV can be carried out. However, it is essential to ensure that the sow is completely unconscious and it is sometimes difficult to be sure of this without having to administer large doses of anaesthetic or other drugs which will give rise to marked respiratory and central nervous depression in the piglets. Techniques of this nature are,

therefore, best avoided except by the experienced veterinary anaesthetist.

Involution of the uterus after delivery of the piglets may, if the animal is not hypoxic or hypercapnic, be helped by i.v. 2–10 i.u. oxytocin or, if bleeding is a problem i.v. 1.0–1.5 mg ergometrine tartrate, but this latter drug may produce cardiac arrhythmias if the $PaCO_2$ is elevated when it is given.

DOGS

For elective caesarian section to deliver live pups it is essential that the minimum of depressant drugs should be in the pups by the time of their delivery, and that the bitch shall be conscious as soon as possible after operation so that she will accept and be able to look after her offspring. It is also necessary, however, that the bitch shall not appreciate pain during the operation, that the surgeon shall be provided with adequate operating conditions and the bitch with adequate postoperative analgesia. Although there were several studies published prior to 1975 (Wright, 1939; Freak, 1962; Mitchell, 1966; Goodger & Levy, 1973) there have been many new agents introduced since then and there is a tremendous variation in perioperative management. The problems presented and the general principles of management, however, have not changed since the earlier days.

The bitch may be fit and healthy at the time of operation (as she should be for an elective operation) or she may be exhausted from a prolonged obstructed labour. Even after several hours of starvation her stomach may not be empty and if she has already delivered one or more puppies spontaneously *per vaginum* she may have voluntarily ingested placental material. Thus the likelihood of vomiting at induction of general anaesthesia must be recognized as a potential hazard. Premedication with a low dose of morphine (0.1 mg/kg) or papaveretum ('Omnopon' 0.2 mg/kg) will usually provoke vomiting and ensure an empty stomach but may cause some depression in the pups. However, as long as low doses are used this will seldom be a problem and in any case, if it occurs it may be overcome by giving the pups naloxone. There is little quantitative information regarding the dose of naloxone which may be needed but a s.c. dose of 0.04 mg/kg is suggested as being an appropriate initial dose. Similarly, the use of xylazine or medetomidine for their emetic properties may cause prolonged and serious respiratory depression in the offspring but this can be overcome by the use of atipamezole (up to 10 μg/kg s.c.). Sleepiness of the pups caused by premedication of the bitch with acepromazine cannot, however, be counteracted for there is no specific antagonist to the phenothiazine derivatives.

In the supine animal pressure on the caudal vena cava from the gravid uterus causes circulatory disturbances; pressure on the posterior vena cava can interfere with venous return to the heart and result in arterial hypotension. This pressure can be avoided by a wedge of plastic foam material placed under the right side of the supine bitch. Major circulatory changes also occur once intraabdominal pressure has been reduced by removal of the gravid uterus or the pups and the ability of the bitch to compensate for these disturbances may have been reduced by the drugs used for general anaesthesia or the sympathetic blockade induced by some techniques of local analgesia. It is, therefore, advisable to set up an intravenous infusion prior to the induction of anaesthesia and this may be essential if the bitch is already toxic or very exhausted. Respiratory function usually improves greatly after delivery of the puppies and the concentration of any inhalation anaesthetic being administered at this time may need to be reduced if overdose is to be avoided.

Some of the agents used during anaesthesia may interfere with the involution of the uterus. In women, halothane is particularly likely to lead to postoperative uterine haemorrhage after caesarean section but the difference in placental attachment makes this complication much less likely in bitches. Provided the bitch is not hypercapnic an i.v. ecbolic such as oxytocin (2–10 IU), or ergometrine (up to 0.5 mg) depending on the size of the bitch, may be given after delivery of the pups to promote involution of the uterus and control any uterine haemorrhage.

Although there are considerable differences in the rate at which drugs cross the placenta, it is always safest to assume that any drug given to the bitch will exert an influence on the pups in the postdelivery period. As long as the respiratory depression is not too severe the pups will rapidly eliminate any of the less soluble inhalation agents which may have come to them from the mother but elimination of parenterally administered anaesthetic agents may be much more difficult due to the immaturity of the newborn pups' detoxicating mechanisms. For example, it has been estimated that renal function may take as long as 1 to 2 weeks before reaching adult levels (Baggot, 1992).

Anaesthetic-induced depression of the offspring can be avoided by the use of local analgesia. Epidural block is particularly suited to caesarean section but it should only be used in quiet, easily restrained bitches. If heavy sedation is required for the restraint of the animal the pups will be affected and the method will offer no - advantages over a well managed general anaesthetic.

In bitches of reasonable temperament, premedication before general anaesthesia may be limited to an anticholinergic agent, but minimal doses of opiates may be used and if they cause vomiting the stomach should be empty when anaesthesia is induced.

Induction of general anaesthesia with an inhalation agent has the advantage of rapid elimination by the puppies and, when carried out by an experienced anaesthetist, can be both rapid and excitement-free. The main disadvantage of inhalation induction is that vomiting may occur before endotracheal intubation is possible, so suction apparatus should be available to enable the airway to be cleared rapidly if the bitch is unable to do so by coughing. Halothane, enflurane, isoflurane, sevoflurane and desflurane can all be used for caesarian section with satisfactory results but (the now obsolete) methoxyflurane usually produced marked depression of the pups for some time after their delivery.

In large or bad tempered bitches an intravenous agent may be used for induction of anaesthesia. Propofol in doses of 4 to 6 mg/kg is probably the agent of choice but methohexital (up to 2.5 mg/kg) and thiopental (up to 5 mg/kg) can be used without risk of serious depression of the pups. If endotracheal intubation is not possible at these low dosages anaesthesia may be deepened with an inhalation anaesthetic administered by facemask.

When i.v. agents have been used it is advisable to wait a few minutes (about 15 minutes when propofol is used) before delivering the pups in order to allow blood levels of induction agent to decline. Dodman (1979) when reviewing the literature on the subject, pointed out that after a barbiturate induction of anaesthesia there is often sufficient barbiturate remaining to cause considerable depression in the bitch at the time of delivery of the pups, yet the pups are surprisingly lively. Accumulation of the barbiturate in the foetal liver, as shown by Finster *et al.* (1972) or further dilution of the drug before it reaches the foetal brain may explain this. A recent review, together with survival rates for the bitches was published by Moon *et al.* (1998).

Techniques involving the use of neuromuscular blocking agents can be used very satisfactorily for caesarian section, as these drugs do not cross the placenta in sufficient quantities to paralyse the muscles of the offspring. However, there is apparently no real advantage to be gained from the use of neuromuscular blockers.

Where apparatus for the administration of inhalation anaesthesia is not available, serious consideration should be given to the use of light sedation together with some method of local analgesia such as epidural block or local infiltration of the line of incision and topical application of local analgesic to the broad ligaments.

Postoperative pain relief for the bitch is essential but care must be taken to ensure that drugs used for this purpose are not excreted in the milk in concentrations which may affect suckling pups. The provision of adequate pain relief may pose problems when opioid antagonists have been used to produce more rapid awakening of the bitch.

CATS

The requirements of anaesthesia for caesarian section in the cat, and the problems likely to be encountered, are similar to those already discussed above for dogs. Although cats may vomit on induction of anaesthesia, inhalation of vomit is less likely than in bitches for cats have more active laryngeal reflexes. Nevertheless, endotracheal intubation should be carried out as soon as anaesthesia is induced and, when a non-cuffed tube is used, a pharyngeal pack introduced around the tube.

Many cats presented for caesarian section or hysterectomy are carrying dead kittens and the uterus may be infected. Ideally, in such cases a balanced electrolye solution should be infused before anaesthesia is induced but, unless the queen is exhausted or otherwise very ill, this is often delayed until after careful anaesthetic induction.

Premedication before caesarian section is usually limited to the administration of anticholinergics, and an inhalation induction of anaesthesia with low-solubility agents leads to the quickest recovery of both mother and kittens. With care, such an induction can be smooth, but many anaesthetists prefer to induce unconsciousness with small doses of thiopental, methohexital, propofol or Saffan before going on to the inhalation anaesthetic. Only minimal quantities of any intravenous agent should be used and inhalation agents should be employed to maintain the lightest possible levels of anaesthesia.

If total i.v. anaesthesia has to be used for caesarian section, Saffan is probably the best available. Although the Saffan steroids cross the placental barrier and will affect the kittens, no noticeable respiratory depression results. If it is necessary to use Saffan alone for this operation it is probable that it should be used in conjunction with local analgesia so that the lightest levels of general anaesthesia can be employed.

Diazepam or midazolam with ketamine (<5 mg/kg) can be used for induction of anaesthesia but in general neuroleptanalgesic methods are contraindicated in cats and after ketamine recovery is too prolonged if the offspring are alive and need maternal care soon after delivery. The advent of medetomidine, however, has changed this situation in that after its use for premedication (in doses of up to 80 μg/kg) the dose of ketamine can be reduced to low levels (< 2 mg/kg), while the effects of medetomidine itself can be antagonized with atipamezole.

Epidural analgesia can provide excellent analgesia and muscle relaxation, but in cats the need for deep sedation to control the head end of the animal severely limits its usefulness. All sedatives in current use will depress the kittens and their condition will be no better than after well-administered general anaesthesia.

Maternal postoperative analgesia may be provided by the use of small doses of morphine (0.05 mg/kg i.m.), i.m. pethidine (meperidine) 10 mg/kg, or butorphanol (0.2 mg/kg). Any suckling kittens must be carefully watched for signs of undue sleepiness that indicate high drug levels in the mother's milk.

REFERENCES

Baggot, J.D. (1992) Drug therapy in the neonatal animal. In: *Principles of Drug Disposition in Domestic Animals: the Basis of Veterinary Clinical Pharmacology.* Philadelphia: W.B. Saunders.

Dodman, N.H. (1979) Anaesthesia for caesarian section in the dog and cat: a revision. *Journal of Small Animal Practice* **20**: 449–460.

Finster, M., Morishima, H.O., Mark, L.C., Perel, J.M, Dayton, P.G. and James, L.S. (1972) Thiopental concentrations in the fetus and newborn. *Anesthesiology* **36**: 155–158.

Freak, M.J. (1962) Abnormal conditions associated with pregnancy and parturition in the bitch. *Veterinary Record* **74**: 1323–1325.

Goodger, W.J. and Levy, W. (1973) Anaesthetic management of caesarean section. *Veterinary Clinics of North America: Small Animal Practice* **3**: 85–99.

Mitchell, B. (1966) Anaesthesia for caesarean section and factors influencing mortality rates of bitches and puppies. *Veterinary Record* **79**: 252–257.

Moon, P.F., Erb, H.N., Ludders, J.W., Gleed, R.D. and Pascoe, P.J. (1998) Perioperative management and mortality rates of dogs undergoing cesarian section in the United States and Canada. *Journal of the American Veterinary Medical Association* **213**: 365–369.

Wright, J.G. (1939) Caesarian hysterotomy-hysterectomy. *Veterinary Record* **51**: 1331–1346.

Intrathoracic surgery

19

INTRODUCTION

The anaesthetic management of the pneumothorax created by the wide opening of the chest wall and/or diaphragm for surgical access to the contents of the thoracic cavity involves 'controlled respiration' or 'IPPV' (Chapter 8). Although in veterinary practice ventilation of the lungs by manual squeezing of the reservoir bag of the anaesthetic breathing circuit is still carried out in centres where little intrathoracic surgery is undertaken, or where neuromuscular blocking drugs are seldom used, the use of mechanical ventilators is now widespread. Surgeons find it easier to work with the regular movement produced by these devices and their use makes it possible to stabilize the tidal and minute volumes of respiration, the airway pressures and the duration of the inspiratory and expiratory periods, in a way which cannot be achieved by manual 'bag squeezing'. Apart from the fact that IPPV is obligatory while the pleural cavity is open to the atmosphere, the actual anaesthetic methods employed for intrathoracic surgery are largely governed by the personal preferences and experience of the anaesthetist. The main anaesthetic problems centre around the elimination of any pneumothorax remaining after closure of the thoracotomy incision and here the close cooperation between the surgeon and anaesthetist is essential for their satisfactory resolution.

CLOSURE OF THE CHEST

The anaesthetic technique used while the chest is being closed varies with the nature of the operation but should always include drainage of the pleural cavity. In the past, after a limited operation not involving injury to the lung the chest was often closed without drainage. An attempt was made to achieve full re-expansion of any collapsed area of the lung tissue and to maintain full control of the breathing with the lungs held in full expansion as the last suture was tied to make the chest airtight. Sometimes a cannula was left in the pleural cavity until the thoracotomy wound was completely closed and this cannula was withdrawn quickly while the lungs were held in what was presumed to be full expansion. However, the methods employed never succeeded in removing all the residual air from the pleural cavity, portions of the lung remained collapsed and often became a focus of infection. The air trapped in the pleural cavity caused movements of the chest wall to be transmitted to the lung by negative intrapleural pressure and pleural exudation occurred as a result of this.

Proper drainage of the pleural cavity with removal of all the residual air overcomes all of these problems but if, on occasion, the chest has to be closed without drainage the amount of air trapped in the pleural cavity can be minimized by inserting a catheter through an intercostal space and applying suction after the chest wall is closed. The catheter is then pulled out with a sharp tug. Alternatively, when the thoracotomy wound has been closed a large-bore catheter connected to a suction apparatus is introduced into the pleural cavity and suction applied until there is a negative pressure present in the system. The catheter may become blocked by the lung and the method is therefore not very satisfactory. It is, however, commonly used in cats where, after closure of the thorax, a 13 swg intravenous catheter may be introduced into the pleural cavity, the needle part being withdrawn after penetration of the skin and the blunt ended catheter forced through the intercostal muscles and parietal pleura.

When there is any risk of injury to the lung which could cause a leak, or there is any likelihood of continuing haemorrhage into the pleural cavity the chest *must* be drained. Underwater drainage is undoubtedly the most reliable and informative procedure and for this the drain tube is connected to a container of water or a weak aqueous solution of chlorhexidine. The drain tube dips about 2.5 cm below the surface of the fluid and should have an internal diameter of about 0.5 cm. The container must have an internal diameter of not less than 15 cm. The system acts as a non-return valve and allows air or fluid to be expelled from the pleural cavity but prevents the indrawing of air during inspiration. When the closure of the chest is complete, inflation of the lung, or spontaneous respiratory movements of the animal, forces air out of the pleural cavity whenever the pressure in the pleural sac is greater than about 2.5 cmH$_2$O (0.25 kPa), i.e. the depth which the tube dips below the surface of the water. Provided that the container is kept at least 80 cm below the level of the animal's body, water cannot be aspirated into the chest, for no effort of the animal can lift the water up this distance. The large diameter of the container should ensure that no matter how high the level rises in the tube the end of the tube will always be below the fluid surface (Fig. 19.1).

When the animal breathes spontaneously the water level in the drainage tube rises on inspiration (as the cavity between the lung and chest wall increases) and falls on expiration. When the lung occupies the whole of the pleural space the pressure does not show marked fluctuations

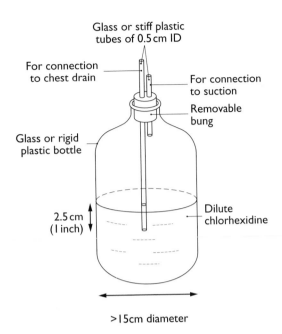

FIG. 19.1 Underwater-seal drain bottle. The bottle, tubing and bung can be autoclaved before use or the whole apparatus may be purchased, sterile and ready for use from a commercial source.

during the respiratory cycle. If, however, the lung is not fully expanded large variations of pressure occur. Observation of the water level in the glass or transparent plastic tube thus provides useful information as to the state of expansion of the lungs – the greater the amplitude of the swing of the water level in the tube the poorer is the expansion of the lung. The drain should be allowed to remain in the pleural cavity until the lung is fully expanded as shown by minimal amplitude of the swing with a completely unobstructed drain. It is then pulled out with a sharp tug during expiration, and a skin suture, which has been laid for the purpose, tied tightly to occlude the hole in the skin.

After any operation which has involved stripping of the visceral layer of the pleura there will be an air leak from the raw surface of the lung. In such circumstances suction may have to be applied to the far side of the underwater seal apparatus to control the pneumothorax. This suction must be maintained until there is no bubbling of air, indicating that the leak has been sealed off by inflammatory reaction. It may not be possible to remove the drain for up to 48 hours after operation and during this time the animal must be kept well sedated. Experience has shown that in cats this sedation is best achieved by the use of Saffan given either as a continuous infusion or by intermittent injection, while in dogs combinations of morphine and diazepam give excellent results particularly when combined with the instillation of 3 to 5 ml/10 kg of 0.25 % bupivacaine into the pleural cavity. Whatever sedation and analgesia is used it is important that restlessness is overcome without at the same time producing respiratory depression. After any thoracotomy the animal must be examined both physically and radiologically for evidence of lung collapse. Collapse of a lung, or of a lobe of a lung, may necessitate immediate intrabronchial suction to remove any material occluding the bronchus to the lung or lobe. Whenever possible, an immediate postoperative chest radiograph should be taken to confirm full expansion of the lungs, the absence of pneumothorax and the position of any drainage tubes. It also serves as a reference against which later films can be assessed.

The drain can be used in any animal and sterile units ready for connection to the pleural catheter are commercially available. The outlet tube from the air above the surface of the liquid in the container can be connected to a source of suction. Suction is usually only necessary when there is a continuous air leak in the thoracic cavity but, if the leak is gross, the application of suction can be life-saving. Suction must be provided from a high-volume, low-pressure apparatus.

For horses, cattle, sheep, goats, pigs and ambulant large dogs it is sometimes more convenient to use a Heimlich valve (Fig. 19.2). These are also available from commercial sources. This valve should be attached to the animal's chest wall by a skin suture and drain tubes tied tightly to the valve inlet – a Y-piece can be used if more than one drain is in use. The Heimlich valve gives no indication as to the state of expansion of the lungs and regular, frequent inspection is needed to check that it is working properly.

All drainage tubes introduced into the pleural cavity should be of adequate bore and made from siliconized material which does not soften too much at body temperature. Small-bore chest drains are almost worse than useless – they occlude

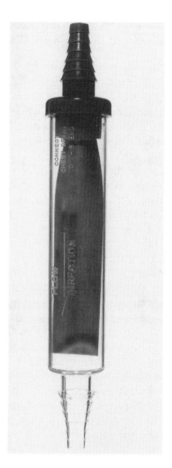

FIG. 19.2 Heimlich chest drain valve.

easily if they become slightly kinked around a rib and are readily blocked by the expanded lung or a small blood clot. For cats a 2.5 mm internal bore tube is the narrowest which should be used, but even in the smallest of dogs and puppies 7.5 mm bore diameter tubing should be used. Commercially available, sterile chest drainage tubes are designed for use in man and may have more side holes than the one or two convenient for use in small animals.

Dogs and cats can be turned from side to side to promote drainage of either air or blood but in large animals such as horses it is often necessary to insert two chest drains – one ventrally for the drainage of blood and one dorsally for the drainage of air. These can be connected through a Y-tube to a Heimlich drain (Fig. 19.3).

The time for removal of the drain should be a matter for consultation between the surgeon and

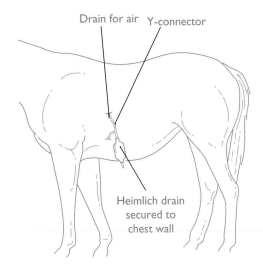

FIG. 19.3 Two chest drains for blood or fluid drains connected to a Heimlich valve by a Y-piece connector for drainage of both air and fluid from a standing horse.

anaesthetist. It is essential that it should be removed as soon as it is of no further use but should a pleural effusion or pneumothorax develop after it has been taken out, another intercostal drain should be introduced immediately under local infiltration analgesia.

ANAESTHETIC MANAGEMENT FOR SPECIFIC SURGICAL PROCEDURES

SIMPLE THORACOTOMY FOR NON-PULMONARY LESIONS

Thoracotomies for most non-pulmonary lesions present few special problems. Large neoplasms within the thorax can cause an animal considerable respiratory difficulty but removal of the space-occupying lesions eases the respiration at once. In removing some of the more extensive mediastinal tumours the surgeon may open both pleural cavities but with the maintenance of controlled ventilation no trouble is encountered during operation. Carcinomata of the bronchi may release catecholamines when manipulated by the surgeon. It may be necessary to drain both pleural cavities and the two intercostal drains can be connected to the same underwater seal or Heimlich drain by a Y-connector.

OESOPHAGEAL SURGERY

The problems in oesophageal surgery arise from the danger of regurgitation of food and/or saliva which have been retained in the oesophagus. Prompt endotracheal intubation in the prone animal with the head raised will usually prevent this mishap from occurring. Thoracotomy for oesophageal surgery presents no special anaesthetic problems that have not already been discussed.

REPAIR OF RUPTURES OF THE DIAPHRAGM

Although the majority of diaphragmatic ruptures are best repaired through an abdominal incision the pleural cavity is, of course, opened to the atmosphere during the course of the operation. The anaesthetic management of these cases is not always easy.

Diaphragmatic rupture produces respiratory inefficiency which results both from reduced breathing capacity and from an unbalanced distribution of blood and air within the lungs. The presence of abdominal viscera and effusion within the chest reduces the vital capacity; the absence of displacement of effective diaphragmatic movement limits the enlargement of the thoracic cavity. Twisting or displacement of the lung lobes causes partial obstruction of the bronchi, leading to the uneven distribution of the inspired air. The blood passing through overventilated areas of the lung will lose more CO_2 than it would under normal conditions, but cannot become more than fully oxygenated. In the under ventilated areas of lung both O_2 uptake and CO_2 elimination are impaired. Because of these effects the mixed blood returning from the lungs to the systemic circulation usually has a $PaCO_2$ near to normal, but its PaO_2 is low, i.e. the main threat to the animal's life is hypoxia. Anything which distresses the animal and thus increases its O_2 requirements may prove fatal. When most of the thoracic cavity is occupied by abdominal viscera and/or effusion, the animal can only survive by making maximal breathing efforts and the use of respiratory depressant sedative or analgesic drugs is most unwise. Heavy sedation for diagnostic radiography is particularly contraindicated. In dogs, phenothiazine ataractics like acepromazine together with small doses of an opioid such as pethidine (meperidine) generally produce sufficient, safe sedation, and in cats small (10 mg) doses of pethidine are useful. All animals must be kept under close observation after any sedative or analgesic premedication to detect the development of respiratory distress.

Anaesthesia for animals with diaphragmatic rupture may be managed in a variety of ways. No hard and fast rules can be given and each individual case must be treated on its own merits. All cases must be handled very quietly and gently before anaesthesia is induced, and a smooth induction of anaesthesia with an intravenous agent is advisable. Some animals do not resent the application of a face-mask on or near the face and they may usefully be given oxygen to inhale for 2 to 3 minutes before the induction of anaesthesia ('preoxygenation'). In dogs, whenever it can be done without undue disturbance of the animal, an intravenous fluid infusion should be set up before anaesthesia, otherwise it is set up as soon as possible during the course of the operation. This drip is often needed to remedy the fall in arterial blood pressure seen when re-expansion of the lungs alters the haemodynamic state of the body (presumably due to the re-opening of areas of the pulmonary vascular bed). Endotracheal intubation is, of course, essential in all cases.

At the end of the operation no attempt should be made to forcibly expand regions of lung tissue which have been in a collapsed state for more than a day, for this leads to pulmonary oedema. The use of a chest drain allows some over expansion of healthy, non-collapsed lung to fill the pleural cavity and encourages collapsed regions to re-expand over a period of time. Chest drainage also allows removal from the pleural cavity of fluid which often appears in the first 24 to 48 hours of the postoperative period.

Postoperative pain, which limits breathing to rapid, very shallow movements of the chest wall, is best controlled by the injection of pethidine or morphine, given as required, in doses appropriate for the size and species of animal concerned. Infiltration of the abdominal incision with 0.25 % bupivacaine is also very effective in alleviating pain.

THORACOTOMY FOR PULMONARY SURGERY

One of the major problems in pulmonary surgery is the prevention of spillage of secretions or pus from the affected part to the remainder of the lung. In man this problem is overcome by drainage or isolation of the affected part of the lung with some form of blocker (usually incorporating a tube for drainage) or, alternatively, endobronchial tubes, either single or double lumen, provide means of protecting the sound lung which can then be ventilated selectively. In animals, due to the shape of the chest and bronchial tree, most of these techniques are impossible and reliance has to be placed on preoperative preparation with antimicrobials and expectorants to make the lung relatively 'dry'. Non-irritating anaesthetic agents also play a part in reducing the volume of secretions, while any remaining can be removed by bronchoscopic aspiration carried out at frequent intervals through the endotracheal tube.

During lobectomy or pneumonectomy, ventilation after severance of the bronchus and prior to its closure presents surprisingly little difficulty and although IPPV results in some frothing of blood this does not usually obscure the surgeon's view of the bronchial stump. Should it prove to be impossible to obtain adequate lung expansion while the bronchus is wide open the surgeon may be asked to occlude the bronchial opening with a finger or thumb while the lung is inflated between the laying of bronchial sutures. Provided the minute volume is kept constant the removal of a lobe or even of one lung does not result in a significant rise in $PaCO_2$ and indeed the $PaCO_2$ may actually fall, indicating an improvement in the dead space/tidal volume ratio. There is usually a fall in $PaCO_2$ as soon as the chest is opened and measures which have been recommended to minimize patchy alveolar collapse during constant minute volume IPPV, such as intermittent manual hyperinflation and continuous manual inflation, are quite ineffective and may be harmful. The PaO_2 usually remains above 80 mmHg (10.6 kPa) when the inspired gases contain at least 50% of oxygen even when only one lung is available for ventilation.

Frequent suction is needed to clear the bronchial tree in bronchiectasis cases and the use of halothane/oxygen or isoflurane/oxygen without nitrous oxide has been found to be advantageous in avoiding hypoxaemia when ventilation of the lungs is interrupted for the passage of the suction catheter. Oxygenation by diffusion continues when ventilation is stopped at the end of inspiration but the $PaCO_2$ rises until ventilation recommences.

In certain cases, such as operations for the removal of congenital cysts of the lung, it is advisable to allow spontaneous respiration to continue until the pleural cavity is opened. This avoids the risk of overdistension of the cysts with collapse of normal lung tissue.

Replacement of blood loss during the operation and the maintenance of fluid balance should follow the usual practice for major surgery but after the removal of lung tissue animals seem to make better progress if they are slightly short of fluid. Over-transfusion with blood or the administration of excessive amounts of other fluids is associated with pulmonary oedema and this is particularly disastrous after resection of any significant amounts of lung tissue. It should be noted that in dogs, traction on the hilum of the lung can cause arterial hypotension; this is not an indication for the administration of fluids – blood pressure returns quickly to normal when traction ceases.

Postoperatively, animals which have had a lung lobe removed should be nursed lying on the sound side until they are able to sit up; this encourages re-expansion of lung remaining on the side of operation and facilitates drainage of any pneumothorax. After pneumonectomy the animal should be nursed on the side of operation. The first dose of postoperative sedative analgesic should be given intravenously in order that the patient's needs may be more accurately assessed. A routine chest radiograph is advisable before removal of the intercostal drainage tube but it must be recognized that positioning for this may distress the animal and under these circumstances it may be necessary to rely upon auscultation of lung sounds to check that the lungs are fully expanded. Instillation of 3 to 5 ml/10 kg of 0.25 % bupivacaine into the pleural cavity on the operated side will usually provide most useful postoperative analgesia for up to 6 hours.

CARDIAC SURGERY

Cardiac surgery involves more than simple thoracotomy. The drugs used may affect the heart and alter the vascular tone generally. Equally, disorders of the circulatory system may modify the absorption, excretion and action of anaesthetic drugs. The problems that arise are often peculiar to each lesion but certain general principles of anaesthetic management can be enunciated.

All animals should be handled quietly to avoid excitement and reduce the effect on the heart of endogenous catecholamine secretion. A *small* dose of acepromazine is often valuable to calm and facilitate handling of all species of animal.

If an i.v. agent is to be used for the induction of anaesthesia two points must be noted. First, slowing of the circulation due to the disease process causes a considerable lag between the administration of the drug and the development of its effect. This makes it very easy to give too much, for it may give the impression of drug resistance. Secondly, these drugs may depress the myocardium and produce peripheral vasodilatation. In animals where cardiac output is fixed (e.g. by valvular stenoses), the vasodilatation may produce a very marked fall in arterial blood pressure. The i.v. drug should always be administered very slowly and in very dilute solutions. However, clinical experience indicated that the dangers of i.v. drugs have been overemphasized. The quiet, smooth induction of anaesthesia more than makes up for its supposed disadvantages which are, in any case, much less obvious with the small doses needed in properly premedicated patients.

Provided it does not excite the animal, O_2 should be administered through a face-mask before anaesthesia is induced, but in every case it should be given as soon as consciousness is lost. A perfect airway is always essential and a large-bore endotracheal tube must be introduced as soon as possible.

Pericarditis and cardiac tamponade are very crippling conditions because they limit the cardiac output and depress tissue respiration by the widespread action of raised venous pressure. Associated ascites and pleural effusions reduce the vital capacity and venous back pressure may damage the liver. Careful preanaesthetic preparation of these cases is necessary. Pleural and peritoneal effusions must be tapped and fluid retention reduced by the use of diuretics. Cardiac tamponade must be relieved by paracentesis under local infiltration analgesia.

Much has been written concerning anaesthesia of healthy animals of various species for experimental cardiac surgery but little of this is relevant to clinical veterinary practice. Clinical cases presented for cardiac surgery for the correction of acquired or congenital lesions almost invariably have circulatory disturbances which complicate their management, and in many, failure of medical treatment is the reason why operation is contemplated. Few veterinary centres will ever receive enough cases to enable the expertise necessary for their successful treatment to be developed and the assistance of an experienced medical cardiac surgery team should be sought to give the animal the best chance of survival. However, some of the simpler lesions may be amenable to correction under moderate hypothermia by veterinary surgical teams. Even when cardiopulmonary bypass techniques involving an expert medical perfusionist are needed it is usual for a veterinary anaesthetist to be involved in the patient's general management. The veterinary clinical anaesthetist should, therefore, be familiar with the principles of bypass techniques, and of moderate hypothermia, for circulatory arrest.

It is probable that most cardiac surgery will be carried out in dogs and the techniques of anaesthesia used in these animals will be described below. They are not difficult to adapt for other species of animal should the need arise. It must be emphasized, however, that in veterinary practice cardiac surgery is seldom likely to be an economic proposition and it is often undertaken out of an academic interest in the advancement of knowledge relating to circulatory disorders generally.

Ultrasonography

This technique of investigation can be carried out without risk to an animal that can be handled quietly and the administration of drugs is usually quite unnecessary.

Cardiac catheterization

Most animals presented for cardiac surgery are first investigated by cardiac catheterization.

Radiopaque catheters, visible by fluoroscopy, can be advanced from a peripheral vein into the right heart and pulmonary artery. By wedging the tip in a pulmonary artery, an indication of left atrial pressure can be obtained. In addition, a needle connected to a fine tube can be passed through the catheter when it is in the right atrium to pierce the atrial septum and measure the pressure in the left atrium directly. The left ventricle can be entered directly if a catheter is introduced from a peripheral artery.

Information is obtained by pressure measurement, by measurement of cardiac output and by blood gas analysis on samples of blood taken from known positions of the catheter tip. Angiography is usually carried out on the same occasion using large film rapid changers or cineradiography. Anaesthesia must not interfere with any of these diagnostic procedures.

After full premedication anaesthesia may be induced by the careful i.v. injection of small doses of thiopentone, diazepam/ketamine, or midazolam/propofol, followed by i.v. pancuronium, atracurium or vecuronium, and endotracheal intubation as soon as relaxation of the jaw muscles is obtained. To maintain blood gases as near normal as possible, IPPV is carried out with gas mixtures containing 20% O_2 in such a way as to maintain the $PaCO_2$ between 35 and 40 mmHg (4.7 and 5.3 kPa). The use of IPPV overcomes alterations of PaO_2 which may result in an uncontrolled way when the animal is breathing spontaneously. The procedure is usually undertaken in a darkened room and the wise anaesthetist withdraws briefly during the radiation period.

Cardiac catheterization is not without risk. Severe arrhythmias and circulatory instability are relatively common. The anaesthetist must be prepared to deal with these as they arise, for example by giving 1–2 mg/kg of lignocaine (lidocaine) i.v. as a bolus to treat tachyarrhythmias.

Hypothermia

Provided that it has no work to do, heart muscle itself is not harmed by short periods of circulatory arrest but brain cells are extremely sensitive to oxygen lack and at normal body temperatures of 37–38 °C cannot survive if the circulation stops for more than 3 to 5 minutes. Reducing the temperature of brain cells depresses their metabolism and enables them to withstand the effects of longer periods of circulatory arrest. For example, at 30 °C the brain will survive and function after a circulatory arrest of 10 minutes.

Body temperature measurement

During the rapidly changing conditions of body cooling and rewarming associated with hypothermia techniques, a temperature measurement made in the mouth or rectum fails to provide an adequate index of temperature in other regions of the body. There is ample evidence, however, that the oesophageal temperature at heart level is a most reliable measure of heart and blood temperature. For this reason a suitable calibrated thermometer probe introduced correctly into the oesophagus, should always be used for temperature measurement.

Reactions to cold

The reactions of the body in response to chilling were well described many years ago by Dripps (1956). In a conscious animal cutaneous vasoconstriction is the first reaction of the body to a cold environment. Adrenaline (epinephrine) is released from the adrenal glands and this, besides causing vasoconstriction, stimulates cellular metabolism mobilizing glycogen and increasing heat production. Other responses include release of thyrotrophic hormone and adrenal corticoids, both of which result in greater heat production. If these reactions prove insufficient to maintain normal body temperature shivering occurs and a tremendous increase in heat production results. Shivering is by far the most effective means of maintaining body temperature.

As the body cools, the heart rate slows and it is about halved when body temperature reaches 25 °C. This slowing is apparently due to cooling of the pacemaker and is accompanied by a prolongation of systole and isometric contraction. Changes in the ECG include prolongation of the P–R interval and a lengthening of the QRS complex. Elevation of the S–T segment or the appearance of a wave rising steeply from the S wave heralds the onset of ventricular fibrillation. The onset of ventricular fibrillation during hypothermia is influenced by a number of factors:

1. The type of anaesthesia.
2. Mechanical stimulation. Stimulation of the heart by catheters in the ventricles or by surgical manipulations may induce fibrillation.
3. Under-ventilation of the lungs, with a consequent rise in $PaCO_2$ and a fall in pH, predisposes to fibrillation.
4. Changes in ionic equilibrium of the blood. The relative concentrations of potassium and calcium are particularly important here.
5. Sympathetic discharge. There is some evidence suggesting that blocking sympathetic nerves to the heart protects this organ from fibrillation under hypothermia.
6. Blood pressure. Abrupt falls in ABP giving rise to decreased coronary blood flow can, during hypothermia, precipitate ventricular fibrillation.

The blood flow in the brain, kidney and splanchnic region is reduced as body temperature falls. The femoral vascular bed dilates down to oesophageal temperatures of about 34 °C, then vasoconstriction occurs and later at 20–25 °C a second vasodilatation takes place. One of the common uses of hypothermia is in circumstances requiring clamping of the aorta for a considerable time. After occlusion lasting more than about 30 minutes, the vasodilatation which follows the release of the clamp is large and lasts as long when the body is cold as when it is warm. Vasoconstrictor substances or blood transfusion may be necessary to counteract this effect.

A fall in body and brain temperature results in a decrease in cerebral oxygen consumption. At 25 °C brain O_2 uptake is about one-third of that at 37 °C and over this range O_2 consumption is a linear function of temperature. A matter of major importance is the degree of protection afforded to nervous tissue from the effects of circulatory arrest by hypothermia. At 25 °C the circulation can be stopped for 15 minutes without apparent damage to brain cells and for various reasons this time of 15 minutes seems to be maximum which can be achieved by surface cooling (between 28 and 25 °C the incidence of ventricular fibrillation rises steeply). The EEG begins to change as body temperature falls to 36–34 °C. The potential recorded shows a decreased amplitude and large δ-waves appear, particularly in the frontal area, at about 30 °C. The electrical activity then declines until between 18 and 20 °C no activity is recorded.

Moderate hypothermia has several potentially harmful effects (Deakin *et al.*, 1988). The O_2 dissociation curve is shifted to the left resulting in an increased affinity of haemoglobin for O_2 at a given partial pressure of O_2. This reduced O_2 delivery to tissues is partly offset by an increase in free dissolved O_2 by as much as 20% at 30 °C. Hypothermia increases muscle tone and, at moderate degrees of hypothermia, will trigger shivering which can increase O_2 consumption several fold but is prevented by the use of neuromuscular blocking drugs.

Techniques for the production of hypothermia

Techniques for producing hypothermia include body surface cooling, body cavity cooling, intragastric cooling and blood stream cooling.

Before hypothermia can be produced by surface cooling the animal's natural defences to cold must be obtunded. Otherwise, attempts to reduce body temperature are likely to increase rather than reduce cellular metabolism. The efficacy of body surface cooling therefore depends on maintaining a coincident vasodilatation of the superficial blood vessels and preventing shivering. Fortunately, the anaesthetic agents which affect one reaction generally modify the other. Chlorpromazine hydrochloride appears to be the best drug to produce vasodilatation and prevent shivering; acepromazine does not seem to result in the production of as marked cutaneous vasodilatation. Once anaesthesia is induced neuromuscular blocking drugs can be given to make shivering impossible.

Hypothermia by body surface cooling is induced by immersing the animal in a water bath at 15 to 20 °C and circulating the water around the body while the trunk and limbs are massaged to maintain the cutaneous circulation. The animal is removed from the bath when the oesophageal temperature is about 30 °C and dried with towels. One of the principal dangers of body surface cooling by this immersion method is the 'after-drop' when the animal has been removed from the bath.

The 'after-drop' reduces oesophageal temperature by up to 2 °C and it is important to allow for this because ventricular fibrillation is common at temperatures below 28 °C. The 'after-drop' occurs because when the animal is removed from the bath the skin and neighbouring tissues are extremely cold. In fact they are much colder than the circulating blood and as the blood reaches these parts it continues to cool long after active cooling measures have been stopped.

In many cases the animal has rewarmed sufficiently by the end of the operation but if it has not done so it may be partially immersed in a bath of warm water. If surgery is not complete, anaesthesia may be continued when the body temperature is above 35 °C.

Surface body cooling is a messy, inconvenient procedure, but it does not involve use of any complicated apparatus and it can be applied by even inexperienced personnel with a fair degree of safety to animals of below about 70 kg.

Intragastric cooling is a slower but much more sophisticated process. A very good, relatively inexpensive apparatus utilizes an intragastric balloon which is introduced into the stomach via the oesophagus after the induction of general anaesthesia. Cold water is circulated through this balloon and reduction of body temperature to below 28–29 °C usually takes some 1 to 2 hours. This may seem a relatively long time but during the cooling process ECG leads and blood pressure transducers can easily be attached and vascular cannulations made while the surgical procedure is started. Rewarming can be commenced at any time during surgery (without interrupting its progress) by circulating warm water through the balloon, and rewarming is more rapid than can be achieved by any other method.

Bloodstream cooling is normally regarded as being part of the cardiopulmonary bypass technique but hypothermia can be produced in this way with relatively simple equipment. An external circuit containing a transfusion warming coil and a roller peristaltic pump is primed with a plasma substitute such as Haemaccel and the coil is immersed in a bath of water maintained at 4–5 °C. Cannulae are inserted into the animal's femoral or carotid artery and femoral or jugular vein and the animal is given 3 mg/kg heparin (using heparin without a preservative). The cannulae are then connected to the external circuit so that arterial blood is run through the coil and pumped back into the vein. The animal cools quite rapidly and the external circulation is stopped when the desired oesophageal temperature has been reached. Heparin has a half-life of about 1 hour and to maintain heparinization of the animal it is necessary to give half the initial dose for each hour of operation.

Rewarming can easily be achieved by recommencing the external circulation with the water in the water bath maintained at 40 °C. Once the animal has rewarmed the external circulation is stopped and the heparinization reversed by the administration of protamine sulphate at the rate of 1.5 to 2.0 times the initial dose of heparin.

Technique of cardiopulmonary bypass

Cardiopulmonary bypass enables the heart and lungs to be excluded from the circulation while an adequate blood supply to the rest of the body is maintained. In order to exclude the heart and lungs from the circulation, the vena cavae or the right atrium are cannulated and the blood is allowed to flow through these cannulae to the pump-oxygenator or 'heart-lung' machine. Having passed through the oxygenator to a reservoir it is pumped back into the circulation via a cannula in either the aorta, or carotid or femoral artery. The heart-lung machine is provided with a means of altering the temperature of the blood being returned to the patient as required by the circumstances (e.g. cooling during the bypass procedure, or rewarming at the end of bypass). It is also provided with a number of pumps which are used to aspirate blood from the heart cavities and pericardium for return to the patient's circulation via the oxygenator during the bypass procedure.

The pumps used for heart-lung machines are usually roller pumps which occlude and milk siliconized tubing against a track and thus cause the blood contained in the tubing to flow along it. The mechanical part of the pump does not come into contact with the blood and this minimizes haemolysis.

Modern oxygenators are designed to expose a thin film of blood to a flowing gas mixture separated from it by a plastic film. This allows oxygenation to take place and carbon dioxide to be removed with minimal blood damage. Whatever the actual design, the gas input is usually a mixture of O_2 and CO_2 at a flow adjusted to maintain satisfactory levels of gaseous exchange. The machines must, of necessity, have a large surface area for gaseous exchange and this leads to considerable cooling of the blood so some form of heat exchanger is always incorporated in the design.

In order that blood may be pumped through the heart-lung machine without clotting the patient must be anticoagulated with heparin before bypass. The management of the anticoagulation is greatly assisted by the use of the activated clotting time (ACT) where 2–3 ml of blood are added to 12 mg celite which reduces the normal whole blood clotting time to 90–130 s. Adequate heparinization is achieved by prolonging the ACT to at least three times baseline levels. At the end of the procedure heparinization is reversed with protamine sulphate given carefully to avoid undesirable side effects such as hypotension.

Before the patient can be connected to the heart-lung machine air must be excluded from the system by filling with fluid ('priming of the system'). A typical prime allows the administration of 30 to 50 ml/kg of 5% dextrose or Ringer's lactate solution from the circuit to the patient when bypass commences. The resulting haemodilution reduces the viscosity of the blood and enables better body perfusion to be achieved. The high flow rates used today in cardiopulmonary bypass and meticulous attention to blood replacement prevent any acidosis from suboptimal perfusion of some tissues developing, so that it is not necessary to administer sodium bicarbonate to correct acidosis at the end of the procedure.

Anaesthesia for open heart surgery may be administered in many ways and it is probable that each centre carrying out this type of surgery has its own favoured technique. All methods are chosen to cause minimal changes in heart rate or blood pressure, and to have no direct depressant effect on the myocardium. Recently, the technique of low flow cardiopulmonary bypass in small dogs has been recorded (Lew *et al.*, 1997) with 6 out of 6 dogs being successfully weaned from bypass.

Premedication consists of administering effective doses of sedative drugs. Agents such as diazepam, midazolam, morphine, hyoscine and papaveretum may be used in full doses and often a small dose of atropine is included with them. Heavy sedation helps to allay fear, induction of anaesthesia is smoother and total drug dosage during anaesthesia is reduced. It is probable that propofol is the best induction agent, administered until the eyelash reflex is just abolished. Some small reduction of arterial pressure occurs but is seldom of significance if the rate of administration of the intravenous agent is slow. IPPV is commenced after injection of a neuromuscular blocking drug (e.g. atracurium, vecuronium), has abolished spontaneous breathing.

An intraoesophageal thermometer probe is placed middle of the thoracic oesophagus and other temperature probes are placed in the nasopharynx and on the tympanic membrane. An i.v. infusion is established and closed bladder drainage is set up with a self-retaining urinary catheter or, in male animals, with a catheter retained in position with a stitch. A catheter for arterial pressure monitoring is introduced and another for CVP measurement is passed via the jugular vein. ECG leads using needle electrodes are attached and the ECG is monitored continuously thereafter. The arterial and venous catheters are attached to their respective manometer lines, including 3–way taps for easy withdrawal of blood samples.

For the maintenance of anaesthesia IPPV is usual with minimal infusions of propofol (2.5 to 3.0 mg/kg) which can be added to the pump-oxygenator during total bypass. During total bypass lung ventilation is stopped and the lungs held at an airway pressure of about 10 cmH2O (1 kPa) to prevent collapse. Typically, the oxygenator gases consist of 97% O_2 with 3% CO_2 and an inhalation agent such as isoflurane or halothane may be included to assist in vasodilatation. Nitrous oxide is usually reintroduced for IPPV after coming off bypass as soon as the arterial blood saturation is satisfactory.

In addition to the management of anaesthesia, the anaesthetist plays an important role in monitoring respiratory and circulatory function and the correction of any departures from optimum as may occur. The preperfusion period is often the most hazardous. The heart lesion is uncorrected and induction of anaesthesia may produce a further deterioration in the animal's condition. When the mediastinum is opened and the heart and great vessels are manipulated by the surgeon the effectiveness of the heart's action may be temporarily impaired. Arrhythmias are easily provoked by contact between the heart and suction catheters and swabs or retractors may obstruct the venous return or the flow in the pulmonary artery. Constant observation of the arterial pressure wave-forms as displayed on an oscilloscope, and of the ECG are, therefore, essential. Before going on bypass the surgeon may have to be asked to stop activities until the heart has recovered normal rhythm.

Arrhythmias of all kinds may be seen, but are often only transient, resolving spontaneously when the cause is removed. Bradycardia may be due to hypoxia, which must be eliminated as a cause before atropine is given. In the absence of sinus rhythm isoprenaline may be needed; an incomplete heart block is also treated with this drug. Myocardial irritability may be due to hypokalaemia and is often corrected by the very slow intravenous injection of potassium chloride, but if this does not produce the desired result lignocaine may have to be given. It is most important to have facilities for rapid estimation of blood electrolytes readily available. Vary rarely, cardiac irritability may be the result of metabolic acidosis needing treatment with i.v. sodium bicarbonate.

During perfusion the haematocrit falls because of the diluting effect of the pump prime and the aim is to keep it between 20 and 25% by addition of blood to the pump circuit as needed. Some redistribution of body fluids occurs and urinary output usually increases so that additional priming fluid has to be added. Diuretics (e.g. frusemide) are given if the urinary output is unsatisfactory and potassium is given to replace that lost in the urine.

Lung ventilation is recommenced immediately before perfusion is stopped. Caval snares are released and blood fills the heart and enters the lungs. The surgeon uses this blood to ensure that air is displaced from the left heart before allowing the systemic circulation to depend on the left ventricular contraction. Proper cardiac filling is, of course, essential and blood is transfused from the pump circuit or by i.v. infusion until atrial pressures are adequate. Initially atrial filling pressures may have to be increased slowly to 15 mmHg (2 kPa) or until no further improvement in arterial pressure occurs, and inotropic support (adrenaline) may be needed but usually over a period of about 30 minutes a much lower atrial filling pressure of 5–6 mmHg (0.7–0.8 kPa) becomes effective.

Perfusion is controlled by the perfusionist to produce an adequate tissue blood supply without excessive flow rates which result in destruction of red blood cells and cause a greater incidence of postoperative bleeding. It is possible to reduce the perfusion rate needed by inducing hypothermia and, consequently, cardiopulmonary bypass with moderate hypothermia (reduction of central body temperature to 30–32 °C) is commonplace. Many surgical units use additional profound hypothermia of the myocardium, cooling it to 15–18 °C .

There are many variations for the technique of perfusion but typically after heparinization (about 3 mg/kg) and introduction of the necessary catheters and snares, cardiopulmonary bypass is begun without arrest of the patient's own circulation. Systemic cooling is instituted and once the desired body temperature is reached IPPV is discontinued and a left ventricular vent is placed through the apex of the ventricle. The caval snares are then drawn tight and the aorta is cross-clamped to produce total bypass. The heart is electrically fibrillated with low voltage alternating current shock and the aortic root perfused with cold cardioplegic solution to cause rapid arrest of the heart in diastole. At the same time external cardiac cooling through the pericardial sac is commenced via a recirculation cooling system using cold saline. The cardioplegic solution contains buffered potassium, calcium and magnesium salts with heparin and procaine. The cardiac muscle normally becomes quite flaccid at 15–18 °C giving about 30 minutes operating time.

Rewarming is accomplished by removing the aortic clamp and allowing blood, warmed in the pump-oxygenator, to perfuse the animal, including the coronary circulation. The myocardium recovers in 10–20 minutes and goes into coarse fibrillation. The application of a direct current shock of about 45 J applied directly to the heart restores normal rhythm and the caval snares are released. Supportive bypass is maintained while the right atrial pressure is adjusted to about 5 mmHg (0.7 kPa) by fluid replenishment as needed. Bypass is then discontinued and protamine sulphate is given over a 10 minute period while blood is transfused from the heart-lung machine into the animal to maintain the right atrial pressure. Any tendency to arterial hypotension in spite of an adequate right atrial pressure is treated by the infusion of a weak solution of adrenaline (1: 50 000 in Hartmann's solution) given at the rate of 2–3 drops per minute or administered by an infusion pump.

Postoperative care

All animals subjected to open heart surgery with cardiopulmonary bypass should be treated in an intensive care situation with continuous nursing attention for at least the first 24 hours postoperation. During this time arterial and venous pressures, heart and respiratory rates, PaO_2 and $PaCO_2$ should be recorded at 30 minute intervals while a continuous watch is kept on the ECG and urinary output.

Surgical bleeding is not uncommon and treatment may require reopening of the chest. Although the pericardium is seldom sutured, cardiac tamponade should be suspected when ABP is low, the CVP is high and the urinary output poor. If clotting studies produce normal results, any animals continuing to bleed from the skin wound or into the chest require surgical re-exploration.

Poor tissue perfusion, low output states and massive blood replacement together with lung collapse may all lead to acid–base changes necessitating the administration of sodium bicarbonate.

Emboli may be introduced into the circulation at any time during bypass and surgery. They may be particles of silicone antifoam from the oxygenator, air or oxygen, or tissue debris. The most important results of such embolism are neurological and it can produce anything from transient monoplegia to total brain death.

Sedation and pain relief are particularly important for the facilitation of nursing care for the first 24 hours after surgery and i.v. frusemide (1 mg/kg) may have to be given to prompt a satisfactory urinary output of 0.5 to 1 ml/kg/hour.

Chest drains are usually removed some 24 to 36 hours after operation and if oedema develops it may be necessary to administer concentrated plasma to counteract the effects of haemodilution at the time of bypass.

Insertion of pacemakers

Pacemakers are devices which ensure that the heart beats sufficient times per minute regardless of the intrinsic rhythmic activity. They are inserted for different types of conduction deficits and usually only when an animal is showing symptoms. Most pacemakers used in veterinary practice are obtained from human cadavers prior to cremation of the body.

Temporary pacemakers have wires passed through the veins to rest in the right ventricle. There are some needle electrodes which can be inserted through the chest wall but these are for emergency use only. Oesophageal pacing is also possible. Permanent pacemakers are frequently inserted under general anaesthesia. The pacing wire passes via the jugular vein and tricuspid valve to the right ventricle where it is anchored to the trabeculae by some kind of hook. A subcutaneous pocket is then constructed for the 'pacemaker box' or it is placed in the abdominal cavity. They are powered by various types of battery. Less commonly permanent pacemakers are implanted into the epicardium via a min-thoracotomy.

Pacemakers have one of three modes of operation. They may be fixed rate and have the advantage of simplicity, but are now seldom used (Fig.19.4). Demand pacemakers have the ability to suppress cardiac pacemaker activity if the heart rate is adequate but cut in if the rate falls below a pre-set minimum; they are the most common kind. Sequential pacemakers are complex, with atrial and ventricular electrodes, usually fired by the P wave of the ECG; as yet, they have not been extensively used in veterinary medicine.

Anaesthesia for fitting of pacemakers usually presents no difficulty but the surgeon should avoid diathermy and the pulse should be monitored by a precordial or oesophageal stethoscope, or a peripheral pulse monitor which is not obliterated by electrical interference. It is advisable to have an isoprenaline or dopamine infusion ready

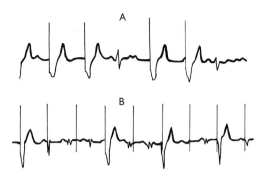

FIG. 19.4 A: ECG with demand pacemaker. These have an internal ability to suppress their activity if the heart rate is adequate but 'cut in' if the spontaneous heart rate falls below a preset minimum. **B**: ECG with a fixed rate pacemaker. These are seldom used today; ECG complexes are usually abnormal during pacemaker function because of depolarization commencing at an ectopic site.

for use should bradycardia develop in the anesthetized animal before the pacemaker can be made operational.

Many anaesthetists do not usually put temporary pacemakers in animals with stable 3rd degree A–V block because these animals seem to maintain stable haemodynamics when anaesthetized. Should pharmacologic support be needed, dopamine at about $10\,\mu g/kg/min$ usually produces a satisfactory increase in the heart rate. When facilities are available, however, most anaesthetists put a pacemaker in animals with sick sinus syndrome or in cases where there is concern about the stability of the slow rhythm before anaesthesia is induced.

REFERENCES

Deakin, C.D., Knight, H., Edwards, J.C., Monro, J.L., Lamb, R.K., Keeton, B. and Salmon, A.P. (1988) Induced hypothermia in the postoperative management of refractory cardiac failure following paediatric surgery. *Anaesthesia* **53**: 848–853.

Dripps, R.D. (1956) *The Physiology of Induced Hypothermia. National Research Council Publications No. 451.* Washington DC: National Research Council.

Lew, L.J., Fowler, J.D., Egger, C.M., Thompson, D.J., Rosin, M.W. and Pharr, J.W. (1997) Deep hypothermic low flow cardiopulmonary bypass in small dogs. *Veterinary Surgery* **26**: 281–289.

Prevention and management of anaesthetic accidents and crises

20

INTRODUCTION

When the profound physiological changes initiated by drugs used in anaesthesia are considered it is surprising that serious accidents and emergencies are not more common. Familiarity with techniques and drugs can lead to a nonchalant attitude but the anaesthetic may be a greater hazard to the life of the animal than is the operation. During anaesthesia some accidents occur suddenly and the reason for the mishap must be recognized immediately so that the appropriate remedy can be applied at once. Other incidents are less dramatic and their results may only become apparent during the postoperative period. Moreover, one kind of emergency may lead to another. Few serious emergencies are truly sudden in onset: they are usually the result of summation of various problems which may have been overlooked. Most disasters can be avoided by critical assessment of potential hazards of the particular situation and by suitable monitoring that enables potential problems to be recognized before they progress to seriously life-threatening situations. Prevention is not always possible and serious problems can ensue if the anaesthetist is not always ready to apply the appropriate remedy in any difficult situation which may arise. Anaesthesia is still an art, and there is no substitute for experience, but even inexperienced anaesthetists can deal successfully with most mishaps if aware of the nature of the more common accidents and emergencies.

The final result of most serious or fatal anaesthetic accidents is that of tissue hypoxia. Brain cells are particularly easily damaged, and even mild hypoxia may result in a loss of intelligence and change in temperament following anaesthesia, whilst a more prolonged insult results in coma, and possibly death. Hypoxia of the myocardium will reduce myocardial contractility and may, particularly if coupled with hypercapnia, sensitize the heart to other stimuli and finally produce cardiac arrest or fibrillation. Lack of oxygen will also damage the liver, kidneys and even somatic muscle, both directly and by increasing the toxic effects of any anaesthetic used, but the results of such damage may not become obvious until well into the postoperative period. Haemoglobin desaturation of arterial blood reduces the O_2 supplies to all tissues and is, therefore, very important to the anaesthetist.

HAEMOGLOBIN DESATURATION

The diagnosis and treatment of falls in O_2 transport by haemoglobin in arterial blood (desaturation) requires rapid, effective correction during anaesthesia. New technologies such as pulse oximetry have revolutionized its early recognition. When it occurs the immediate response consists of rapid performance of the well-known 'Airway, Breathing and Circulation' check routine (see p. 517) and, where possible, provision of an increase in inspired O_2. Next, attention should be focused on differential diagnosis of more defined causes of hypoxia.

Arterial desaturation can be detected directly by observation of the colour of the patient's mucous membranes as well as by monitors such as the pulse oximeter. The clinical sign of cyanosis is dependent on a number of factors other than arterial desaturation. These include anaemia, ambient lighting and superficial pigmentation. Cyanosis may not be seen at all in anaemic or shocked animals. The coexistence of cyanosis with a pulse oximeter reading that indicates adequate saturation may be due to local stasis of blood in the peripheral tissues (which is usually distinguishable from central cyanosis by examination of the colour of the tongue). The colour of lighting sources in the room can also give a false impression of cyanosis or normality. This is well known: shops use longer wavelength light to make counter displays of meat look pinker and fresher.

Reasons for arterial desaturation which the anaesthetist needs to consider are given below.

APPARATUS

Routine following of a checklist such as that given below before administration of any general anaesthetic will prevent mishaps occurring from malfunctioning or misuse of equipment.

Anaesthetic machines

Before administering any anaesthetic, but especially those involving general anaesthetic methods:

1. First:

(i) Note any labelling or service information attached to any machine by service engineers and, if appropriate, switch on electrical supply.

(ii) Switch on and note whether any O_2 analyser (if fitted) is calibrated and if so, whether it is functioning correctly.

2. Gas supplies:

(i) Check the connections to an O_2 supply. If connected to a pipeline confirm correct connection with a 'tug test', ie a sharp pull at the connection, and inspect for any attempt to connect incorrectly by nursing or other staff.

(ii) If connected to a pipeline, switch on spare O_2 cylinder ('tank' in North America) and check that the contents are adequate. For non-pipeline machines switch on the 'in use' cylinder and check its contents, turn off the cylinder, repeat the check on the reserve cylinder and after turning it off re-open the 'in use' cylinder.

(iii) If N_2O use is intended check that the machine is connected to a N_2O supply. For non-pipeline machines check the contents of the N_2O cylinder.

(iv) If intended to use an air supply (pipeline or cylinder) check the machine is connected to it.

(v) If a CO_2 supply is attached to the machine confirm that it is turned off.

(vi) Make sure that blanking plugs are fitted to all empty or unused cylinder yokes.

3. Flowmeters:

(i) Check that all flowmeters move freely throughout their range.

(ii) Confirm that with O_2 flowing at 5 l/min any O_2 analyser fitted reads 100%.

(iii) Make sure that all flowmeters are turned off.

4. Emergency O_2 bypass control:

(i) When the bypass control is operated see that flow occurs without significant drop in the pipeline or cylinder pressure.

(ii) Check that the flow ceases when the control is released.

(iii) If fitted, note that the O_2 analyser reads 100% when the oxygen is flowing.

5. Vaporizers:

(i) Check that the vaporizers for the required volatile agents are present, locked to the back-bar, correctly seated and adequately filled.

(ii) Make sure that the filling ports of the vaporizers are tightly closed and that the controls of each vaporizer move throughout their range.

(iii) If the back bar is protected by pressure relief valve, with an O_2 flow of 5 l/min occlude the common gas outlet, note that the flowmeter bobbin dips and that there is no leak from the filling ports of the vaporizers.

6. Breathing systems:

(i) Ensure that the breathing system is correctly assembled with all the connections tight.

(ii) Listen for any leaks when gas is flowing and the system is pressurized by occlusion of the common gas outlet.

(iii) Check that the pressure relief valve(s) open and close fully.

(iv) By breathing through the system confirm that in any circle system the unidirectional valves operate correctly.

(v) When endotracheal intubation is contemplated check that tubes of appropriate sizes are available and that their cuffs do not leak when inflated with air.

7 Ventilators:

(i) Make sure that the ventilator is correctly assembled and that all the connections are tight. Set the controls and switch on to check that adequate pressure is generated in the inspiratory phase.

(ii) Ensure that an alternative means of ventilation (e.g. manual squeezing of a reservoir bag) is readily available.

(iii) Check that the pressure relief valve operates correctly when the patient port is occluded.

(iv) Ensure that any disconnection alarm which is present is operating correctly (if necessary consult the manufacturer's instructions).

8. Scavenging:

Make sure that any scavenging system is correctly attached and functioning.

Ancillary equipment

(i) Confirm that all laryngoscopes likely to be needed are in working order.

(ii) Check that suction apparatus is available and able to generate adequate negative pressure rapidly.

(iii) Check that appropriate monitoring equipment is present, switched on and calibrated with appropriate alarm limits set.

Checks such as these occupy very little time and should be repeated before each anaesthetic administration.

AIRWAY

Obstruction or excessive resistance within the patient breathing circuit of the apparatus will have the same result as obstruction of the patient's own airway. A spontaneously breathing, lightly anaesthetized animal commonly responds to respiratory obstruction by making frequent violent attempts to breath, but the short vigorous inspiratory efforts make the situation worse as they increase the resistance created by the obstruction. Unfortunately, these vigorous movements can be taken by the inexperienced anaesthetist to mean that anaesthesia is too light and the result may be an attempt to increase anaesthetic depth. The response to obstruction in a deeply anaesthetized animal is usually much quieter, ventilation simply becomes inadequate to maintain respiratory homeostasis.

If a breathing system including a reservoir bag is in use for a spontaneously breathing animal, the best guide to the patency of the airway is the excursion of this bag, but if one is not present in the system, diagnosis of airway obstruction may be difficult. Although complete obstruction is usually fairly easy to detect, a partial obstruction is often not so obvious and may result in the insidious onset of hypoxia and hypercapnia.

In animals connected to a ventilator, observation of its pressure or volume measuring dials often enables obstruction of the airway to be quickly recognized and some machines have devices which warn of obstructions or changes in gas flow into or out of the lungs.

In the non-intubated animal respiratory obstruction is usually due to the base of the tongue or the epiglottis coming into contact with the posterior wall of the pharynx. This type of obstruction is overcome by extending the head on the neck and pulling the tongue forwards out of the mouth. In pigs over-extension of the head on the neck will also cause respiratory obstruction and in these animals care should be taken to keep the head in a normal position ('sniffing for food') in relation to the neck. Horses have a naturally good airway and seldom, if ever, suffer from respiratory obstruction of this nature.

Brachycephalic dogs may develop respiratory obstruction due to the ventral border of the soft palate coming into contact with the base of the tongue. Many brachycephalic breeds are almost unable to breathe through their nostrils and obstruction can only be overcome by endotracheal intubation. The main problem in these breeds occurs during recovery, when the semiconscious dog will not tolerate an endotracheal tube. Ideally, anaesthetic agents which ensure a very rapid return to consciousness should be used to reduce this danger, but spraying of the larynx with a local analgesic (4% lignocaine) at the end of the anaesthetic may enable the endotracheal tube to be tolerated for a longer period.

Large blood clots may accumulate in the pharynx after tonsillectomy, tooth extraction or endotracheal intubation when the tube has been passed through the nostril. These blood clots must be found and removed at the end of operation. Animals unconscious after nose and throat operations should be placed in a position of lateral decubitus during the recovery period and kept under observation until fully conscious and able to safeguard their own airway by coughing and swallowing.

Camelids (e.g. llamas) are often compulsory nasal breathers and the posterior nares can become blocked by the soft palate if this comes to lie dorsal to the epiglottis. This can occur at any time in non-intubated llamas, but more often it is encountered after extubation. Inducing the animal to swallow causes the palate to resume its normal position. An animal can usually be induced to swallow by lightening anaesthesia and introducing a small-bore stomach tube into the oropharynx.

The fact that an endotracheal tube is in the trachea does not necessarily mean that the airway is clear. Endotracheal tubes may kink, particularly if the head is flexed on the neck (Fig. 20. 1); they may become blocked with mucus and in the case of cuffed tubes a faulty cuff may actually occlude the end of the tube, or the pressure inside the cuff may obliterate the tube lumen (Fig. 20.2). During anaes-

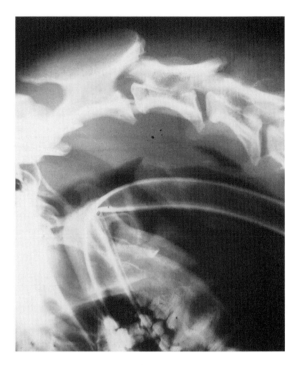

FIG. 20.1 Acute flexion of a dog's neck for radiography leading to kinking of the cuffed endotracheal tube with complete obstruction of the airway.

thesia with N_2O cuffs can become overdistended by diffusion of N_2O into a cuff that has originally been inflated with air.

An overlong endotracheal tube may pass down one bronchus (usually the right) effectively obstructing the airway to the other lung. Obstruction may also be due to an animal biting on the tube.

An uncommon but serious cause of respiratory obstruction in horses is impaction of the epiglottis in the glottic opening. This may occur during 'blind' intubation in young horses and also in sheep, when a soft, flexible epiglottis is forced backwards into the glottic opening by the forcible passage of an endotracheal tube. Unless the epiglottis is dislodged to its normal position by the withdrawal of the tube at the end of anaesthesia, it can give rise to serious respiratory obstruction in the recovery period until either coughing occurs, or the cause of the obstruction is recognized and overcome by hooking the epiglottis out of the airway with a tube passed through the nostrils.

In horses, oedema of the upper respiratory passages develops during general anaesthesia if the

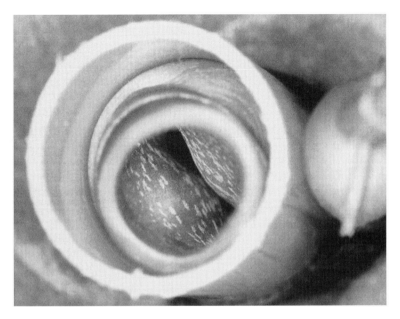

FIG. 20.2 Occlusion of a soft-walled endotracheal tube by overinflation of the cuff forcing the wall inwards until the lumen is almost obliterated. This picture was obtained by inflating the cuff with the tube inside the barrel of a plastic syringe.

head is in a dependent position or if the jugular veins are partially occluded for any length of time. This can result in serious respiratory obstruction in the recovery period that can only be relieved by endotracheal intubation, preferably with a nasal tube.

Animals suffering from laryngeal paralysis or tracheal collapse may obstruct during the recovery period when the increased effort of breathing tends to draw the sides of the larynx and/or trachea together. As with the brachycephalic breeds of dogs, it may be necessary to leave an endotracheal tube in place longer than would otherwise have been necessary.

LARYNGEAL AND BRONCHIAL SPASM

Laryngeal spasm

Laryngeal spasm appears to be seen much more commonly than bronchial spasm, but both conditions can occur together during general anaesthesia. Laryngeal spasm can, in theory, occur in all animals but it is most common in cats and pigs when attempts are made to force them to breathe high concentrations of inhalation anaesthetics dur-

ing induction of anaesthesia before the protective laryngeal reflexes have been subdued.

Another common complication of anaesthesia in cats is laryngeal 'crowing' – the crowing noise being caused by partial spasm of the vocal cords due to their irritation by a blob of mucus, saliva, blood or vomit. The incidence of this post-extubation complication has fallen since the introduction of endotracheal tubes manufactured from substances more inert than red rubber. When it persists after aspiration of foreign material from the vocal cords, i.v. or oral steroid (e.g. dexamethasone 0.3 mg/kg) may relieve it.

In horses laryngeal spasm is rare, but obstruction occurs when the soft palate becomes displaced from its normal position under the epiglottis. This situation often arises following extubation and it is important that the horse swallows when the endotracheal tube is removed for, as in camelids, this act restores the soft palate to its normal position. Endotracheal tubes are best not removed until gentle manipulation of the tube or laryngeal region of the neck is seen to induce the horse to swallow.

When laryngeal spasm is very troublesome the best treatment is to administer a neuromuscular blocking agent in order to relax the spasm, and then to intubate with an endotracheal tube. Attempts at intubation by forcible passage of the tube without the aid of neuromuscular blockers will usually be unsuccessful and will prolong the spasm. Although deepening of anaesthesia itself may relax the spasm this can be hazardous. Repeated attempts at forcible intubation through a closed glottis can result in oedema of the mucous membrane necessitating tracheostomy. Spraying of the larynx with 4% lignocaine hydrochloride does not produce instant relaxation of the cords and may result in postanaesthetic problems from their desensitization causing difficulties in swallowing.

Bronchial spasm

'Bronchial spasm' or constriction of the bronchioles is uncommon but occasionally seen in all kinds of animal. Ruminants appear to be particularly liable to develop this complication due to unsuspected regurgitation and inhalation of ruminal fluids. Bronchial spasm may also be initiated reflexly during light anaesthesia by stimuli from the site of operation and there is some evidence suggesting that passage of blood with a low P_2O_2 and high $PaCO_2$ through the brain causes bronchoconstriction.

The first warning sign that bronchial spasm is imminent is usually a bout of coughing and if an endotracheal tube is not in use the larynx closes. Complete respiratory arrest follows. The chest is rigid and the lungs can only be inflated by great pressure on a rebreathing bag. While this may produce an adequate inspiratory volume, the passive recoil of the lungs and chest wall may be inadequate to provide adequate expiratory volume. If a second breath is delivered before complete expiration the phenomenon of 'stacking' occurs, with increased thoracic gas volume, alveolar distension and increased risk of barotrauma and reduced cardiac output. Thus the animal with severe bronchospasm should be ventilated with a slow rate allowing a prolonged expiratory time.

In the extreme situation virtually no expiration occurs and pressure on the chest wall may be life-saving. When untreated, cyanosis sets in and is soon replaced by a grey pallor of the mucous membranes. If not in robust condition the animal may die, but usually the severe hypoxia releases the spasm and the animal gasps. The gasp is followed by normal spontaneous respiration and the animal recovers. Unfortunately, bronchial spasm may recur if the stimulus responsible for the first attack is still present. In all cases the anaesthetist must ensure that the upper airway is clear and that whenever possible the first gasp of the animal will be of an O_2 enriched atmosphere.

If it is necessary to treat bronchospasm with drugs because other procedures have been unsuccessful, adrenaline is the drug of first choice as being the one most likely to relieve the spasm. In small animal patients an i.v. loading dose of 2.5 to 5 ml of 1:10 000 followed by an infusion may be used; these doses need to be scaled up appropriately for larger animals.

ASPIRATION OF MATERIAL FROM THE OESOPHAGUS AND STOMACH

This accident occurs more frequently than is commonly realized for material from the oesophagus and stomach may reach the pharynx as a result of vomiting or passive reflux. In either case the primary problem is respiratory obstruction, possibly accompanied by bronchospasm if foreign material has penetrated deeply enough into the lungs. Inhalation pneumonia may manifest itself over the next few days.

In those animals that can vomit, it is an active process either during induction or recovery. It is often preceded by swallowing or 'gagging' movements (sharp rhythmic contractions of the abdominal and thoracic muscles); these contractions increase intra-abdominal pressure and force gastric or oesophageal contents into the pharynx. When active vomiting occurs during the induction of anaesthesia, the protective mechanisms of laryngeal closure, coughing and breath holding are usually present and the accident should not have dire consequences, All that is necessary is to clear the pharynx of vomited material, by swabbing or suction, and to allow the animal to cough vigorously before proceeding with further administration of the anaesthetic. The dog, however, has very weak protective reflexes and in a few cases, particularly when vomiting occurs during the recovery period and the dog is still sleepy, these reflexes fail to protect the airway so that inhalation of vomited material occurs. In such cases it may even prove necessary to re-anaesthetize the dog in order to use vigorous suction to clear the tracheobronchial tree.

It is obvious that if anaesthetics are not given to animals whose stomachs might contain food then aspiration is unlikely to occur, but this is a counsel of perfection which cannot always be realized. Clearly, it can never be achieved in ruminants and in simple stomached animals the stomach may contain material many hours after the eating of a meal, particularly if an accident has occurred in the meanwhile or if the animal has gone into labour.

Passive regurgitation is most commonly seen in ruminant animals but it also occurs in horses, pigs, dogs and cats. It usually happens when the animal is in a head-down position, or lying horizontally on its side, and relaxation is induced by deep anaesthesia or the use of neuromuscular blocking drugs. In these circumstances the protective reflexes are not active and aspiration occurs all too readily. In deeply anaesthetized ruminants any increase in intra-abdominal pressure will force fluid ingesta up the oesophagus into the pharynx, and this type of regurgitation is frequently seen in adult cattle becoming recumbent after induction of anaesthesia. To prevent regurgitation in cases of equine surgical colic the stomach should be decompressed by the passage of a stomach tube prior to the induction of anaesthesia. It is almost impossible to pass a tube into the stomach of an anaesthetized horse.

In cases of oesophageal dilation or obstruction there may be an accumulation of fluid in the oesophagus, while the stomach may contain fluid material if there is an obstruction of the pylorus or small intestine. The most certain way of preventing the aspiration of material from the oesophagus and stomach is to perform endotracheal intubation with a cuffed tube immediately anaesthesia has been induced. In the case of small animals, keeping the head raised after induction of anaesthesia, together with rapid intubation of the trachea and cuff inflation will completely prevent the danger of inhalation from passive regurgitation, but this is obviously not practicable in ruminants.

Often, the first sign that aspiration has occurred is the unexpected appearance of cyanosis, dyspnoea and tachycardia. The severity of the consequences depends on the quantity of fluid aspirated and extent of the lung regions involved. Immediate treatment consists of thorough aspiration of the tracheobronchial tree – although this is more easily advised than performed. Oxygen should be administered and attention directed towards the relief of bronchiolar spasm. If, after operation, the animal develops bronchopneumonia the appropriate treatment must be instituted (antimicrobials, corticosteroids etc.).

Tracheostomy

The obvious treatment of respiratory obstruction is to locate it and remove the cause, but this is not always possible and occasionally in cases of upper respiratory obstruction an emergency tracheostomy is required to save the animal's life.

In a cat, a 14 gauge needle or catheter, placed percutaneously directly into the trachea, if possible through the cricothyroid membrane when the obstruction is cranial to this, provides an adequate short-term airway. In small dogs (up to 5 kg) 10 gauge catheters or needles may be used in a similar manner. In all but these small animals the size of such airways is totally inadequate for more than one or two minutes but may be sufficient to sustain life whilst a surgical tracheostomy is carried out. Curved plastic tracheostomy tubes or cannulae (Fig. 20.3) are available in sizes suitable for surgical placement in most dogs. They are inserted through the cricothyroid membrane, between two tracheal rings or by slitting a tracheal ring longitudinally. Once such a tube is in place in a dog or other small animal, the patient should be under constant observation as the tube may become dislodged or blocked by folds of skin, secretions, or flexure of the neck.

In the horse, tracheostomy is much easier to carry out, and if necessary can provide a safe airway for a long period of time. In emergency, or for short term use, narrow curved tubes (Fig. 20.4) are suitable. On superficial examination these tubes may appear to provide far too small an airway, but they are fully effective in such situations. For more prolonged use a tracheostomy tube which can be

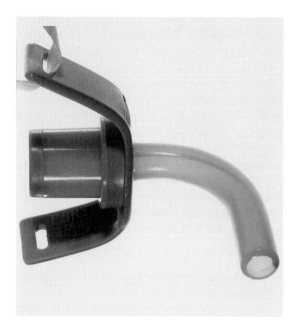

FIG. 20.3 Disposable tracheostomy tube. This type of tube is suitable for dogs, cats, sheep, goats and small calves.

removed and cleaned is employed. These are often formed of interlocking pieces for ease of removal and replacement.

It must be pointed out that the need for an emergency tracheostomy is rare. In the cat it may be required because of severe, persistent laryngeal spasm but in most other species of animal it is made necessary by pathological obstructions of the airway which prevent endotracheal intubation. In many cases, therefore, the requirement can be foreseen and equipment for tracheostomy kept readily available.

BREATHING

APNOEA

Apnoea during anaesthesia is very common and its successful treatment depends on the original cause. Although respiratory arrest is obvious, it is often preceded by respiratory insufficiency, which is much more difficult to assess. In either case, the immediate requirement is that oxygenation of the tissues should be maintained, so as soon as the problem is diagnosed the anaesthetist should carry out the following routine:

1. Check the airway and, if necessary take steps to clear it.

2. Apply artificial respiration (ensuring there is no anaesthetic in the inspired gas).

3. Check the pulse.

Assuming that the circulation is adequate, in the majority of cases steps 1 and 2 should prevent further hypoxia and hypercarbia, and give the

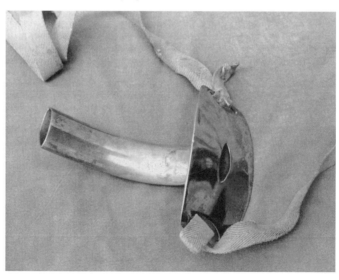

FIG. 20.4 A laryngotomy tube for a horse. These tubes are intended for insertion through the incision should obstruction develop after a laryngoventriculectomy, but they may be used as emergency tracheostomy tubes because they can be easily slipped through an incision between the tracheal rings.

anaesthetist time to assess the problem and apply further measures accordingly. The commonest reason for the failure to resuscitate an apnoeic animal is delay in instituting artificial ventilation. It must be emphasized that there are no circumstances in which such ventilation is contraindicated in the treatment of apnoea.

The efficiency of artificial ventilation in an emergency depends on the apparatus available and size of the patient. Where anaesthetic systems utilizing reservoir bags are being employed it is possible to ventilate by squeezing the bag, but otherwise resuscitation is more difficult. Self-filling bag/valve units such as the Ambu bag (Fig.20.5) are useful to ventilate small animals via a non-rebreathing valve attached to a facemask or endotracheal tube. Ventilation is with room air but, if it is available, extra oxygen may be added to the inspired gas. These units are excellent in emergencies away from operating room areas, and should be part of any portable resuscitation kit for small animals. Where only an endotracheal tube may be available a dog or cat can, in an emergency, be ventilated by a person blowing gently down the tube (expired air ventilation). Expired air ventilation produces only just adequate inspired PO_2 and is very tiring to perform. Clearly, the small human

forced expired volume cannot be expected to produce effective ventilation in large animal species.

In the absence of any apparatus, small animals can be ventilated by blowing down the nostrils while the mouth is held closed, but the person performing this must produce a seal with his or her lips around the animal's nostrils. Another method of artificial ventilation, i.e. intermittent pressure on the animal's chest wall, may well be preferred. This is totally inadequate in providing ventilation for any length of time but may keep the animal alive for a few minutes. Often, compressing the chest triggers a reflex spontaneous respiration, which is more effective than the attempt to ventilate in this manner.

Stimulation of the animal in various ways may result in a reflex spontaneous breath. Such a reflex is the 'chest deflation reflex' described above. Movement of the tube in the trachea may also make the animal breathe. Most reflexes, however, are associated with painful input, the most obvious one being the respiratory response to the commencement of surgery. Janssens *et al.* (1979) suggest the use of acupuncture to stimulate respiration and recommends the placing of a needle in the nasal septum. Certainly in cats and dogs that area is extremely sensitive, and its stimulation

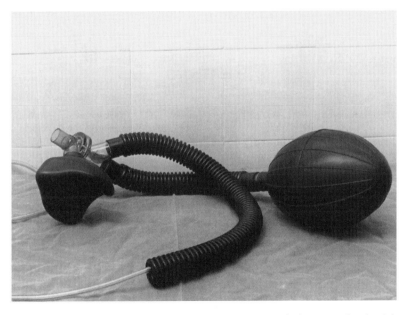

FIG. 20.5 Ambu self-inflating bag for IPPV. If available, O_2 can be given to enrich the inspired air by delivering it through the small-bore plastic tubing.

may trigger reflex respiration, but in lightly anaesthetized animals it may also trigger cardiac arrest. In horses, stimulation of respiration by twisting the ear appears more effective. It must be emphasized that adequate artificial respiration must be continued whilst these attempts to stimulate respiration are being made.

The common causes of apnoea are listed in Table 20.1. As treatment further to initial immediate artificial ventilation is dependent on the cause of failure, it is essential that the anaesthetist is capable of making the diagnosis. The most common cause of apnoea is respiratory obstruction or (commonly in horses) too great resistance within the patient breathing system. Once the resistance is removed, spontaneous ventilation resumes. On induction and recovery from anaesthesia the animal may hold its breath for a few seconds, particularly if an endotracheal tube is in place. Examination of the level of unconsciousness shows very light anaesthesia and spontaneous respiration resumes rapidly once the endotracheal tube is removed.

Central nervous depression is the most serious common cause of apnoea under anaesthesia. It is particularly serious as it may be accompanied by circulatory inadequacies, so that the pulse should be carefully monitored until recovery occurs. Depression may be caused by overdoses of anaesthetic or analgesic agents or by cerebral hypoxia. The animal will be deeply unconscious but estimation of the depth can be very difficult for the inexperienced anaesthetist. Hypoxia and hypercapnia, from whatever cause, can lead to a jerky respiratory movements with jaw and limb movements, leading the unwary into thinking that anaesthesia is light. Gasping respirations of the Cheyne-Stokes last-gasp type may precede apnoea, and again the overall movement of the animal which accompanies these may be misleading. Despite movement, there is, at this stage, no tone in the muscles and all reflexes show that anaesthesia is, in fact, deep.

Drug overdoses are best treated by maintaining IPPV until the drug can be eliminated or its action antagonized. However, reliance should never be placed on the use of analeptic or antagonistic drugs alone. Where volatile agents are implicated they are removed from the circulation by ventilation, and rapid recovery occurs. Parenteral agents, however, are more difficult to remove from the circulation. Where only a small dose of the anaesthetic has been given i.v. anaesthesia usually lightens as redistribution of the agent occurs, but where a relative or gross overdose has been administered and no antagonists are available the only method of increasing excretion may be to increase the renal output by means of an i.v. infusion of dextrose, a balanced electrolyte solution or a diuretic such as frusemide (furosemide).

Respiratory depression due to opioid drugs may be counteracted by specific antagonists. Diprenorphine (Revivon) is the specific antagonist to etorphine but should not be used to treat etorphine intoxication in man, because it has agonist properties. Naloxone (Narcan) is the drug in current use to antagonize the effect of all opioid agonist drugs. Its long-acting derivative, naltrexone, has not been studied in veterinary anaesthesia but could prove useful should a long-acting pure antagonist be required.

Naloxone is most effective against the pure opioid agonists, and is less effective against partial agonists such as buprenorphine. It may be given to pups delivered from a bitch given a morphine-like drugs during labour. In dogs and cats the initial i.v. bolus of naloxone is 200 μg and this can be repeated every 2 to 3 mins, up to a total dose of 2 mg, until the desired response is obtained. Large doses, or doses given too rapidly after each other, will result in hypertension and arrhythmias.

TABLE 20.1 **Causes of hypoxia in absence of respiratory obstruction**	
Causes of hypoxaemia	**Remedy**
Failure of O_2 supply	Ensure no disconnection from the anaesthetic system, no empty cylinder when supply is not from pipeline
Accumulation of N_2 in breathing system	Flush breathing system with pure O_2 or fresh anaesthetic gas mixture
Sticking of valves in circle systems	Check operation of directional valves and if necessary replace breathing system

In horses naloxone has been used in i.v. bolus doses of 0.005–0.02 mg/kg but its use in equine anaesthesia is still controversial because its efficacy as an adjunct has not been established and by antagonizing the horse's endogenous opioids a horse which is in pain may become restless.

Overdoses of the α_2 adrenoceptor agonists can be treated with antagonists such as yohimbine or atipamezole.

The place of analeptic drugs in the treatment of respiratory failure during anaesthesia is debatable and it is undoubtedly true that the experienced anaesthetist only rarely finds it necessary to recourse to them. Their duration of action is relatively short and that of a single dose may be too transient to restore complete respiratory activity. Thus it is necessary to maintain a careful watch until signs of recovering consciousness are evident and should breathing again become alarmingly shallow or cease, repeated doses should be given (or naltrexone used with caution because its effects in veterinary patients are currently uninvestigated).

Doxapram hydrochloride (Dopram V) increases the respiratory minute volume by acting on the respiratory centre and, in general, doses considerably larger than those used clinically must be used before general stimulation results in convulsions. Its use is safe at i.v. doses of 2 mg/kg in a wide range of species. For clinical purposes an initial intravenous dose of 1 mg/kg is usually employed and further doses given if required. Doxapram may also be used by the sublingual route to stimulate respiration in the new-born. Despite the claims as to the specificity of the action on the respiratory centre, in practice clinical doses are usually found to decrease the level of unconsciousness of the anaesthetized animal. Whilst this is useful if apnoea is due to central depression, this drug must be used with care in large animals such as horses, where the awakening may be violent.

Normal levels of carbon dioxide in the blood are necessary to maintain spontaneous respiration. However, the role of carbon dioxide in resuscitation in veterinary anaesthesia has been grossly abused. Although a slight increase in carbon dioxide stimulates respiration in the conscious animal, this reflex is considerably reduced in anaesthetized individuals. Under anaesthesia increases in $PaCO_2$ cause increasing central nervous depres-

sion, which will itself eventually result in apnoea. Hypercapnia also sensitizes the heart to arrhythmias and may precipitate cardiac arrest. In the majority of case apnoea is preceded by respiratory insufficiency and by the time that respiration ceases, hypercapnia already exists. The only circumstances where CO_2 is required to stimulate respiration is to treat hypocapnia following vigorous hyperventilation. If CO_2 is required to correct hypocapnia it is best added to the inspired gas either from cylinders on the anaesthetic machine, or by increasing the deadspace of the patient circuit, as in this way it is possible to continue ventilation and prevent hypoxia from occurring. IPPV should never be stopped to allow accumulation of CO_2 in the breathing system

Failure to antagonize the effects of neuromuscular blocking drugs used during anaesthesia will result in respiratory failure. Treatment consists of the continuation of IPPV until the effects of the blocker have worn off or been adequately antagonized. Pain in the postoperative period, particularly that involved in movement of the thoracic and abdominal muscles, may cause hypoventilation. If opioid analgesics in limited doses are used in such circumstances, the increased ventilation through pain relief is usually greater than any respiratory depression as a direct result of the drug. Other causes of inadequate ventilation include pathological changes such as space-occupying lesions of the lung or pleural cavity, and bleeding into the substance of the lung.

Normal $PaCO_2$ is essential for the maintenance of normal tissue perfusion and hypocapnia leads to a decrease in cerebral blood flow. However, severe hypocapnia does not occur in spontaneously breathing animals and the cerebral circulation is only likely to be affected when IPPV is carried out in such a way as to remove excessive amounts of CO_2.

Assuming ventilation to be adequate, the commonest causes of hypoxaemia during general anaesthesia include an inadequate supply of O_2 to the breathing system from failure of supply (empty cylinder, disconnection), accumulation of nitrogen or nitrous oxide in a low-flow system or faulty valves preventing the proper circulation of gases around the system (Table 20.1). Such accidents occur quite commonly, and should be suspected if an animal which has previously been well becomes cyanotic despite an adequate respiratory minute volume and an apparently adequate circulation. Treatment consists of the administration of O_2, preferably utilizing a simple non-rebreathing patient system. However, as long as an animal is breathing spontaneously simply disconnecting it from the machine and allowing it to breathe room air will usually provide the necessary O_2 whilst the fault is being located.

Diminished excretion of CO_2 from the lungs results in respiratory acidosis. This state is commonly seen when the total gas flow rate in a non-rebreathing system is too low, or when the soda lime in an absorber is exhausted. It also occurs when the airway is obstructed, or when respiratory movements are hampered by the position of the animal's body on the bed or operating table. Usually, when the duration of anaesthesia is short there is insufficient time for severe acidosis to develop, but long duration anaesthesia can lead to a serious fall in blood pH. Death occurs when the arterial blood pH falls below about 6.7.

The signs of respiratory acidosis are not always obvious. Hypoxaemia may have been avoided by an increase in the inspired O_2 so that the animal's mucous membranes remain pink and its pulse slow and of good volume (sometimes noted as a 'bounding pulse'). Although in normal animals an increase in the $PaCO_2$ causes a frank increase in the tidal volume, in the anaesthetized animal this may not occur. The ABP first rises, then returns to normal and finally falls. Circulatory failure, when it occurs, is rapid and is due to heart failure. When severe respiratory acidosis has developed an animal may collapse at the end of operation, for excess CO_2 is rapidly excreted as respiratory depression decreases with lightening of anaesthesia and the circulatory reflexes are not active enough to compensate for the rapid change in blood pH. The condition may be erroneously diagnosed as shock, but unlike shock is characterized by a slow pulse and, usually, in otherwise fit animals, spontaneous recovery.

CIRCULATORY FAILURE

Circulatory failure may be due to volume or primary cardiac insufficiency. The main concern is failure of organ perfusion and ABP is often used as an assessment of this because modern technology has made pressure measurement easy in most animals. However, ABP does not necessarily correlate with O_2 transport which is more related to blood flow. Fortunately, the brain, heart and kidneys are protected by autoregulation and blood flow remains constant in spite of large changes in ABP. Cerebral and coronary flow remain constant down to a MAP of 60 mmHg and renal blood flow does not fall until MAP falls below about 70 mmHg. Unexpected arterial hypotension during anaesthesia must always be investigated and remedial measures taken to avoid serious consequences for the animal.

As is well known, ABP is determined by the cardiac output (CO) and the systemic vascular resistance (SVR). The CO is dependent on the stroke volume (SV) and heart rate (HR). Arterial hypotension results from a change of one or more of these factors and diagnosis and treatment of hypotension must be based on these fundamental considerations.

INADEQUACY OF THE CIRCULATING FLUID VOLUME

Inadequacy of the circulating fluid volume to fill the existing vascular bed may be due to an absolute reduction in blood or body fluid volumes, or to an increase in vascular space as a result of peripheral vasodilatation. In either case if compensatory mechanisms are impaired the effect is to decrease venous return and reduce preload. Reduction in preload decreases ventricular end-diastolic filling with consequent decrease in SV and hence in CO. Hypovolaemia is one of the most common causes of hypotension during anaesthesia, operating either alone or in conjunction with other aggravating factors. Venodilatation causes reduced preload when compensatory mechanisms are impaired – for example when sympathetic venomotor tone is diminished by neuroaxis blockade.

A very common cause of circulatory failure under anaesthesia is surgical haemorrhage. There may be a sudden effusion of blood or, more commonly, an almost imperceptible loss over the course of a long operation. Unless blood loss is actually measured by swab weighing or some other technique, it is very difficult to estimate the amount of haemorrhage occurring and many surgeons do not appreciate the extent of the blood loss they cause. Many of the drugs used in anaesthesia abolish the normal physiological response to haemorrhage and the tachycardia response seen in young, healthy animals may not occur in the elderly or sick.

For practical clinical purposes all animals can be considered to have a circulating blood volume of about 88 ml/kg and when a loss of 10% of this (i.e. 8–9 ml/kg) has occurred it needs to be replaced. Replacement of lost blood volume with non-blood substances is often desirable if a moderate degree of haemodilution can be tolerated. An acceptable minimal level of haemoglobin seems to be around 7 g/dl which offsets the reduced O_2 content of the blood with reduced viscosity (Concensus Conference, 1988). However, the heart must be capable of increasing CO to cope with tissue demands and so animals suffering from restricted CO (e.g. aortic stenosis, valvular incompetence) must be maintained at a higher haemoglobin concentration.

The crystalloid *v.* colloid debate has often been argued (e.g. Davies, 1989), but the best course is probably to combine the two and replace extracellular deficits with crystalloid solutions and large blood losses with a colloid (albumin, polygeline or hydroxyethyl starch) and/or blood. Crystalloid solutions, in a ratio of 3 ml to replace 1 ml of blood loss result in euvolaemia after approximately 1 hour because the crystalloids usually distribute themselves to the extracellular fluid after about 20 minutes. Some tissue oedema occurs and the final equilibration results in less than one-quarter of the infused fluid remaining in the circulation; any diuresis evoked by the lower colloid pressure will reduce this contribution still further. Thus, an animal which has had its circulating fluid deficit replaced adequately by crystalloids soon after haemorrhage may have a circulating fluid deficit and be suffering from arterial hypotension some hours later, despite having suffered no further haemorrhage.

Fluid deficits which may have arisen in the preoperative period may lead to hypotension when blood vessels are dilated by anaesthetic drugs.

When the fluid loss is primarily an electrolyte loss, such as seen in vomiting dogs and cats or equine colic cases, circulatory changes can be so severe that the animal appears shocked. However, in cases where the deficit is primarily of water, it is more difficult to recognize and assess but unless this is done these animals will become hypotensive following the administration of vasodilator drugs, or following an apparently small blood loss. Also, elderly animals do not tolerate degrees of haemorrhage which might not give rise to concern in young, fit subjects. In all these instances deficits should, whenever possible, be corrected before anaesthesia is induced, the only exceptions being cases of intestinal obstruction where it is prudent to restore only the circulatory fluid volume if the surgeon is not to be inconvenienced.

Peripheral vasodilatation due to drugs administered before and during anaesthesia, or, more seriously, due to endotoxins may lead to circulatory failure but in their absence major changes in the peripheral circulation can occur in response to autonomic reflex activity. For example, sudden hypotension during operation sometimes occurs without warning in an animal whose cardiovascular and autonomic systems are healthy and where there has been but little loss of blood. The pulse becomes imperceptible, respiration ceases and the veins (notably in the tongue) are dilated. The pupils remain normal in size and this may be the only indication that the heart has not stopped beating. This alarming reaction appears to be initiated reflexly by certain surgical manipulations. For example, it may be seen during caesarian hysterotomies in cattle and sheep when traction is exerted on the mesovarium or on the broad ligament of the uterus. It may also be seen in dogs and cats when swabs or retractors are allowed to press upon the coeliac plexus, or when the stomach and liver are handled by the surgeon. Traction on the eyeball also invokes parasympathetic mediated hypotension. When it arises the surgeon should stop and not recommence operating until recovery has occurred. These reactions may be avoided by gentle surgery and the anaesthetist should note that gentle surgery is only possible when the patient's muscles are adequately relaxed.

SHOCK

Shock is best regarded as a caricature of physiological responses to insults such as haemorrhage or prolonged decrease in circulating fluid volume. In shock the outline of the body's defensive features to these insults remains recognizable but it is exaggerated and distorted to a degree that becomes both absurd and damaging. The major factors in its initiation and maintenance are, therefore, as in arterial hypotension, decreased cardiac output, increased vascular resistance and decreased circulating blood volume. Unless corrected, each of these feeds back directly, or through the autonomic nervous system, to worsen the state of the circulation until there is insufficient perfusion of tissues, i.e. the animal becomes 'shocked'.

Realization that the development of shock can be prevented by the correction of the conditions leading to it resulted in its being classified on aetiological grounds:

1. *Hypovolaemic* – due to haemorrhage (surgical or traumatic), fluid loss (vomiting, diarrhoea).

2. *Vasculogenic* – changes in systemic resistance or venous capacitance due to sepsis, anaphylaxis, loss of vasomotor tone from central nervous lesions or anaesthetic agents.

3. *Cardiogenic* – when the heart ceases to be an effective pump. This can result from such things as severe cardiac depression from drugs, arrhythmias, ruptured chorda tendineae, cardiac tamponade, or failure of venous return due to aortocaval compression in tension pneumothorax. Ventricular strain may be caused by prolonged increase in systemic vascular resistance and the heart muscle itself can be contused by thoracic trauma.

This classification, while useful in recognition of the factors which has been responsible for shock developing, have little bearing on the shock syndrome itself. The conditions giving rise to the shock state may be amenable to suitable prompt treatment but delay in initiating treatment, or failure to respond to treatment for some other reason, leads from a final common pathway to inevitable death. The actual processes which lead to this irreversibility are complex and still the subject for debate.

It seems likely that irreversibility begins when ischaemic hypoxia changes to stagnant hypoxia in certain tissues, and prolonged vasoconstriction is thought to be a key factor. For instance, after severe haemorrhage, sympathetic activity and catecholamine secretion produce vasoconstriction and ischaemic hypoxia in the splanchnic bed, liver and kidneys. This regional vasoconstriction enables the circulation to be maintained through the unconstricted cerebral and coronary vessels in spite of any reduction in CO. Transfusion at this stage improves CO, relieves hypotension and much of the vasoconstriction, allowing tissue perfusion to be restored. If transfusion is delayed the constricted arterioles become less and less responsive to adrenaline (epinephrine), apparently due to the accumulation of metabolites in the tissues. The venules retain their responsiveness to adrenaline and when the arterioles relax the capillaries become engorged as flow stagnates. Capillary engorgement then raises the hydrostatic pressure so that fluid exudes from the capillary beds and oligaemia becomes more severe. Anoxic changes become serious, local haemorrhages appear and transfusion is of no avail because it merely engorges further the stagnant capillary bed. The venous return and CO continue to fall and the heart ceases to beat as the coronary flow is reduced.

Changes in the abdominal viscera and sympathetic activity are of importance in irreversibility as is the endotoxin of Gram-negative bacilli. This toxin is absorbed from the damaged (anoxic) bowel, acts on the nervous system, produces a relentless abdominal sympathetic-induced vasoconstriction, and then it cannot be detoxicated because of failure of the reticuloendothelial enzyme in the hypoxic spleen and liver. Endotoxin action certainly has an important adrenergic component because its lethal effect is countered by adrenolytic compounds and it potentiates the pressor responses to catecholamines.

Vasopressors are much more likely to be harmful than beneficial in shocked animals. The only measures which consistently reduce mortality are those which increase blood volume or reduce vasoconstriction and this has led to the suggestion that vasodilators may have a place in the treatment of shock. Although not to be used when the blood volume is already reduced and no substitute for correct fluid therapy it is claimed by some that anti-adrenergic drugs and other methods of inhibiting sympathetic activity improve survival after haemorrhage or trauma provided that further transfusion is given to cover the increased capacity of the vascular system. It is extremely doubtful if the adrenal cortex plays any part although hydrocortisone (itself a vasodilator) given in massive doses of 50 mg/kg doses has been used. Such massive doses are impracticable for large animals, but phenylbutazone, in doses of 15 mg/kg may be as effective as corticosteroids in the treatment of endotoxic shock. Unfortunately, the best results are only obtained when these drugs are given before shock actually develops. Flunixin (1 mg/kg i.v.) may counter endotoxaemia in equine colic cases. During shock the endogenous opioid β endorphin is released from the pituitary and it has been suggested that it may contribute to hypotension since this is alleviated by the administration of naloxone. Although the use of naloxone may be efficacious it may also restore pain sensitivity which is usually reduced in shock.

The infusion of small volumes of hypertonic saline may be beneficial in shocked animals. This approach has been reviewed by Gasthuys (1994) and is quite distinct from volume replacement therapy. Hypertonic solutions are easily prepared and are non-viscous, so that rapid infusion is possible in spite of their high osmolality (for 7.2 % solution 2400 mosm/litre). They cause movement of fluid from the intracellular compartment to the interstitium and the circulation and, consequently, this form of therapy must be followed by large quantities of isotonic solutions or other fluids such as whole blood given i.v. The effects of i.v. hypertonic saline solutions, sometimes mixed with colloids such as dextran, have been reported in cats (Muir & Sally, 1989), dogs (Mermel & Boyle, 1986; Rocha et al., 1990; Kein et al., 1991; Dupe et al., 1993), pigs (Maningas et al., 1986; Hellyer et al., 1993;), sheep (Smith et al., 1985) and horses (Bertone et al., 1990; Dyson & Pascoe, 1990; Allen et al., 1991; Arden et al., 1991; Moon et al., 1991). Infusion of these hypertonic solutions is not without its drawbacks. A potentially dangerous initial decrease in arterial blood pressure has been noted (Kein et al., 1991). Extreme neuronal dehydration and hypernatri-

aemia can induce marked neurological dysfunction (Kleeman, 1979), i.v. hypertonic solutions can cause phlebitis and saturated (25%) or semi-saturated (15%) NaCl solutions produce haemolysis (Rocha et al., 1990). Care must be taken in the interpretation of these reports since some relate to infusions in normovolaemic as opposed to hypovolaemic or shocked animals.

Much work has been done to establish the best methods of estimating the state of the circulation. Undoubtedly the most useful determinations are measurement of ABP, CVP, capillary refill time, the state of distension of peripheral veins and the urinary output. Treatment of established shock is seldom effective and it is, therefore, most important to intervene during the progression of the conditions which lead to it. Early transfusion to restore the vascular volumes and expeditious operation to arrest bleeding, removal of damaged tissue and, if necessary, fixation of broken bones, will prevent irreversible shock from developing.

DISTURBANCES OF CARDIAC RHYTHM

Tachycardia is usual in young animals, but in adults the pulse rate increases in shock or after the administration of anticholinergics. It must be emphasized, too, that in animals under the influence of neuromuscular blocking agents tachycardia may indicate an insufficient depth of anaesthesia.

Many factors determine whether an animal will develop arrhythmias during anaesthesia but some may well have existed prior to anaesthesia. Holter monitoring for 24 hours has demonstrated that a large proportion of conscious asymptomatic animals show arrhythmias. Pre-existing arrhythmias are usually benign and include sinus arrhythmia in healthy young animals and sinus bradycardia in trained athletic animals.

If the anaesthetic agent is known to depress the functional capacity of the heart muscle it is natural to assume that the direct action of the drug on the myocardium is the cause, but it is more probable that serious arrhythmias are caused by the action of autonomic nerves to the heart. The nervous system is often hyperactive immediately before anaesthesia, especially if the animal is frightened, and stimulation of sympathetic nerves to the heart may cause ventricular extrasystoles (VES) or even ventricular fibrillation if the heart muscle is sensitized by anaesthetic agents. CO_2 may accumulate in the body; this accumulation and/or mild degrees of hypoxia can cause stimulation of the sympathetic nervous system, so arrhythmias are common when respiration is depressed or obstructed.

Cardiac arrhythmias during anaesthesia are common and most are benign but in an emergency situation the anaesthetist must know how to treat those which have haemodynamic consequences or those that are potentially dangerous. Although attempts have been made to grade arrhythmias such as VES this has not so far proved to be productive in terms of prognosis. During anaesthesia a classification system based on an ECG may be useful because ECG monitoring is now very common in veterinary anaesthesia. Before contemplating administration of anti-arrhythmic drugs it is essential to consider the possibility that the arrhythmia might have an anaesthetic (hypercapnia, hypoxic) or surgical (haemorrhage, traction on tissues) cause. Cardiac arrhythmias only require pharmacological treatment when:

(a) they cannot be corrected by removing the suspected cause,
(b) they are haemodynamically relevant, and
(c) when the type of arrhythmia is likely to progress to a life-threatening condition.

First, hypercapnia, hypoxia, arterial hypotension, inadequate anaesthesia and electrolyte disorders should be corrected. Next, the use of potentially arrhythmogenic drugs should be terminated. Only if these treatments are ineffective should the use of antiarrhythmic drugs be started. Currently, in medical anaesthesia there is a growing concern about the safety of many antiarrhythmic agents because these drugs have the potential to fail, increase the severity of the arrhythmias or produce other circulatory disturbances (Podrid, 1991).

Bradyarrhythmias

Bradyarrhythmias are the result of an abnormal prolongation of the transmission of the electrical signal to the ventricles or to an decreased automaticity of the sinoatrial node. They may result in reduced CO and very slow HR may lead to escape beats. The optimum therapeutic approach is to increase HR using atropine or glycopyrrolate. If bradycardia occurs in animals having epidural or spinal analgesia it is probable that i.v. ephedrine as a bolus, possibly followed by an infusion, is the regimen of choice.

Supraventricular arrhythmias

Supraventricular extrasystoles originate at or above the bundle of His so that the QRS complex of the ECG is narrow. They may represent the physiological response to light anaesthesia, sympathomimetic stimulation, direct myocardial trauma or loss of circulating blood volume. Exclusion of an anaesthetic and/or surgical aetiology suggests that treatment with a Ca^{++} channel blocker such as verapamil may be indicated. However, verapamil may cause sinus bradycardia, sinus arrest, AV block, ventricular arrhythmias and even ventricular asystole. It also has a marked negative inotropic effect and interacts with other drugs, principally digoxin and β blockers. While interaction of Ca^{++} channel blockers with digoxin is synergistic, the combination with β blockers aggravates the negatively inotropic properties of both drugs and can lead to asystole.

Atrial fibrillation is easily detected by the absolute arrhythmia and if chronic before anaesthesia does not require any therapeutic intervention unless it causes very high heart rates. Digoxin or β blockers may be useful if atrial fibrillation appears unexpectedly during anaesthesia.

Ventricular arrhythmias

Premature VES are very common and result in wide QRS complexes in the ECG because depolarization spreads across the ventricle from cell to cell rather than through the His-Purkinje system. Common causes during anaesthesia include hypercapnia, electrolyte imbalance, direct myocardial trauma and high levels of circulating catecholamines. Predisposing factors are medication with digitalis and ventricular dilatation. Isolated VES do not need specific antiarrhythmic treatment but if there is a significant rise in HR or ventricular tachycardia occurs, therapy is essential. Lignocaine (lidocaine) is the drug of choice.

Heart block

Heart block is due to the faulty transmission of the electrical signal from the sinoatrial node to the ventricles. Usually this occurs at the atrioventricular node (AV block) or in the His bundle (left or right bundle branch blocks). First degree AV block shows as an increased time interval between the P wave of the ECG and the beginning of the QRS complex. Second degree AV block is characterized by the failure of some of the atrial depolarizations to reach the ventricles, whilst in third degree AV block none of the atrial depolarizations reach the ventricles. Second degree AV blocks are classified as Mobitz I and Mobitz II blocks. In Mobitz I blocks there is an increasing time between the P waves and the QRS complex until for a single atrial depolarization a complete block occurs. This type of heart block is known as the Wenckebach phenomenon. Mobitz II blocks have a constant PR interval; however, there is a failure of some of the atrial depolarizations to reach the ventricles.

Animals with Mobitz I or first degree block do not need special treatment but Mobitz II is much more serious and any animal showing this condition before anaesthesia should be thoroughly investigated and equipment for cardiac pacing should be available if anaesthesia is needed.

CARDIAC ARREST

The causes of cardiac arrest, when the heart ceases to function as a pump, are numerous and in any one case it is likely that several factors may be implicated but in the majority of cases hypoxia and hypercapnia contribute significantly to its occurrence. Cardiac arrest of neurogenic origin, usually stimulation of the vagus nerves, is the exception to the general rule of multiple causation. Where the surgeon stimulates the vagus nerves, either directly or by initiating a reflex such as the oculocardiac, the heart may stop with no prior warning. Such an arrest can only be detected by continuous palpation of the pulse or with an ECG, as the suddenness of the cessation of circulation as the heart ceases to beat means that the tissues are well oxygenated, the mucous membranes remain pink, and spontaneous respiration may continue for 2 to 3 minutes until the respiratory centres become anoxic. By the time respiration has ceased and the pupil has dilated, cerebral hypoxia makes successful resuscitation much more difficult. The horse and the cat are the species of animal most sensitive to vagal arrest of the heart and they should be protected by the administration of anticholinergics prior to surgery in the head and neck regions.

Cessation of the cardiac pumping action may follow complete cardiac arrest (asystole), ventricular fibrillation, or electromechanical dissociation (EMD). Electromechanical dissociation is similar to asystole except that there is a regular electrical rhythm demonstrated on the ECG coupled with the progressive failure of ejection of blood from the ventricles. EMD occurs with overdose of anaesthetic drugs, hypovolaemia, acute cardiac decompensation, hypoxaemia or severe acidosis. These three types of cardiac failure can be differentiated by observation of the ECG and palpation of a peripheral pulse. Diagnosis of cardiac arrest must be rapid because during anaesthesia it may have been preceded by respiratory or circulatory insufficiency so that the brain may already be hypoxic when the circulation ceases. Diagnosis is based on the absence of a palpable peripheral pulse, absence of heart sounds and ashen-coloured mucous membranes coupled with an absence of bleeding from any surgical wound. These signs are closely followed by wide dilatation of the pupils and either agonal gasping or apnoea. Respiration will continue until the respiratory centres become anoxic.

When any or all of these signs are observed the traditional ABC protocol should be instituted without delay. **A** refers to airway and it is most important to ensure that the airway is clear. The presence of an endotracheal tube does not necessarily mean that the airway is clear and its patency and positioning should be checked. Endotracheal intubation is the best way of ensuring a patent airway in an animal which has not got a tube in position. **B** refers to breathing and IPPV is usually needed to ensure an adequate alveolar gas exchange. A high inspired concentration of O_2 is most desirable. **C** indicates attention to the circulation which in this situation means repetitive compression of the heart or intact chest.

Conservative treatment is not only useless but also wastes valuable time. The only way of restoring an effective circulation is the immediate institution of resuscitative measures. Once an effective circulation with O_2 delivery to the tissues has been established, the immediate danger to the life of the animal is over.

It is always worth trying the effect of a manual thump over the precordial region of the chest because this sometimes results in resumption of cardiac contractions and does not delay the institution of other measures. There are two ways of attempting to provide an effective circulation to the brain and myocardium. One, and first that should be tried, is compression of the intact chest; the second is direct compression of the surgically exposed heart. The use of cardiac stimulant drugs should not be considered until the myocardium is once more well oxygenated and, therefore, they have no place in the initial treatment.

There should be a simple, set routine for the treatment of circulatory arrest, which is known to all those working in the theatre, recovery unit or elsewhere. Table 20.2 sets out such a routine.

TABLE 20.2 Cardiac resuscitation routine

Stage 1: Establishment of an artificial circulation
1. Notify the surgeon and note the time
2. Clear and maintain the airway
3. Carry out IPPV (if possible with O_2)
4. External compression of the chest; if ineffective perform internal cardiac massage
5. Where possible, place and maintain in head-down position

Stage 2: Infuse fluid to restore or maintain circulating volume
This may be left until after Stage 3

Stage 3: Improve condition of the heart
Administer adrenaline (epinephrine) in appropriate doses for the type of animal concerned, preferably i.v. but if impossible into the tracheobronchial tree or directly into the left ventricle

Stage 4: Post-resuscitation
1. Continue IPPV
2. Counteract acidosis by pulmonary hyperventilation
3. Prevent cerebral oedema – corticosteroids, diuretics
4. Continue circulatory support with adrenaline infusion into a central vein (dopamine, dobutamine can be used)

As soon as circulatory arrest is detected the administration of any anaesthetic must be stopped; a clear airway must be ensured and IPPV preferably with pure O_2 instituted. At the same time external chest compression (see below) should be started to improve the venous return to the heart; whenever possible the animal should be placed in a head down position. The effectiveness of chest compression may be judged by the presence of a palpable carotid pulse caused by each compression and a reduction in the diameter of the pupil. If chest compression does not prove to be effective, then direct cardiac compression of the surgically exposed heart must be considered.

Effective external chest compression is possible in most animals although it is probable that except in cats and similar small animals this will not compress the heart itself. In cats and small dogs the chest walls over the region of the heart are compressed between the fingers and thumb of one hand. Larger animals are quickly placed on their side on a hard, unyielding surface. The upper chest wall over the region of the heart is then forced inward and allowed to recoil outwards, movement of the lower chest being restricted by the hard surface on which the animal is lying. It is an advantage if the lower chest wall can be supported. In dogs and other small animals pressure on the uppermost chest wall with the hand is adequate, but in adult horses and cattle or similarly sized animal the knee or foot is applied to the chest wall over the region of the heart. The rate of compression should be about 60 compressions/min in dogs, or 30/min in adult horses and cattle. A remarkably effective circulation can be maintained (Fig. 20.6); respiratory movements may return, although they are usually inadequate to provide proper gaseous exchange in the lungs and IPPV should not be stopped. The size of the pupils should decrease and the level of unconsciousness should lighten. The authors have seen a horse start to recover consciousness and to move its limbs while thoracic compression was being performed. The way in which external chest compression produces blood flow in the body is debated. It was initially thought that when the chest was compressed the heart was squeezed, so ejecting blood into the aorta. This may be so in small animals,

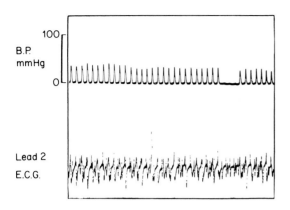

FIG. 20.6 Tracing showing carotid arterial pressure produced by chest compressions in a dog suffering from coarse ventricular fibrillation. Provided the myocardium is well oxygenated electrical defibrillation should restore spontaneous heart beat.

particularly in cats or animals of a similar size and in narrow chested dogs, where it is usually possible to feel the resistance to compression of the ventricles through the compliant chest wall, but this is unlikely to occur in larger animals. It seems more likely that another mechanism is also involved in the latter, and this may be the only mechanism in larger animals. External chest compression induces intrathoracic pressure changes, pushing blood in a retrograde and forward fashion, but due to the presence of valves and collapse of veins, retrograde flow is stopped early on and blood is allowed to flow into the aorta. The flow of blood through the lungs is thought to be due to a cascade effect between the right and left sides of the heart but emptying of the blood from the lungs is also caused by pulmonary ventilation. Whatever the reason for forward blood flow through the aorta it appears that external chest compression may not be very protective of the brain as if this is performed for more than 3–4 min it is often followed by significant neurological deficits, possibly because the induced cerebral blood flow supplies glucose but insufficient O_2 for its metabolism, so that anaerobic metabolism produces large amounts of lactate and other products. As against this, if resuscitation is delayed for more than 3 to 4 min the glucose substrate will become exhausted.

Because the technique of external chest compression is often not followed by a satisfactory outcome several procedures have been advocated for improving the pulmonary pump mechanism. The first is to bind the abdomen with an Esmarch bandage to limit the caudal displacement of the diaphragm and hence increase the intrathoracic pressure during chest compression. The second is to alternate compression of the chest and abdomen but this gives rise to risk of damage of the liver. A third suggestion is to limit the collapse of the lungs during compression by ventilating with IPPV as the chest compression is applied. None of these has been shown to improve survival in veterinary clinical practice.

Cardiac fibrillation may be present as the cause of circulatory arrest or may be precipitated in an asystolic heart by the effects of drugs or even chest compression. The best and most specific treatment is to pass an electric shock through the myocardium so that when the contraction it causes passes off the whole muscle remains in a relaxed state of asystole: following this it is hoped that normal contractions will start spontaneously. Electrical defibrillation attempts will do no harm to a heart that is in asystole and may even induce it to start beating, so applying a shock, or shocks, is now regarded as one of the first measures to be undertaken in cases of cardiac failure during anaesthesia. Compact and relatively inexpensive apparatus is available for external defibrillation (electrodes placed on the chest wall (Fig. 20.7) and internal use electrodes placed on the myocardium itself). All these pieces of apparatus are designed for man and they are suitable for use in small animals but their output may be inadequate for larger animal use unless repeated shocks are given. This may not be so much of a problem in horses for ventricular fibrillation, when it does occur, tends to be very short lived

For defibrillation through the intact chest wall, with good electrical contact assured by conducting gel, shocks of about 1 J are necessary in cats, from 1 to 8 J in dogs and 400 J (repeated shocks at 15 second intervals) in horses and cattle. When the electrodes are applied over saline-soaked pads directly on the myocardium shocks of about 0.2 J/kg appear to be effective in most cases. Attempts at electrical defibrillation are much more likely to be effective if the myocardium is showing coarse fibrillation and is well oxygenated before the shock is applied.

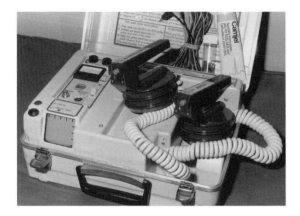

FIG. 20.7 Defibrillator for external use. For reasons of safety in use both the electrodes have switches in their insulated handles. These switches need to be pressed simultaneously to deliver the shock. This particular model of defibrillator has its own monitor ECG.

If an effective circulation cannot be produced by external chest compression coupled with electrical defibrillation, the heart must be exposed by a thoracotomy incision. Obviously, facilities for IPPV must be available before this can be done. No time should be lost in 'scrubbing up' or in preparing the operation site before making an intercostal incision and when the heart is exposed the ventricles must be squeezed rhythmically. The squeezing should be carried out with a motion from the apex towards the base of the heart (rather like the reverse of hand-milking of a cow's teat). The rate of compression should not be too rapid for the chambers of the heart need to have time to fill between compressions and a slight head-down inclination of the body assists this. In every case care must be taken to avoid rupture of the heart by the fingertips. In small animals the ventricles can be compressed by the grasp of one hand but in larger animals both hands must be used. The effectiveness of the circulation produced by this may be gauged by the maintenance of a small pupil size and the presence of a palpable carotid pulse when the ventricles are squeezed.

Often, when the chest is opened because external chest compression is judged to be ineffective it is found that venous return is not sufficient to fill the heart between compressions, indicating that the reason for cardiac failure was hypovolaemia, and in these circumstances direct cardiac compression is also ineffective until a rapid i.v. infusion has corrected the deficit in the blood volume.

Once an apparently satisfactory artificial circulation has been established there is no longer any necessity for haste and there is time for a considered approach. Ideally, as soon as the primary resuscitative measures have been commenced intravenous fluids should be given to expand the circulatory volume. Where cardiac failure is of unknown origin, 5% dextrose is used, but if haemorrhage caused the problem, then a plasma volume expander such as a gelatine or starch solution is to be preferred. However, in veterinary anaesthesia there may be no venous line in place and so this may be a counsel of perfection as venepuncture is usually very difficult at this time. Attempts to set up an intravenous infusion should not interfere with resuscitation and, if venepuncture is impossible, placement of an intravenous line should be deferred until the situation is more stable.

In the past bicarbonate was often administered at this stage to counteract the acidosis which occurs as a result of hypoxia. However, today the consensus of opinion appears to be that acidosis should be counteracted by deliberate hyperventilation of the lungs. This avoids the risk of alkalosis due to too much bicarbonate provoking arrhythmias and resulting in intractable ventricular fibrillation. Although various substances such as calcium chloride were formerly used, adrenaline (epinephrine) is now generally considered to be the cardiac stimulant of choice. Treatment with adrenaline will do no further harm to a fibrillating heart and indeed it may even be successful in restoring a normal rhythm. It acts on α and β sympathetic receptors thus not only stimulating the myocardium but also increasing the peripheral resistance and hence improving coronary perfusion. An initial dose of $10\,\mu g/kg$ should be given and as the action of this drug is short-lived further doses are often needed every 3–4 min or an i.v. infusion may be used (1:50 000 in Hartmann's solution). If i.v. injection cannot be achieved, the initial dose may be given through a catheter passed through the endotracheal tube and wedged in a bronchus. Attempts to inject directly into the ventricles are inadvisable since coronary vessels may be damaged.

When an electrical defibrillator is not available lignocaine hydrochloride in doses of 1 mg/kg may be injected i.v. and massage continued to force it into the coronary vessels. At this dose lignocaine (lidocaine) depresses cardiac excitability and prolongs the refractory period of heart muscle, but it also decreases myocardial contractility. Although worth trying, experience has shown that its use is only seldom successful in stopping ventricular fibrillation.

Ventilation of the lungs with O_2 should be continued until all evidence of circulatory failure has vanished. At this stage, there will be a metabolic acidosis due to the products of anaerobic metabolism in the peripheral tissues being returned to the circulation.

Bradycardia with heart block is common following restoration of the circulation after prolonged myocardial hypoxia. This bradycardia is usually refractory to treatment with atropine and many cases do not respond to sympathomimetic drugs so electrical pacing of the heart may offer the only hope of successful treatment. However, it is always worth trying the effects of 1 in 50 000 adrenaline before considering electrical pacing. External pacing of the heart uses voltages of 100–150 V and frequently leads to skin burns at the site of the electrodes, so internal pacing using 3–5 V from a wire electrode passed from the jugular vein into the right ventricular chamber is to be much preferred.

If, in spite of transfusion to a satisfactory right atrial filling pressure as shown by a CVP of 6 to 7 mmHg, and distension of peripheral veins, the spontaneous heart beat is incapable of maintaining an adequate CO and ABP, inotropic support should be given. Dopamine is claimed to have the advantage of improving renal blood flow by stimulation of renal receptors and is a relatively safe inotropic drug. Dobutamine, on the other hand, is a pure β_1 agonist which is said to work primarily by improving stroke volume rather than by increasing the heart rate. Isoprenaline, another β agonist, also improves cardiac output but causes a marked tachycardia. Adrenaline (1:50 000 in Hartmann's solution) given at a rate of 0.02 ml/kg/min or as necessary to maintain a systolic pressure of about 120 mmHg is, however, the inotropic drug of choice. Once inotropic support has been started it cannot be withdrawn abruptly and careful weaning is necessary, usually over a period of several hours.

Cerebral oedema is not uncommon due to hypoxia during the circulatory arrest and animals which have apparently been successfully resuscitated may lapse into unconsciousness from this several hours later. To limit this oedema, the resuscitated animal should be given large i.v. doses of corticosteroids (e.g. 1 mg/kg methylprednisolone, every 6 hours for four doses) and diuretics such as frusemide (which also decreases CSF production and enhances its clearance).

The greater the time elapsing before restoration of adequate spontaneous circulation, the poorer the prognosis. The heart is more resistant to the effects of hypoxia than is the brain so that if the heart does not readily respond to resuscitative measures it is likely that cerebral function will be so compromised as to make normal life impossible. Usually, it is unrewarding to attempt resuscitation of an animal that has had no effective circulation for more than 5 minutes unless it was very hypothermic when circulatory arrest occurred.

Following successful restoration of the heart beat by open chest cardiac massage the beat should be observed for several minutes before the chest is closed. This time is used to secure any bleeding points. In spite of the lack of sterile precautions in opening the chest and massaging the heart, sepsis is rare in animals which recover.

EMERGENCY RESUSCITATION EQUIPMENT

In the operating room, most animals are routinely intubated and facilities for airway and ventilation control are readily available on the anaesthetic machine. An emergency trolley for use in the operating room should carry syringes and needles of all commonly used sizes, a fluid administration set and i.v. cannulae, several bags of infusion fluids, and drugs – appropriate for the treatment of cardiac arrest in the various species of animal already – drawn up into labelled, capped syringes, with the doses, in terms of volumes of solution, required for the size of animal written on the syringe labels (in an emergency there is little time to calculate the doses from those given on data sheets in mg/kg or the dilutions needed).

Whenever possible the kit should include a cardiac defibrillator and electrocardioscope. In general, drugs on the emergency trolley should be kept to a minimum, e.g. lignocaine, atropine, and naloxone. Other drugs such as vasopressors, cardiac stimulants, β blockers and diuretics are best kept on a second shelf or in a drawer of the trolley so that identification problems do not arise at the time of greatest emergency.

Because the success of resuscitation depends greatly on the speed and efficiency with which it is applied it is advisable to have a basic resuscitation kit wherever animals are recovering from anaesthesia. The actual requirements depend on the species of animal concerned and on the particular circumstances. Airway problems are likely to be important and the kit should contain endotracheal tubes, laryngoscope, and a self-inflating bag, (e.g. an Ambu bag, Fig.20.5). Some drugs such as adrenaline and naloxone should be included with a suitable range of needles and syringes, and a bag of intravenous infusion fluid together with an administration set may be thought worthwhile.

HYPOTHERMIA AND HYPERTHERMIA

Although body temperature may rise during anaesthesia, hypothermia is much more commonly encountered. Whenever return to consciousness is unexpectedly delayed hypothermia should be suspected. Waterman (1981) reviewed the causes, effects and prevention of hypothermia. Basically, the causes consist of a reduction in heat production by the animal, usually coupled with an increased heat loss. It is very difficult to influence production, but Waterman recommends several methods of reducing heat loss. She suggests that care should be taken not to wet the animal excessively to reduce evaporative heat losses, placing the animal on a warm surface, preferably a water blanket heated to 38 °C (Fig 20.8) and keeping the drapes over the animal as dry as possible. Ambient room temperature should be kept high but not so high as to make for impossible working conditions (20 to 22 °C is usually satisfactory). Respiratory heat losses are increased when the animal breathes cold dry gas from non-rebreathing systems. Although such loss-

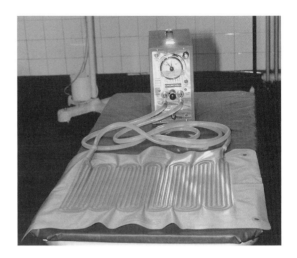

FIG. 20.8 Circulating pump and water blanket for small animal patients.

es are reduced by the use of the use of rebreathing circuits, the use of these systems may entail excessive resistance to respiration for small animals where heat loss is particularly significant. In these small animals a suitable humidifier can be used to reduce heat losses (Dodman & Brito-Babapulle, 1979). Particularly in small animals, all infused fluids should be heated to 38 °C using an electric fluid warmer or by letting them flow through a coil of tubing immersed in a bath of warm water.

With the smallest of animals hypothermia is a very serious problem, but it may be the cause of slow recovery from anaesthesia in any cat, dog, foal, calf or lamb. Should it occur it is easily treated by warming the patient, but many hypothermic animals will shiver violently in the recovery period and, as well as increasing heat production this causes a considerable increase in oxygen consumption, so that the administration of O_2 should be considered in addition to the provision of warmth.

Hyperthermia, or heat stroke, is an unusual complication of anaesthesia. It may, however, occur in a warm environment if small animals are anaesthetized using a low-flow system in a high environmental temperature. Systems with CO_2 absorption prevent the loss of heat by panting and evaporation from the respiratory tract. Treatment is to change the anaesthetic system to one which delivers cold, dry gases, to cool the animal with ice-packs and cold water applications and, if necessary, to administer drugs producing vasodilatation. Active treatment should be discontinued when the body temperature is still 1 °C above normal or it may overshoot in a most disconcerting way. Hyperthermia will, of course, also occur in pathological sensitivity reactions such as porcine malignant hyperthermia.

ANAPHYLAXIS AND ANAPHYLACTOID REACTIONS

An adverse drug reaction is the occurrence of any drug effect not of therapeutic, diagnostic or prophylactic benefit to the animal. Anaphylaxis (an anaphylactic reaction) is an exaggerated response to a substance to which the individual has become sensitized, in which histamine, serotonin and other vasoactive substances are released from basophils and mast cells in response to an IgE mediated reaction. An anaphylactoid reaction is clinically indistinguishable from anaphylaxis but is not mediated by sensitizing IgE antibody. Previous exposure is needed for anaphylaxis but not for an anaphylactoid reaction. Whether a reaction is designated anaphylactic or anaphylactoid may depend on how it has been investigated and how the results of tests are interpreted. Recurrence of symptoms can occur up to 8 hours after the initial manifestation, apparently due to recruitment of inflammatory cells such as eosinophils.

Clinical manifestations of anaphylaxis can appear within seconds of exposure to the antigen but may be delayed for 30 to 60 min. The diagnosis is based solely on clinical grounds because there is no quick diagnostic test. Vasodilatation together with an increase in vascular permeability produces oedema, hypotension and decreased tissue perfusion. Cardiac arrest can occur with but little warning. Laryngeal oedema and bronchospasm may interfere with pulmonary ventilation. Facial oedema may occur and periorbital oedema has been seen in horses and dogs, while cattle have shown, in addition, multiple cutaneous uticarial plaques.

Treatment involves the 'ABC' of resuscitation (p. 517). High concentrations of O_2 should be administered and any IPPV support needed should be given with prolonged expiratory times to allow the lungs to empty in spite of the presence of bronchospasm. The drug of choice is adrenaline (epinephrine), preferably given i.v. in doses of 1 µg/kg/min but an i.m. injection of 10 µg/kg is initially probably as good. Further treatment to support the blood pressure entails the i.v. infusion of adrenaline 0.5 µg/kg/min, or as needed. All animals with anaphylaxis should receive steroids and antihistamines (e.g. 1 mg/kg of methylprednisolone, promethazine 0.2 to 1.0 mg/kg) because although these drugs are not helpful in the immediate management of the condition they may reduce the severity of the late-phase response. There is a synergistic effect between adrenaline and the infusion of i.v. fluids given rapidly to expand the intravascular volume.

When an anaphylactic episode has been encountered during anaesthesia the animal's owner should be notified and given a written statement to present to any veterinarian contemplating anaesthetizing the animal at a future date. This statement should, where possible, indicate the suspected allergen, or at least specify all the agents used in the procedure when the reaction occurred.

TABLE 20.3 **Based on booklet of the Association of Anaesthetists of Great Britain and Ireland and British Society of Allergy and Clinical Immunology (1995)** *Suspected Anaphylactic Reactions Associated with Anaesthesia* **(revised edition)**	
Type A anaphylaxis	**Type B anaphylaxis**
Dose related	Not dose related – may be precipitated by a very small dose. More severe on re-exposure
Extension of pharmacological response	Signs unlike normal pharmacological response. Typical of drug allergy
Common	Uncommon

OTHER CAUSES OF ANAESTHETIC ACCIDENT

POSTURE

All anaesthetized animals should be moved with great care to ensure that they are adequately supported at all times. In small animals, mishandling of the patient can, for example, result in the protrusion of a calcified intervertebral disc. The arthritic animal, if mishandled, may be in considerable pain for several days following anaesthesia for purposes unconnected with joint problems. The problems in large animals may be even more serious. If the hindlegs of horses and cattle are abducted during anaesthesia obturator paralysis may result in the animal being unable to regain the standing position on recovery. The facial nerve of the horse is easily damaged by pressure on the face from the buckle of a head-collar or the edge of an operating table. Ischaemic muscle damage in horses has already been considered and these animals appear to suffer intense pain from this condition.

The position during operation must always be given careful consideration; pressure points may need to be protected by suitable padding, and limbs should never be held abducted but always restrained forward or backwards to avoid nerve damage. The cornea can be protected by closing the eyelids, if necessary with adhesive bandage, but because this precludes observation of the eyeball position, and elicitation of the lid or corneal reflexes, it is always better to keep the level of anaesthesia light enough for the eyelids to remain open during general anaesthesia and tear formation to be preserved.

ANAESTHETIC EXPLOSIONS AND FIRES

Probably the main cause of explosions in operating rooms used to be static electricity coupled with the use of explosive inhalational agents. Today, with the almost universal use of non-inflammable, non-explosive agents, fires in the operating areas are generally associated with the use of diathermy and alcoholic skin disinfectants by surgeons. It must be remembered that many substances will burn in oxygen and, therefore, that no oil or grease must be used on O_2 cylinder connections; moreover, N_2O will support combustion.

INTRAVENOUS INJECTIONS

The commonest mishap is accidental injection of an irritant solution such as guaiphenesin or thiopentone into perivascular tissues. When this happens the injected irritant solution should be diluted by immediate injection of a large volume of saline into the site. Hyaluronidase may be dissolved in the saline and this enzyme will hasten absorption of the irritant drug. No other treatment is required. It is often suggested that a local analgesic such as lignocaine (lidocaine) should be injected into the site of extravasation because these solutions have a low pH that counteracts the high pH of solutions such as thiopentone but it is likely that any beneficial effect noted is due to the vasodilatation they produce. Solutions of them containing vasoconstrictors such as adrenaline do not have any beneficial effect.

Venous thrombosis is common in small animals after the i.v. injection of 5% thiopental but, as it does not appear for 5 to 10 days, it may be missed unless the anaesthetist has occasion to give another injection after that time. Whenever possible, thiopental should be used as a 2.5% or even more dilute solution, and care should be taken that venous flow is not obstructed when the injection is made. Venous obstruction caused by acute flexion of the elbow or unnatural position of the limbs will result in i.v. irritant solutions being retained in the vein and this may give rise to thrombosis. In horses similar considerations apply to guaiphenesin and care should be taken to ensure that it is not retained in the jugular vein due to the obstruction of this vein.

Permanent obliteration of vessels results from repeated, clumsy attempts at venepuncture, the use of unnecessarily large needles or cannulae and allowing large haematomata to form at the site of venepuncture. In animals superficial veins are not too plentiful and their preservation is important.

LOCAL ANALGESIA

Generally manifest toxic reactions to analgesic drugs arise when the drugs are absorbed into the circulation at a greater rate than that at which they can be broken down by the body. Rapid absorption occurs from any hyperaemic or inflamed tissue and the rate of absorption is increased by the use of solutions which contain spreading agents such as hyaluronidase. Accidental intravascular injection may occur even though no blood can be aspirated into the syringe before injection. The rate of absorption is decreased by the addition of vaso-constrictor drugs to the system.

Local analgesics both stimulate and depress the activity of the central nervous system. They have the same membrane stabilizing effect on the heart and nervous tissue of the brain as on the peripheral nervous system. Overt symptoms of central nervous system toxicity appear before the cardiovascular effects become apparent. In large doses local analgesics affect cardiac conduction and contractility. ECG changes include an increase in PR interval, atrioventricular dissociation and prolongation of the QRS complex. As plasma concentrations increase, pacemaker activity decreases, causing sinus bradycardia and, eventually, asystole.

Often, toxic effects manifested by stimulation will vary according to the region of the brain affected. Cortical stimulation produces generalized clonic convulsions, while stimulatory effects in the medulla cause an increase in the rate and depth of respiration, tachycardia and vomiting in those animals where this is possible. Typical general anaesthesia with respiratory and vasomotor depression usually follows. It is uncertain whether death is due to cardiac or to respiratory failure, but it seems probable that i.v. injection of the agent causes sudden primary cardiac failure, while rapid absorption from tissues results in depression of the central nervous system and respiratory failure.

The minimum lethal doses of the various local analgesic agents for the different species of animal encountered in veterinary practice are largely unknown. It is probable that insufficient attention is given to the quantities of local analgesics injected in clinical veterinary anaesthesia. In every case where collapse has occurred after the use of a local analgesics IPPV should be commenced at once. Analeptic drugs should be withheld since they increase the O_2 requirements of the brain. Convulsions should be controlled by the i.v. injection of hypnotic doses of short or ultra-short acting barbiturates and it is probable that thiopental will be the drug most readily available for this purpose. Hypotension due to peripheral or central vasomotor failure should be treated by the intravenous injection of vasopressor drugs. Primary cardiac failure must be treated by chest compression or direct cardiac massage (p. 518).

EPIDURAL ANALGESIA

Drugs used to produce spinal analgesia can cause a reaction affecting both the meninges and spinal nerves. Clinical signs resulting from damage to nerves appear rather rapidly after the effects of the nerve block should have passed off. The region of the spinal cord subjected to the greatest concentration of the drug shows the most marked pathological changes. Where the main lesion is in the meninges clinical signs appear later and reaction to the drug takes the form of an aseptic meningitis which may be mild or severe. These complications do not appear to be due to faulty technique. Injection of the drug into the substance of the spinal cord produces a severe myelitis and neuritis. Damage to the CNS is rarely reversible and management requires prevention, not treatment.

In man, post lumbar puncture headache is a well recognized complication and it has been observed that sheep subjected to spinal analgesia behave in a manner suggesting they too suffer from headache. The headache is believed to be due to low cerebrospinal fluid pressure caused by leakage of the fluid through the needle puncture in the dura mater. It does not occur after epidural blocks.

Infection of the epidural space is fortunately rare but has been reported after caudal epidural block in cattle. The prognosis appears to be better in those cases in which the infection is within the dura for it usually remains localized. Strict aseptic precautions should be employed whenever a spinal or epidural block is attempted.

The rapid injection of a large volume of fluid into the epidural space may cause arching of the back and opisthotonus. This reaction is presumably due to a rapid increase in pressure in the epidural space and is usually of short duration. No treatment is required.

DANGERS TO THE ANAESTHETIST

Modern drugs are very potent and it is most important that the anaesthetist does not come under their influence. Drugs such as ketamine, the α_2 adrenoceptor agonists or their antagonists, which are normally injected into animals, may be absorbed through the human skin or mucous membranes and when handling them appropriate care should be taken. Splashing onto the skin, the lips or eyes should be avoided, but if it does occur, immediate, copious irrigation of the site with water is essential to avoid their effects. Gloves should be worn when handling some of the α_2 adrenoceptor agonists or their antagonists and etorphine. Syringes and needle cases should *never* be held in the mouth (this appears to be a common practice under field conditions but cannot be excused) because their exterior surfaces may have been contaminated with the drug while it was being drawn up and air expelled from the syringe.

Dangers of exposure of the anaesthetist and operating room personnel to inhalation agents have already been discussed. In the UK the Department of Health (1976) has advised that reasonable measures should be taken to reduce the risk of serious contamination of the atmosphere with volatile substances. Similar, but much more elaborate recommendations, have been made in the USA by the National Institute of Occupational Safety and Health (1977).

Sensible, simple measures which can be taken in veterinary practice to reduce atmospheric pollution in operating rooms include:

1. Vaporizers should always be filled outside the operating room and proper filling apparatus should be used, but if this is not possible funnels can reduce the risk of spillage of the liquid anaesthetic.

2. Vaporizers should be turned off when not in use.

3. Anaesthetic agents should not be used for cleaning purposes (especially of clothes!) or skin disinfection.

4. Whenever it is safe and convenient to do so, low flow systems of administration should be used.

5. Scavenging of waste gases and vapours should be encouraged.

6. Whenever practicable, endotracheal intubation should be practised to prevent undue atmospheric pollution as may occur from the use of ill-fitting face-masks.

7. All breathing circuits, especially those designed for low-flow use, should be checked, regularly, for leaks.

There are many scavenging devices suitable for veterinary purposes but care must be taken to ensure that their use does not have an adverse effect on the patient. It must also be remembered that activated charcoal containers used to remove vapours such as halothane from the exhaled gases do not absorb N_2O.

REFERENCES

Allen, A., Schertel, E., Muir, W.W. and Valentine, A. (1991) Hypertonic saline/dextran resuscitation of dogs with experimentally induced gastric dilatation-volvulus shock. *American Journal of Veterinary Research* **52**: 92–96.

Arden, W.A., Reisdorff, E., Loeffler, B.S., Stick, J.A., and Walters, D. (1991) Effect of hypertonic-hyperoncotic fluid resuscitation on cardiopulmonary function during colon torsion shock in ponies. *Veterinary Surgery* **20**: 329–333.

Bertone, J.J., Gossett, K.A., Shoemaker, K.E.; Bertone, A.I. and Schneiter, H.L. (1990) Effect of hypertonic vs. isotonic saline solution on responses to sublethal *E. coli* endotoxemia in horses. *American Journal of Veterinary Research* **51**: 999–1007.

Concensus Conference (1988) Perioperative red blood cell transfusion. *Journal of the American Medical Association* **260**: 2700–2703.

Davies, M.J. (1989) Crystalloid or colloid: does it matter? *Journal of Clinical Anesthesia* **1**: 464–471.

Department of Health (1976) HC(76)38 or SHHD/DS (76). 65. London: DHSS.

Dodman, N.H. and Brito-Babapulle, L.A. (1979) The role of humidification in anaesthesia. *Proceedings of the Association of Veterinary Anaesthetists of Great Britain and Ireland* **8**: 141–147.

Dupe, R. Bywater, R.J. and Goddard, M. (1993) A hypertonic infusion in the treatment of experimental shock in calves and clinical shock in dogs and cats. *Veterinary Record* **133**: 585–590.

Dyson, D.H. and Pascoe, P.J. (1990) Influence of preinduction methoxamine, lactated Ringer solution, of hypertonic saline solution infusion or postinduction dobutamine infusion on anesthetic-induced hypotension in horses. *American Journal of Veterinary Research* **51**: 17–21.

Gasthuys, F. (1994) The value of 7.2% hypertonic saline solution in anaesthesia and intensive care: myth or fact? *Journal of Veterinary Anaesthesia* **21**: 12–14.

Hellyer, P.W., Meyer, R.E. and Olson, N.C. (1993) Resuscitation of anesthetized endotoxaemic pigs by the use of hypertonic saline solution containing dextran. *American Journal of Veterinary Research* **54**: 280–286.

Janssens, L., Altman, S. and Rogers, P.A.M. (1979) Respiratory and cardiac arrest under general anaesthesia: treatment by acupuncture of nasal philtrum. *Veterinary Record* **105**: 273–276.

Kein, N.D., Kramer, G.C. and White, D.A. (1991) Acute hypotension caused by rapid hypertonic saline infusion in anesthetized dogs. *Anesthesia and Analgesia* **73**: 597–602.

Kleeman, N.S. (1979) CNS manifestations of disordered salts and water balance. *Hospital Practice* 60–73.

Maningas, P.A., DeGuzman, L.R., Tilman, M.S. *et al.* (1986) Small volume infusion of 7.5% NaCl in 6% Dextran 70 for the treatment of severe hemorrhagic shock in swine. *Annals of Emergency Medicine* **1**: 1131–1137.

Mermel, G.W. and Boyle, W.A. (1986) Hypertonic saline resuscitation following prolonged hemorrhage in the awake dog. *Anesthesiology* **65**(3A): 91.

Moon, P.F., Snyder, J.R., Haskins, S.C., Perron, P.R. and Kramer, G.C. (1991) Effects of a highly concentrated hypertonic saline-deltran volume expander on caroiopulmonary function in anesthetized normovolemic horses. *American Journal of Veterinary Research* **52**: 1611–1618.

Muir, W.W. and Sally, J. (1989) Small-volume resuscitation with hypertonic saline solution in hypovolemic cats. *American Journal of Veterinary Research* **50**: 1883–1889.

NIOSH (1977) DHEW Publication No 77–140. Washington DC: US Government Printing Office.

Podrid, P.J. (1991) Safety and toxicity of antiarrhythmic drug therapy: benefit versus risk. *Journal of Cardiovascular Pharmacology* **17**: (Suppl 6): S65–S73.

Rocha, E., Silva, M., Irineu, I., and Porfirio, M. (1990) Hypertonic saline resuscitation: saturated salt-dextran solutions are equally effective, but induce hemolysis in dogs. *Critical Care Medicine* **18**: 203–211.

Waterman, A.E. (1981) Maintenance of body temperature during anaesthesia. *Proceedings of the Association of Veterinary Anaesthetists of Great Britain and Ireland* **9**: 73–85.

Appendices

Appendix I

i.t.	Intratracheal
i.v.	Intravenous; intravenously
K^+	Potassium; potassium ion
kPa	Kilopascal (1 kPa = approximately 7.5 mmHg)
l	Litres
l/kg	Litres per kilogramme body weight
LVF	Left ventricular failure
MABP	Mean arterial blood pressure
mg	Milligrammes
Mg^{++} or Mg^{2+}	Magnesium; magnesium ion
mg/kg	Milligrammes per kilogramme body weight
ml	Millilitres
ml/kg	Millilitres per kilogramme body weight
mmH_2O	Millimetres of water
mmHg	Millimetres of mercury
mol	Mole = amount of substance
N_2	Nitrogen
N_2O	Nitrous oxide
Na^+	Sodium; Sodium ion
NO	Nitric oxide
O_2	Oxygen
°C	Degrees Celsius
PAWP	Pulmonary artery wedge pressure
PCO_2	Carbon dioxide tension
PEEP	Positive end-expiratory pressure
PEFR	Peak expiratory flow rate
PiO_2	Inspired O_2 tension or concentration
PO_2	Oxygen tension
psi	Pounds per square inch
PVC	Posterior vena cava
$P\bar{v}CO_2$	Venous CO_2 $\bar{v}$= mixed venous tension)
$P\bar{v}O_2$	Venous O_2 $\bar{v}$ = mixed venous tension)
PVR	Peripheral vascular resistance
SBP	Systolic blood pressure
s.c.	Subcutaneous; subcutaneously
s.w.g.	Standard wire gauge
TLC	(i) Total lung capacity or (ii) Tender loving care
UK	United Kingdom
VIC	Vaporizer in the (breathing) circuit
VOC	Vaporizer outside the (breathing) circuit
V/Q	Ventilation: perfusion ratio
$V_{D(Anat)}$	Respiratory anatomical deadspace volume
$V_{D(Physiol)}$	Respiratory physiological deadspace volume
VEs	Ventricular extrasystoles
VF	Ventricular fibrillation
V_t	Tidal volume of respiration
µg	Microgrammes
µg / kg	Microgrammes per kilogramme bodyweight
µl	Microlitres
µl / kg	Microlitres per kilogramme bodyweight

Appendix II

In many countries there are maximum concentrations of inhalation anaesthetics in the atmosphere to which workers may be exposed, either recommended or governed by regulations, and applying to all places of work. These concentrations vary from country to country and as yet there appear to be no specified limits for sevoflurane or desflurane.

1. The UK

In the UK, Occupational Exposure Standards (OES) were introduced in January 1996 for the four main anaesthetic agents: N_2O 100 ppm; halothane 10 ppm; isoflurane 50 ppm and enflurane 50 ppm.[1] These form part of the Control of Substances Hazardous to Health Regulations 1994 (COSHH)[2] with limits based on an 8 hour time-weighted average (TWA). These limits were set as a consequence of alleged adverse effects associated with human exposures.

[1] Health Services Advisory Committee (1995) *Anaesthetic Agents. Controlling Exposure Under COSHH.* London: HMSO.
[2] Control of Substances Hazardous to Health(COSHH) (1994) *Regulations. Approved Code of Practice.* London: HMSO.

2. The USA

Maximal levels of exposure have been suggested by the National Institute of Occupational Safety and Health (NIOSH).[3] These are 2 ppm for halogenated anaesthetic agents and 25 ppm for N_2O.[4,5]

[3] Whitcher, C. (1975) Development and evaluationof methods for the elimiantion of waste anaesthetic gases and vapors in hospitals. *NIOSH No. 75–137.* Washington DC: Department HEW Publications.
[4] Rogers, D. (1996) Exposure to waste anesthetic gases. *American Association of Occupational Health Nurses Journal* **34**: 574–579.
[5] Yagiela, J.A. (1991) Health hazards and nitrous oxide: a time for reappraisal. *Anesthetic Progress* 38: 1–11.

Appendix III

US Name	UK Name
Acetominophen	Paracetamol
Alfadolone	Alfadolone
Alfaxalone	Alphaxalone
Bupivacaine	Bupivacaine
Buprenorphine	Buprenorphine
Butorphanol	Butorphanol
Cromylin sodium	Sodium cromoglycate
Dibucaine	Cinchocaine
Epinephrine	Adrenaline
Ergonovine	Ergometrine
Flunixine	Flunixine
Furosemide	Frusemide
Guaifenesin	Guaiphenesin
Isoprenterenol	Isoprenaline
Lidocaine	Lignocaine
Methohexital	Methohexital (methohexitone)
Meperidine	Pethidine
Pentobarbital	Pentobarbital (pentobarbitone)
Phenobarbital	Phenobarbital (phenobarbitone)
Quinalbarbitone	Secobarbital
Salbutamol	Salbutamol
Scopolamine	Hyoscine
Succinylcholine	Suxamethonium
Tetracaine	Amethocaine
Thiopental	Thiopental (thiopentone)

Index

Entries in **bold** indicate main discussion, entries in *italic* denote illustrations and tables.